ANTICONVULSANTS

MEDICINAL CHEMISTRY
A Series of Monographs

EDITED BY

GEORGE DESTEVENS

Pharmaceuticals Division, CIBA-GEIGY Corporation
Summit, New Jersey

ANTICONVULSANTS

Edited by

Julius A. Vida

Bristol Myers Company
International Division
New York, New York

ACADEMIC PRESS   New York   San Francisco   London   1977
A Subsidiary of Harcourt Brace Jovanovich, Publishers

ACADEMIC PRESS, INC.
111 Fifth Avenue, New York, New York 10003

United Kingdom Edition published by
ACADEMIC PRESS, INC. (LONDON) LTD.
24/28 Oval Road, London NW1

Library of Congress Cataloging in Publication Data

Main entry under title:

Anticonvulsants.

    (Medicinal chemistry series ; no.)
    Includes bibliographies and index.
    1.   Epilepsy—Chemotherapy.   2.   Anticonvulsants—
Therapeutic use.   3.   Anticonvulsants—Testing.
4.   Neuropharmacology.   I.   Vida, Julius A.,   Date
II.   Series: Medicinal chemistry, a series of
monographs ; no.
RC374.C48A57   616.8'53'061   76-19492
ISBN 0–12–721840–8

TO MY WIFE, MARTHA

CONTENTS

LIST OF CONTRIBUTORS

Numbers in parentheses indicate the pages on which the authors' contributions begin.

JOHN D. ALVIN (113), School of Pharmacy, University of Pittsburgh, Pittsburgh, Pennsylvania

MILTON T. BUSH (113), Vanderbilt Medical School, Nashville, Tennessee

BRIAN B. GALLAGHER (11), Departments of Pharmacology and Neurology, Schools of Medicine and Dentistry, Georgetown University, Washington, D.C.

ELISABETH H. GERRY (151), Kendall Company, Lexington, Massachusetts

LEMONT B. KIER (577), Department of Chemistry, Massachusetts College of Pharmacy, Boston, Massachusetts

WALLACE J. MURRAY (577), Department of Medicinal Chemistry and Pharmacognosy, College of Pharmacy, University of Nebraska Medical Center, Omaha, Nebraska

NICHOLAS P. PLOTNIKOFF (293), Abbott Laboratories, North Chicago, Illinois

FRANK D. POPP* (329), Department of Chemistry, Clarkson College of Technology, Potsdam, New York

JOHN F. REINHARD (57), Department of Pharmacology, Massachusetts College of Pharmacy, Boston, Massachusetts

JOHN F. REINHARD, JR. (57), Laboratory of Neuroendocrine Regulation, Department of Nutrition and Food Science, Massachusetts Institute of Technology, Cambridge, Massachusetts

JULIUS A. VIDA (1, 151), Bristol Myers Company, International Division, New York, New York

HAROLD E. ZAUGG (293), Abbott Laboratories, North Chicago, Illinois

*Present address: Department of Chemistry, University of Missouri, Kansas City, Missouri.

PREFACE

From 1960 to 1974 no new anticonvulsant drug was marketed in the United States (with the exception of diazepam, which was marketed primarily as a minor tranquilizer). With the approval in 1974 of car-bamazepine, the marketing in 1975 of clonazepam, and the anticipated marketing in 1977/1978 of sodium dipropylacetate, eterobarb, mexiletine, and possibly others, a resurgence of interest in anticonvulsant drugs is apparent in the United States. Interest in anticonvulsant drugs never ceased outside the United States as witnessed by the introduction of many new drugs to the international market since 1961.

Many years have passed since the publication of the excellent chapter, Anticonvulsant Drugs, by W. J. Close and M. A. Spielman in "Medicinal Chemistry" (W. H. Hartung, ed., Wiley, New York, 1961). Although many other interesting books have appeared on the subject (e.g., "Basic Mechanisms of the Epilepsies," H. H. Jasper, A. A. Ward, and A. Pope, eds., Little, Brown, Boston, Massachusetts, 1969; "Anticonvulsant Drugs," D. M. Woodbury, J. K. Penry, and R. P. Schmidt, eds., Raven, New York, 1972; "Anticonvulsant Drugs, International Encyclopedia of Pharmacology and Therapeutics," J. Mercier, ed., Pergamon, Oxford, 2 volumes, 1973), none was intended specifically for the medicinal chemist.

In the late 1960's and early 1970's the need for a new book became apparent to many of us working jointly for the Kendall Company in Cambridge, Massachusetts. Drs. John F. Reinhard, Milton T. Bush, Brian B. Gallagher, and myself, among others, were involved, respectively, in the laboratory evaluation, drug disposition, clinical evaluation, and synthesis and design of anticonvulsant drugs. Although hundreds of compounds have been synthesized since 1959, no systematic treatise on anticonvulsant drugs has been written since the chapter by Close and Spielman. I proposed writing this book to the aforementioned researchers and, later, to others. The idea appealed to all, for which I am grateful.

Although this work was written specifically for the medicinal chemist, biochemists, neurologists, and pharmacologists should also find it of interest. Chapter 1 provides an overview and Chapter 2 a neuropharmacological background. Chapter 3 details the laboratory evaluation of compounds and Chapter 4 deals with drug disposition. Chapters 5 through 8 describe the chemistry and biological activities of the various classes of anticonvulsant compounds. Specifically, Chapter 5 contains the cyclic ureides, Chapter 6 the benzopyrans, Chapter 7 other heterocyclic drugs, and Chapter 8 the noncyclic anticonvulsants. Since compilation of data depends on availability in the literature, it was not possible to treat each topic uniformly. Since the chapter by Close and Spielman covered the literature through 1958, ours begins with 1959 and extends to 1976.

I am grateful to the following people for their help: Mrs. Mary-Lou O'Shea (formerly with Kendall Co., presently with NIAMDD) and Dr. William R. Wilber (formerly with Kendall Co., presently with Rohm and Haas Co.) for literature searches; Mrs. Claire Gibbons and Miss Debbie Hudson (Kendall Co.), Mrs. Sandra Meech and Mrs. Sharon Yaddow (Bristol Laboratories), and the secretaries of the contributors for typing parts of the manuscript; Dr. J. Kiffin Penry and Mr. Lawrence D. Smith (National Institutes of Neurological and Communicative Disorders and Stroke, National Institute of Health) for providing data and literature printouts; Dr. Paul Szentmiklosi and Mrs. Alexandra Andor (Medimpex, Budapest) for providing data on decimemide; Mr. Louis Chauvet (Orsymonde S.A., Paris) for providing data on doxenitoin; my former classmate, Mrs. Martha Windholz (Merck, Sharp & Dohme Research Laboratories), for providing literature data; Mrs. Suzanne Woodbury (Georgetown University) for providing data and illustrations; Dr. Jonas A. Gylys (Bristol Laboratories) for reading part of the manuscript; Dr. George deStevens (Ciba-Geigy Corporation) and Dr. Warren J. Close (Abbott Laboratories) for their encouragement; and particularly Dr. Maxwell Gordon (Bristol Laboratories) for his help and encouragement.

I wish to express my thanks to all of the contributors to the book. My special thanks are due Dr. Brian B. Gallagher for his constructive review of parts of the manuscript. Above all, my thanks are due my wife for her assistance and understanding during the genesis of this book.

Julius A. Vida

1

ADVANCES IN ANTICONVULSANT DRUG DEVELOPMENT

Julius A. Vida

The first effective anticonvulsant drug, sodium bromide, was introduced by Charles Locock (1857). In the absence of other drugs, bromide therapy of epileptics became popular. The disadvantages of bromide therapy were discovered, however, quite early: The bromides have an unfavorable therapeutic ratio. Prolonged treatment of epileptic patients with sodium bromide or other bromide preparations causes chronic toxicity manifested by sedation, psychic disturbances, skin rashes, increased glandular secretion, and gastric distress.

The second and still one of the most important drugs for the treatment of epilepsy, phenobarbital, was introduced by Alfred Hauptmann (1912). Phenobarbital is generally considered to be the drug of choice for the treatment of generalized tonic–clonic seizures. It is also the drug of choice for the management of epileptic children. Phenobarbital, however, has the disadvantage of being hypnotic, a property that often prevents the clinician from using sufficient doses to ensure full protection against epileptic seizures. The second barbiturate drug, mephobarbital, was introduced 20 years later for the treatment of grand mal epilepsy (Blum, 1932; Weese, 1932).

Six years later a landmark discovery was made by Merritt and Putnam (1938). In the course of a systematic pharmacological screening program of potential anticonvulsant compounds they discovered that diphenylhydantoin displayed anticonvulsant properties. Although this drug displays a number of side effects, it is one of the most important drugs for treating grand mal; it is not useful, however, for the treatment of absences (petit mal seizures).

After the discovery of diphenylhydantoin, the search for new anticonvulsant drugs intensified. These investigations were aimed at finding new potent

anticonvulsant drugs devoid of sedative and toxic properties. Diphenylhydantoin was followed by other hydantoins, e.g., mephenytoin (Loscalzo,
1945; Kozol, 1946) and ethotoin (Livingston, 1956; Schwade *et al.*, 1956),
and a barbiturate, metharbital (Peterman, 1948).

Barbiturates
  Metharbital
    (1-methyl-5,5-diethylbarbituric acid)
  Mephobarbital
    (1-methyl-5-ethyl-5-phenylbarbituric acid)
  Phenobarbital
    (5-ethyl-5-phenylbarbituric acid)

Hydantoins
  Diphenylhydantoin
    (5,5-diphenylhydantoin)
  Mephenytoin
    (3-methyl-5-ethyl-5-phenylhydantoin)
  Ethotoin
    (3-ethyl-5-phenylhydantoin)

The next therapeutic class of compounds were the oxazolidinediones, e.g.,
trimethadione (Everett and Richards, 1944) and paramethadione (Davis and
Lennox, 1947), followed by the succinimides, e.g., phensuximide (Chen *et
al.*, 1951), methsuximide (Zimmerman, 1953), and ethosuximide (Vossen,
1958; Zimmerman and Burgemeister, 1958). These drugs were quickly
accepted and incorporated into clinical practice, for these classes of compounds were the first effective drugs for the management of absences (petit
mal seizures). The use of the oxazolidinedione and succinimide drugs is
limited, however, because of their side effects.

Oxazolidinediones
  Trimethadione
    (3,5,5-trimethyloxazolidine-2,4-dione)
  Paramethadione
    (3,5-dimethyl-5-ethyloxazolidine-2,4-dione)

Succinimides
  Methsuximide
    (*N*-2-dimethyl-2-phenylsuccinimide)
  Phensuximide
    (*N*-methyl-2-phenylsuccinimide)
  Ethosuximide
    (2-ethyl-2-methylsuccinimide)

A highly promising anticonvulsant drug, phenacemide, was the first
noncyclic ureide to gain acceptance (Gibbs *et al.*, 1949). Initially, this drug
was considered to be effective in the treatment of grand mal, petit mal, and
psychomotor seizures. Later it was used primarily for psychomotor seizures.
Ultimately, however, it became evident that the toxic effects of phenacemide
outweighed its advantages as an anticonvulsant. Acetazolamide, a carbonic

anhydrase inhibitor, was postulated to be effective against epilepsy (Berg-strom *et al.*, 1952) and has been found to be effective in the treatment of petit mal seizures (Lombroso *et al.*, 1954; Merlis, 1954; Holowach and Thurston, 1958). The drug has limited therapeutic usefulness, however, since tolerance to its anticonvulsant effect develops rapidly.

Phenacemide   Acetazolamide   Primidone

In the 1950's a new drug, primidone, was found to be clinically effective in the treatment of grand mal, psychomotor, and focal epilepsy (Handley and Stewart, 1952). Since primidone is a deoxybarbiturate, its effectiveness was initially ascribed to its conversion to phenobarbital. Later it was shown, however, that phenylethylmalonamide (PEMA), as well as phenobarbital, is formed metabolically from primidone. The observed anticonvulsant effectiveness of primidone is due partly to its own activity and partly to that of the two metabolites, phenobarbital and phenylethylmalonamide (Gallagher and Baumel, 1972). In the last few years primidone has gained in popularity as an effective anticonvulsant drug.

Although chlordiazepoxide, the first marketed (1960) drug of the benzodiazepine class, was shown to possess marked anticonvulsant properties in experimental animals (Sternbach *et al.*, 1960, 1964) it was not introduced into clinical practice for the treatment of convulsive seizures in the United States. Diazepam, another member of the benzodiazepine class, was found to be more selective in its anticonvulsant action in experimental animals (Randall *et al.*, 1961). In 1968 diazepam was approved as an adjunct anticonvulsant drug in the United States. Injectable diazepam has proved to be very useful in the management of status epilepticus (Mattson, 1972). Another

Diazepam   Nitrazepam   Clonazepam

benzodiazepine used as an anticonvulsant outside the United States is nitrazepam (Völzke *et al.*, 1967; Peterson, 1967; Sörensen and Dreyer, 1970). Clonazepam has been extensively investigated for its usefulness in anticonvulsant therapy (Gastaut, 1969; Blum *et al.*, 1973; Rossi *et al.*, 1973). Clonazepam has been marketed in the United States since July 1975 for the treatment of akinetic, myoclonic, and petit mal variant seizures.

Carbamazepine, a tricyclic compound structurally related to the imipramine type of antidepressants, was marketed in the United States in the early 1960's for the treatment of trigeminal neuralgia. Later carbamazepine was investigated and found to be effective in the treatment of epileptic patients with grand mal and psychomotor seizures (Cereghino *et al.*, 1974). The drug is now in general use for the treatment of convulsive disorders.

A number of amides and phenylacylureas have been employed outside the United States as anticonvulsant drugs. These include beclamide (*N*-benzyl-3-chloropropionamide), which has been marketed in a number of European countries and South America (Hoenig *et al.*, 1956; Sharpe *et al.*, 1958; Kaye *et al.*, 1959; Wilson and Walton, 1959; Puech *et al.*, 1962).

$$\text{—CH}_2\text{NHCOCH}_2\text{CH}_2\text{Cl}$$

Beclamide

$$\text{CONH}_2$$

Carbamazepine

Chlorphenacemide has been marketed in Austria, and ethylphenacemide (pheneturide) has been marketed in Poland, Spain, and the United Kingdom (Vas and Parsonage, 1967).

Fenaclone was marketed in the Soviet Union for the treatment of grand mal epilepsy (Maskovskij, 1972). This drug resembles a central nervous system (CNS) stimulant more than a CNS depressant since it is devoid of sedative properties and occasionally actually prevents sleep.

$$\text{—CHCONHCONH}_2 \quad | \quad \text{Cl}$$

Chlorphenacemide

$$\text{—CHCONHCONH}_2 \quad | \quad \text{C}_2\text{H}_5$$

Ethylphenacemide

$$\text{—CH}_2\text{CH}_2\text{NHCCH}_2\text{CH}_2\text{Cl} \quad \| \quad \text{O}$$

Fenaclone

All amides and phenylacetylureas are used in the treatment of grand mal and psychomotor seizures.

There are a number of other drugs that are used in Europe for the treatment of epileptic patients.

Chlormethiazole [5-(2-chloroethyl)-4-methylthiazole], an effective drug in the treatment of status epilepticus (Glatt, 1966; Harvey *et al.*, 1975), has been marketed in Scandinavia and the United Kingdom.

Sodium dipropylacetate
(sodium valproate)

Chlormethiazole

Doxenitoine

A new type of drug, sodium dipropylacetate, has been marketed in Europe since the middle 1960's for the treatment of generalized and partial convulsive disorders (Carraz *et al.*, 1964). It has been reported that this drug, the first open-chain acid, exerts its action by significantly increasing brain γ-aminobutyric acid (GABA) levels (Simler *et al.*, 1968; Godin, *et al.*, 1969). This drug is expected to reach the United States market in 1977.

Doxenitoine was evaluated in the United States (Millichap *et al.*, 1955) but marketed only in France. This drug, a deoxyhydantoin, bears the same structural resemblance to diphenylhydantoin as does primidone to phenobarbital. Reports suggest that the drug has a wider margin of safety than diphenylhydantoin.

Ethadione (3-ethyl-5,5-dimethyloxazolidine-2,4-dione), an effective drug against absences, has been marketed in Belgium, France, and Scandinavia.

Fluoresone

Methindione

Ethadione

Fluoresone (4-fluorophenyl ethyl sulfone) has been marketed in France as an adjunct in the treatment of epilepsy.

Methindione was introduced in the Soviet Union for the treatment of grand mal epilepsy and pyschomotor seizures (Hörig *et al.*, 1974). The profile of this drug is similar to that of carbamazepine. Methindione possesses some antianxiety activity but it is not sedative. If used in combination with phenobarbital (or primidone), the dose of the latter might be substantially reduced without loss of effectiveness.

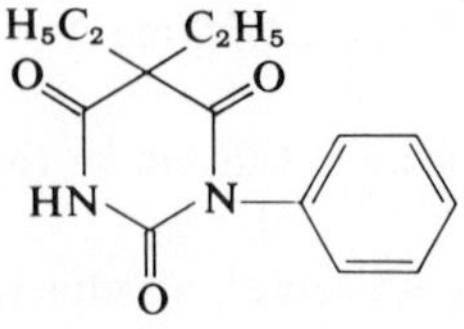

Phetarbital 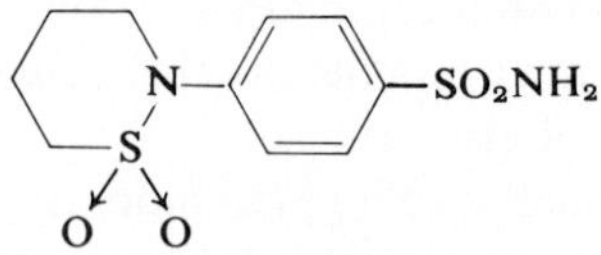   Sulthiame

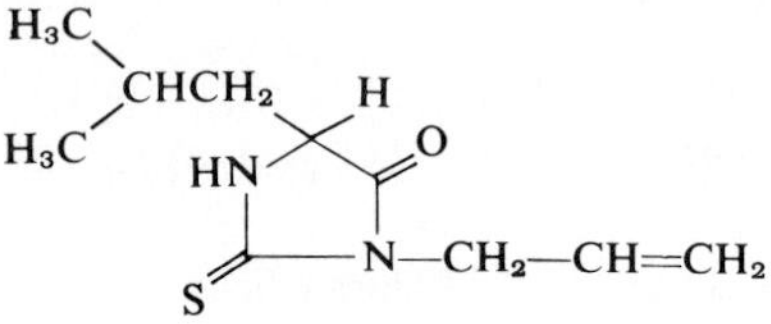

Albutoin

Phetarbital (1-phenyl-5,5-diethylbarbituric acid), an effective drug in controlling absences (Millichap, 1960), has been marketed in Hungary and the United Kingdom.

Sulthiame was introduced in Europe in the 1960's for the treatment of epilepsy (Engelmeier, 1960; Flugel *et al.*, 1960; Raffauf, 1960). Subsequent clinical trials have revealed that sulthiame is useful as an adjunct drug in the treatment of psychomotor seizures.

Albutoin (3-allyl-5-isobutyl-2-thiohydantoin) was reported to be a useful drug in the treatment of grand mal and psychomotor seizures (Davis and Schwade, 1959; Millichap and Ortiz, 1967; Green *et al.*, 1969). In a subsequent trial a great percentage of adults displayed nausea, vomiting, and abdominal pain during albutoin therapy (Cereghino *et al.*, 1972). Due to

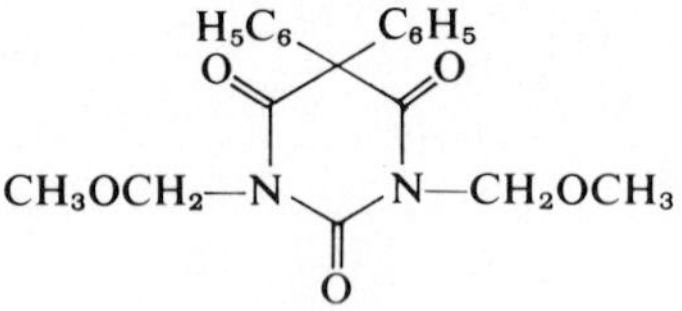

Eterobarb 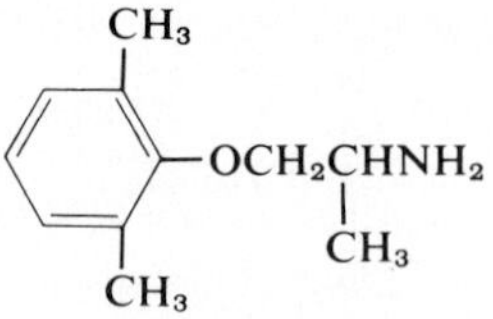   Mexiletine

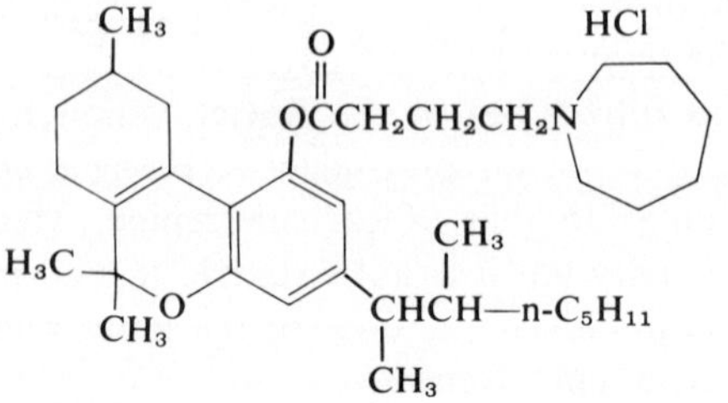

SP-175

TABLE I　ANTIEPILEPTIC DRUGS MARKETED IN THE UNITED STATES

Year Introduced	Trade name	Generic name	Company
1912	Luminal	Phenobarbital	Winthrop
1935	Mebaral	Mephobarbital	Winthrop
1938	Dilantin	Diphenylhydantoin	Parke-Davis
1946	Tridione	Trimethadione	Abbott
1947	Mesantoin	Mephenytoin	Sandoz
1949	Paradione	Paramethadione	Abbott
1950[a]	Thiantoin	Phenthenylate	Lilly
1951	Phenurone	Phenacemide	Abbott
1952	Gemonil	Metharbital	Abbott
1952[b]	Hibicon	Benzchlorpropamide	Lederle
1953	Milontin	Phensuximide	Parke-Davis
1954	Mysoline	Primidone	Ayerst
1957	Celontin	Methsuximide	Parke-Davis
1957	Peganone	Ethotoin	Abbott
1960[c]	Elipten	Aminoglutethimide	CIBA
1960	Zarontin	Ethosuximide	Parke-Davis
1968[d]	Valium	Diazepam	Roche
1974	Tegretol	Carbamazepine	Geigy
1975	Clonopin	Clonazepam	Roche

[a] Withdrawn 1952.
[b] Withdrawn 1955.
[c] Withdrawn 1966.
[d] Approved by the Food and Drug Administration as adjunct.

gastric distress encountered during therapy, albutoin requires further clinical evaluation.

A new investigational drug, eterobarb, a bismethoxymethyl derivative of phenobarbital, has undergone extensive clinical trials in the United States (Gallagher *et al.*, 1973, 1974; Smith *et al.*, 1974). This drug possesses a wide range of anticonvulsant activity, similar to that of phenobarbital, but appears to be much less sedative. The drug is expected to reach the market in 1977.

Mexiletine (KÖ 1173) is reported to have activity similar to that of diphenyl-hydantoin (Allen *et al.*, 1970). This drug is currently under investigation in Europe and the United States.

Several candidates of the benzopyran class appear on the horizon. Preliminary reports indicate that some candidates are potent anticonvulsants and will be chosen for clinical trials (Plotnikoff *et al.*, 1975). The structure of the most promising compound (SP-175) is shown.

Table I, compiled by the National Institute of Neurological and Communicative Disorders and Stroke, Section on Epilepsy,* lists the antiepileptic drugs marketed in the United States.

* The author is grateful to Dr. J. Kiffin Penry for kindly supplying the list.

REFERENCES

Allen, J. D., Kofi Ekue, J. M., Shanks, R. G., and Zaidi, S. A. (1970). *Br. J. Pharmacol.* **39**, 183P.

Bergstrom, W. H., Carzoli, R. F., Lombroso, C., Davidson, D. T., and Wallace, W. M. (1952). *Am J. Dis. Child.* **84**, 771.

Blum, E. (1932). *Dtsch. Med. Wochenschr.* **58**, 696.

Blum, J. E., Haefely, W., Jalfre, M., Polc, P., and Schärer, K. (1973). *Arzneim. Forsch.* **23**, 377.

Carraz, G., Fau, R., Chateau, R., and Bonnin, J. (1964). *J. Ann. Med.-Psychol.* **122**, 577.

Cereghino, J. J., Brock, J. T., and Penry, J. K. (1972). In "Antiepileptic Drugs" (D. M. Woodbury, J. K. Penry, and R. P. Schmidt, eds.), p. 283. Raven, New York.

Cereghino, J. J., Brock, J. T., Van Meter, J. C., Penry, J. K., Smith, L. D., and White, B. G. (1974). *Neurology* **24**, 401.

Chen, G., Portman, R., Ensor, C. R., and Bratton, A. C. (1951). *J. Pharmacol. Exp. Ther.* **103**, 54.

Davis, J. P., and Lennox, W. G. (1947). *Res. Publ., Assoc. Res. Nerv. Ment. Dis.* **26**, 423.

Davis, J. P., and Schwade, E. D. (1959). *Fed. Proc., Fed. Am. Soc. Exp. Biol.* **18**, 380.

Engelmeier, M. P. (1960). *Dtsch. Med. Wochenschr.* **85**, 2207.

Everett, G. M., and Richards, R. (1944). *J. Pharmacol. Exp. Ther.* **81**, 402.

Flugel, F., Bente, D., and Itil, T. (1960). *Dtsch. Med. Wochenschr.* **85**, 2199.

Gallagher, B. B., and Baumel, I. P. (1972). *In* "Antiepileptic Drugs" (D. M. Woodbury, J. K. Penry, and R. P. Schmidt, eds.), pp. 361–366. Raven, New York.

Gallagher, B. B., Baumel, I. P., and Mattson, R. H. (1973). *Neurology* **23**, 405.

Gallagher, B. B., Baumel, I. P., Woodbury, S. G., and DiMicco, J. A. (1974). *Program Am. Epilepsy Soc., Annu. Meet.* p. 8.

Gastaut, H. (1969). *Excerpta Med. Int. Found. Congr. Ser.* **193**, 5.

Gibbs, F. A., Everett, G. M., and Richards, R. K. (1949). *Dis. Nerv. Syst.* **10**, 47.

Glatt, M. M. (1966). *Prescribers J.* **5**, 90.

Godin, Y., Heiner, L., Mark, J., and Mandel, P. (1969). *J. Neurochem.* **16**, 869.

Green, J. R., Miller, L. H., and Burnett, P. D. (1969). *Neurology* **19**, 1207.

Handley, R., and Steward, A. S. R. (1952). *Lancet* **2**, 742.

Harvey, P. K. P., Higgenbottam, T. W., and Loh, L. (1975). *Br. Med. J.* **2**, 603.

Hauptmann, A. (1912). *Muench. Med. Wochenschr.* **59**, 1907.

Hoenig, J., Crotty, I. M., and Chisholm-Batten, W. R. (1956). *J. Ment. Sci.* **102**, 105.

Holowach, J., and Thurston, D. L. (1958). *J. Pediatr.* **53**, 160.

Hörig, C., Koch, H., Mayr, E., Richter, J., and Selchau, M. (1974). *Pharmazie* **29**, 634.

Kaye, N., Jones, I. H., and Warrior, G. K. (1959). *Br. Med. J.* **1**, 627.

Kozol, H. L. (1946). *Am. J. Psychiatry.* **103**, 154.

Livingston, S. (1956), *J. Pediatr.* **49**, 728.

Locock, C. (1857). *Lancet* **1**, 527.

Lombroso, C. T., Davidson, D. T., Jr., and Grossi-Bianchi, M. L. (1954). *Epilepsia* **3**, 123.

Loscalzo, A. E. (1945). *J. Nerv. Ment. Dis.* **101**, 537.

Maskovskij, M. D. (1972). "Lekarstvennye Stredstva," Part I, p. 117. Medicina, Moscow.

Mattson, R. H. (1972). *In* "Antiepileptic Drugs" (D. M. Woodbury, J. K. Penry, and R. P. Schmidt, eds.,) pp. 497–518. Raven, New York.

Merlis, S. (1954). *Epilepsia* **3**, 117.

Merritt, H. H., and Putnam, T. J. (1938). *J. Am. Med. Assoc.* **111**, 1068.

Millichap, J. G. (1960). *Br. Med. J.* **1**, 111.

Millichap, J. G., and Ortiz, W. R. (1967). *Neurology* **17**, 163.

Millichap, J. G., Goodman, L. S., and Madsen, J. A. (1955). *Neurology* **5**, 700.
Peterman, M. G. (1948). *J. Am. Med. Assoc.* **138**, 1012.
Peterson, W. G. (1967). *Neurology* **17**, 878.
Plotnikoff, N. P., Zaugg, H. E., Peterson, A. C., Andersen, D. L., and Anderson, R. F. (1975). *Life Sci.* **17**, 97.
Puech, J., Robin, C., Richet, L., and Tetart, A. (1962). *Presse Med.* **70**, 1015.
Raffauf, H. J. (1960). *Dtsch. Med. Wochenschr.* **85**, 2203.
Randall, L. O., Heise, G. A., Schallek, W., Bagdon, R. E., Banziger, R. F., Boris, A., Moe, R. A., and Abrams, W. B. (1961). *Curr. Ther. Res.* **3**, 405.
Rossi, G. F., DiRocco, C., Maira, G., and Meglio, M. (1973). *In* "The Benzodiazepines" (S. Garrattini, E. Mussini, and L. O. Randall, eds.), pp. 461–488. Raven, New York.
Schwade, E. D., Richards, R. K., and Everett, G. M. (1956). *Dis. Nerv. Syst.* **17**, 155.
Sharpe, D. S., Dutton, G., and Mirrey, J. R. (1958). *Br. Med. J.* **1**, 1044.
Simler, S., Randrianarisoa, H., Lehman, A., and Mandel, P. (1968). *J. Physiol. (Paris)* **60**, 547.
Smith, D. B., Goldstein, S. G., and Roomet, A. (1974). *Program Am. Epilepsy Soc., Annu. Meet.* p. 16.
Sörensen, N., and Dreyer, R. (1970). *Med. Welt* **33**, 1407.
Sternbach, L. J., Kaiser, S., and Reeder, E. (1960). *J. Am. Chem. Soc.* **82**, 475.
Sternbach, L. J., Randall, L. O., and Gustafson, S. R. (1964). *In* "Psychopharmacological Agents" (M. Gordon, ed.), Vol. I, pp. 137–224. Academic Press, New York.
Vas, C. J., and Parsonage, M. J. (1967). *Acta Neurol. Scand.* **43**, 580.
Völzke, E., Doose, H., and Stephan, E. (1967). *Epilepsia* **8**, 64.
Vossen, R. (1958). *Dtsch. Med. Wochenschr.* **83**, 1227.
Weese, H. (1932). *Dtsch. Med. Wochenschr.* **58**, 697.
Wilson, J., and Walton, J. N. (1959). *Br. Med. J.* **1**, 1275.
Zimmerman, F. T. (1953). *Am. J. Psychiatry* **109**, 767.
Zimmerman, F. T., and Burgemeister, B. B. (1958). *Neurology* **8**, 769.

2

NEUROPHARMACOLOGY AND TREATMENT OF EPILEPSY

Brian B. Gallagher

I. INTRODUCTION

This chapter is not intended to be an exhaustive review of the literature relative to either the neuropharmacology or the treatment of epilepsy. Rather it is intended to provide an overview of the clinical aspects of epilepsy for those who work in related disciplines in order that the relevance of their work to the clinical problem will become apparent. In recent years, a number of comprehensive reviews of epilepsy and anticonvulsant drugs have been published which contain detailed references. As much as possible, the reader is referred to these publications for further information.

The epilepsies are a group of diverse disorders or diseases with a common central nervous system manifestation: the occurrence of seizures. It is difficult to be more concise than Hughlings Jackson in defining a seizure as "a state produced by an abnormal excessive neuronal discharge within the central nervous system" (Penfield and Jasper, 1954). It is common practice to refer to seizures that result from a known and identified central nervous system dysfunction as symptomatic, while those seizure disorders in which an identifiable etiology cannot be established are termed idiopathic. This merely reflects the relative inefficiency of our diagnostic procedures and a lack of knowledge concerning subtle structural and biochemical derangements in the central nervous system that result in the occurrence of seizures. At least two studies agree that the cause of a given seizure disorder is reasonably identifiable in approximately one-fourth of patients with recurrent seizures. Lennox (1960) analyzed data compiled by Gibbs and Gibbs in a population of 7668 epileptic patients; an etiology was presumed to be identified in 1978 (25.8%) subjects. The predominant cause was postnatal trauma (11.3%), followed by infectious (5.5%), paranatal trauma (4.5%), brain tumors (1.9%), circulatory defect (1.5%), congenital defect (0.6%), and other causes (0.5%). Hauser and Kurland (1975) in a comprehensive and detailed study of epilepsy in Rochester, Minnesota, from 1935 to 1967 report identification of the cause of seizures in 120 patients in a population of 516 (23.3%) epileptics diagnosed during that time interval. Trauma and vascular disorders were the most frequent cause (each 5.2% of total population) followed by brain tumor (4.1%), congenital defects (3.9%), infectious (2.9%), birth anoxia (1.4%), and degenerative neurological diseases (0.6%). Assuming that these data are generally applicable to all patients with recurrent seizures, cause cannot be identified in about three-fourths of the population, and at present etiology is a poor basis for classification of seizures. However, causal factors should always be searched for if only to identify those people with progressive or treatable diseases.

The age at which recurrent seizures originate is important for several reasons. The majority of symptomatic and idiopathic seizures begin in childhood with estimates ranging from 65 to 75% of seizure disorders originating in the first 20 years of life. Consequently, the physical, psychological, and social consequences of recurrent seizures and chronic medication are extremely pertinent to the treatment of epilepsy. The prevalence of epilepsy has been estimated to be at least 5 per 1000 people. Hauser and Kurland (1975) found a prevalence of 5.4 per 1000 population in Rochester, Minnesota, in 1965. Brewis *et al.* (1966) report a rate of 5.5 per 1000 population in England, and other authors report lower or higher values. At least 90% of these patients are not candidates for surgical treatment and many of those who qualify for surgery require continuing medical management. The medical therapy of epilepsy is a multifaceted problem involving the use of anticonvulsant drugs, psychotropic drugs, psychiatric treatment, social, psychological, and developmental rehabilitation, and adjustment to a chronic disorder that requires continuous diagnostic and neurological assessment of the patient.

II. CLASSIFICATION OF SEIZURES

The clinical manifestations of seizures include a bewildering array of sensory, motor, and autonomic phenomena. The observable presentation of these disturbances in central nervous system function are, at present, the only basis on which a working classification of seizures can be constructed that will serve the purpose of standardizing communication about seizures. Such a descriptive classification of seizures has been developed by the International League Against Epilepsy (Gastaut, 1970) and has received general acceptance. This is not a classification of epilepsies. A patient has *epilepsy*, which may manifest itself in several patterns of *seizures*. The international classification attempts to describe such seizures in relation to six aspects: (1) the clinical seizure type; (2) electroencephalographic seizure type (EEG pattern during a seizure); (3) electroencephalographic intericital expression (EEG pattern between clinical seizures); (4) anatomical substrate; (5) etiology; and (6) age.

For our purposes the clinical seizure type and age are the most informative, and the interested reader may refer to Gastaut (1970) or Masland (1975) for more detailed presentations. Four major categories of seizures are recognized:

> Partial seizures (seizures that originate locally or from a "focus" of abnormal neurons)
>> Generalized seizures (bilateral symmetrical seizures without local onset)
>> Unilateral or predominantly unilateral seizures
>> Unclassified seizures (i.e., inadequate or incomplete data)

A. PARTIAL SEIZURES

Partial seizures are those in which the clinical manifestations initially indicate local activation of a functional and/or anatomical group of neurons. These are further subdivided as partial seizures with elementary symptoms (generally without impairment of consciousness), partial seizures with complex symptoms (generally with impairment of consciousness), and partial seizures secondarily generalized.

1. Partial Seizures with Elementary Symptoms

Partial seizures with elementary symptoms include focal motor seizures. These often begin with tonic contraction of the involved muscles followed by clonus. The seizure may originate in facial, extremity, or trunkal musculature with unilateral innervation. It may remain confined to the muscles originally involved or may spread to other muscle groups. When such a seizure spreads in an orderly sequence it is called a Jacksonian focal motor seizure, and the spread has been referred to as a Jacksonian march. Such seizures reflect paroxysmal activity in the contralateral frontal motor cortex. Frequently, focal motor seizures may involve several or numerous muscle groups simultaneously. In contrast to these tonic and/or clonic seizures a frequent motor manifestation consists of postural deviations of head, eyes, extremity, or trunk. These are usually tonic coordinated movements that are termed adversive when the paroxysmal activity originates in the contralateral frontal cortex, and the postural deviation consists of a turning movement away from the side of the focus. When the turning movement is toward the side of the focus the seizure is said to be ipsiversive. Postural deviations are frequently complex, they may occur unilaterally or bilaterally, and their interpretation in relation to localization of the site of origin of the epileptic discharge is complicated (Ajmone-Marsan and Goldhammer, 1973).

In addition to motor patterns, partial seizures with elementary symptoms may consist of speech arrest (aphasia) or vocalization. Sensory involvement may accompany the motor symptoms or may occur by itself. Special sensory seizures may consist of visual phenomena such as flashing lights, a bright or dark spot, or colors, auditory events including buzzing or ringing noises, vertigo or dizziness, and olfactory and gustatory sensations frequently described as unpleasant. Somatosensory seizures consist of localized or spreading paresthesias (tingling, "pins and needles," formication), dysethesias (burning, unpleasant sensations), or a feeling that there is movement when none occurs. Autonomic manifestations also occur in partial elementary seizures and include pupillary dilatation, esophageal contractions, tachycardia, nausea and vomiting, abdominal or visceral pain, flushing, etc. More frequently, these autonomic events are associated with partial complex seizures. Compound partial elementary seizures consist of combinations of several of the previously described symptoms and, as a general rule, consciousness is maintained throughout these seizures, although focal motor seizures with loss of consciousness may occur.

2. Partial Seizures with Complex Symptoms

Partial complex seizures are usually associated with an alteration or impairment of consciousness and various degrees of amnesia. If the patient is not amnesic for the onset of the seizure, the symptoms occurring at the onset will be recalled and are referred to as an "aura." The aura is an ictal, not preictal, event. In the international classification, six categories of partial complex seizures are identified: (1) with impaired consciousness alone; (2) with cognitive symptomatology; (3) with affective symptomatology; (4) with psychosensory symptomatology; (5) with "psychomotor" symptomatology (automatisms); (6) compound forms (combination of 1-5).

These are the seizures of the temporal lobe, and the designation as "complex" is particularly apt. They are the most frequent seizure pattern (Penry, 1975) and have a particularly high incidence in adults. Accurate descriptions of the entire seizure complex are difficult to obtain because they rely, to a considerable extent, on the patient's ability to report subjective feelings which are often lost with impaired consciousness and amnesia. It is not unusual to witness an entire complex seizure lasting 1-2 minutes and have the patient then report that he or she was entirely unaware that a seizure had occurred. One obvious implication of this fact is that a patient's accounting of seizure frequency may be erroneous, and this is a potential problem in clinical trials of new anticonvulsant drugs.

Impairment of consciousness is frequently the first manifestation of partial complex seizures (Ajmone-Marsan and Ralston, 1957). Ongoing activity may be interrupted; the patient appears to stare and is unresponsive or confused. All of these manifestations of the seizure may occur to various degrees. Speech may not occur or may be incoherent, inappropriate, or nonsensical. Impairment of cognition reflects alteration in awareness of thoughts or perception. Examples of this are the phenomena of déjà vu, in which a new situation is perceived as a repetition of a previous situation; déjà vecu, in which a new experience is perceived as having been previously encountered; and jamais vu, in which a familiar experience or situation is suddenly strange and unfamiliar. A thought or phrase may repeat itself incessantly ("forced thinking") or the patient may experience a feeling of depersonalization, as if he is separate from himself, or a feeling of strangeness or unreality. Affective symptoms frequently accompany partial complex seizures. Fear is the sensation most frequently perceived (Williams, 1956) and many patients find it difficult to describe. It is often associated with abdominal sensations (tightness, "butterflies in the stomach") which may be perceived as rising up through the chest immediately prior to loss of consciousness. The feeling of fear may be extremely intense (Daly, 1958), but most often it is of brief duration and described by patients as having an unreal or unfocused quality. Pleasurable and/or sexual sensations are rarely described as an ictal event. Feelings of sadness and loneliness have been reported (Weil, 1959), and there is general agreement that directed anger or rage during a seizure is so unusual that its actual occurrence is doubtful (Goldstein, 1974). Psychosensory symptoms, when they occur, may be extremely dramatic hallucinations or illusions. Visual illusions consist of distortions of shape or size of objects in the visual field or of body parts. Visual hallucinations may be relatively unformed (flashing lights, a single object moving through the visual field, colors, etc.) or they may be extremely formed and complicated scenes. Auditory hallucinations, in a similar manner, may vary from unformed noises or sounds to voices, poetry, music, nursery rhymes, etc. Olfactory hallucinations are often but not always unpleasant and when they are encountered should always raise the suspicion of a tumor (Feindel, 1975). "Psychomotor" symptoms refer to automatisms. As with the other categories of partial complex symptoms, these motor manifestations cover a wide range of patterns from simple repetitive movements (lip smacking, swallowing, patting a leg, picking at one's clothes, etc.) to highly complex integrated acts of behavior that may obscure the fact, to the casual observer, that consciousness has been altered. Attempts to restrain patients during automatisms often lead to a resistance from the patient that may be quite aggressive until the attempt at restraint is halted. Misinterpretation of this fact contributes in part to the erroneous association of epilepsy and aggression.

The sixth category of partial complex seizures, compound forms, is in fact the usual presentation of these seizures. It has been suggested that the temporal sequences in which the disturbances of cognition, consciousness, affect, psychosensory, and motor function appear may be analogous to the progression of motor manifestations in the Jacksonian march in partial elementary seizures (Stevens, 1957).

3. Partial Seizures Secondarily Generalized

Partial seizures secondarily generalized are seizures that begin with any of the previously described manifestations of partial seizures and evolve into a generalized seizure with tonic and/or clonic manifestations that are either symmetrical or asymmetrical.

B. GENERALIZED SEIZURES

These seizures, bilateral symmetrical seizures without local onset, are defined in the international classification as

> seizures in which the clinical features do not include any sign of symptom referable to an anatomical and/or functional system localized in one hemisphere, and usually consist of initial impairment of consciousness, motor changes which are generalized or at least bilateral and more or less symmetrical and may be accompanied by an "en masse" autonomic discharge; in which the electroencephalographic patterns from the start are bilateral, grossly synchronous and symmetrical over the two hemispheres; and in which the responsible neuronal discharge takes place, if not throughout the entire grey matter, then

at least in the greater part of it and simultaneously on both sides (Masland, 1975).

Eight categories are recognized: (1) absences (petit mal); (2) bilateral massive epileptic myoclonus: (3) infantile spasms; (4) clonic seizures; (5) tonic seizures; (6) tonic–clonic seizures (grand mal); (7) atonic seizures; and (8) akinetic seizures.

1. Absences

Absences are nonconvulsive seizures without local onset and are subdivided into two categories: those in which impairment of consciousness is the sole manifestation and those in which other clinical signs occur with the impairment of consciousness. The former are referred to as simple absences and the latter as complex absences. A variety of names have been attached to these seizures: petit mal, minor attacks, and pyknolepsy. Since the term "petit mal" has been indiscriminately applied by some to any brief seizure, it is hoped that the designation of absence seizure will focus attention on the cardinal feature of these seizures and avoid confusion in the future.

The simple absence seizure consists of an abrupt interruption of consciousness of short duration (usually less than 20 seconds) during which the patient appears to stare and any ongoing motor activity is suspended. There may be some blinking or jaw movements at a rate of about three per second. The patient is unresponsive and unreceptive to stimuli. There is amnesia for the duration of the attack, which terminates abruptly and not uncommonly with a smile. There is usually no postictal confusion, and activity that was in progress before the seizure is resumed. The patient may be unaware that a seizure has occurred. Variation in the intensity of the interruption of consciousness may occur, permitting some perception of stimuli and the environment.

Complex absence seizures are those associated with automatisms or more motor involvement than eye blinking, head nodding, or jaw twitching. Clinically, these can be extremely difficult to differentiate from partial complex seizures. The electroencephalogram with its classical three per second spike and slow-wave discharge during the ictal periods is invaluable in such cases. Absence seizures are also very susceptible to precipitation by photic stimulation and hyperventilation. There is another group of seizures with many characteristics of absence seizures which are difficult to classify. These are the atypical absences (petit mal variant or Lennox–Gastaut syndrome). Consciousness is interrupted and various degrees of tonic motor activity accompany the absence. The seizures may be extremely brief and frequent and are associated with significant central nervous system impairment. The electroencephalogram is diffusely slow with a typical spike and wave discharges that occur at frequencies other than three per second.

2. Bilateral Massive Epileptic Myoclonus

Sudden flexor contractions of major muscle groups, usually bilateral, characterize these brief but severe seizures. Objects held in the hand during an attack may be thrown, and dropping to the ground occurs when the legs are involved. Such seizures may occur as isolated events or as a series of myoclonic jerks that may progress to a generalized tonic–clonic seizure. They also may follow a generalized tonic–clonic seizure. Photic stimulation and the transition from sleep to wakefulness are potent precipitating factors for these seizures. Usually, consciousness is retained and the patient is aware of the attack. These seizures are seen frequently in younger people but may occur at any age.

3. Infantile Spasms (West's Syndrome)

Exceedingly brief tonic flexion contractions that are symmetrical character- ize these seizures. Trunkal muscles are involved, causing the infant to flex at the waist and neck ("salaam seizure") with the legs and arms usually also flexed. Occasionally, extension occurs. Infantile spasms predominantly begin in the first year of life and are associated with a characteristic electroence- phalographic abnormality designated as hypsarrhythmia by Gibbs and Gibbs (1952). The hypsarrhythmic electroencephalogram consists of high-amplitude, asynchronous, disorganized spikes, slow waves, and sharp discharges occur- ring in many patterns. The syndrome is usually associated with severe central nervous system damage and, although an etiology is often not found, it has been reported to occur in metabolic derangements (phenylketonuria, lipidosis, pyridoxine deficiency), Sturge–Weber syndrome, diffuse encephalo- pathies, and a variety of other central nervous system pathologies. The usual course of the disorder consists of a reduction or cessation of the spasms during the next two to four years with the majority of individuals affected having significant mental retardation.

4. Clonic Seizures

Clonic seizures also occur especially in children and are characterized by loss of consciousness and postural tone followed by bilateral clonic contrac- tions which may be either symmetrical or asymmetrical. During the course of the seizure, the particular muscle groups involved may vary considerably.

5. Tonic Seizures

Tonic contraction of trunkal and extremity musculature, usually of brief duration (less than 1 minute), characterizes tonic seizures. Consciousness is always impaired but to various degrees. Vocalization usually occurs as a result of contraction of thoracic muscles forcing air past a tonic larynx. Tonic leg flexion results in falling, while tonic extension of the lower extremities may keep the patient erect. A variety of autonomic changes may accompany these seizures, and postictal stupor usually is not prolonged. These seizures frequently occur in conjunction with atypical absences in the Lennox–Gastaut syndrome and are particularly seen in children.

6. Tonic–Clonic Seizures (Grand Mal)

The seizure, which may be preceded by several or many myoclonic jerks, begins with abrupt loss of consciousness and tonic contraction of all muscle groups, causing the patient to fall. The initial contraction may be flexor and is rapidly followed by more prolonged extension. Tonic contraction of the jaw may cause injury to the tongue. Vocalization occurs with contraction of thoracic muscles, while the arms extend in front of the body and leg extension leads to opisthotonus. During transition from the tonic to the clonic phase, rapid vibratory tremors are seen which progress to violent flexor contractions and relaxation. The clonic contractions gradually become more widely spaced until the seizure ends. Profound autonomic changes occur during the seizure, principally in the tonic phase. The pupils dilate, blood pressure and pulse rate may double, respirations cease, the skin initially flushes and then becomes cyanotic, and bladder pressure rises considerably. Salivation and bronchial secretion increase, resulting in "foaming at the mouth" during the clonic and postictal phases. Apnea persists until the postictal period. The postictal period may begin with another tonic contraction especially in the facial muscles while autonomic activity continues. Cardiac arrhythmias may occur at this time, and hyperventilation occurs associated with a change from cyanosis to pallor. Bladder sphincter muscles relax and the bladder empties. In association with the tonic facial contraction, hyperventilation, and salivation, saliva is forcibly ejected (stertorous phase). The autonomic changes subside; the patient becomes flaccid and remains unconscious. Gradually, consciousness returns and the patient often is extremely confused before regaining consciousness. After recovery the patient usually has a severe headache and sore muscles and is tired. Although the ictal phase seems prolonged to most observers, it is usually no more than 1–2 minutes in duration. The patient is amnesic for the ictal and postictal periods, and at times the amnesia may extend to significant pre- and postictal intervals. Although tonic–clonic seizures may occur at all ages, they are more frequently encountered after puberty.

7. Atonic Seizures

In atonic seizures an abrupt loss of consciousness occurs in association with loss of muscle tone. No movements are involved and the attacks may be very brief or more prolonged. They occur especially in children.

8. Akinetic Seizures

Akinetic seizures are defined in the international classification as brief seizures in which there is loss of movement without atonia. Loss of consciousness is not as profound as it is in atonic seizures, and postural control is maintained. These seizures also occur particularly in children.

C. UNILATERAL OR PREDOMINANTLY UNILATERAL SEIZURES

Unilateral seizures are tonic–clonic or clonic seizures which may or may not be associated with loss of consciousness and which principally are restricted to one side of the body with paroxysmal electroencephalographic activity in the contralateral hemisphere. They are most frequently seen in children and may vary in the side involved in successive seizures. Gastaut *et al.* (1962) have described unilateral tonic–clonic seizures, unilateral tonic seizures, unilateral clonic seizures, unilateral infantile spasms, unilateral massive myoclonus, and unilateral atonic seizures.

D. UNCLASSIFIED SEIZURES

These are seizures in which the relevant information is insufficient to allow classification in the other categories.

This somewhat detailed description of the clinical characteristics of seizures is intended to emphasize the diverse manifestations of paroxysmal discharges in the central nervous system. It would be naive to expect a single anticonvulsant drug to be effective in all of these seizures. In fact, some of them do not respond to any of the currently available anticonvulsants and many respond only poorly or erratically.

1. Febrile Seizures

Febrile seizures are a most interesting entity. They are usually brief, generalized tonic and/or clonic seizures occurring between the ages of about 6 months and 5 years with a peak incidence during approximately the second year of life. They usually occur during the rising phase of a fever, and generally only a single seizure occurs although as many as one-third of the affected children may have two or three seizures occurring in a single febrile episode. During the vulnerable age, each fever potentially may precipitate a seizure. The incidence of febrile seizures is amazingly high with an average of about 30 per 1000 children under 5 years old. In this age group, the average incidence of all seizures is about 50 per 1000. There is a strong familial relationship for febrile seizures and an even greater incidence of abnormal electroencephalograms among siblings of children with febrile seizures. There is evidence to support the notion that susceptibility to febrile seizures is determined by an irregular autosomal dominant gene (Lennox-Buchthal, 1975). Furthermore, there is similar evidence that absence seizures and at least some partial seizures are influenced by a genetic factor consistent with irregular autosomal dominance (Bray and Wiser, 1965; Andermann and Metrakos, 1973). This is an extremely important concept that offers some explanation for the fact that seizures occur in some individuals and not in others with apparently similar central nervous system insults. Further, it implies a biochemical basis for variation in seizure threshold which, if known, would be of considerable significance to the design of new anticonvulsant drugs and perhaps eventually to the prevention of epilepsy.

2. Status Epilepticus

Status epilepticus, a medical emergency when the seizures result in anoxia, refers to the repetitive occurrence of seizures without complete recovery between attacks and can manifest itself with any of the seizure patterns described. Generalized seizures are more frequently involved in status epilepticus than are partial complex seizures, which have only infrequently been reported. Fatalities do occur and are higher among those people with an identifiable etiology. It is obviously important to identify an etiology, if possible, because the treatment must be aimed at any correctable problem (infection, metabolic derangement, toxic chemical reaction, etc.) as well as at suppression of the seizures. The various clinical presentations of status epilepticus have been described in detail by Roger *et al.* (1975). Treatment is discussed later in Section VI,H.

III. NEUROCHEMISTRY

To a certain extent development of the neurochemistry of epilepsy has paralleled the development of biochemical techniques applicable to such a heterogeneous structure as the central nervous system. The earliest studies focused principally on energy metabolism in relation to oxygen supply, glucose metabolism, and oxidative phosphorylation. The relationship of available energy supply to the maintenance of ionic gradients across neuronal membranes logically developed from this, and more recently the role of glial cells in the maintenance of ionic homeostasis has been emphasized. The role of possible neurochemical transmitter substances has received more attention as techniques have been developed for more refined investigation. It is reasonable to assume that cellular control mechanisms will receive increasing attention in the future.

A. ENERGY METABOLISM

The principal substrate for energy metabolism in the brain is glucose, which must be continually supplied by cerebral blood flow. In order to meet this demand the brain receives about 20% of the total cardiac output and utilizes 20% of the total body oxygen consumption along with more than 50% of the total body glucose consumption. Energy derived from the oxidation of glucose is stored as phosphocreatine and utilized as adenosine triphosphate (ATP). As much as 50% of the available energy supply may be used for the maintenance of intracellular–extracellular cation gradients. The oxidation of two carbon fragments in the central nervous system is mediated by the classical citric acid cycle; however, a unique metabolic pathway, the γ-aminobutyric acid (GABA) shunt, exists (Fig. 1). Thus, in addition to the usual oxidative pathway from α-ketoglutarate to succinate, an alternate pathway consists of transamination of α-ketoglutarate to glutamate, decarboxylation of glutamate to GABA, transamination of GABA to succinic semialdehyde followed by dehydrogenation to succinate. Glutamic acid occupies a key position in central nervous system metabolism. Transaminations with pyruvate or oxaloacetate provide access to the citric acid cycle via α-ketoglutarate. Decarboxylation by glutamic acid decarboxylase, a B_6 vitamer-dependent apoenzyme, produces GABA, which is felt to be an important inhibitory modulator or transmitter substance. As the substrate for the reversible formation of glutamine, glutamate is also important for ammonia metabolism. A variety of manipulations of glutamic acid metabolic pathways produce increased or decreased seizure susceptibility. For example, depletion of the B_6 vitamer pyridoxal 5-phosphate by a number of methods (dietary depletion, inactivation, competitive antagonism) has been shown to produce convulsions in animals and man. In this situation depletion of GABA occurs because the affinity of glutamic acid decarboxylase for the B_6 vitamer is considerably less than that of the transaminase. Hypoglycemia is a well-established cause of seizures, and the potential role of glutamic acid in cerebral energy metabolism is emphasized by the fact that only glutamic acid can replace glucose in the maintenance of energy metabolism.

B. ELECTROLYTES

The normal neuronal resting membrane potential results from the maintenance of an intracellular electrolyte concentration that is high in K^+ and low in Na^+ relative to the extracellular fluid concentration. Energy is utilized by an electrolyte transport system in the neuronal membrane, Na–K–Mg-ATPase, to maintain these gradients. With excitatory postsynaptic depolarization sufficient to generate an action potential, Na^+ moves intracellularly and

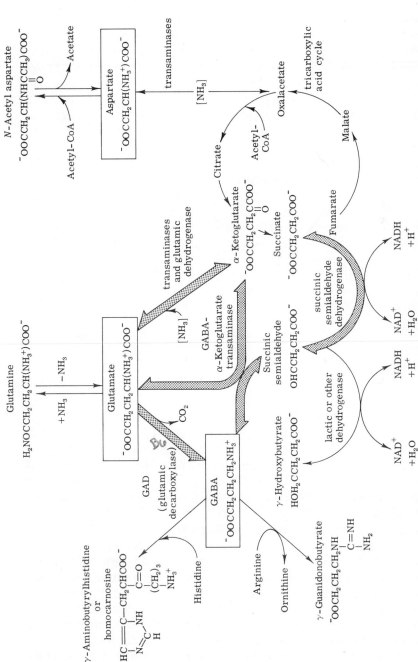

Fig. 1. Outline of chief known reactions of GABA, glutamate, and aspartate in the nervous system. The reactions pertinent to GABA metabolism are emphasized by the large arrows (Roberts, 1974).

K$^+$ flows out. During repolarization, Na$^+$ extrusion is coupled with K$^+$ uptake and the utilization of ATP to reestablish the membrane potential. Inhibitory postsynaptic potentials hyperpolarize the neuron and an action potential is not generated. Deficiencies in the supply of available ATP or functioning of the Na–K–Mg-ATPase system would lead to intracellular accumulation of Na$^+$, lowering of membrane potential, and enhanced excitability. This has been shown experimentally with ouabain, adrenalectomy, hypoglycemia, extracellular K$^+$ perfusion, and a variety of other procedures.

Depolarization of the presynaptic ending is felt to be associated with release of neurochemical transmitters that are specific for the neuron involved. There is presumptive evidence that acetylcholine, GABA, norepinephrine, dopamine, 5-hydroxytryptamine, glycine, and glutamic acid may be neurotransmitters in the brain or spinal cord. Any events that alter the synthesis, release, sensitivity to, or inactivation of neurotransmitters affect the excitation or inhibition mediated by the compound. There are numerous examples of such influences on seizure threshold. Organic phosphates bind to and inactivate an acetylcholinesterase which is important in inactivation of released acetylcholine. These compounds also produce seizures that are antagonized by 2-pyridine aldoxime, a compound that reverses the inactivation of acetylcholinesterase.

IV. NEUROPHYSIOLOGY

When an anatomically localized group of neurons, discharging synchronously at a rapid rate, produces sufficient excitation to involve adjacent normal neurons in the paroxysmal discharge, a seizure occurs. The clinical manifestations of the seizure are determined by the direction, extent, and speed with which the paroxysmal discharge spreads from the focus of abnormal neurons. Most neurons in the central nervous system consist of a cell body with two types of specialized extensions (Fig. 2). Dendrites are the receptive elements, which extend and branch over considerable distances. The efferent structure is the axon, which also extends for variable distances before branching to terminate on dendrites and cell bodies of other neurons. In addition, the axon may send recurrent collateral branches back to its own and other cell bodies. Each connection between neurons is a specialized structure called the synapse. Depolarization of the axon terminal or presynaptic membrane results in the release of a chemical transmitter substance which then influences the postsynaptic membrane to produce a localized change in membrane potential. If the change is in the direction of increasing polarization, an inhibitory postsynaptic potential has occurred. An excitatory postsynaptic potential results from a localized decrease in membrane potential. If the total

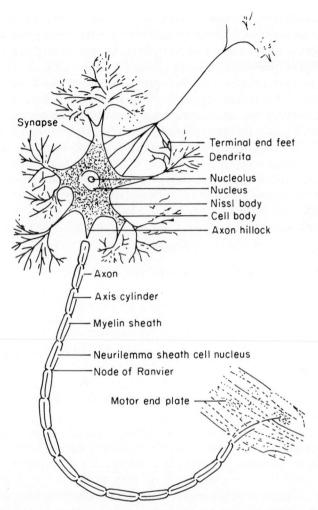

Fig. 2. Typical central nervous system motor neuron. [Reproduced from Woodburne (1957) by permission of Oxford University Press.]

number of excitatory postsynaptic potentials arriving at a cell body at one time is sufficient to cause a critical amount of depolarization in the region where the axon originates from the cell body, an action potential is propagated down the axon to its synapses. If the major input to the cell is inhibitory, the neuron is hyperpolarized and resistant to propagation of an action potential. An action potential is the result of the neuronal membrane becoming permeable to sodium ions, which causes a sudden rise in intracellular sodium concentration. The increase in intracellular sodium changes the potential difference between the inside and outside of the cell from negative to positive. When sodium entry stops, active extrusion of sodium begins accompanied by membrane permeability to potassium, which moves out of the cell, resulting in repolarization. The whole process is complete in slightly more than 1 msec. With inhibitory postsynaptic potentials, hyperpolarization is the result of permeability to potassium ions in the postsynaptic membrane.

Considering this elementary description of synaptic transmission, it can be appreciated that three broad categories of events may determine the occurrence of a seizure: (1) an increase in excitatory synaptic influences; (2) a decrease in inhibitory synaptic influences; and (3) an alteration in normal neuronal membrane characteristics. Hence, an effective anticonvulsant drug should stabilize neuronal membranes, augment inhibitory processes, or suppress excitation.

V. MECHANISM OF ANTICONVULSANT
DRUG ACTION

Hypotheses concerning the mechanism(s) of action of anticonvulsant drugs have been derived from observations of their effects in a variety of neurophysiological systems. These systems include isolated peripheral nerve, neuromuscular junction preparations, spinal cord preparations, and repetitive electrical activity within and between various central nervous system structures induced by focal, electrical, or chemical stimuli. Other models utilize seizure induction in intact animals with chemical or electrical stimulation. Consequently, the observations of anticonvulsant drug effects in most of these models are made with normal neuronal systems or normal neurons that have been made to discharge in an abnormal manner. If anticonvulsant drugs exert their principal effects on normal neurons, these model systems are appropriate. However, if the critical action of an anticonvulsant drug involves an effect on abnormal neurons in the epileptic focus, observations in normal neuronal systems may not be pertinent. Evidence does exist to support the hypothesis that phenytoin does indeed exert its major anticonvulsant effects on normal neurons; however, it is less clear how or where most other anticonvulsants act. The experimental systems that have been developed for the study of epileptic phenomena have been described in critical detail in the volume edited by Purpura *et al.* (1972).

The effect of anticonvulsant drugs on conduction and synaptic transmission in peripheral nerve reflects some of the properties of these drugs observed in the central nervous system. Normal conduction in peripheral nerve is unaffected by either phenobarbital or phenytoin, except at very high concentrations. However, hyperexcitability induced in peripheral nerve by either chemical or electrical stimulation is suppressed by phenobarbital and phenytoin. This indicates that both of these drugs have the capacity to stabilize neuronal membranes in the peripheral nervous system, in contrast to trimethadione, which does not exhibit such an effect. Phenobarbital and phenytoin differ in their action on synaptic transmission in peripheral nerve and in the central nervous system. These effects have been illustrated in model systems for synaptic transmission in the spinal cord described by Esplin (1972). The system (Fig. 3) consists of an afferent limb, the dorsal root, and an efferent limb, the ventral (motor) root. The afferent and efferent limbs are connected in several ways. There is a direct synapse of the afferent terminals on the motoneuron of the efferent limb which is called the monosynaptic pathway. There is also a polysynaptic pathway in which one or more interneurons are interspaced between the afferent terminals and the efferent motoneuron. Synaptic connections may be excitatory or inhibitory. Excitatory transmission is studied by electrically stimulating the dorsal root and recording the response from the ventral root, which consists of an early component representing monosynaptic transmission and a later component reflecting transmission through polysynaptic pathways. Barbiturates decrease excitatory postsynaptic potentials without altering the resting membrane potential. This effect is a result of an increase in the stability of the motoneuron, which requires greater depolarization to initiate an action potential. Barbiturates also prolong synaptic recovery time. Hydantoins have no influence on monosynaptic transmission of single stimuli but do produce some depression of polysynaptic transmission. Trimethadione and carbamazepine do not affect monosynaptic transmission, while acetazolamide does cause suppression. In

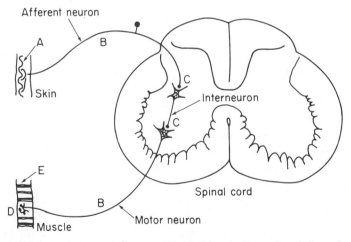

Fig. 3. Diagram of simple reflex arc in spinal cord. (Reproduced from Ruch and Fulton by permission of W. B. Saunders Company.)

contrast to its effect on monosynaptic pathways, acetazolamide has no effect on polysynaptic pathways and, in the same manner, carbamazepine, which does not influence monosynaptic transmission, does increase the latency and reduce the response in polysynaptic pathways. The benzodiazepines suppress both types of transmission.

Inhibitory transmission in the spinal cord can be observed by first stimulating an adjacent dorsal root, followed by stimulation of the dorsal root corresponding to the ventral root from which the response is recorded. Diminution in the response observed with initial stimulation of an adjacent dorsal root compared to the response observed without such stimulation reflects inhibition. Inhibition mediated by transmitter acting on the postsynaptic membrane may occur in several ways. Direct inhibition refers to transmission through a pathway in which a single interneuron exists between the afferent limb and the motoneuron. This type of inhibition is unaffected by phenytoin. When multiple interneurons are involved in the inhibitory pathway, the inhibition is polysynaptic. When inhibition originates from axon collaterals of motoneurons synapsing on interneurons called Renshaw cells, which in turn synapse on the same or adjacent motoneurons, it is called recurrent postsynaptic inhibition. In low doses phenobarbital augments monosynaptic responses, and this may be related to a depression of polysynaptic inhibition. The benzodiazepines do not affect postsynaptic inhibition.

Another type of response that can be elicited with the spinal cord system is called facilitation. This is an augmentation of the response to maximal afferent stimulation that occurs if the stimulus has been immediately preceded by an afferent stimulus at the minimal intensity required to elicit a response. The conditioning stimulation allows more excitatory synapses to be discharged by the maximal stimulation and thus the response is greater. Phenytoin is without effect on monosynaptic facilitation.

Considerable attention has been directed toward the effect of anticonvulsant drugs on repetitive stimulation in the spinal cord. Following low-frequency repetitive stimulation, there is a depression of the monosynaptic response which is further depressed by trimethadione. When the stimulation is applied at frequencies fast enough to induce tetany, the phenomenon of posttetanic potentiation is observed. This is an augmentation of the monosynaptic response following tetanizing stimulation that is attributed to hyperpolarization of presynaptic terminals, which increases the terminal action potential and, as a consequence, a larger postsynaptic motoneuron pool is activated. It is thought that the phenomenon of posttetanic potentiation may explain the spread of seizure activity from the focus, and in particular it may be critical for the development of the tonic phase of generalized tonic–clonic seizures. Phenytoin is extremely effective in blocking posttetanic hyperpolarization and posttetanic potentiation of the monosynaptic response. It does this in doses that do not exert other effects on peripheral nerve or spinal cord synaptic transmission. Phenobarbital also suppresses posttetanic potentiation, but high doses are required and the effect is not as selective as that seen with phenytoin. Acetazolamide, trimethadione, and the benzodiazepines do not affect posttetanic potentiation; however, carbamazepine is effective in blocking this phenomenon.

Repetitive stimulation of structures in the brain can produce an afterdischarge, which is a sustained repetitive neuronal discharge persisting after the stimulation is terminated. The discharge may remain localized or spread to other areas. The frequency and intensity of the applied stimulation are factors critical to the development of an afterdischarge, as is the region to which the stimulus is applied. The cerebellum is most resistant to the development of afterdischarges, while the hippocampus has the lowest threshold. Progressively higher thresholds to afterdischarges are seen in reticular formation, motor cortex, amygdala, neostriatum, specific thalamic nuclei, nonspecific thalamic nuclei, and occipital cortex. Phenytoin is very effective in shortening the duration of afterdischarges in cortex, limbic system, and diencephalon; however, higher doses are required to elevate the threshold to electrical stimulation. Phenobarbital is also effective in shortening the duration of afterdischarges in cortex, subcortex, and brainstem. In cortex, phenobarbital has a biphasic effect on threshold to electrical stimulation, with low doses reducing and high doses elevating the threshold. Trimethadione is capable of raising the threshold to electrical stimulation in most areas of the central nervous system, and it appears to be highly effective in doing so in the thalamus. It is not very effective in reducing the spread of discharges in cortex but does effectively block spread from cortex to thalamus. The effect of trimethadione on thalamus and spread of corticothalamic discharges may be related to its effectiveness against absence seizures. Carbamazepine also may suppress activity in a specific thalamic nucleus, and in addition it is effective in suppressing afterdischarges in cortex and limbic structures. The benzodiazepines are extremely effective in elevating the threshold to electrical stimulation in the reticular activating system, which may be related to their potent sedative activity. They also effectively shorten the duration and reduce the spread of repetitive discharges in cortex and limbic system.

It is worth noting that neurochemistry, neurophysiology, seizures, and anticonvulsant drugs all have one compound of common interest, γ-aminobutyric acid. Its structure is quite similar to the highly potent anticonvulsant phenylacetylurea. γ-Aminobutyric acid is clearly involved in central nervous system inhibition, and compounds that inhibit the action of GABA, such as bicuculline, produce seizures as do compounds that inhibit the production of GABA, such as hydrazides or antagonists of pyridoxal 5-phosphate. The anticonvulsant dipropylacetic acid elevates brain GABA concentration.

γ-Aminobutyric acid is an important inhibitory substance in the cerebellum, and there is evidence to suggest that stimulation of the cerebellum may be involved in the anticonvulsant activity of phenytoin (Julien and Halpern, 1972). The role of GABA in epilepsy has been consistently emphasized by Tower (1969), and it might be an important starting point for the future development of new anticonvulsant drugs.

VI. THERAPEUTIC USE OF ANTICONVULSANT DRUGS

A. BROMIDES

Salts of bromides were inadvertently recognized by Locock in 1857 as having anticonvulsant properties. The principal problem with the clinical utilization of bromides as anticonvulsant compounds is that the effective plasma concentration of bromide ion (10–20 mEq/liter) coincides closely with toxic plasma concentrations (15 mEq/liter). Bromide salts, taken in large doses, produce severe gastrointestinal irritation and vomiting, which limits acute toxic reactions. The more important clinical toxicity occurs with chronic dosing, which may lead to significant accumulation of bromide as a result of its extremely long half-life of about 12 days in man. Chronic bromide toxicity, or bromism, includes central nervous system manifestations of confusion, loss of memory, irrational behavior, delusions, hallucinations, and eventually coma. These may be associated with a diffuse dermatitis, conjunctivitis, and anorexia. Bromides are administered as an equal mixture of the salts of sodium, potassium, and ammonium or as the sodium salt alone in doses ranging from 1 to 5 gm/day. Plasma concentrations should be followed closely, and individual differences in efficacious and/or toxic concentrations may occur. It has been postulated that the anticonvulsant activity of bromide involves an effect on synaptic transmission either involving presynaptic inhibition (Muchnik and Gage, 1968) or by hyperpolarization of inhibitory postsynaptic potentials (Woodbury, 1969). The use of bromides is usually limited to special circumstances in which more effective anticonvulsants cannot be used such as multiple drug allergies or porphyria (Magnussen *et al.*, 1975).

B. BARBITURATES

1. Phenobarbital

Phenobarbital, the first modern anticonvulsant drug, was reported to be clinically effective as an anticonvulsant by Hauptman in 1912. To this day it remains one of the major anticonvulsant drugs. It has the widest spectrum of

H_5C_6 C_2H_5

Phenobarbital

H_5C_6 C_2H_5

Mephobarbital

H_5C_6 C_2H_5

Eterobarb

H_5C_6 C_2H_5

Primidone

activity in different seizure patterns, and many anticonvulsant drugs are structural derivatives of this barbiturate. Usual doses are in the range of 2–3 mg/kg and rarely exceed 5 mg/kg. Doses in excess of 250 mg/day are almost always associated with toxicity in the form of sedation, lethargy, and mental dullness, which is the principal toxic effect of the drug. The other major toxic reaction is restless, irritable, hyperactive behavior with short attention span, especially in children. Nevertheless, the ubiquitous clinical use of phenobarbital attests to its relative safety with chronic administration.

The long plasma half-life of phenobarbital in man, 3–6 days, results in extremely stable plasma concentrations and permits once daily dosing, which is a distinct advantage. The necessity of multiple daily doses of a drug taken chronically readily predisposes to forgetting doses and irritation with the inconvenience of continually having to remember to take medication. These inconveniences lead to noncompliance with prescribed doses and failure to obtain seizure control. Similarly, with such a long half-life it is totally unnecessary to use time-release formulations, which are most likely poorly absorbed. Finally, it is important to recognize that the time to reach approximately 95% of the steady-state plasma concentration of a drug that is disposed with first-order kinetics is a direct function of its half-life. Thus, phenobarbital requires 12–24 days to approximate its steady-state concentration. Failure to recognize this principle can lead to overdosing and erroneous conclusions about the efficacy of the drug. The time to steady-state concentration can be shortened, perhaps at the expense of some toxicity, by increasing the initial doses and subsequently reducing the dose to the desired amount as the appropriate concentration is approached. These principles have been discussed in detail elsewhere (Fingl, 1972).

Considerable experience has accumulated relating serum concentrations of phenobarbital to efficacy and toxicity. A good correlation exists between toxicity and serum concentration; however, wide individual differences are seen. In general, once an efficacious concentration is obtained for an individual patient, it remains effective; i.e., pharmacodynamic tolerance to the anticonvulsant activity is not common or extensive with phenobarbital. Some patients are controlled with concentrations below 10 μg/ml of serum. Sedative toxicity is absolutely minimal or nonexistent at such concentrations after initial tolerance to sedation is established. In contrast to the anticonvulsant activity, pharmacodynamic tolerance to sedation with phenobarbital does occur to a considerable extent (Butler *et al.*, 1954). The majority of patients who benefit from phenobarbital without excessive sedation do so with concentrations ranging from 10 to 30 μg/ml. As concentrations exceed 30 μg/ml, sedation is increasingly encountered. It is unusual to find no evidence of sedation or slowness in patients with concentrations greater than 50 μg/ml.

In addition to sedation and hyperactive behavior, some patients may experience an increase in seizure frequency with excessively high phenobarbital concentrations. While this is unusual it must always be kept in mind. Since this effect of phenobarbital has not been well documented in the literature several case reports from the author's experience follows to illustrate the point.

a. Case Report 1 (K. B.)

A 31-year-old white woman had her first seizure at the age of 11½ years. Her seizures begin without an aura and consist of staring, arrest of ongoing behavior, head turning in either direction, and varied automatisms usually with walking. Brief confusion follows the seizure, and she is aware that a segment of time has been lost. She has never had a generalized tonic–clonic seizure. Her seizures varied in frequency from none to about 35 per day, and she rarely experienced more than one consecutive day without seizures except during her only pregnancy in 1971, when her seizures decreased to one or two per week. With the birth of her normal child, the seizures resumed their previous frequency. Electroencephalograms initially revealed a mixture of left temporal lobe spikes and generalized three to three and one-half per second spike and slow-wave discharges. As an adult, the left temporal lobe focus predominated and three per second spike and slow-wave patterns were only occasionally seen with hyperventilation. She had failed to respond to all of the available anticonvulsant drugs in various combinations and had experienced numerous episodes of anticonvulsant toxicity.

In 1974, she entered a double-blind study comparing 3 months of treatment with phenobarbital to 3 months of treatment with eterobarb. At the beginning of the study, she was taking phenytoin 400 mg/day and primidone 1 gm/day. Seizures were occurring at the rate of 20–30 per day. The serum concentration of phenytoin was 17 μg/ml, that of phenobarbital was 46 μg/ml, and that of primidone was 10 μg/ml. At this time, she was moderately slow in speech and thought and was experiencing trouble with irritability and a short temper.

During the first 3-month period, she received eterobarb in doses up to

720 mg/day and averaged about 90 seizures per week. Her phenobarbital concentration averaged 60 μg/ml (range 44–77 μg/ml). During the second 3-month period, she averaged 87 seizures per week with a mean phenobarbital serum concentration of 38 μg/ml (range 31–51 μg/ml) achieved with phenobarbital doses up to 200 mg/day. When the study was completed and the data examined it became apparent that seizure frequency correlated well with serum phenobarbital concentration. Subsequently, she was gradually withdrawn from barbiturates. Initially, her seizures shortened in duration and then in frequency so that about 1 month after barbiturate withdrawal they were only apparent to herself and occurred at the rate of one to two per month. She continued to improve during the next one and a half years. She became an alert, relaxed, and happy person and her facial acne cleared completely.

b. *Case Report 2 (R. G.)*

A 32-year-old black woman has had seizures since the age of 12 years. Her seizures are generalized tonic–clonic without an aura, followed by 1–2 hours of postictal confusion. Electroencephalograms demonstrated a left frontal spiking focus. The patient's sister, paternal aunt, and paternal uncle also have seizures. She usually experienced one or two seizures per month in spite of treatment with various doses and combinations of phenytoin, phenobarbital, and primidone to the point of toxicity on several occasions. Pregnancy and the use of alcohol had resulted in a considerable increase in seizure frequency in the past.

In December 1973, she began a double-blind crossover study comparing 3 months of treatment with eterobarb to 3 months of treatment with phenobarbital. At the beginning of the study, she was receiving primidone 750 mg/day, which produced serum concentrations of 18 μg/ml phenobarbital and 20 μg/ml primidone. During the first 3-month period she received phenobarbital in doses of 120–160 mg/day and had an average serum concentration of 31 μg/ml (range 25–38 μg/ml). She experienced three seizures. During the next 3 months she received eterobarb in daily doses ranging from 360 to 480 mg with an average phenobarbital concentration of 53 μg/ml (range 40–78 μg/ml). She experienced six seizures. She continued taking the eterobarb for an additional month and had three more seizures. Her medication was then changed to phenytoin 200 mg/day and phenobarbital 180 mg/day, which produced serum concentrations of 28 μg/ml phenytoin and 45 μg/ml phenobarbital. During the next month, she had fifteen seizures. She was hospitalized in a state of severe confusion. During the next 10 days her phenytoin was gradually discontinued and phenobarbital was reduced to 120 mg/day. Her phenobarbital concentration eventually stabilized at 16 μg/ml. During the following year, she had three seizures, all of which were less severe than any she had previously experienced.

When phenobarbital treatment is to be discontinued, it must be accomplished gradually. Abrupt or too rapid withdrawal from phenobarbital is almost always associated with an increase in seizure frequency and is particularly likely to provoke a generalized tonic–clonic seizure. The exacerbation usually occurs at about one half-life after abrupt withdrawal of the drug (Gallagher *et al.*, 1975). In general, withdrawal should be accomplished in three or four equal reductions of the total dose spaced at intervals of at least two half-lives (i.e., approximately 1 week apart). Gradual withdrawal is not essential when drugs such as primidone, eterobarb, or mephobarbital are substituted for phenobarbital, since these are each metabolized in part to phenobarbital.

Phenobarbital is metabolized by the mixed-function oxidase enzyme system of the hepatic endoplasmic reticulum. Hydroxylation occurs primarily at the para position of the 5-phenyl group; however, smaller amounts of the drug are hydroxylated in the ethyl moiety and dihydroxylated on the phenyl ring. These polar metabolites of phenobarbital are excreted by the kidney as such or may be conjugated to glucuronate or sulfate prior to excretion. Phenobarbital is a potent inducing agent for the mixed function oxidase enzyme system, and this forms the basis for some important drug interactions. It should be remembered that most epileptic patients have been exposed to large amounts of various anticonvulsant drugs for many years and may be maximally induced. Consequently, induction is not seen consistently when drugs having this property are administered. Induction or increased clearance of drug administered concomitantly with phenobarbital, whether or not true induction has occurred (Mannering, 1971), has been reported for a number of compounds. These include endogenous substances such as steroids, bilirubin, glucuronic acid, and the precursors of porphyrins. Among the drugs that may be cleared more rapidly in the presence of phenobarbital are bishydroxycoumarin, digitoxin, diphenylhydantoin, griseofulvin, DDT, antipyrine, and many others. The net effect of induction is a function of the activity of the metabolites and the parent compound.

2. Mephobarbital

The N-methylated derivative of phenobarbital has anticonvulsant activity (Craig and Shideman, 1971) and is metabolized rapidly and probably completely to phenobarbital. It either is not absorbed well (Butler and Waddell, 1958) or possibly undergoes biliary excretion more extensively than phenobarbital (Klaasen, 1971). In either event, there is no appreciable accumulation of mephobarbital in serum of epileptic patients treated with this drug, and consequently it offers no advantage in comparison to phenobarbital and has the disadvantages of extreme variability in phenobarbital serum concentration and greater expense for the patient. There has not been any convincing documentation that phenobarbital derived from mephobarbital is less sedating than equal amounts of phenobarbital not metabolically derived.

3. Eterobarb

The N,N'-dimethoxymethyl derivative of phenobarbital appears to be an interesting anticonvulsant compound. To date, it has been examined in four open investigations, with both patient and physician aware of the medication received, and in three double-blind trials comparing eterobarb to phenobarbital (Gallagher *et al.*, 1975; Gallagher and Woodbury, 1976). In addition, the sedative activity of phenobarbital administered as such or metabolically derived from eterobarb has been compared in a group of normal volunteers using a battery of psychological tests (Smith *et al.*, 1974).

The studies concerning efficacy uniformly found superior seizure control with eterobarb in patients with generalized tonic–clonic seizures as well as in those with partial complex seizures with or without secondary generalization. These studies were all conducted with concomitant measurement of serum anticonvulsant concentrations. A consistent finding was higher phenobarbital concentrations in the patients treated with eterobarb without a corresponding increase in sedation. In fact, some patients were less sedated even though serum phenobarbital concentration rose during eterobarb treatment. The psychological study in normal volunteers was also consistent with an interpretation of decreased sedative activity for a given serum concentration of phenobarbital derived from eterobarb compared to that from phenobarbital administered as such. The doses employed ranged from 2 to 11 mg/kg with most patients receiving between 240 and 480 mg/day.

The metabolism of eterobarb in man is of some interest. The compound is absorbed rapidly when administered orally and exhibits a "first-pass" effect; i.e., the parent compound passes from the gastrointestinal tract through the portal circulation to the liver and never appears in the systemic circulation. Oral and intravenous administration appear almost identical in the pattern of metabolite appearance and removal (Matsumoto and Gallagher, 1976).

The two principal metabolites are monomethoxymethylphenobarbital and phenobarbital. Monomethoxymethylphenobarbital disappears with a half-life of 4–6 hours and does not appear unchanged in urine. Urine collected during the first 24 hours after administration of the drug contains a much larger amount of polar metabolites, presumably of phenobarbital, than are found after comparable doses of phenobarbital. The principal polar metabolites are *p*-hydroxyphenobarbital and glucuronide conjugates of *p*-hydroxyphenobarbital. Biliary secretion has not been studied; however, it may occur since significant quantities of the drug were not recovered in urine with collections for up to 9 days after dosing.

In animal studies (Baumel *et al.*, 1976) the monomethoxymethyl metabolite does possess anticonvulsant activity. It is not clear that this is sufficient to account for convincing superiority of eterobarb as an anticonvulsant in man. It has been suggested (Gallagher *et al.*, 1975) that the attenuated sedative activity may allow higher concentrations of phenobarbital to be tolerated and that anticonvulsant activity continues to rise with increasing concentrations, at least for some patients. Elucidation of the mechanism by which sedative activity is attenuated should have extremely important implications for the design of new anticonvulsants as well as for the mechanism of pharmacodynamic tolerance to barbiturates.

4. Deoxybarbiturate (Primidone)

Primidone was synthesized in 1949 (Bogue and Carrington, 1953) and introduced to clinical use in 1952 by Handley and Stewart. It is the 2-deoxy derivative of phenobarbital and represents another derivative with a spectrum of anticonvulsant and toxic activity different from that of phenobarbital.

In animals and man, primidone is metabolized to phenylethylmalondiamide (PEMA) and phenobarbital (Gallagher and Baumel, 1972). Recent studies with ^{14}C-labeled primidone found no evidence of polar metabolites of primidone or PEMA in urine from epileptic patients (Zavadil and Gallagher, 1976). Primidone is excreted unchanged in urine in significant amounts, and this may result in crystalluria with acute overdose. Quantitatively, the principal metabolite is PEMA, which is also excreted unchanged in urine. Phenylethylmalonamide has a half-life of about 40 hours in epileptic patients, and on the basis of animal studies it is a weak anticonvulsant that has the capacity to potentiate the anticonvulsant activity of phenobarbital in concentrations that have no other demonstrable activity (Gallagher and Baumel, 1972). Primidone itself is an extremely potent anticonvulsant in animals with a spectrum of activity similar to that of phenytoin (Baumel et al., 1973). The oxidation of primidone to phenobarbital occurs with an enzyme system localized in hepatic microsomes which has all the characteristics of the mixed-function oxidase enzyme system. The reaction occurs at a low rate and can be induced by other anticonvulsants such as diphenylhydantoin and carbamazepine (DiMicco and Gallagher, 1975). This is responsible for several interesting clinical observations concerning the use of primidone. If the drug is given alone there is a lag period of 2–4 days before phenobarbital can be detected in serum and the steady-state ratio of primidone to phenobarbital is about 1:1. If it is given in conjunction with diphenylhydantoin or carbamazepine (and probably other anticonvulsants) the steady-state ratio of primidone to phenobarbital in serum is about 1:3. Most of these observations concerning the metabolism and activity of primidone have been made in the last five years. Prior to that time primidone was usually used when phenobarbital and diphenylhydantoin failed to control seizures. Primidone would then be substituted for phenobarbital in doses ranging from 500 to 1500 mg/day. With these doses in the presence of diphenylhydantoin significant concentrations of phenobarbital accumulate, usually in the range of 20–40 μg/ml of serum. To a great extent, such large amounts of phenobarbital obscure the anticonvulsant activity of primidone itself. Since this activity has not been well documented in previous literature, a typical case report illustrating the point follows.

Case Report (H.C.)

A 42-year-old black man with a history of generalized seizures in infancy following head trauma was well until the age of 30 years. At that time he developed episodes of staring, altered consciousness, lip smacking, and auto-matisms with his hands, lasting 30 seconds to 1 minute. Electroencephalograms intermittently contained right temporal lobe spikes while all other studies, including pneumoencephalograms, cerebral arteriograms, and brain scans were normal. He was initially seizure free for four years while receiving phenytoin 300 mg/day. From 1968 through 1972, he experienced 16 seizures. In March 1973 he had another seizure, and phenobarbital 60 mg/day was added to the phenytoin. Four more seizures occurred in the next month, and phenobarbital was increased to 90 mg/day. By September 1973 he had experienced an addi-tional two seizures. Serum concentration of phenytoin was 20 μg/ml, while that of phenobarbital was 32 μg/ml. In November 1973 phenytoin concentration was 20 μg/ml and that of phenobarbital was 25 μg/ml. Because of drowsiness the dose of phenobarbital was reduced to 60 mg/day. In January 1974 the serum concentrations of phenytoin and phenobarbital were each 17 μg/ml. By March 1974 he had experienced three more seizures. Primidone was gradually sub-stituted for phenobarbital. From March 1974 until October 1975 he has remained seizure free. Multiple serum concentrations of phenytoin and phenobarbital have never exceeded 23 μg/ml, while primidone concentration has varied from 2 to 6 μg/ml. The average serum phenobarbital concentration during this 19-month interval was 12 μg/ml.

The toxic reactions associated with primidone are quite interesting. When primidone is administered in doses of 250 mg or more to patients who have not been receiving phenobarbital (or a drug metabolized to phenobarbital), an acute toxic syndrome is frequently encountered. The symptoms include severe dizziness, a sense of inebriation, nausea, vomiting, drowsiness, and double vision, which may last from 6 to 24 hours. Tolerance to this syndrome develops when primidone therapy is gradually increased from low doses. Phenobarbital produces a tolerance to this acute toxic reaction to primidone (Gallagher and Baumel, 1972), and it is possible that the metabolism of primidone to phenobarbital is essential for the development of such tolerance. We have studied one patient who oxidized primidone at such a low rate that phenobarbital never accumulated and she never developed tolerance to the toxic reaction. The chronic toxicity of primidone is essentially identical to that of phenobarbital.

C. HYDANTOINS

1. Phenytoin (Diphenylhydantoin)

This drug may also be considered a structural analogue of phenobarbital. It has been the most intensely studied anticonvulsant drug, yet its fundamental mechanism of action has not been clearly established. Because it does not have the sedative properties of barbiturates it was considered to be less toxic than phenobarbital. This is certainly not the case, and the wide range of toxic effects of phenytoin has been reemphasized recently (Glaser, 1972). Its

Phenytoin
(diphenylhydantoin)

Mephenytoin

Ethotoin

Doxenitoine
(deoxyhydantoin)

greatest efficacy is for generalized tonic–clonic seizures and it is also useful in most of the partial seizures. Phenytoin is metabolized by the hepatic mixed-function oxidase system. The principal metabolite is p-hydroxyphenytoin, and smaller amounts of a dihydrodiol, a catechol, and O-methylcatechol are also formed. The polar metabolites are excreted as such or as conjugates of glucuronate. Excretion of unchanged phenytoin is negligible, and as a consequence inhibition of metabolism or genetically determined impairment of ability to oxidize phenytoin leads to toxicity if the drug is administered in conventional doses. A wide range of toxic reactions occurs with chronic exposure to phenytoin, especially at high serum concentrations. As with phenobarbital, efficacy may be encountered at any serum concentration. With concentrations below 15 μg/ml, toxicity is usually not a problem. Toxicity increases in incidence and severity with further elevation of the serum concentration so that almost every person has some manifestations of toxicity with concentrations greater than 30 μg/ml. Toxic reactions frequently reflect disturbances in the vestibular–cerebellar systems and are manifested by ataxia, nystagmus, diplopia, and tremor. Wide individual differences are encountered in the degree to which these disturbances appear, and they cannot be relied on as an absolute indication of excessively high serum concentrations of phenytoin. Direct measurement of serum concentration must be performed. With chronic exposure to high phenytoin concentrations a cerebellar degeneration may occur which usually is not completely reversible. A diffuse encephalopathy, characterized by an alteration in mental function ranging from slowness in thought, confusion, delirium, or coma, also may develop. Frequently this is associated with an increase in seizure frequency and there may be focal neurological signs. This syndrome is reversible in most instances with reduction in the serum phenytoin concentrations. Other toxic reactions include a peripheral neuropathy, nausea and vomiting, a megaloblastic anemia probably secondary to folic acid deficiency, hypocalcemia and osteomalacia secondary to vitamin D deficiency, hirsutism, acne, and gingival hyperplasia. The gingival hyperplasia is most frequently encountered in children and is highly undesirable cosmetically and for dental hygiene. The allergic reactions to the drug are those usually encountered with any compound.

Numerous drugs and endogenous substances have been shown to interact with phenytoin metabolism. Both increased and decreased clearance rate of phenytoin have been documented. The interested reader is referred to the excellent reviews by Kutt (1975) and by Buchanan and Sholiton (1972).

2. Mephenytoin

Mephenytoin is the 5-ethyl-5-phenyl-3-methyl derivative of hydantoin. It was introduced for clinical use in 1945 after the 5-ethyl-5-phenyl derivative of phenytoin (Nirvanol) proved to be excessively toxic. Mephenytoin is rapidly *N*-demethylated and hence exhibits the same spectrum of toxicity found with Nirvanol. As a result its clinical use is restricted to situations in which a hydantoin might be useful (generalized tonic and/or clonic seizures and some partial seizures) and in which the other hydantoins have failed or produced toxic reactions that preclude their utilization. Mephenytoin may cause fatal exfoliative dermatitis, hepatitis, or aplastic anemias. Like ethotoin it has sedative properties that exceed those of phenytoin and it is capable of producing all of the toxic and allergic reactions associated with hydantoins. The usual doses are identical to those used with phenytoin.

3. Ethotoin

Ethotoin, the 5-phenyl-3-ethyl derivative of hydantoin, is a useful adjunctive anticonvulsant in certain instances. It is less toxic than phenytoin and may be used in doses up to about 3 gm/day. It has sedative properties that are greater than those of phenytoin. Ethotoin is most useful in patients whose seizures respond to phenytoin only at concentrations that involve some toxicity. Under these circumstances the addition of ethotoin frequently permits a reduction in the dose of phenytoin without loss of seizure control, and usually some reduction in toxicity is achieved.

4. Deoxyhydantoin (Doxenitoine)

Doxenitoine (5,5-diphenyltetrahydroglyoxalin-4-one) is the 2-deoxy derivative of phenytoin. Therefore, it bears the same structural relationship to phenytoin as primidone does to phenobarbital. The compound has been studied in a variety of animal models of epilepsy and in patients undergoing electroconvulsive shock for treatment of depression (Goodman *et al.*, 1954). Doxenitoine was effective in blocking the tonic component of maximal electroshock seizures in mice and rats. The compound was less potent than phenytoin: mice, ED_{50} doxenitoine 32 mg/kg (range 29.6–34.6); rats, ED_{50}

doxenitoine 36 mg/kg (range 28.4–46.0); mice, ED_{50} phenytoin 11.0 mg/kg (range 7.6–16.0); rats, ED_{50} phenytoin 27.5 mg/kg (range 20.4–37.1). However, doxenitoine was less toxic than phenytoin, which resulted in higher protective index scores, and it also possessed a wider spectrum of anticonvulsant activity than phenytoin. In patients undergoing electroshock therapy, oral doses of doxenitoine (800–2400 mg) successfully blocked tonic seizure activity in six of nine patients studied and it shortened the duration of the tonic component in the other three patients. With chronic administration of doxenitoine, both the tonic and the clonic components of the electroshock seizures were prevented. Phenytoin does not block the clonic component of such seizures.

The anticonvulsant activity of doxenitoine was subsequently examined in epileptic patients. In the first clinical trial (Millichap *et al.*, 1955), the seizure frequency of 22 institutionalized children and adults, while being treated with diphenylhydantoin plus other anticonvulsant drugs, was compared to that during an 18-month period of doxenitoine treatment alone. Four of the 22 patients had greater than 50% reduction in seizure frequency and 12 patients had their seizures completely controlled. The average dose used was 800 mg/day (20 mg/kg) and the maximal dose was 1400 mg/day. Ten of the 22 subjects had side effects, which were principally symptoms of gastric irritation. Importantly, only 1 of the 9 patients with normal gingivae developed hyperplasia during the 18 months and 3 of 9 patients with gingival hypertrophy at the onset of treatment experienced a recession.

Another study was reported by Boudin *et al.* (1959). They administered doxenitoine in doses of 500–800 mg/day along with constant doses of each patient's other anticonvulsant drug. There were 29 outpatients studied for various durations (greater than 1 year, 4 patients; 6 months to 1 year, 6 patients; 3 months to 6 months, 16 patients; and 1 month to 3 months, 3 patients). They obtained the results shown in the following tabulation:

Generalized seizures	$\frac{3}{9}$ complete control
	$\frac{2}{9}$ partial control
	$\frac{4}{9}$ no effect
Temporal lobe seizures	$\frac{3}{11}$ complete control
	$\frac{3}{11}$ partial control
	$\frac{1}{11}$ complete control for 1 month followed by return of seizures
	$\frac{1}{11}$ no effect
	$\frac{3}{11}$ indeterminate
Absence seizures	$\frac{2}{9}$ complete control
	$\frac{2}{9}$ partial control
	$\frac{2}{9}$ transitory control
	$\frac{2}{9}$ no effect
	$\frac{1}{9}$ indeterminate

They encountered vestibular dysfunction resembling hydantoin toxicity in one patient who accidently consumed 1600 mg/day. Drowsiness was dose related in 4 patients and transient gastric irritation was noted in 2 patients. The authors concluded that doxenitoine was an effective anticonvulsant without serious toxicity.

The metabolism of doxenitoine has been studied in rats by Glasson *et, al.* (1963). They utilized single doses of [2-^{14}C]doxenitoine. They found eight apparent metabolites in urine. They were unable to find phenytoin as a metabolite, and they did find a 5-phenylhydroxy metabolite with and without conjugation to sulfate and glucuronate. They also found the parent compound in urine, and they failed to recover as much as 40% of the radioactivity, suggesting the possibility of ring cleavage at C-2, where the label was placed. It is still possible that with chronic administration in man the compound might be oxidized to phenytoin.

D. ACETYLUREAS

Several acetylurea compounds have been used as anticonvulsants, as have structurally related derivatives. Structure–activity relationships have been established, and it is interesting to note that some of these compounds have both antipentylenetetrazole and antimaximal electroshock activity. The prototype drug is phenylacetylurea (phenacemide), in which a phenyl group exists at R_1 and the other three positions are occupied by hydrogen. Anticonvulsant activity is lost without a phenyl group at R_1. Substitution of a methyl group at R_2 increases sedative activity and retains the anticonvulsant properties. A methyl substitution at R_3 increases activity against pentylenetetrazole seizures, while methyl substitutions at R_3 and R_4 abolish this action. Sedation is increased with an ethyl group at R_2 and pentylenetetrazole antagonism is reduced. Finally, a phenyl substitution at R_2 abolishes anticonvulsant activity (Everett and Richards, 1952).

$$R_1 \diagdown \atop R_2 \diagup CH-\overset{\overset{\displaystyle O}{\|}}{C}-N-\overset{\overset{\displaystyle O}{\|}}{C}-NH-R_4 \atop \underset{R_3}{|}$$

1. Phenacemide

Phenylacetylurea is a straight-chain anticonvulsant compound with significant efficacy for generalized tonic and/or clonic seizures, absence seizures, and many partial seizures. Unfortunately, it is also one of the most toxic anticonvulsant drugs. The principal toxic reactions that occur frequently involve mood changes such as depression, irritability, agitation, and aggressive or violent behavior. Psychotic reactions also occur. Phenacemide has also produced fatalities associated with hepatitis, aplastic anemia, and renal failure. Its use should be restricted to the most refractory clinical situations, and patients taking the medication should be closely supervised and have frequent blood tests to monitor renal, liver, and bone marrow function.

$$\langle\!\!\!\!\!\!\!\!\bigcirc\!\!\!\!\!\!\rangle\text{—CH}_2\text{—CO—NH—CO—NH}_2$$

Phenacemide

The anticonvulsant activity of phenacemide has been reported by several investigators. Gibbs *et al.* (1949) studied 90 patients who were resistant to other anticonvulsants and found a 50% or greater reduction in seizure frequency for one-half of the group while the other half was not improved. Most of their patients had partial complex seizures. They encountered a 20% incidence of personality change and 12% of the patients developed anorexia. Carter *et al.* (1950) administered phenacemide in doses ranging from 0.5 to 6 gm/day to 88 epileptic patients. Duration of treatment varied from 2 weeks to 17 months and most of patients continued to receive their previous medications. Twenty-five patients were lost from the study, principally because of toxicity. Of the remaining 63 patients, 32% had a significant reduction in seizure frequency and 68% were unchanged. The best results were in patients with absence seizures; however, at the end of the $1\frac{1}{2}$-year study 86% of the patients had stopped taking the drug because of toxicity. Davidson and Lennox (1950) observed the effects of phenacemide in 178 patients, of whom 75% were children. Seizures were completely controlled in 3%, reduced in frequency 50% or more in 22%, and reduced in frequency less than 50% in 24% of the group. Carter *et al.* found efficacy for all patterns of seizures in those who responded, and they reported improved behavior in 26 patients as well as deteriorated behavior in 26 patients. Perry and Simonds (1951) found improved seizure control in 25 of 34 patients observed for 3–8 months.

2. Ethylphenacemide (Pheneturide)

Pheneturide is an anticonvulsant used in Europe. Orloff *et al.* (1951) reported the results of administering pheneturide without other anticonvulsants to ten institutionalized patients in doses of 1–7 gm/day. Only one patient had beneficial effects without toxicity. The compound appears to elevate serum concentrations of other anticonvulsant drugs, and it is usually administered as a combination formulation of pheneturide 200 mg, phenytoin 40 mg, and phenobarbital 15 mg. The clinical studies with the combination tablet will not be reviewed because data relating to serum concentration are lacking and this information is critical for an interpretation of the results.

3. Beclamide (*N*-Benzyl-3-chloropropionamide)

Beclamide is another straight-chain anticonvulsant compound that has been studied in epileptic patients. Most of the reports give little or no detail and are not enthusiastic about the compound. Livingstone (1953) administered the drug in combination with other anticonvulsants to 43 patients and by itself to 6 patients. Only a small number of patients experienced temporary improvement, but no data were presented. In the same manner, Peterman (1954), without presenting data, states that the compound was effective in only 2 of 68 patients. Kaplan and Maslanka (1952) briefly reported greater than 50% reduction, principally for generalized tonic–clonic seizures, in 16 of 31 patients. In contrast to the previous studies, Hawkes (1952) obtained beneficial results in 39 of 59 patients observed for two years. The drug was used alone in all but 11 patients. Complete seizure control or at most rare seizures occurred in 23 of the 39 patients, while the other 16 who improved experienced one to four seizures per month. Toxicity was not a problem in this group of patients.

$$\text{C}_6\text{H}_5{-}\text{CH}{-}\text{CO}{-}\text{NH}{-}\text{CO}{-}\text{NH}_2 \qquad \text{Cl}{-}\text{CH}_2{-}\text{CH}_2{-}\text{CO}{-}\text{NH}{-}\text{CH}_2{-}\text{C}_6\text{H}_5$$
$$\qquad\quad \overset{|}{\text{CH}_2{-}\text{CH}_3}$$

Ethylphenacemide   Beclamide

4. Atrolactamide (2-Hydroxy-2-phenylpropionamide)

Atrolactamide was administered to 300 drug-resistant epileptic patients by Stamps *et al.* (1952). Doses ranged from 4 to 12 gm/day. For generalized tonic–clonic seizures 98 of 115 patients experienced 50% or greater reduction in seizure frequency with 49 of these having complete seizure control for two years. Eleven of 20 patients with atypical absences achieved the same seizure control with 3 patients completely seizure free. With partial complex seizures, greater than 50% reduction was reported for 118 of 140 patients with 26 seizure free. Seventeen of 33 patients with absence seizures and 10 of 13 patients with partial elementary seizures achieved 50% or more reduction in seizure frequency. While no adverse effects were noted on behavior, 16 patients experienced sedation, 11 developed a leukopenia, 6 were ataxic, 4 had a skin rash, and 2 had aplastic anemia, and 1 case of diplopia and 1 urticarial

$$\text{C}_6\text{H}_5\overset{\displaystyle\text{OH}}{\underset{\displaystyle\text{CH}_3}{-\overset{|}{\underset{|}{\text{C}}}-}}\text{CO}{-}\text{NH}_2$$

Atrolactamide

reaction were noted. This apparently was a highly effective drug, but on subsequent use patients experienced more toxicity. However, these reports are not in the literature as far as this author is aware.

E. CARBAMAZEPINE

Carbamazepine is a major anticonvulsant drug with significant efficacy for all partial seizures as well as for generalized tonic and/or clonic seizures. Carbamazepine is an iminostilbene derivative and as such represents a new chemical class of anticonvulsants. However, the three-dimensional structure of the compound is quite similar to that of the barbiturates and hydantoins. Metabolism of carbamazepine in man has not been completely determined; however, it appears to at least involve epoxide formation at the 10–11 double bond with subsequent formation of a 10,11-dihydroxy metabolite. The carbamyl group also may be removed from the nitrogen at position 5. The dihydroxy and iminostilbene metabolites also appear to be conjugated with at least glucuronic acid. The metabolites identified in urine thus far do not account for the total disposition of the drug. Conventional anticonvulsant doses in adults usually vary from 600 to 1200 mg/day, and there is little accumulation of the parent compound with these doses. Serum concentrations of carbamazepine are generally less than 10 μg/ml, and toxicity is frequently associated with higher concentrations. Consequently, the compound is either incompletely absorbed or disposed of by means that have not yet been elucidated.

Carbamazepine

The anticonvulsant efficacy of carbamazepine is indisputable. Carbamazepine has anticonvulsant activity in a variety of experimental models of epilepsy. It blocks the hindlimb extensor component after maximal electroshock, elevates the threshold to minimal electroshock, and blocks pentylenetetrazole seizures at doses and serum concentrations in the range encountered with its clinical use (Julien and Hollister, 1975). It also effectively suppresses penicillin-induced spikes and electrically induced cortical afterdischarges, while it is relatively ineffective against estrogen-induced paroxysmal discharges and suppresses posttetanic potentiation in spinal cord preparations at high doses.

The drug appears to be of some benefit in approximately 70% of most patient populations that have been studied with partial complex or generalized tonic–clonic seizures. There are numerous reports that the compound also possesses significant beneficial psychotropic effects; however, every well-controlled study designed to identify such effects has failed to find any significant psychotropic effect. The idea that carbamazepine should have effects on behavior undoubtedly arises from its structural relationship to the tricyclic antidepressant drugs. Perhaps the major problem in identifying a causal relationship between behavioral changes and carbamazepine treatment is the fact that the compound has relatively little toxicity and considerable efficacy. As a result, the behavioral changes that result from increased seizure control and/or reduced toxicity from the anticonvulsant drug that was replaced by carbamazepine may be misinterpreted as a direct effect of carbamazepine. These are exceedingly difficult factors to control in a clinical trial, and there are numerous problems in the interpretation of psychological tests in epileptic patients receiving multiple anticonvulsant drugs.

Toxicity with carbamazepine is relatively minor. The most serious effect is its capacity to suppress bone marrow function and possibly to produce an aplastic anemia which may be fatal. Considering the thousands of patients who have been treated with the drug, this is a rare event. Some suppression of the white blood cell count is seen in a large percentage of patients receiving carbamazepine, and this should not be an indication for discontinuing treatment unless the total count falls below 3000/mm^3 or a significant thrombocytopenia or anemia develops. If the peripheral blood counts are routinely followed in patients receiving the drug, it is most likely that serious toxicity can be completely avoided. The most frequent side effects involve mild drowsiness, diplopia, and gastric irritation. These are usually dose related and occur in about 5% of the population. The relatively low incidence of toxicity makes carbamazepine an extremely valuable anticonvulsant drug, and this should be carefully noted in relation to the development of new anticonvulsant drugs. Toxic side effects with most anticonvulsant drugs are a major clinical problem. Seizures occur intermittently while toxicity, when present, is a liability 24 hours a day.

F. SUCCINIMIDES

1. Phensuximide

Three succinimides are available for clinical utilization. Two of the compounds have phenyl substitutions at the C-2 position of the succinimide ring. For phensuximide, this is the only substitution, and there is general agreement that the compound has little or no clinical usefulness.

Methsuximide   Phensuximide   Ethosuximide

2. Methsuximide

Methsuximide, with methyl and phenyl substitutions at the C-2 position, is a slightly more useful compound. It has some efficacy for absence seizures (Zimmermann and Burgemeister, 1954), and in this author's experience it is also useful with some myoclonic seizures. Methsuximide is metabolized extremely rapidly in man. Glazko and Dill (1972) report a half-life of about $2\frac{1}{2}$ hours with initial exposure to the drug and a much faster rate of clearance after 4 weeks of administration of the drug. This is consistent with our own unpublished observations. We have identified the parent compound in serum from epileptic patients only during the first week of exposure to the drug. Consequently, its anticonvulsant activity may be a function of one or more metabolites. However, animal experiments indicate that methsuximide accumulates at greater concentration in tissues than in plasma, with highest tissue to plasma ratios in fat and brain (Glazko and Dill, 1972).

3. Ethosuximide

The most useful succinimide is ethosuximide (2-ethyl-2-methylsuccinimide). This is a highly effective drug in the treatment of absence seizures and has some usefulness as an adjunctive medication in the treatment of partial complex seizures. The rate of metabolism and excretion of ethosuximide in man is of interest because age is an important factor. The average half-life in children is 30 hours, while that for adults is 60 hours (Chang *et al.*, 1972). In contrast to methsuximide, tissue concentration of ethosuximide is about equal to the plasma concentration. The complete metabolic pathway of ethosuximide has not been elucidated in man. Hydroxylation of the 1-ethyl carbon occurs, and some of this metabolite is excreted as a conjugate of glucuronate. The hydroxylated metabolite is less potent than the parent compound in blocking pentylenetetrazole seizures. There is good evidence that maximal efficacy with ethosuximide is achieved for most patients with serum concentrations greater than 40 μg/ml. This does not mean that some patients do not obtain complete seizure control with lower concentrations (Sherwin and Robb, 1972; Penry *et al.*, 1972). Toxicity is not a major problem with ethosuximide. The most frequently encountered side effects are dose-related symptoms of gastric irritation, headache, dizziness, and tiredness. Non-dose-related toxicity usually involves skin rashes of various degrees of severity and bone marrow suppression. There are reports of behavioral changes associated with ethosuximide treatment, and there is evidence that patients with mixed seizure patterns may experience an increase in the frequency of nonabsence seizures during ethosuximide treatment (Gastaut *et al.*, 1973).

G. OXAZOLIDINEDIONES: TRIMETHADIONE AND PARAMETHADIONE

Although a variety of substitutions at the 3 and 5 positions of the oxazolidenedione nucleus have been examined, only two compounds are available for clinical use in the treatment of absence seizures. These are trimethadione and paramethadione (3,5-dimethyl-5-ethyloxazolidine-2,4-dione). Both compounds undergo fairly rapid *N*-demethylation. The plasma half-life of trimethadione is about 16 hours in normal subjects (Booker, 1972) and undoubtedly is shorter in epileptic patients who have been chronically treated with the drug. The *N*-demethylated metabolite, dimethadione, ionizes at physiological pH and is not further metabolized. Dimethadione is slowly excreted with a half-life ranging from 5 to 10 days. Consequently, plasma concentrations of dimethadione require about 1 month to approach equilibrium. Dimethadione is almost as potent an anticonvulsant as the parent compound and, because it accumulates extensively, the major anticonvulsant effect is related to dimethadione. Trimethadione and dimethadione antagonize pentylenetetrazole seizures extremely effectively over a wide range of doses. The fundamental mechanism of action is not known; however, extensive neurophysiological observations have been made with this compound and these have been summarized by Kutt (1975). Since dimethadione accumulates to concentrations in the range of 1 mg/ml of serum and is almost entirely ionized, it is capable of producing an extra- and intracellular acidosis (Butler *et al.*, 1966) by displacing bicarbonate. There is general agreement that serum concentrations of dimethadione should be at least 700 μg/ml for maximal effectiveness (Booker, 1972; Jensen, 1962).

A variety of toxic reactions have been associated with the oxazolidinediones. One of the more dramatic reactions is hemeralopia or the glare effect. This consists of a temporary loss of visual acuity during a change from low

Trimethadione   Paramethadione

illumination to high illumination. This is a retinal phenomenon which most likely involves impaired brightness discrimination (Sloan and Gilger, 1947). Trimethadione has been reported to increase the frequency of generalized tonic–clonic seizures in some patients. The usual dermatological effects have been reported with the oxazolidinediones.

Hematological toxicity is the most frequent reaction encountered. About 20% of patients experience a decrease in their white blood cell count that does not fall below 3000 cells/mm^3. Unfortunately, others experience a further leukopenia which may progress to a fatal pancytopenia. There are also some rare but potentially dangerous allergic reactions to the oxazolidinediones. A reversible nephrotic syndrome has been clearly associated with trimethadione (Barnett *et al.*, 1948), and there have been two reports of a myasthenic syndrome related to trimethadione therapy (Booker *et al.*, 1970; Peterson, 1966).

H. BENZODIAZEPINES

1. Chlordiazepoxide, Diazepam, and Oxazepam

This class of anticonvulsant drugs illustrates many of the features that have been encountered with the previously described compounds. There are five drugs that have been used clinically: chlordiazepoxide, diazepam, oxazepam, nitrazepam, and clonazepam. They all have a broad spectrum of pharmacological action, which is reflected in their clinical use as tranquilizers, muscle

Oxazepam   Chlordiazepoxide

Diazepam   Nitrazepam   Clonazepam

relaxants, and anticonvulsants. Diazepam may be considered the prototype drug of this class, and it has a wide range of neurophysiological effects. It is quite effective in suppressing electrically induced afterdischarges in many central nervous system structures (Hernandez-Peon *et al.*, 1964; Schallek *et al.*, 1964). It also blocks pentylenetetrazole-induced seizures in very low doses (Kopeloff and Chusid, 1967) and is a potent anticonvulsant in the experimental model of epilepsy that utilizes topical application of estrogens to cortex (Julien *et al.*, 1975). The anticonvulsant activity of the benzodiaze- pines may reflect multiple effects at several levels in the central nervous system.

Regardless of their potent activity in experimental models, their clinical usefulness is impeded by toxicity, tolerance, and, for some, rapid metabolism and distribution effects. Chlordiazepoxide is used principally as a tranquilizing agent. It does have some anticonvulsant activity and may be useful in some individual cases. Diazepam is also used as a tranquilizer and has been pro- moted as a primary treatment for status epilepticus. When given intravenously, this highly lipid soluble compound enters the central nervous system with great rapidity; however, rapid redistribution lowers the brain concentration within 15–30 minutes and status epilepticus may return (Mattson, 1972). In this author's experience, the best results are obtained when diazepam is used in conjunction with phenobarbital intravenously in the treatment of status epilepticus. When diazepam is administered orally, it is much less effective because tolerance develops to the anticonvulsant effect within weeks or several months. This may occur in as many as 50% of those treated. For those who maintain the anticonvulsant effect, toxic side effects are a major limiting factor. The most bothersome is sedation, which can interfere with higher mental functioning to a considerable extent. Hypotonia or muscle relaxation also occurs and may lead to problems with coordination and balance, which are particularly noticeable in children.

In man, diazepam undergoes N-demethylation followed by hydroxylation at C-3 to produce oxazepam. The metabolites are anticonvulsant and N-demethyldiazepam has a longer half-life than the parent compound. The hydroxylated metabolites are conjugated with glucuronate and excreted rapidly principally as N-demethyl-3-hydroxydiazepam glucuronide. The terminal metabolite from diazepam, oxazepam, is commercially available and used primarily as a tranquilizer.

2. Nitrazepam

Nitrazepam is 7-nitro-5-phenyl-$3H$-1,4-benzodiazepin-2($1H$)-one. It has been used as a hypnotic and anticonvulsant with reported efficacy for akinetic, myoclonic, partial elementary, and partial complex seizures. The problems with toxicity and tolerance described for diazepam are shared by this compound.

3. Clonazepam

Clonazepam is the most recent benzodiazepine anticonvulsant. It differs from nitrazepam only in the substitution of a chloride group in the unsubstituted phenyl ring. It is more potent than the other compounds and has been efficacious in a variety of partial and generalized seizures. The same disadvantages of toxicity and tolerance occur with this drug. It is reported to be highly effective in the treatment of status epilepticus (Gastaut *et al.*, 1971).

I. SULFONAMIDES

These compounds contain a free SO_2NH_2 group and have the common action of inhibiting carbonic anhydrase. Their anticonvulsant activity has been attributed to this action, which implies an indirect activity because carbonic anhydrase is found only in glial cells in the central nervous system.

Acetazolamide

Sulthiame

1. Acetazolamide

Acetazolamide is the most widely used sulfonamide in the treatment of seizures. The drug is rapidly absorbed and is excreted without further metabolism in man. The plasma half-life is about 1.5 hours, and a single dose is completely recovered in urine within 24 hours (Maren, 1967). The inhibition of carbonic anhydrase results in an accumulation of carbonic acid and CO_2 in the central nervous system. This has been associated with increases in extracellular sodium and intracellular potassium (Woodbury and Esplin, 1959), which may account for the anticonvulsant effect. In experimental models of epilepsy acetazolamide is extremely potent in blocking the tonic component of maximal electroshock seizures and is a weak antagonist of pentylenetetrazole-induced seizures. Clinically, however, acetazolamide has efficacy for absence seizures but generally not for tonic–clonic seizures. Tolerance appears to develop rapidly to the anticonvulsant effect. It has been used to treat seizures that occur or increase in frequency in association with the menstrual cycle. The drug is usually administered in doses of about 10 mg/ kg for a period of 3–4 days before, during, and 3–4 days after the menstrual period. This avoids the problem of tolerance and, in the author's experience, it is most likely to be effective in women who experience symptoms of fluid retention with menstruation.

Toxicity is not a major problem with acetazolamide. Occasional patients complain of dizziness or dysethesias. The usual allergic reactions occur, and the drug should not be used in patients with liver disease because it can decrease the excretion of ammonia by elevating urine pH.

2. Sulthiame

Sulthiame is another carbonic anhydrase-inhibiting sulfonamide with anticonvulsant activity. In experimentally induced seizures, its spectrum of activity is similar to that of acetazolamide but it is less potent. It is rapidly absorbed and has a longer half-life than acetazolamide (about 8 hours). It is used as an adjunct to other anticonvulsants and is not a potent anticonvulsant drug itself. Doses used generally range from 400 to 1000 mg/day. It is a less effective inhibitor of carbonic anhydrase than acetazolamide, which suggests that it may have other anticonvulsant actions. It has been suggested that its ability to increase the serum concentration of other anticonvulsants by inhibition of metabolism or displacement from protein binding might account for some of the anticonvulsant activity (Hansen *et al.*, 1968).

Toxicity is a major problem with sulthiame. The side effects encountered frequently include hyperventilation, paresthesias, headache, ataxia, gastric irritation, and, in some patients, lethargy.

J. DIPROPYLACETIC ACID

$$\begin{array}{c} H_7C_3 \\ \diagdown \\ \diagup \\ H_7C_3 \end{array} CH-COONa$$

Sodium salt of
dipropylacetic acid

This simple branched-chain fatty acid has anticonvulsant activity when administered as a salt or as an amide. It has a broad spectrum of anticonvulsant activity in experimental models of epilepsy. Both electrical and pentylenetetrazole-induced seizures are antagonized. It is ineffective against strychnine, picrotoxin, or cocaine seizures, however, the amide does antagonize these seizures and is more potent in its effects on electrical and pentylenetetrazole seizures. This is consistent with clinical experience with the two compounds. The salt of the acid is effective in the treatment of generalized seizures, especially absences (DeBiolley and Sorel, 1969), while the amide is reported to be effective in partial seizures (Favel *et al.*, 1973). However, since the amide is metabolized to the acid this may not represent a differential effect. Simon and Penry (1975) have reviewed the published clinical experience with sodium dipropylacetate, which involves a total population of 1116 patients who received the drug most often as an adjunctive medication. When the results were considered without regard to seizure pattern 46% of the patients experienced at least 75% fewer seizures, 25% had at least 33% fewer seizures, and 29% failed to achieve a 33% reduction in seizure frequency. When the data were analyzed in relation to seizure pattern, a broad range of anticonvulsant activity was apparent. A decrease in seizure frequency greater than 33% was found in 39 of 48 patients with partial elementary seizures, in 81 of 127 patients with partial complex seizures, in 191 of 218 patients with absence seizures, and in 205 of 279 patients with generalized tonic–clonic seizures. In the treatment of absence seizures, sodium dipropylacetate appears to be comparable to ethosuximide. The most frequently encountered toxicity involved gastric irritation and sedation, which is most likely to occur when the drug is combined with barbiturates. Doses generally range from 0.5 to 3.0 gm/day, and at present there is little information relating to serum concentrations. Loiseau *et al.* (1975) found the compound to be absorbed rapidly, with peak plasma concentration occurring in about 1 hour. The plasma half-life is in the range of 7–10 hours and enterohepatic circulation does occur. As with most other anticonvulsants, wide individual differences in serum concentration occur with a given dose of sodium dipropylacetate. In general, concentrations of 50–100 μg/ml appear to be well tolerated. In experimental animals sodium dipropylacetate elevates cerebellar and wholebrain concentration of GABA (Godin *et al.*, 1969; Simler *et al.*, 1973), presumably by inhibiting GABA-transaminase, and this effect may be directly related to its anticonvulsant action.

REFERENCES

Ajmone-Marsan, C., and Goldhammer, L. (1973). *In* "Epilepsy. Its Phenomena in Man" (M. A. B. Brazier, ed.), pp. 236–258. Academic Press, New York.

Ajmone-Marsan, C., and Ralston, B. L. (1957). "The Epileptic Seizure: Its Functional Morphology and Diagnostic Significance." Thomas, Springfield, Illinois.

Andermann, E., and Metrakos, J. D. (1973). *Epilepsia* **13**, 348–349.

Barnett, H. L., Simons, D. J., and Wells, R. E., Jr. (1948). *Am. J. Med.* **4**, 760–764.

Baumel, I. P., Gallagher, B. B., DiMicco, J. A., and Dionne, R. (1973). *J. Pharmacol. Exp. Ther.* **180**, 305–314.

Baumel, I. P., Gallagher, B. B., DiMicco, J. A., and Dionne, R. (1976). *J. Pharmacol. Exp. Ther.* **196**, 180–187.

Bogue, J. Y., and Carrington, H. C. (1953). *Br. J. Pharmacol. Chemother.* **8**, 230–235.

Booker, H. E. (1972). *In* "Antiepileptic Drugs" (D. M. Woodbury, J. K. Penry, and R. P. Schmidt, eds.), pp. 403–407. Raven, New York.

Booker, H. E., Chun, R. W. M., and Sanguino, M. (1970). *J. Am. Med. Assoc.* **212**, 2262–2263.

Boudin, G., Garbizet, J., and Labrain, C. (1959). *Therapie* **14**, 994–999.

Bray, P. F., and Wiser, W. C. (1965). *Pediatrics* **36**, 207–211.

Brewis, M., Poskanzer, D. C., Rolland, C., and Miller, H. (1966). *Acta Neurol. Scand.*, *Suppl.* **24**, 42.

Buchanan, R. A., and Sholiton, L. J. (1972). *In* "Antiepileptic Drugs." (D. M. Woodbury, J. K. Penry, and R. P. Schmidt, eds.), pp. 181–192. Raven, New York.

Butler, C. R., and Waddell, W. J. (1958). *Neurology* **8**, Suppl. 1, 106–112.

Butler, T. C., Mahaffee, C., and Waddell, W. J. (1954). *J. Pharmacol. Exp. Ther.* **111**, 425–435.

Butler, T. C., Kuroiwa, Y., Waddell, W. J., and Poole, D. T. (1966). *J. Pharmacol. Exp. Ther.* **152**, 62–66.

Carter, S., Sciarra, D., and Merritt, H. H. (1950). *Dis. Nerv. Syst.* **11**, 139–141.

Chang, T., Burkett, A. R., and Glazko, A. J. (1972). *In* "Antiepileptic Drugs" (D. M. Woodbury, J. K. Penry, and R. P. Schmidt, eds.), pp. 425–429. Raven, New York.

Craig, C. R., and Shideman, F. E. (1971). *J. Pharmacol. Exp. Ther.* **176**, 35–41.

Daly, D. (1958). *Amer. J. Psychiatry* **115**, 97–108.

Davidson, D. T., and Lennox, W. G. (1950). *Dis. Nerv. Syst.* **11**, 167–173.

DeBiolley, M. D., and Sorel, L. (1969). *Electroencephalogr. Clin. Neurophysiol.* **27**, 452.

DiMicco, J. A. and Gallagher, B. B., (1975). *Fed. Proc.* **34**, 726.

Esplin, D. W. (1972). *In* "Experimental Models of Epilepsy" (D. P. Purpura *et al.*, eds.), pp. 223–248. Raven, New York.

Everett, G. M., and Richards, R. K. (1952). *J. Pharmacol. Exp. Ther.* **106**, 303–313.

Favel, P., Cartier, J., Gratadou, J. P., and Gratadou, G. (1973). *Epilepsia* **14**, 329–334.

Feindel, W. (1975). "Handbook of Clinical Neurology" (P. J. Vinken and G. W. Bruyn, eds.), Vol. 15, pp. 87–106. Am. Elsevier, New York.

Fingl, E. (1972). *In* "Antiepileptic Drugs" (D. M. Woodbury, J. K. Penry, and R. P. Schmidt, eds.), pp. 7–21. Raven, New York.

Gallagher, B. B., and Baumel, I. P. (1972). *In* "Antiepileptic Drugs" (D. M. Woodbury, J. K. Penry, and R. P. Schmidt, eds.), pp. 361–371. Raven, New York.

Gallagher, B. B. and Woodbury, S. G. (1976). In "Epileptology Proceedings of the Seventh International Symposium on Epilepsy," (D. Jane, ed.), 1975, pp. 117–122. Georg Thieme, Stuttgart.

Gallagher, B. B., Baumel, I. P., Woodbury, S. G., and DiMicco, J. A. (1975). *Neurology* **25**, 399–404.

Gastaut, H. (1970). *Epilepsia* **11**, 102–113.

Gastaut, H., Roger, J., Faidherbe, J., Ouahchi, R., and Franck, G. (1962). *Epilepsia* **2**, 56–68.

Gastaut, H., Courjou, J., Poire, R., and Weber, M. (1971). *Epilepsia* **12**, 197–214.

Gastaut, H., Roger, J., and Lob, H. (1973). *Int. Encycl. Pharmacol. Ther.* Sect. 19, Vol. 2, pp. 562–566.

Gibbs, F. A., and Gibbs, E. L. (1952). "Atlas of Electroencephalography" Addison-Wesley, Reading, Massachusetts.

Gibbs, F. A., Everett, G. M., and Richards, R. K. (1949). *Dis. Nerv. Syst.* **10**, 47–49.

Glaser, G. H. (1972). *In* "Antiepileptic Drugs" (D. M. Woodbury, J. K. Penry, and R. P. Schmidt, eds.), pp. 219–226. Raven, New York.

Glasson, B., Benakis, A., and Ernst, C. (1963). *Therapie* **18**, 1483–1491.

Glazko, A. J., and Dill, G. A. (1972). *In* "Antiepileptic Drugs" (D. M. Woodbury, J. K. Penry, and R. P. Schmidt, eds.), pp. 455–464. Raven, New York.

Godin, Y., Heiner, L., Mark, J., and Mandel, P. (1969). *J. Neurochem.* **16**, 869–873.

Goldstein, M. (1974). *Arch. Neurol. (Chicago)* **80**, 1–35.

Goodman, L. S., Swinyard, E. A., Brown, W. C., and Schiffman, P. O. (1954). *J. Pharmacol. Exp. Ther.* **110**, 405–410.

Handley, R., and Stewart, A. S. R. (1952). *Lancet* **262**, 742–744.

Hansen, J. M., Kristensen, M., and Skorsted, L. (1968). *Epilepsia* **9**, 17–22.

Hauptman, A. (1912). *Muench. Med. Wochenschr.* **59**, 1907–1909.

Hauser, W. A., and Kurland, L. T. (1975). *Epilepsia* **16**, 1–66.

Hawkes, C. D. (1952). *Arch. Neurol. Psychiatry* **67**, 815–820.

Hernandez-Peon, R., Rojas-Ramirez, J. A., O'Flaherty, J. J., and Mazzuchelli-O'Flaherty, A. L. (1964). *Int. J. Neuropharmacol.* **3**, 405–412.

Jensen, B. N. (1962). *Dan. Med. Bull.* **9**, 74–79.

Julien, R. M., and Halpern, L. M. (1972). *Epilepsia* **13**, 387–400.

Julien, R. M., and Hollister, R. P. (1975). *Adv. Neurol.* **11**, 263–276.

Julien, R. M., Fowler, G. W., and Danielson, M. G. (1975). *J. Pharmacol. Exp. Ther.* **192**, 647.

Kaplan, L. A., and Maslanka, S. (1952). *Dis. Nerv. Syst.* **13**, 88–89.

Klaasen, C. D. (1971). *Br. J. Pharmacol.* **43**, 161–166.

Kopeloff, L. M., and Chusid, J. C. (1967). *Int. J. Neuropsychiatry* **3**, 469–471.

Kutt, H. (1975). *In* "Handbook of Clinical Neurology" (P. J. Vinken and G. W. Bruyn, eds.), Vol. 15, pp. 621–663. Am. Elsevier, New York.

Lennox, W. G. (1960). "Epilepsy and Related Disorders," Vol. 1, p. 353. Little, Brown, Boston, Massachusetts.

Lennox-Buchthal, M. A. (1975). *In* "Handbook of Clinical Neurology" (P. J. Vinken and G. W. Bruyn, eds.), Vol. 15, pp. 246–263. Am. Elsevier, New York.

Livingstone, S. (1953). *J. Pediatr.* **43**, 673–674.

Locock, C. (1857). *Lancet* **1**, 527.

Loiseau, P., Brachet, A., and Henry, P. (1975). *Epilepsia* **16**, 609–615.

Magnussen, C. R., Dohety, J. M., Hess, R. A., and Tschudy, D. P. (1975). *Neurology* **12**, 1121–1125.

Mannering, G. J. (1971). *In* "Fundamentals of Drug Metabolism and Drug Disposition" (B. N. LaDu, H. G. Mandel, and E. L. Way, eds.), pp. 206–252. Williams & Wilkins, Baltimore, Maryland.

Maren, T. H. (1967). *Physiol. Rev.* **47**, 595–781.

Masland, R. L. (1975). *In* "Handbook of Clinical Neurology" (P. J. Vinken and G. W. Bruyn, eds.), Vol. 15, pp. 1–29. Am. Elsevier, New York.

Matsumoto, H., and Gallagher, B. B. (1976). *In* "Quantitative Analytical Studies in Epilepsy" (P. Kellaway and I. Petersen, eds.), pp. 137–145. Raven, New York.

Mattson, R. H. (1972). *In* "Antiepileptic Drugs" (D. M. Woodbury, J. K. Penry, and R. P. Schmidt, eds.), pp. 497–518. Raven, New York.

Millichap, J. G., Goodman, L. S., and Madsen, J. A. (1955). *Neurology* **5**, 700–705.

Muchnik, S., and Gage, P. W. (1968). *Nature (London)* **217**, 373.

Orloff, M. J., Feldman, P. E., Shaiova, C. H., and Pfeiffer, C. C. (1951). *Neurology* **1**, 377–385.

Penfield, W., and Jasper, H. H. (1954). "Epilepsy and the Functional Anatomy of the Human Brain," p. 20. Little, Brown, Boston, Massachusetts.

Penry, J. K. (1975). *Adv. Neurol.* **11**, 1–10.

Penry, J. K., Porter, R. J., and Dreifuss, F. E. (1972). *In* "Antiepileptic Drugs" (D. M. Woodbury, J. K. Penry, and R. P. Schmidt, eds.), pp. 431–442. Raven, New York.

Perry, G. F., and Simonds, S. (1951). *Dis. Nerv. Syst.* **12**, 200–205.

Peterman, M. G. (1954). *J. Pediats.* **44**, 624–629.

Peterson, H. DeC. (1966). *N. Engl. J. Med.* **274**, 506–507.

Purpura, D. P., Penry, J. K., Woodbury, D. M. and Walter, R. (1972). "Experimental Models of Epilepsy," Raven, New York.

Roberts, E. (1974). *Biochem. Pharmacol.* **23**, 2637.

Roger, J., Log, H., and Tassinari, C. A. (1975). *In* "Handbook of Clinical Neurology" (P. J. Vinken and G. W. Bruyn, eds.), Vol. 15, pp. 145–188. Am. Elsevier, New York.

Schallek, W., Zabransky, F., and Kuehn, A. (1964). *Arch. Int. Pharmacodyn. Ther.* **149**, 467–483.

Sherwin, A. L., and Robb, J. P. (1972). *In* "Antiepileptic Drugs" (D. M. Woodbury, J. K. Penry, and R. P. Schmidt, eds.), pp. 443–448. Raven, New York.

Simler, S., Ciesielski, L., Maitre, M., Randrianarisoa, H., and Mandel, P. (1973). *Biochem. Pharmacol.* **22**, 1701–1708.

Simon, D., and Penry, J. K. (1975). *Epilepsia* **16**, 549–573.

Sloan, L. L., and Gilger, A. P. (1947). *Am. J. Ophthalmol.* **30**, 1387–1405.

Smith, D. B., Goldstein, S. G., and Roomet, A. (1974). *Program Am. Epilepsy Soc., Annu. Meet.* Abstract, p. 16.

Stamps, F. W., Marshall, W. H., Orloff, F. A., Gibbs, F. A., and Pfeiffer, C. C. (1952). *J. Pharmacol. Exp. Ther.* **106**, 418.

Stevens, J. R. (1957). *Arch. Neurol. Psychiatry* **77**, 227–236.

Tower, D. B. (1969). *In* "Basic Mechanisms of the Epilepsies" (H. H. Japser, A. A. Ward, and A. Pope, eds.), pp. 611–638. Little, Brown, Boston, Massachusetts.

Weil, A. A. (1959). *Arch. Neurol. (Chicago)* **1**, 101–111.

Williams, D. (1956). *Brain* **79**, 29–67.

Woodburne, R. T. (1957). "Essentials of Human Anatomy," p. 26. Oxford University Press, New York.

Woodbury, D. M. (1969). *In* "Basic Mechanisms of the Epilepsies" (H. H. Jasper, A. A. Ward, and A. Pope, eds.), pp. 672–675. Little, Brown, Boston, Massachusetts.

Woodbury, D. M., and Esplin, D. W. (1959). *Res. Publ., Assoc. Res. Nerv. Ment. Dis.* **37**, 24–56.

Zavadil, A. and Gallagher, B. B. (1976). *In* "Epileptology Proceedings of the Seventh International Symposium on Epilepsy," (D. Jane, ed.), 1975, pp. 129–139. Georg Thieme, Stuttgart.

Zimmerman, F. T., and Burgemeister, B. B. (1954). *Arch. Neurol. (Chicago)* **72**, 720–725.

3

EXPERIMENTAL EVALUATION OF ANTICONVULSANTS

John F. Reinhard and John F. Reinhard, Jr.

I. INTRODUCTION

Within recent years there has been a resurgence of interest in the development of better drugs for the management of epilepsy. Relevant studies have been reviewed critically by Woodbury and co-workers (1972) and experimental models of the disease have been evaluated by Purpura and collaborators (1972). From these studies one can draw at least three basic conclusions: first, that experimental approaches designed to elucidate the mechanisms underlying the epileptic state have been disappointing in that the disease remains enigmatic; second, that the levels of biogenic amines are likely to be involved intimately in the epileptic state since they are profoundly altered by anticonvulsants (Meyer and Frey, 1973; Schreiber and Schlesinger, 1971); and third, that further progress will be possible through the development of new chemical entities with greater selectivity of action, particularly on neurohumoral mechanisms involving biogenic amines and possibly other endogenous substances (Costa *et al.*, 1975).

Largely on an empirical basis a number of excellent drugs have been made available for the treatment of epilepsy. Their therapeutic usefulness, however, is often limited by their inherent toxicity. The challenge is to produce new drugs with greater selective activity than those currently available, but with markedly reduced toxicity. To meet this challenge, carefully coordinated interdisciplinary teamwork is essential.

This volume is addressed to the chemists who must synthesize these new drugs, and this chapter is addressed to the pharmacologists who must evaluate their activity and toxicity. In our experience rapid feedback of preliminary pharmacological information serves as a guide to further synthetic effort, and the speed with which valid information is communicated largely determines the efficiency of the operation.

Preliminary screening of a compound is usually conducted in the mouse and begins with a few relatively simple procedures. The compound is tested for its ability to inhibit maximal electroshock seizures (MES), to raise the threshold for clonic pentylenetetrazole seizures (Met), and to produce toxic effects, e.g., neurological deficit (TD_{50}) and lethality (LD_{50}).

The dose of a compound that elicits an anticonvulsant response in 50% of the animals (ED_{50}), compared to that required for a standard of reference (e.g., diphenylhydantoin or other known therapeutic agents), provides information relating to potency, and the test itself yields additional information referable to the area of potential therapeutic value, e.g., grand mal in the case of the MES test and petit mal for the Met test (Woodbury, 1972). The ratio of the TD_{50} and ED_{50} values p.i. (protective index) provides a rough measure of safety. These few preliminary tests can often be used to decide whether a compound merits further consideration.

However, ED_{50} values can be misleading unless determined at the time of peak activity, which presumably correlates with brain concentration of the drug or an active metabolite; moreover, they can be influenced significantly by a variety of factors, including route of administration, species and strain of animal, sex, and the season of the year. Two additional factors, namely, duration of the anticonvulsant effect and repeated daily dosing, have an important bearing on the ED_{50} and can be estimated readily by means of the MES or Met test. In our hands results of such determinations, especially if both oral and parenteral routes of administration are employed, have provided clues relating to accumulation or tolerance as well as to absorption of a compound from the gastrointestinal tract and, as such, can influence decision making.

Once a compound has passed these tests of activity and safety, it may be evaluated further by means of a battery of additional tests designed to disclose other areas of potential therapeutic usefulness. At each stage of the evaluation a question arises whether the compound has sufficient merit to warrant further consideration. The question is important since the compound must compete with drugs already available, and the decision to proceed may hinge on negative as well as positive features, such as the absence of hypnotic activity and tolerance, time of onset, and duration of activity.

In order to make valid comparisons the investigator is completely dependent on "hard" pharmacological data for selected standards of reference. Logically, such data are determined in side-by-side comparison studies under the investigator's experimental conditions. But starting doses often pose a problem, and considerable time could be spared by having such doses at hand. In our experience such information is not often readily available, and acquiring it may involve an exhaustive search of the literature.

It occurred to us, therefore, that a useful purpose would be served if a compilation were made of published data for antiepileptic drugs in the following categories: hydantoin derivatives, barbiturates and related compounds, oxazolidinediones, succinimides, benzodiazepines, and a miscellaneous group consisting of phenacemide and sulthiame. For each category our search of the literature has uncovered pertinent information for a variety of commonly employed test procedures including effective doses, species of animal, route of administration, and the reference source. This information has been summarized in tabular form for ready reference. The body of the text is intended to supplement the tables and comprises explanatory notes, in some instances additional material supplied by the investigator, and interpretive comments.

It seemed important at the outset to provide a brief description of each of the methods referred to in the text and, when possible, to show how various genetic and environmental factors operate to influence the outcome and the interpretation of data generated by the tests. Finally, we have attempted to correlate findings in the experimental animal with therapeutic potential.

II. METHODS

A. MAXIMAL ELECTROSHOCK SEIZURES (60 Hz MES)

Commonly this test is conducted initially in adult male albino mice. Current (60 Hz) is delivered through corneal electrodes at 50 mA for 0.2 second (Toman *et al.*, 1946). A salient feature of the seizure pattern is the appearance of tonic extension of the hindlimbs. Pretreatment with an effective anticonvulsant drug results in the abolition of the hindlimb component of the seizure pattern. Generally, five logarithmically spaced doses of a candidate anticonvulsant are administered to animals in groups of ten, to cover 0–100% protection, and the dose required to protect 50% of the animals (ED_{50}), together with its 95% confidence limits, may be determined graphically by the method of Litchfield and Wilcoxon (1949). If species other than the mouse are employed, different current strengths are required, e.g., 150 mA for rats, 300 mA for rabbits, and 400 mA for cats (Toman *et al.*, 1946). It is customary to conduct preliminary range-finding studies to determine the time of peak effect of anticonvulsants and to estimate their safety by reference to the dose required to produce neurological deficit (TD_{50}) rather than death. Thus, a protective index is defined by the ratio TD_{50}/ED_{50} (Swinyard, 1949). Certain factors can affect the outcome of MES tests: (1) Age of the animals is one factor. Electroshock seizure activity is lower in old than in young rats (Gellhorn and Ballin, 1948); lower activity is correlated with increased cerebral levels of γ-aminobutyric acid (GABA)

(Worum and Porszasz, 1968). For effects of age on ED_{50} values of diphenyl-hydantoin (DPH) and phenobarbital, see Petty and Karler (1965). (2) Strain differences are important. For example, certain strains of mice, such as the DBA, C57, and CFW strains, are highly susceptible to postseizure lethality following electroshock convulsions. On the other hand, ICR and CF#1 strains showed low or no mortality whatever (Torchiana and Stone, 1959). (3) Current strength must be sufficient to induce maximal seizures in 95–100% of the animals in the strain used; thus, a current strength of 150 mA produced maximal seizures in only 50% of adult Royal Hart male albino rats, but 500 mA induced seizures in all of the animals (Rauth and Gray, 1968). The test has predictive value for drugs of potential therapeutic value in the management of grand mal (Woodbury, 1972).

B. MINIMAL ELECTROSHOCK SEIZURE THRESHOLD (MET, 60 Hz EST)

Current is delivered to mice through corneal electrodes, as in the previous test, in single shocks between 6 and 9 mA/0.2 second. Shocks are repeated every 24 hours until a threshold response is obtained. This consists of at least 7 seconds of facial, lower jaw, or forelimb clonus without loss of the upright position. After thresholds have become stabilized, candidate anti-convulsant drugs are administered and the animals are challenged with a current 20% above the previously determined threshold for each animal. The end point of the test is complete protection from the minimal seizure. The ED_{50} values are determined as described in the previous section (Swin-yard, 1949). A lower threshold is assumed to indicate a greater degree of excitability following epileptogenic stimulation of the brain.

Female rats appear to have greater convulsability than males as shown by significantly decreased EST values. This sex difference has been attributed to a hormonal effect, since estradiol has a striking excitatory action. Independent of sex, however, is the finding that low EST values are associated with higher brain acetylcholine content and cholinesterase activity (Wooley et al., 1961).

C. HYPONATREMIC ELECTROSHOCK SEIZURE THRESHOLD (HET, 60 Hz EST)

This is a threshold test, similar to the one described above but in animals rendered sensitive to seizures by acute hyponatremia [induced by intra-peritoneal (ip) injection of isosmolar glucose solution], and measures the ability of drugs to restore the experimentally reduced MET toward normal. The endpoint is based on a quantal response to a 50% increase in current above the expected reduced level (56% below normal). The test is performed in both rats and mice (Goodman *et al.*, 1953b).

D. MINIMAL ELECTROSHOCK SEIZURE THRESHOLD (6 Hz EST OR PsM)

Unidirectional rectangular pulses (0.2 msec) are delivered to mice through corneal electrodes for 3 seconds at a frequency of six pulses per second. The end point is the minimal current required to elicit a seizure pattern in which the animal appears stunned without loss of the upright position; forelimbs are crossed, and hindlimbs spread. Such seizures have been described as "psychomotor" (PsM). A threshold is determined for each animal 24 hours before use in the evaluation of a candidate anticonvulsant drug. The test measures the ability of a drug to elevate the predetermined threshold (Swinyard, 1972).

Goodman *et al.*, (1953b) emphasize that the test is not predictive for compounds of therapeutic potential against psychomotor seizures in man. For example, phenobarbital was shown to be more than 15 times as potent as primidone, yet the latter is clinically more effective in controlling this seizure pattern.

E. METRAZOLE SEIZURE THRESHOLD TEST

1. Subcutaneous

Pentylenetetrazole (Metrazole) is injected subcutaneously (sc) at a dose of 85 mg/kg for mice and 70 mg/kg for rats. Clonic convulsive seizures with loss of the upright position constitute the end point of the test. Failure of pre-treated animals to exhibit this end point is taken to indicate anticonvulsant activity (Swinyard *et al.*, 1952).

Newborn mice are relatively insensitive to pentylenetetrazole. The dose required for convulsions in 50% of the animals (CD_{50}) decreases with advancing age from approximately 180 mg/kg sc at day 1 to 60 mg/kg sc when the animal is adult. The drug appears to act at both cortical and subcortical levels. The increased intensity of effect with increasing age presumably reflects changes in the permeability of the blood–brain barrier (Ferngren, 1965) or may reflect the development of certain neural tracts. It is of interest that pentylenetetrazole, but not electroshock, causes a significant, non-sex-related decrease in serum cholesterol 24 hours after a single injection. This decrease has been attributed to a specific inhibition of sterol biosynthesis (Alexander *et al.*, 1969). The test has predictive value for compounds of potential value in petit mal (Woodbury, 1972).

2. Intravenous

Pentylenetetrazole 15 mg/ml is injected intravenously (iv) into mice continuously at a rate of 0.005 ml/second. The end point is at least 3 seconds of persistent clonic seizure activity (McQuarrie and Fingl, 1958). Swinyard and Castellion (1966) use the dose required for 100% increase in threshold to determine the ED_{50}.

F. MAXIMAL METRAZOLE SEIZURES (MMS)

This test, generally performed in mice, measures the ability of drugs to alter the pattern of chemoshock seizures induced by rapid iv injection of the CD_{97} dose of metrazole (mice, 38 mg/kg). The end point is the same as for the MES test i.e., abolition of the hindleg tonic extensor component of the maximal seizure (Goodman *et al.*, 1953b). The test measures potential for grand mal.

G. AUDIOGENIC SEIZURES

Studies are usually conducted using specially inbred strains of mice selected for audiogenic seizure susceptibility (Plotnikoff and Green, 1957; Fink and Swinyard, 1959). Mice are placed in a seizure chamber and exposed to an auditory stimulus supplied by one or more doorbells. Sequential events are running, jumping, circling, convulsing, and finally immobility resembling catalepsy. Plotnikoff and Green (1957) use a scoring system in which points are assigned to each of the above events. The dose of a candidate anticonvulsant required to reduce the total response to 50% of the control value is recorded as the PD_{50} (or ED_{50}) plus or minus its standard error.

Collins and Horlington (1969) reported on a sequential screening test using the F_1 generation obtained by crossing DBA/1 males with SNR albino female mice. The test compound is administered intraperitoneally at a dose corresponding to 20% of the LD_{50}. Forty-five minutes later the animals are placed singly in a chamber and exposed to a sound stimulus (117 ± 2 dB re 0.2×10^{-4} μbar). The investigators measured sound pressure level with the aid of a Bruel and Kjaer 2604 amplifier and a 4136 microphone. The end point is a running response within 20 seconds following the sound stimulus. Anticonvulsant activity was recorded only if the running component of the seizure pattern was completely suppressed. The test appears to have one serious limitation: No allowance was made for peak time, which conceivably could vary considerably from the 45-minute time limit imposed, depending on the drug. Halberg and Jacobsen (1958) indicated that lighting conditions to which mice are exposed during a 24-hour period can alter the seizure pattern. Schreiber and Schlesinger (1971) reported that in DBA/25 mice seizure susceptibility is inversely proportional to levels of 5-hydroxytryptamine (5-HT), norepinephrine (NE), and GABA. The animals were most susceptible to seizures from the twelfth to the twenty-sixth day of life; moreover, a significant circadian rhythm was observed, with greatest seizure susceptiblity occurring during the night (1900 to 0700 hours).

Nellhaus (1958) reported excellent results with a special breed of rabbit (Beverans), which has peak audiogenic susceptibility during the second month of life. Certain advantages are claimed for these rabbits: Their seizure incidence is nearly 100%, with no risk of death, and they are capable of exhibiting seizures to sensory stimuli other than sound, suggesting a less specific basis for their seizure susceptibility. In marked contrast, although inbred strains of mice show a high incidence of audiogenic seizures, the risk of death is also high. Susceptibility to seizures in rats is disappointingly low, not more than 50%.

Compounds capable of inhibiting maximal audiogenic seizures have therapeutic potential in grand mal (Woodbury, 1972).

H. INTERMITTENT PHOTIC STIMULATION

Killam *et al.* (1967) have been in the forefront of investigators utilizing the baboon (*Papio papio*) as an experimental model for photomyoclonic epilepsy. The syndrome evoked by light in the baboon resembles that seen in man. Intermittent light stimulation (ILS) at a frequency of 25 per second results in paroxysmal activity during the period of light stimulation and as self-sustained discharges. The syndrome consists of clonus of the eyelids initially, followed by clonus of the facial musculature and jaws, and finally violent jerking movements involving the entire body. A number of anticonvulsant drugs are capable of blocking the appearance of photic seizures. Naquet *et al.* (1970) reported a marked rise in blood glucose levels 20–40 minutes following ILS, suggesting an association between ILS-induced seizure activity and hyperglycemia. Killam (1969) reported that the light-sensitive baboon has a low threshold to the convulsant effects of pentylenetetrazole. An exhaustive account of the baboon as an animal model has been presented by Naquet *et al.* (1970). Barnes (1954) reported on the electroencephalographic response of the unanesthetized rabbit to flickering light and its suppression by anticonvulsant drugs. The method has predictive value for compounds of therapeutic potential in grand mal (Woodbury *et al.*, 1972).

I. TOPICAL CONVULSANTS

1. Alumina Cream

Although various species have been employed, the monkey (*Macaca mulatta*) appears to be an animal of choice for the development of chronic recurring seizures resembling the human Jacksonian type. Kopeloff *et al.* (1954) apply alumina cream to the sensorimotor cortex of the monkey by means of linen of fiber disks of 0.2- to 0.25-ml capacity. The method appears to be extremely reliable since Jacksonian epilepsy was produced in 50 out of 51 monkeys within 5–9 weeks (peak time). Moreover, the response persists for a period of years, providing ample opportunity for the evaluation of anticonvulsant drugs. Such animals were also much more sensitive to pentylenetetrazole seizures, the convulsive threshold being 2.8–6.3 mg/kg, compared to a value of 8.5–29 mg/kg intravenously for control monkeys. Faeth *et al.* (1955) reported that the amount of alumina cream is critical. If less than 0.1 ml was injected only 10% of the animals exhibited seizures.

2. Cobalt

Like alumina cream, cobalt may be utilized to produce cortical lesions. Mancia and Lucioni (1966) inject 10 mg of cobalt powder subcortically by means of a needle and stylus. For a complete review of topical convulsant metals, including tungsten, see Ward (1972). The test should have predictive value for compounds of potential usefulness in generalized seizures of the grand mal type as well as epilepsy characterized by clonic activity or myoclonus (Woodbury, 1972).

J. FLUROTHYL SEIZURES

As reported by Boissier *et al.* (1968), 0.05 ml of a 1% solution of flurothyl in PEG-400 is injected intravenously into mice. Seizures appear within a matter of seconds and occur in three phases: a myoclonic phase conisting of jerking movements, a tonic phase, and finally a return to the myoclonic phase. Seizures in animals are reportedly similar to those occurring in man. Inhibition of flurothyl-induced maximal tonic–clonic seizures suggests potential activity against grand mal type of epilepsy (Woodbury, 1972).

K. PICROTOXIN SEIZURES

Barrata and Oftedal (1970) reported convulsions in the rabbit following an intravenous dose of 2.5 mg/kg of picrotoxin. The electrocorticogram (ECoG) showed spike-and-wave formations, reaching a peak 19 minutes following injection. The dosage employed by these investigators was approximately three times the minimum convulsant dosage (0.8 mg/kg iv) reported earlier by Werner and Tatum (1939). Vernadakis and Woodbury (1969) reported that picrotoxin was not a direct stimulant in the rat, but acted by selectively blocking presynaptic inhibition without affecting postsynaptic inhibition. The subcutaneous CD_{50} in this species is approximately 0.9 mg/kg in 4-day-old rats and increases to 3.4 mg/kg at 48 days. The method appears to be useful as a model for detecting compounds with therapeutic potential in petit mal since both diazepam and nitrazepam which are clinically useful in this type of epilepsy inhibit the spike-and-wave pattern within 4–5 minutes. (Barrada and Oftedal, 1970).

L. BEMEGRIDE SEIZURES

Van Duijn and Visser (1972) implant extradural electrodes in the sensorimotor, auditory, and visual cortex of the cat under anesthesia. Two days later bemegride is injected at a rate of 2 ml/minute until tonic–clonic seizure occurs. Threshold is taken as the time from the beginning of the injection to the onset of a multispike phase in the electrocorticogram. Two days later a candidate anticonvulsant is injected subcutaneously and, after 45 minutes, bemegride is again injected until a clonic–tonic seizure occurs. Anticonvulsant activity is indicated if the threshold is increased significantly. This method has the advantage of enabling evaluation of compounds in the alert animal without the need for interfering narcotic or neuromuscular-blocking drugs. The method has disclosed activity of benzodiazepines (Van Duijn and Visser, 1972; Van Duijn, 1973) and should have predictive value for compounds of potential value in petit mal since its site of action in the brain (cortex) is thought to be the same as that of pentylenetetrazole (Hahn, 1960). Its disadvantage, however, is that it does not take into account the time of peak activity.

M. STRYCHNINE SEIZURES

This test is not sufficiently selective for evaluating anticonvulsants since its action is primarily on the cord. Strychnine selectively blocks postsynaptic inhibition and can presumably be used to investigate the nature of inhibitory transmitters (Vernadakis and Woodbury, 1969).

III. HYDANTOINS

A. DIPHENLYHYDANTOIN

1. Maximal Electroshock Seizures

a. Effect of Age. The intraperitoneal dose of DPH (as shown in Table I) required to protect 50% of mice or rats, as indicated by abolition of the hindlimb tonic extensor phase of the maximal seizure pattern, does not appear to change significantly with advancing age. Petty and Karler (1965) have reported ED_{50} values of 8.1 and 14 mg/kg for young and old mice, respectively, and 5.0 and 5.1 mg/kg for young and old rats, respectively. This is of interest in view of the finding of Worum and Porszasz (1968) that, in the case of Wistar albino rats, electroshock seizure activity appears to decrease with age, corresponding to increasing cerebral concentrations of γ-aminobutyric acid.

b. Peak Time. For results to be meaningful, candidate drugs must be evaluated for anticonvulsant activity at the time of their maximum effectiveness. Customarily this peak time is determined by electroshock (MES) challenge at intervals ($\frac{1}{2}$ hour, 1 hour, 2 hours, and 3 hours) following drug administration. In this connection it is important to note that different groups of animals are required at the intervals selected. If the same animals are shocked repeatedly, the tonic extensor component is abolished and false positive results are obtained (Toman, *et al.*, 1946). Peak time can be expected to vary depending on the species of animal, the route of administration, and perhaps other factors as well. In the case of DPH, peak time is approximately 2 hours in the mouse and $\frac{1}{2}$ hour in the rat following intraperitoneal injection (Petty and Karler, 1965). Drugs such as DPH, which protect mice against MES, can be expected to control grand mal seizures in man (Millichap, 1969).

c. Species Differences. Effective doses of DPH for different species and for different routes of administration have been summarized in Table I. For the most part, "effective doses" represent ED_{50} values, with or without limits of error.

An interesting example of drug interaction was reported by Dashputra and Khapre (1970), who found that, in rats of either sex, chlorothiazide congeners are capable of potentiating the anticonvulsant action of DPH against maximal electroshock seizures. The animals used in this study were of Indian origin and young, ranging from weanlings (50 gm) to young adults (150 gm).

2. Minimal Electroshock Seizure Threshold

Effect of Age. Swinyard (1949) was perhaps the first to report the failure of DPH to elevate the threshold for high-frequency stimulation in the adult animal (rat). This failure has been attributed to the drug's causing a discharge of subcortical excitatory systems, one of which could involve the hypothalamohypophyseal system. Excitation of this system would effect the release of adrenocortical steroids, which antagonize any effects DPH might otherwise have in elevating the electroshock seizure threshold (Vernadakis and Woodbury, 1969).

TABLE I HYDANTOINS

Test	Species	Effective dose (mg/kg)	Route of adminis- tration	References
		Diphenylhydantoin		
MES	Mouse (young)	8.1	ip	Petty and Karler (1965)
	Mouse (mature)	9.0	sc	Goodman *et al.* (1953a)
	Mouse (old)	14	ip	Petty and Karler (1965)
	Rat (young)	5.0	ip	Petty and Karler (1965)
	Rat (mature)	30 (20.0–45.0)[a]	po	Swinyard and Toman (1950)
	Rabbit	60	sc	Toman *et al.* (1946)
	Cat	10	ip	Toman *et al.* (1946)
	Cat	12.5	po	Chen and Ensor (1950)
sc Met	Mouse	Inactive	po	Vida *et al.* (1975)
	Rat	> 3200	po	Swinyard and Toman (1950)
MMS	Mouse	46.6	sc	Goodman *et al.* (1953a)
MET (60 Hz EST)	Rat	Inactive	sc	Swinyard (1949)
HET	Rat	94.5	sc	Swinyard (1949)
Audiogenic Seizures	Mouse	5.0	po	Fink and Swinyard (1959)
	Mouse	13.9	ip	Collins and Horlington (1969)
Bemegride seizures	Mouse	100	sc	Rümke (1967)
Intermittent photic stimulation	Rabbit	Inactive	ip	Barnes (1954)
Neurological deficit	Mouse	80	sc	Swinyard *et al.* (1952)
	Rat	140	sc	Swinyard *et al.* (1952)
	Rabbit	180	ip	Toman *et al.* (1946)
	Cat	40	ip	Toman *et al.* (1946)
Acute toxicity	Mouse	490 (295–808)	po	Fink and Swinyard (1959)
		Mephenytoin[b]		
MES	Rat	4.5	ip	Swinyard (1949)
sc Met	Rat	54.9	ip	Swinyard (1949)
MET (60 Hz EST)	Mouse	35	po	Brown *et al.* (1953)
	Rat	72.5	ip	Swinyard (1949)
HET	Rat	35.2	ip	Swinyard (1949)
Bemegride seizures	Mouse	60	po	Rümke (1967)

TABLE I—*Continued*

Test	Species	Effective dose (mg/kg)	Route of administration	References
Neurological deficit	Mouse	ca. 80	po	Brown *et al.* (1953)
	Rat	50 ± 3	ip	Goodman *et al.* (1948)
Acute toxicity	Mouse	560	po	Barnes and Eltherington (1966)
	Rat	270	ip	Barnes and Eltherington (1966)
	Rabbit	340	po	Barnes and Eltherington (1966)
	Cat	190	po	Barnes and Eltherington (1966)
Ethotoin				
MES	Mouse	350	po	Millichap (1972)
sc Met	Mouse	350	po	Millichap (1972)
Neurological deficit	Mouse	400	po	Millichap (1972)
Acute toxicity	Mouse	> 2000	po	Millichap (1972)

[a] Numbers in parentheses generally represent 95% fiducial limits.
[b] Toxicity figures supplied through the courtesy of Sandoz Pharmaceuticals.

If adrenocortical antagonism of DPH were indeed the basis for its failure to elevate EST in the adult animal, one would expect the opposite to occur in the newborn since, at this time and for the first 2 weeks after birth, the hypothalamohypophyseal system is not yet functioning completely (Jailer, 1951). With this in mind, Vernadakis and Woodbury (1965) postulated that an EST-elevating effect of DPH was present at birth and would be lost as the animal matured. Accordingly, mice and rats were treated with DPH at various ages after birth. The study revealed that DPH did indeed elevate the EST in rats, but only during the first 2 weeks of life. The threshold was not increased in older rats. In mice, DPH markedly increased EST up to 18 days of age but had no such effect in older animals.

3. Hyponatremic Electroshock Seizure Threshold

In contrast to its failure to elevate normal EST, diphenylhydantoin has been shown to increase the experimentally lowered electroshock threshold (Table I).

4. Pentylenetetrazole Seizures

a. Metrazole Seizure Threshold (sc Met) Test. Single doses of DPH fail to prevent the development of clonic seizures in response to subcutaneously administered pentylenetetrazole (Vida *et al.*, 1975) and appear actually to intensify the seizures (Goodman and Lih, 1941). However, the latter investigators were able to show a distinct anticonvulsant effect when DPH was administered orally (po) twice daily (20–30 mg/kg) to mice for 4–7 days. Metrazole (85 mg/kg sc) injected 8 hours after the last dose of DPH produced seizures in virtually 100% of nontreated (control) mice. The same appears to hold for rats as well as mice (Goodman and Lih, 1941).

b. Maximal Metrazole Seizures. Although single doses of DPH fail to prevent clonic seizures following subcutaneous administration of pentylenetetrazole they are highly effective in preventing maximal seizures when this convulsant is given by rapid intravenous injection. Table I lists the ED_{50} of DPH as 46.6 mg/kg sc (Goodman *et al.*, 1953a).

5. Audiogenic Seizures

Fink and Swinyard (1959) employed two end points for their study, one based on the abolition of a maximal seizure response (ED_{50} 5.0 mg/kg po; Table I) and the other based on running movements in response to the audiogenic stimulus. The ED_{50} of DPH for the latter end point was 35 (27.2–44.8) mg/kg po (not shown in Table I). Collins and Horlington (1969) administered DPH to a strain of mice obtained by crossing DBA/1 males with SNR strain albino females. Based on suppression of running movements, these investigators reported an ED_{50} of 13.9 (7.7–25.0) mg/kg ip, as shown in Table I.

6. Intermittent Photic Stimulation

In the investigation of Barnes (1954), electroencephalogram (EEG) responses to a flickering light were reported in the unanesthetized rabbit with or without dimethyl tubocurarine. As shown in Table I, DPH failed to suppress the EEG effects of flicker. The author's conclusion was based on experiments in which a relatively large dose of DPH was injected intraperitoneally daily for 5 days. Flicker responses were tested 2–4 and 24 hours after the last injection.

7. Bemegride Seizures

The dose of DPH shown in Table I (100 mg/kg sc) is not an ED_{50}, but rather the dose required for significant elevation of the CD_{50} of bemegride. In this instance the animals were challenged with the convulsant 24 hours after giving DPH and an anticonvulsant effect was produced. However, when 50 mg/kg sc of DPH was given, and the bemegride injected 96 hours later, the CD_{50} of bemegride was lowered, indicating increased susceptibility to seizures (Rümke, 1967).

8. Neurological Deficit

The values shown in Table I for the mouse and the rat represent doses required for some degree of neurological deficit in 50% of the animals; for the larger animals the figures are approximate. Given that the protective index is defined as TD_{50}/ED_{50} (Goodman *et al.*, 1953b), it can be seen from Table I that DPH has a reasonably good margin of safety in the various tests for which ED_{50} values are available.

9. Acute Toxicity

The figure shown in Table I (490 mg/kg po) represents the LD_{50}, i.e., the dose required to kill 50% of the animals. Taken together with the ED_{50} values for the various test procedures, the therapeutic index (LD_{50}/ED_{50}) provides still further indication that the margin of safety of DPH is well within acceptable limits.

B. MEPHENYTOIN

As shown in Table I, mephenytoin is effective against both maximal electroshock and pentylenetetrazole-induced seizures. As such it qualifies as a drug likely to benefit patients with psychomotor seizures as well as grand mal and focal clonic seizures (Millichap, 1969). With respect to bemegride seizures mephenytoin, like DPH, is either proconvulsant or anticonvulsant, depending on the interval between administration and challenge by chemo-shock. The figure given in Table I (60 mg/kg) is based on a study in which bemegride challenge occurred $1-1\frac{1}{2}$ hours following oral administration and the effect is clearly anticonvulsant. However, when bemegride was administered 48 hours following mephenytoin, the convulsive dose was significantly decreased, indicating a proconvulsant action or withdrawal supersensitivity. These studies by Rümke (1967) also show a corresponding dual effect of mephenytoin with respect to pentylenetetrazole. The acute toxicity figures for mephenytoin, as shown in Table I, were supplied through the courtesy of Sandoz Pharmaceuticals.

C. ETHOTOIN

Data for ethotoin, shown in Table I (Millichap, 1972), were supplied through the courtesy of Dr. G. M. Everett of Abbott Laboratories. Like mephenytoin, ethotoin is effective against both maximal electroshock and pentylenetetrazole-induced seizures. The protective indices are lower than those for mephenytoin versus MES and Met and roughly nine times lower than for DPH versus MES. Although neurological deficit occurs at doses close to those required for anticonvulsant activity, ethotoin is clearly the least toxic on an acute basis, since doses as high as 2000 mg/kg were nonlethal.

IV. BARBITURATES AND RELATED COMPOUNDS

A. PHENOBARBITAL

1. Maximal Electroshock Seizures

Effects of species, strain, route of administration, and age are disclosed in Table II. Rats appear to be somewhat more sensitive to the anticonvulsant effects of phenobarbital than mice, and of the two strains of mice tested CF#1 seems to be the more sensitive. Investigations of Petty and Karler (1965) reveal that young rats are less sensitive to phenobarbital than are mature animals, and old rats show the greatest sensitivity. The steady decrease in ED_{50} values of phenobarbital presumably reflects decreasing seizure activity with age and can be correlated with increasing cerebral concentrations of GABA (Worum and Porszasz, 1968).

Since phenobarbital is well established as an activator of hepatic microsomal enzymes (Conney et al., 1960), and presumably of hepatic mitochondrial enzymes as well (Reinhard and Spector, 1970), repeated daily administration of this drug might be expected to result in decreased brain concentration of phenobarbital. Surprisingly, this does not appear to be the case. After a single dose (5 mg/kg ip) of phenobarbital (Craig and Shideman, 1971), which protected 60% of Sprague-Dawley rats challenged by electroshock, the brain concentration of phenobarbital was 4.60 ± 0.43 μg/kg. After injecting the drug for 10 days (5 mg/kg ip), challenge by electroshock resulted in the same protection (60%) and the brain concentration was not significantly different (5.5 ± 0.4 μg/kg) from that obtained after a single injection.

2. Minimal Electroshock Seizure Threshold

The study by Goodman et al. (1953b) reveals that the mouse is more sensitive to phenobarbital than the rat. The protective index is satisfactory ($TD_{50}/ED_{50} = 2.0$) for the mouse but not for the rat ($TD_{50}/ED_{50} = 0.56$) since 62.5 mg/kg po was required to elevate the threshold (ED_{50}), whereas neurological deficit was produced by a much lower dose (35 mg/kg po; see below, under neurological deficit).

3. Hyponatremic Electroshock Seizure Threshold

Here, again, much larger doses were required to elevate the seizure threshold in the rat than in the mouse, also reflecting a favorable protective index ($TD_{50}/ED_{50} = 1.76$) for the mouse but an unfavorable index ($TD_{50}/ED_{50} = 0.44$) for the rat.

TABLE II BARBITURATES AND RELATED COMPOUNDS

Test	Species	Effective dose (mg/kg)	Route of adminis-tration	References
		Phenobarbital		
MES	Mouse (CF#1)	28.0 (24.8–31.6)[a]	po	Goodman *et al.* (1953b)
	Mouse (CFW)	50 (27.5–90.9)	po	Raines *et al.* (1973)
	Mouse (CF#1)	20.6	sc	Goodman *et al.* (1953a)
	Rat (young)	7.4	ip	Petty and Karler (1965)
	Rat (mature)	4.9 (3.7–6.5)	po	Goodman *et al.* (1953b)
	Rat (mature)	12	ip	Toman *et al.* (1946)
	Rat (old)	1.4	ip	Petty and Karler (1965)
	Rabbit	15	ip	Toman *et al.* (1946)
	Cat	2	ip	Toman *et al.* (1946)
sc Met	Mouse	9.8 (6.7–14.2)	po	Vida *et al.* (1973)
	Mouse	15.5 (12.7–19.0)	po	Goodman *et al.* (1953b)
	Mouse	11	sc	Ferngren (1968)
	Rat	67 (48–93)	po	Goodman *et al.* (1953b)
	Cat	30–60	im	Spehlmann and Colley (1968)
MMS	Rat	9.5 (6.3–14.2)	sc	Goodman *et al.* (1953a)
MET	Mouse	25 (18.5–34.0)	po	Goodman *et al.* (1953b)
(60 Hz EST)	Rat	62.5 (57–68)	po	Goodman *et al.* (1953b)
HET	Mouse	29 (22–38)	po	Goodman *et al.* (1953b)
	Rat	80 (70–91)	po	Goodman *et al.* (1953b)
Audiogenic seizures	Mouse	2.3 (1.6–3.4)	ip	Collins and Horlington (1969)
	Mouse	9.0 (5.5–14.8)	po	Robichaud *et al.* (1970)
	Mouse	4.6 (3.1–6.9)	po	Fink and Swinyard (1959)
Strychnine seizures	Mouse	25.0 (15.4–40.5)	po	Robichaud *et al.* (1970)
Bemegride seizures	Cat	30	sc	Van Duijn and Visser (1972)
Picrotoxin seizures	Mouse	13–32	sc	Ferngren (1968)
Focal seizures (cobalt)	Cat	Unchanged	sc	Van Duijn and Visser (1972)
Intermittent photic stimulation	Baboon	15	im	Stark *et al.* (1970)

(continued)

TABLE II—*Continued*

Test	Species	Effective dose (mg/kg)	Route of administration	References
Flurothyl seizures	Rat	20	ip	Baumel *et al.* (1973)
Alumina-Induced seizures	Cat	10–15	im	Steinmann (1967)
Neurological deficit	Mouse	51 (44–60)	po	Goodman *et al.* (1953b)
	Mouse	100	sc	Swinyard *et al.* (1952)
	Rat	35 (30–41)	po	Goodman *et al.* (1953b)
	Rat	30	ip	Toman *et al.* (1946)
	Rat	90	sc	Swinyard *et al.* (1952)
	Rabbit	35	ip	Toman *et al.* (1946)
	Cat	5	ip	Toman *et al.* (1946)
Acute toxicity	Mouse	270 (216–337.5)	po	Vida *et al.* (1973)
	Mouse	200 (167–240)	po	Fink and Swinyard (1959)
Mephobarbital				
MES	Mouse	16 (11.4–22.4)	po	Vida *et al.* (1973)
	Mouse	20.9	sc	Goodman *et al.* (1953a)
	Mouse	20	po	Swinyard *et al.* (1952)
	Rat	ca. 20	ip	Craig and Shideman (1971)
	Rat	10	sc	Swinyard *et al.* (1952)
	Cat	12.5	po	Chen and Ensor (1952)
sc Met	Mouse	24 (16.9–34.1)	po	Vida *et al.* (1973)
	Mouse	25	po	Swinyard *et al.* (1952).
	Rat	40	po	Swinyard *et al.* (1952)
	Rat	15.3	sc	Swinyard (1949)
MMS	Mouse	11.3	po	Goodman *et al.* (1953a)
MET (60 Hz EST)	Mouse	ca. 30	po	Brown *et al.* (1953)
	Mouse	30	po	Swinyard *et al.* (1952)
	Rat	90	po	Swinyard *et al.* (1952)
HET	Mouse	26	po	Swinyard *et al.* (1952)
	Rat	80	po	Swinyard *et al.* (1952)
Neurological deficit	Mouse	65	po	Brown *et al.* (1953)
	Mouse	60	po	Swinyard *et al.* (1952)
	Rat	38 ± 1.1	sc	Swinyard (1949)
	Rat	80	sc	Swinyard *et al.* (1952)
Acute toxicity	Mouse	ca. 300	po	Vida *et al.* (1973)
Metharbital				
MES	Mouse	30 (18.8–48.0)	po	Vida *et al.* (1973)
sc Met	Mouse	18.0 (11.8–27.4)	po	Vida *et al.* (1973)

TABLE II—*Continued*

Test	Species	Effective dose (mg/kg)	Route of adminis- tration	References
Neurological deficit	Mouse	200	po	Barnes and Eltherington (1966)
	Mouse	150	ip	Barnes and Eltherington (1966)
Acute toxicity	Mouse	ca. 820	po	Vida *et al.* (1973)
	Mouse	500	po and ip	Barnes and Eltherington (1966)
		Primidone		
MES	Mouse	13.0 (8.4–20.2)	po	Goodman *et al.* (1953b)
	Rat	4.9 (3.7–6.5)	po	Goodman *et al.* (1953b)
	Rat	7.1 ± 0.6	po	Chen and Ensor (1950)
	Cat	25	po	Chen and Ensor (1950)
sc Met	Mouse	74 (57–96)	po	Goodman *et al.* (1953b)
	Rat	690 (580–821)	po	Goodman *et al.* (1953b)
MET	Mouse	86 (60–123)	po	Goodman *et al.* (1953b)
	Rat	560 (325–963)	po	Goodman *et al.* (1953b)
HET	Mouse	81 (65–100)	po	Goodman *et al.* (1953b)
	Rat	403 (267–605)	po	Goodman *et al.* (1953b)
Audiogenic seizures	Mouse	1.3 (0.7–2.3)	ip	Collins and Horlington (1969)
Neurological deficit	Mouse	1120 (950–1320)	po	Goodman *et al.* (1953b)
	Rat	630 (504–788)	po	Goodman *et al.* (1953b)
Acute toxicity	Mouse	1060	ip	Collins and Horlington (1969)

[a] Numbers in parentheses generally represent 95% fiducial limits.

4. Pentylenetetrazole Seizures

a. Metrazole Seizure Threshold (sc Met) Test. Data for different strains of mice, as shown in Table II, are not significantly different (Vida *et al.*, 1973; Goodman *et al.*, 1953b). Here, again, larger doses were required for the rat than for the mouse, and the protective index ($TD_{50}/ED_{50} = 3.3$) was favorable for the mouse but not for the rat ($TD_{50}/ED_{50} = 0.52$).

A noteworthy species difference in the effects of phenobarbital on the convulsive threshold of pentylenetetrazole was reported by Rümke (1967). In mice, phenobarbital increased the threshold for convulsive seizures (CD_{50}) when given $1\frac{1}{2}$ hours before the convulsant; i.e., the effect was anti-convulsant. However, if the interval was 2 days, the CD_{50} of pentylenetetrazole was significantly reduced; i.e., a proconvulsant effect was produced. This increase in susceptibility to seizures, suggesting withdrawal supersensitivity, was shown in the mouse but not in the rat.

Age of test animals as well as the time following injection appear to be important determinants in the anticonvulsant effectiveness of phenobarbital. Ferngren (1965), working with newborn and young mice of the NMRI strain, found the ED_{50} of phenobarbital to increase steadily with advancing age. Moreover, except in newborn animals, the time after administration affected the size of the ED_{50} from a high of 10 mg/kg at 30 minutes on day 1 to a low of 6 mg/kg at 90 minutes on day 3. The values for the ED_{50} decreased to 6 mg/kg at 3 minutes and increased to 10 mg/kg after 90 minutes on day 21. Since limits of error are not provided, their differences may not be significant.

b. Maximal Metrazole Seizures.   The low value (9.5 mg/kg sc) shown in Table II reflects the ability of phenobarbital to overcome maximal chemo-shock as well as electroshock seizures in the rat, as would be expected for drugs with therapeutic potential in grand mal.

5. Audiogenic Seizures

Here, again, the maximal seizure pattern, which resembles that produced by electroshock (MES) and pentylenetetrazole (MMS), is antagonized by small doses of phenobarbital, as shown in Table II. A larger dose (20 mg/kg po) was required to abolish the running component of the seizure pattern (Fink and Swinyard, 1959). The low dose (2.3 mg/kg ip) reported by Collins and Horlington (1969) probably reflects the more rapid route of administration.

6. Intermittent Photic Stimulation

The intramuscular (im) dose of phenobarbital listed in Table II (15 mg/kg) for the baboon was fairly long lasting, with seizures in response to 25 Hz photic stimulation being inhibited for 24 hours.

7. Bemegride Seizures

The effective dose shown in Table II (30 mg/kg sc), injected 45 minutes before bemegride, caused a marked increase (232%) in the threshold for bemegride seizures in the cat. Although tonic–clonic seizures occurred in the alert cat, threshold was taken as the time required for the onset of the multispike phase in the electrocorticogram.

8. Focal Seizures (Cobalt)

These experiments are included in the bemegride series reported above (Van Duijn and Visser, 1972). Phenobarbital did not alter electrocortical focal seizure activity induced by cobalt in the alert cat.

9. Strychnine Seizures

The ED_{50} of 25 mg/kg po reported by Robichaud *et al.* (1970) was in response to an intraperitoneal dose of 4 mg/kg of strychnine sulfate in female mice.

10. Picrotoxin Seizures

The figure shown in Table II (13–32 mg/kg sc) is based on a study of the effect of phenobarbital during postnatal development in the mouse. The ED_{50} values for the adult ranged from 7 to 15 mg/kg sc, with the lowest value occurring 30 minutes after injection.

11. Flurothyl Seizures

Baumel *et al.* (1973) found the latent period for flurothyl to be 254 ± 7.0 seconds. This period was increased significantly following intraperitoneal doses of 5 or 10 mg/kg of phenobarbital. However, following 20 mg/kg, latency was increased to 343 ± 12.0 seconds, which was significant. This is the value shown in Table III, a single dose rather than an ED_{50}.

12. Alumina Seizures

In the study reported by Steinmann (1967) epileptogenic seizures were produced in a large series of cats by application of aluminum hydroxide to the pyriform lobe of the brain. The figure shown in Table II (10–15 mg/kg im) represents the optimal effect of a single dose. This author found that a delayed onset of treatment was important in that one-third of the animals exhibited no seizures whatever.

13. Neurological Deficit

The ED_{50} values shown in Table II are generally higher in mice than in rats, indicating a lesser sensitivity to phenobarbital. In sharp contrast, the cat appears to have an extraordinary sensitivity to the drug, with an ED_{50} of only 5 mg/kg ip.

14. Acute Toxicity

The values shown in Table II are for different strains of mice, yet the actual LD_{50} values are not significantly different.

B. MEPHOBARBITAL

1. Maximal Electroshock Seizures

The values shown in Table II represent ED_{50} values, except for the cat. Two different strains of mice were used: Charles River (Vida *et al.*, 1973) and CF#1 (Goodman *et al.*, 1953a; Swinyard *et al.*, 1952). Goodman *et al.* (1953a) reported ED_{50} values as millimoles per kilogram; in our reporting, their data were converted to milligrams per kilogram, as shown in Table II. Mephobarbital is clearly in the potency range of phenobarbital. This is not altogether surprising, since mephobarbital is converted to phenobarbital, at least in the rat. Craig and Shideman (1971), working with male Sprague-Dawley rats, showed that, after repeated daily injections of mephobarbital (10 mg/kg ip) for 10 days, brain levels of phenobarbital were roughly eight times those of mephobarbital 4 hours after the last dose of mephobarbital. After 24 hours phenobarbital was still detectable in the brain, but mephobarbital was not. Presumably, repeated administration of mephobarbital activated the enzyme system responsible for its demethylation. The dose of mephobarbital shown in Table II (Craig and Shideman, 1971) actually protected 100% the rats tested against maximal electroshock seizures.

2. Pentylenetetrazole Seizures

a. Metrazole Seizure Threshold (sc Met) Test.   Values shown in Table II represent ED_{50} values. Here, again, values shown for mice reveal no difference referable to strain (Charles River, Vida *et al.*, 1973; CF#1, Swinyard *et al.*, 1952). Data for the rat (Swinyard, 1949) were computed from TD_{50} and PI values (PI = TD_{50}/ED_{50}). These values are for adult mice. Data for newborn and young mice (NMRI strain) are considerably lower. Ferngren (1965) reported ED_{50} values of 4 and 13 mg/kg sc in newborn and 21-day-old mice, respectively, when challenge occurred 50 minutes following administration of the drug.

b. Maximal Metrazole Seizures.   The ED_{50} shown in Table II (11.3 mg/kg po) was determined in CF#1 mice of both sexes and corresponds to the reported value of 0.046 (0.027–0.077) mmole/kg.

3. Minimal Electroshock Seizure Threshold

The ED_{50} values shown in Table II (Swinyard *et al.*, 1952) are for CF#1 male mice and Sprague-Dawley male rats. The CF#1 male mice were used by Brown *et al.* (1953). The ED_{50} reported by Brown *et al.* (1953) (30 mg/kg po) is given as an approximate figure since it was taken from a bar graph. For this test, it would appear that the mouse is three times as sensitive as the rat.

4. Hyponatremic Electroshock Seizure Threshold

Much lower doses of mephobarbital were required for anticonvulsant activity in mice than in rats. In the study reported by Swinyard *et al.* (1952), allowance was made for species differences in the time required for peak hyponatremic activity: 2 hours for mice and 4 hours for rats.

5. Neurological Deficit

The values shown in Table II represent TD_{50} values. Taken together with ED_{50} values for the various tests reported, protective indices (TD_{50}/ED_{50}) would be well within acceptable limits for the MES, Met, and MMS test, and for MET and HET tests in the mouse but not in the rat.

6. Acute Toxicity

The LD_{50} value shown in Table II is given as an approximate figure since the data were not rectilinear.

C. METHARBITAL

Limited data are available for this drug. Vida *et al.* (1973) reported its effectiveness at relatively low dosage in Charles River male mice. Acute toxicity was also low. Data of Barnes and Eltherington (1966) represent a personal communication from Abbott Laboratories.

D. PRIMIDONE

1. Maximal Electroshock Seizures

Primidone reaches its peak effect 6 hours following oral administration, compared with 3 hours for phenobarbital. Consequently, measurements of ED_{50} shown in Table II for the mouse and rat reported by Goodman *et al.* (1953b) were conducted at this time. This longer time required for peak activity may reflect its partial conversion to phenobarbital. However, as reported by Baumel *et al.* (1973), primidone has anticonvulsant activity that is independent of phenobarbital. It is clearly more potent than phenobarbital with respect to MES. It is also considerably more potent than its other metabolite, phenylethylmalonamide (PEMA), which has an approximate ED_{50} of 125 mg/kg ip in the rat.

2. Metrazole Seizure Threshold (sc Met) Test

Primidone is clearly capable of inhibiting pentylenetetrazole seizures, as shown in Table II. Much larger doses are required, however, than for electroshock seizures. A marked species difference in sensitivity is revealed by the investigation of Goodman *et al.* (1953b) in which the dose of primidone required for the rat was nearly ten times that required for the mouse (690 versus 74 mg/kg).

Frey and Hahn (1960) were able to protect both mice and dogs against pentylenetetrazole-induced clonic seizures. Moreover, in a side-by-side comparison with phenobarbital, equal anticonvulsant activity was obtained at primidone-derived phenobarbital plasma concentrations one-third to one-half those obtained from phenobarbital itself. This finding suggests that primidone has anticonvulsant activity of its own, complementing that of phenobarbital, its active degradation derivative.

3. Minimal Electroshock Seizure Threshold and
Hyponatremic Electroshock Seizure Threshold

In both of these tests, much larger amounts of primidone were required for an anticonvulsant effect in the rat than in the mouse. This species difference in sensitivity was shown earlier in this chapter [Metrazole seizure threshold (sc Met) Test] to be the case for phenobarbital as well. With primidone, however, the difference in sensitivity was far greater, emphasizing again that primidone and phenobarbital are distinctly different drugs.

4. Flurothyl Seizures

Gallagher *et al.* (1970), working with adult male albino rats, were able to show that, at comparable plasma phenobarbital levels, primidone was more effective than phenobarbital in raising the threshold for flurothyl-induced tonic–clonic seizures.

5. Neurological Deficit and Acute Toxicity

If the TD_{50} and LD_{50} values shown in Table II for primidone are compared with those for phenobarbital, it is apparent that the two drugs differ markedly in acute toxicity, primidone being orders of magnitude less toxic than phenobarbital in the experimental animal.

V. OXAZOLIDINEDIONES

A. TRIMETHADIONE

1. Maximal Electroshock Seizures

Although employed primarily for the management of petit mal, trimethadione effectively prevents the tonic extensor phase of the maximal electroshock seizure pattern. However, the large doses required, as shown in Table III, necessarily provide small protective indices. Effective doses shown in the table are large for all species listed. The value for the cat represents a minimal dose required to modify electroshock seizures.

2. Pentylenetetrazole Seizures

a. Metrazole Seizure Threshold (sc Met) Test. Here, again, ED_{50} values are high, as shown in Table III, and protective indices are correspondingly low. Although the test is generally considered an excellent model for predicting drugs of therapeutic potential in petit mal, the case of trimethadione suggests that, in routine screening, compounds should not be excluded on the basis of high ED_{50} values.

Continued daily administration of trimethadione leads rapidly to the development of tolerance, as reported by Frey and Kretschmer (1971). After administration of the drug to mice (NMRI strain, bred in Denmark) for 24 hours, the ED_{50} increased from 470 mg/kg, the value shown in Table III for an acute experiment, to 1550 mg/kg. And when the time between drug

TABLE III OXAZOLIDINEDIONES

Test	Species	Effective dose (mg/kg)	Route of adminis- tration	Reference
		Trimethadione		
MES	Mouse	630	sc	Goodman *et al.* (1953a)
	Mouse	625	sc	Swinyard *et al.* (1952)
	Rat	350	sc	Swinyard *et al.* (1952)
	Rat	350	ip	Toman *et al.* (1946)
	Rabbit	500	ip	Toman *et al.* (1946)
	Cat	200	ip	Toman *et al.* (1946)
	Cat	500	po	Chen and Ensor (1950)
sc Met	Mouse	197.3	po	Goodman *et al.* (1953a)
	Mouse	480	sc	Swinyard *et al.* (1952)
	Mouse	250	ip	Everett and Richards (1944)
	Mouse	470 (400–550)[a]	po	Frey and Kretschmer (1971)
	Mouse	314.9	iv	Frey (1969)
	Mouse	200	sc	Ferngren (1968)
	Rat	300	sc	Swinyard *et al.* (1952)
	Rabbit	500	ip	Everett and Richards (1944)
	Cat	500	ip	Everett and Richards (1944)
iv Met	Mouse	275 (252–300)	iv	Swinyard and Castellion (1966)
MMS	Mouse (F)	270 (206–354)	po	Marshall and Vallance (1954)
	Mouse (M)	361.8	po	Goodman *et al.* (1949)
	Mouse (M)	370 (274–500)	po	Swinyard and Castellion (1966)
MET (60 Hz EST)	Mouse	800	po	Randall (1961)
	Mouse	500	sc	Swinyard *et al.* (1952)
	Rat	300	sc	Swinyard *et al.* (1952)
HET	Mouse	700	sc	Swinyard *et al.* (1952)
	Rat	400	sc	Swinyard *et al.* (1952)
Strychnine seizures	Mouse	500	ip	Everett and Richards (1944)
Intermittent photic stimulation	Baboon	50	im	Stark *et al.* (1970)
	Rabbit	500	ip	Barnes (1954)
Picrotoxin seizures	Mouse	500	sc	Everett and Richards (1944)
Neurological deficit	Mouse	445 ± 27.7	po	Goodman *et al.* (1949)
	Mouse	650	sc	Swinyard *et al.* (1952)
	Rat	400	ip	Toman *et al.* (1946)
	Rat	625	sc	Swinyard *et al.* (1952)
	Rabbit	875	ip	Toman *et al.* (1946)
	Cat	400	ip	Toman *et al.* (1946)

(continued)

TABLE III—*Continued*

Test	Species	Effective dose (mg/kg)	Route of adminis- tration	Reference
Acute toxicity	Mouse	2000	iv	Richards and Everett (1946)
	Rat	2200	sc	Barnes and Eltherington (1966)
	Rabbit	1500	iv	Richards and Everett (1946)
		Paramethadione		
MES	Mouse	153.9	sc	Goodman *et al.* (1953a)
	Rat	238.6	ip	Goodman *et al.* (1949)
	Rat	160	sc	Swinyard *et al.* (1952)
sc Met	Mouse	136.9	ip	Goodman *et al.* (1949)
	Mouse	110	sc	Swinyard *et al.* (1952)
	Rat	140	sc	Swinyard *et al.* (1952)
MMS	Mouse	64.4	sc	Goodman *et al.* (1953a)
MET	Mouse	140	sc	Swinyard *et al.* (1952)
(60 Hz EST)	Rat	150	sc	Swinyard *et al.* (1952)
HET	Mouse	140	sc	Swinyard *et al.* (1952)
	Rat	160	sc	Swinyard *et al.* (1952)
Intermittent photic stimulation	Rabbit	250	ip	Barnes (1954)
Neurological deficit	Mouse	140	sc	Swinyard *et al.* (1952)
	Rat	160	sc	Swinyard *et al.* (1952).

[a] Numbers in parentheses generally represent 95% fiducial limits.

administration and chemoshock exceeded 24 hours, only a few animals were protected. This is surprising since serum concentrations of the drug were two to three times higher than those after drug protection in an acute experiment. In an earlier article, Frey (1969) reported that trimethadione was rapidly metabolized to dimethadione and that any activity appearing later than 4–6 hours after injection was due to dimethadione. Trimethadione is demethylated to dimethadione in the liver. Dimethadione is not further broken down but is excreted as such (Withrow *et al.*, 1968). Of additional interest is the report of Dashputra and Khapre (1970), who found that the anticonvulsant activity of trimethadione versus pentylenetetrazole, like that of DPH versus electroshock, is potentiated by chlorothiazide congeners.

b. Maximal Metrazole Seizures. From the figures shown in Table III it appears that doses of trimethadione required to antagonize the maximal seizure pattern evoked by pentylenetetrazole are considerably smaller than those needed to abolish maximal seizures in response to electroshock. Female mice appear to be somewhat more sensitive than males to the action of trimethadione, although the observed difference may not be significant. The ED_{50} reported by Marshall and Vallance (1954) was determined in female albino mice (Schofield strain) starved overnight.

3. Minimal Electroshock Seizure Threshold and Hyponatremic Electroshock Seizure Threshold

Swinyard *et al.* (1952) utilized CF#1 male mice and Sprague-Dawley male rats; strain and sex are not given in the report by Randall (1941). While trimethadione is effective by these tests, the doses required are large, and the protective indices are small.

4. Strychnine Seizures

The dose shown in Table III (500 mg/kg ip) represents a minimal effective dose (MED) of trimethadione required to oppose the surely lethal effects of a 1.5 mg/kg sc dose of strychnine sulfate.

5. Intermittent Photic Stimulation

The dose of trimethadione shown in Table III is an approximate (presumably a minimally effective) dose required to abolish the effects of photic stimulation in the baboon. The dose shown for the rabbit abolished the flicker-fusion effect following daily administration for 5 days (Barnes, 1954).

6. Picrotoxin Seizures

The tabular value shown represents a minimal effective dose in the mouse.

7. Neurological Deficit and Acute Toxicity

All values for neurological deficit represent TD_{50} values. In general, mice were CF#1 strain and rats were Sprague-Dawley strain. The acute toxicity of trimethadione was clearly low, even following intravenous administration.

B. PARAMETHADIONE

Literature reports for this drug do not appear to be as plentiful as for trimethadione. Data shown in Table III, however, reveal that it is far more potent in every area tested. Toxicity was correspondingly high, as represented by low TD_{50} values. Protective indices are generally unfavorable in that, except for the MMS test, the amount of paramethadione required for anticonvulsant activity produces neurological deficit.

VI. SUCCINIMIDES

A. PHENSUXIMIDE

1. Maximal Electroshock Seizures

The value shown in Table IV (183 ± 5.2 mg/kg po) is the ED_{50} versus 60 Hz 24 mA/0.2 second. The animals exhibited mild ataxia; hence, the

TABLE IV   SUCCINIMIDES

Test	Species	Effective dose (mg/kg)	Route of adminis- tration	Reference
Phensuximide				
MES	Mouse	183 ± 5.2	po	Chen *et al.* (1963)
sc Met	Rat	ca. 125	po	Chen *et al.* (1963)
Acute toxicity	Mouse	1513 ± 61	po	Chen *et al.* (1963)
Methsuximide				
MES	Mouse	84 ± 3.3	po	Chen *et al.* (1963)
sc Met	Rat	> 33 < 63	po	Chen *et al.* (1963)
Neurological deficit	Mouse	ca. 250	po	Glazko and Dill (1972)
	Rat	ca. 250	po	Glazko and Dill (1972)
Acute toxicity	Mouse	ca. 1400	po	Glazko and Dill (1972)
	Mouse	1405 ± 33	po	Chen *et al.* (1963)
Ethosuximide				
MES	Mouse	2070	po	Chen *et al.* (1963)
sc Met	Rat	> 63 < 125	po	Chen *et al.* (1963)
Audiogenic seizures	Mouse	146 (110.5–192.5)[a]	ip	Collins and Horlington (1969)
Acute toxicity	Mouse	1536 ± 40	po	Chen *et al.* (1963)
	Mouse	1372	ip	Collins and Horlington (1969)

[a] Numbers in parentheses generally represent 95% fiducial limits.

effective dose overlaps the dose producing neurological deficit, and one would predict a low protective index for this drug. Swiss Webster mice used in this experiment were deprived of food but not water for 16 hours before the experiment. One questions, therefore, whether the animals were in an abnormal state at the time of drug administration and exposure to the electroshock stimulus. For example, hypoglycemia of any degree could conceivably alter sensitivity of the animals to electroshock.

2. Metrazole Seizure Threshold (sc Met) Test

The value shown in Table IV is an approximate value, representing the amount of drug that protected two out of five young (100–150 gm) Sprague-Dawley rats from convulsing. The degree of protection is rated as 2+ on a scale of 0 to 4+; on this basis a dose of 250 mg/kg protected all of five rats and was given a rating of 4+.

3. Acute Toxicity

The value listed in Table IV represents the LD_{50} in nonfasted mice. The pattern of toxicity involved marked incoordination, loss of grasping and righting reflexes, dyspnea, and death from respiratory failure. There were no hematological abnormalities.

B. METHSUXIMIDE

1. Maximal Electroshock Seizures

Methsuximide is evidently about twice as potent as phensuximide. Although the animals were described as "quiet," the effective dose is stated to be below the dose required to induce neurological deficit.

2. Metrazole Seizure Threshold (sc Met) Test

Here, again, methsuximide shows greater potency than phensuximide. The figure shown in Table IV is based on the finding that a dose of 33 mg/kg protected two out of five rats from convulsing, while 63 mg/kg protected all animals. The rating was 2+ for the lower dose and 4+ for the higher one.

3. Acute Toxicity

The acute oral toxicity of methsuximide is high and of the same order as that for phensuximide. Here, again, the pattern of toxicity was the same.

C. ETHOSUXIMIDE

1. Maximal Electroshock Seizures

Ethosuximide protected mice and rats againt electroshock seizures (Table IV), but only at doses that induced the loss of the righting reflex, i.e., hypnotic doses (Chen *et al.*, 1963).

2. Metrazole Seizure Threshold (sc Met) Test

A dose of 63 mg/kg protected one out of five rats and was rated at the lowest level. A dose of 125 mg/kg protected five out of five animals, and protection was rated as 4+ (Chen *et al.*, 1963).

3. Audiogenic Seizures

The effective dose shown in Table IV is an ED_{50}, based on suppression of the running component of the seizure pattern. The mice used in this study (Collins and Horlington, 1969) were the F_1 generation obtained by crossing DBA/1 males with SNR albino females.

4. Acute Toxicity

It is of interest that the LD_{50} values shown in Table IV are numerically close, despite the difference in route of administration and strain. Presumably Collins and Horlington (1969) employed the strain bred for audiogenic sensitivity, whereas Chen *et al.* (1963) used a non-audiogenic-sensitive strain.

VII. BENZODIAZEPINES

A. CHLORDIAZEPOXIDE

1. Maximal Electroshock Seizures

Banziger's (1965) data, as shown in Table V, were obtained with CF#1 male mice, Wistar strain male rats, and cats of both sexes. The drug was administered orally in 5% aqueous acacia 1 hour before electroshock. Data of Swinyard and Castellion (1966) are based on CF#1 male albino mice. Their studies were done 2 hours after oral administration (peak time), yet the ED_{50} (41 mg/kg) does not differ significantly from Banziger's (1965) figure when limits of error are taken into account. The figure reported by Robichaud *et al.* (1970) was obtained using Manor Farms female mice. Their ED_{50} (49 mg/kg) was within the range reported by Swinyard and Castellion (1966), yet shocking was done at a lower amperage (12 mA/0.2 second). From all of these studies conducted in mice, it would appear that sensitivity of chlordiazepoxide to electroshock was significantly affected by strain or sex differences.

Only a single study is shown in which the rat was used. From this study, however (Banziger, 1965), it is apparent that the ED_{50} (5.8 mg/kg) of chlordiazepoxide was far lower in this species than in the mouse. The effective dose reported by Banziger (1965) for the cat is stated to be less than 10 mg/kg since this dose conferred full protection against electroshock after 1 hour and up to 8 hours, at which time drug activity was still detectable. The cat, like the rat, appears to be extremely sensitive to the anticonvulsant effects of chlordiazepoxide on maximal electroshock seizures. The oral dose of 10 mg/kg produced sedation, indicating a low protective index in this species.

2. Metrazole Seizure Threshold (sc and iv Met) Tests

As a drug primarily associated with the management of petit mal, a high level of activity against clonic seizure activity of chlordiazepoxide would have been predicted. And this indeed appears to be the case since the ED_{50} values versus clonic seizures induced following either subcutaneously administered pentylenetetrazole (Banziger, 1965; Swinyard and Castellion, 1966) or intravenously administered pentylenetetrazole (Swinyard and Castellion, 1966), were extremely low, in the range of 3–8 mg/kg.

Rabbits (Banziger, 1965) and monkeys (Chusid and Kopeloff, 1961) are likewise extremely sensitive to the action of chlordiazepoxide, since ED_{50} values are in the range of 1–4 mg/kg (Table V). The rat is also sensitive to this action of chlordiazepoxide, although far less so than the other species reported.

TABLE V   BENZODIAZEPINES

Test	Species	Effective dose (mg/kg)	Route of adminis- tration	Reference
		Chlordiazepoxide		
MES	Mouse	17.0	po	Gluckman (1971)
	Mouse	29.9 ± 3	po	Banziger (1965)
	Mouse	41.0 (29.5–57.0)[a]	po	Swinyard and Castellion (1966)
	Mouse	49.0 (40–60)	po	Robichaud et al. (1970)
	Rat	5.8 ± 1.7	po	Banziger (1965)
	Rat	12 ± 1.5	po	Christmas and Maxwell (1970)
	Cat	< 10	po	Banziger (1965)
sc Met	Mouse	3.7	po	Gluckman (1971)
	Mouse	8 ± 0.9	po	Banziger (1965)
	Mouse	3.6 (2.5–5.0)	po	Swinyard and Castellion (1966)
	Rat	13 ± 3.7	po	Banziger (1965)
	Rabbit	1.55 ± 0.25	po	Banziger (1965)
	Monkey	1.1–4.4	iv	Chusid and Kopeloff (1961)
iv Met	Mouse	6.2 (4.3–9.0)	iv	Swinyard and Castellion (1966)
	Cat	1.2	—	Straw (1968)
MMS	Mouse	3.1 (2.3–4.2)	po	Swinyard and Castellion (1966)
MET (60 Hz EST)	Mouse	91.7	po	Banziger (1965)
	Rat	> 800	po	Banziger (1965)
MET (6 Hz EST)	Mouse	32.5 (19.1–55.3)	po	Swinyard and Castellion (1966)
Audiogenic seizures	Mouse	4.4 (2.8–6.9)	po	Robichaud et al. (1970)
	Mouse	1.95 (1.4–2.7)	ip	Collins and Horlington (1969)
Strychnine seizures	Mouse	> 100	po	Robichaud et al. (1970)
Neurological deficit	Mouse	152 (91–225)	po	Swinyard and Castellion (1966)
	Mouse	10.7 (9.8–12.2)	po	Fennessy and Lee (1972)
	Mouse	9.3	po	Gluckman (1971)
Acute toxicity	Mouse	720 ± 51	po	Banziger (1965)
	Mouse	680 (540–856)	po	Robichaud et al. (1970)
		Diazepam		
MES	Mouse	3.4	po	Gluckman (1971)

(continued)

TABLE V—*Continued*

Test	Species	Effective dose (mg/kg)	Route of adminis-tration	Reference
	Mouse	6.4 ± 0.8	po	Banziger (1965)
	Mouse	14.0 (8.2–23.8)	po	Robichard et al. (1970)
	Mouse	18.7 (14.5–24.1)	po	Swinyard and Castellion (1966)
	Rat	48 ± 12	po	Christmas and Maxwell (1970)
	Cat	>10	po	Banziger (1965)
sc Met	Mouse	0.28–2.8	iv	Marcucci et al. (1971)
	Mouse	0.27 (0.15–0.47)	po	Swinyard and Castellion (1966)
	Mouse	1.2 (0.91–1.66)	po	Robichaud et al. (1970)
	Mouse	1.37 ± 0.02	po	Banziger and Hane (1967)
	Rat	12 ± 2	po	Banziger (1965)
	Rabbit	0.3 ± p.2	po	Banziger (1965)
	Monkey	0.05–0.10	iv	Kopeloff and Chusid (1967)
iv Met	Cat	0.25	—	Straw (1968)
MMS	Cat	1.0	im	Spehlmann and Colley (1968)
MET (60 Hz EST)	Mouse	86	po	Randall et al. (1970)
	Mouse	64	po	Banziger (1965)
	Rat	42 ± 8.0	po	Banziger (1965)
MET (6 Hz EST)	Mouse	18.7 (10.4–33.7)	po	Swinyard et al. (1966)
Audiogenic seizures	Mouse	ca. 1.5	po	Robichaud et al. (1970)
Strychnine seizures	Mouse	16	po	Randall et al. (1970)
	Mouse	13.0	sc	Robichaud et al. (1970)
Bemegride seizures	Cat	2	sc	Van Duijn and Visser (1972)
Focal seizures cobalt	Cat	Increases seizures	sc	Van Duijn and Visser (1972)
Intermittent photic stimulation	Baboon	0.5–2	im	Stark et al. (1970)
Alumina cream seizures	Monkey	>0.05 < 0.20	iv	Kopeloff and Chusid (1967)
Picrotoxin seizures	Rabbit	0.33	iv	Barrada and Oftedal (1970)
Flurothyl seizures	Mouse	0.125	ip	Boissier et al. (1968)

TABLE V—*Continued*

Test	Species	Effective dose (mg/kg)	Route of adminis- tration	Reference
Neurological deficit	Mouse	1.9	po	Gluckman (1971)
	Mouse	57 (40–81)	po	Swinyard and Castellion (1966)
	Mouse	7.3 (6.9–8.1)	po	Fennessy and Lee (1972)
	Cat	0.2	po	Randall *et al.* (1970)
	Monkey	1.0	iv	Gluckman (1971)
Acute toxicity	Mouse	970 ± 66	po	Randall *et al.* (1970)
	Mouse	220 ± 21	ip	Randall *et al.* (1970)
	Mouse	ca. 750	po	Robichaud *et al.* (1970)
	Mouse	620 + 30	po	Banziger (1965)
	Rat	278 (235–388)	po	Marcucci *et al.* (1968)

Oxazepam

Test	Species	Effective dose (mg/kg)	Route of adminis- tration	Reference
MES	Mouse	28	po	Randall *et al.* (1970)
	Mouse	3.1	po	Gluckman (1971)
	Rat	25 ± 9.6	po	Christmas and Maxwell (1970)
sc Met	Mouse	0.7	po	Randall *et al.* (1970)
	Mouse	0.34–4.85	iv	Marcucci *et al.* (1971)
	Mouse	0.6	po	Gluckman (1971)
MET (60 Hz EST)	Mouse	233	po	Randall *et al.* (1970)
Strychnine seizures	Mouse	100	po	Randall *et al.* (1970)
Neurological deficit	Mouse	4.9	po	Gluckman (1971)
	Cat	1.0	po	Randall *et al.* (1970)
Acute toxicity	Mouse	>4000	po	Randall *et al.* (1970)
	Mouse	>800	ip	Randall *et al.* (1970)
	Mouse	1540 (1419–1670)	po	Marcucci *et al.* (1968)
	Mouse	>1500	ip	Marcucci *et al.* (1971)

Medazepam

Test	Species	Effective dose (mg/kg)	Route of adminis- tration	Reference
MES	Mouse	36	po	Randall *et al.* (1970)
sc Met	Mouse	7	po	Randall *et al.* (1970)
MET (60 Hz EST)	Mouse	238	po	Randall *et al.* (1970)
Strychnine seizures	Mouse	20	po	Randall *et al.* (1970)
Neurological deficit	Mouse	15.4 (13.9–17.4)	po	Fennessy and Lee (1972)

(*continued*)

TABLE V—*Continued*

Test	Species	Effective dose (mg/kg)	Route of adminis- tration	Reference
Acute toxicity	Mouse	1070 ± 108	po	Fennessy and Lee (1972)
	Mouse	360 ± 19	ip	Randall *et al.* (1970)
Prazepam				
MES	Mouse	24.6 (17.3–34.9)	po	Robichaud *et al.* (1970)
sc Met	Mouse	3.2 (2.1–4.8)	po	Robichaud *et al.* (1970)
Audiogenic seizures	Mouse	1.7 (1.1–2.4)	po	Robichaud *et al.* (1970)
Strychnine seizures	Mouse	36.0 (22.5–57.6)	po	Robichaud *et al.* (1970)
Acute toxicity	Mouse	> 2000	po	Robichaud *et al.* (1970)
Lorazepam				
MES	Mouse	2.0	po	Gluckman (1971)
sc Met	Mouse	0.07	po	Gluckman (1971)
Neurological deficit	Mouse	0.9	po	Gluckman (1971)
	Monkey	5	iv	Gluckman (1971)
Acute toxicity	Mouse	3178 (2960–3412)	po	Owen *et al.* (1971)
	Mouse	1001 (933–1073)	ip	Owen *et al.* (1971)
	Mouse (neonatal)	ca. 250	po	Owen *et al.* (1971)
	Rat	> 5000	po	Owen *et al.* (1971)
	Rat	1728 (1594–1873)	ip	Owen *et al.* (1971)
	Rat (neonatal)	ca. 2000	po	Owen *et al.* (1971)
	Dog	> 2000	po	Owen *et al.* (1971)
	Dog	> 25	im	Owen *et al.* (1971)
Nitrazepam				
MES	Rat	35 ± 9	po	Christmas and Maxwell (1970)
sc Met	Mouse	3.3 ± 0.8	po	Christmas and Maxwell (1970)
im Met	Monkey	0.77	iv	Berman *et al.* (1968)
iv Met	Cat	0.125	—	Straw (1968)
Audiogenic seizures	Mouse	0.14 (0.08–0.3)	ip	Collins and Horlington (1969)
Picrotoxin seizures	Rabbit	0.33	iv	Barrada and Oftedal (1970)
Neurological deficit	Mouse	23.5 (21.6–26.8)	po	Fennessy and Lee (1972)

TABLE V—*Continued*

Test	Species	Effective dose (mg/kg)	Route of adminis- tration	Reference
Acute toxicity	Mouse	275	po	Collins and Horlington (1969)
		Clonazepam		
Bemegride seizures	Cat	0.2	sc	Van Duijn (1973)
Focal seizures (cobalt)	Cat	0.2	sc	Van Duijn (1973)
Neurological deficit	Mouse	2.5 (2.1–3.0)	po	Fennessy and Lee (1972)

[a] Numbers in parentheses generally represent 95% fiducial limits.

3. Maximal Metrazole Seizures

As shown in Table V, the low ED_{50} obtained by Swinyard and Castellion (1966) indicates that the mouse is extremely sensitive to the antagonistic effects of chlordiazepoxide against maximal as well as clonic seizures evoked by pentylenetetrazole.

Swinyard and Castellion (1966) have raised the interesting question of why the benzodiazepines are so much more potent against maximal seizures in response to pentylenetetrazole than those evoked by electroshock. Goodman *et al.* (1953a) provided at least a partial answer in pointing out that some agents are more effective in preventing seizure spread than in raising the threshold for convulsive discharge. Antagonism of maximal electroshock seizures, by drugs, such as DPH, involves primarily an inhibition of seizure spread; antagonism of maximal metrazole seizures, by drugs like chlor-diazepoxide, appears to involve both threshold elevation and seizure spread.

4. Minimal Electroshock Seizure Threshold (60 Hz EST)

The dose (91.7 mg/kg) referred to in Table V represents the oral ED_{50} in the mouse without reference to limits of error. Marked species difference is indicated since more than 800 mg/kg was required to elevate seizure threshold in the rat. The author does not state whether this large dose actually elevated the threshold of any of the animals.

5. Audiogenic and Strychnine Seizures

Male mice (12–18 gm) of the O'Grady strain were used in the study by Robichaud *et al.* (1970). The dose required to offset convulsions (Table V) following a 1-minute sound stimulus was shown to be 4.4 mg/kg. The study by Collins and Horlington (1969) utilized the F_1 generation obtained by crossing DBA/1 males with SNR females, and anticonvulsant activity was recorded if the running movement of the seizure pattern was completely suppressed. It is of interest that the doses required to inhibit audiogenic seizures are in the range of those required to antagonize pentylenetetrazole. In marked contrast to these results, the drug appears to have little effect on strychnine-induced seizures.

6. Neurological Deficit and Acute Toxicity

The oral TD_{50} reported for neurological deficit (152 mg/kg) by Swinyard and Castellion (1966) was determined in male albino mice of the CF#1 strain at peak time (120 minutes). Comparison of ED_{50} values for the various tests shown above shows protective indices well within acceptable limits for tests involving MES, low-frequency (lf) EST, Met, and MMS and audiogenic seizures, but not for MET and strychnine. The LD_{50} values were high, and almost identical, despite strain and sex differences. Chlordiazepoxide emerges as an effective anticonvulsant having low acute toxicity, at least in the mouse.

The TD_{50}, determined by motor incoordination in the study by Fennessy and Lee (1972), as shown in Table V, is very small compared with that reported by Swinyard and Castellion (1966). This marked discrepancy can presumably be attributed to the strain of mouse used by Fennessy and Lee (1972), the Commonwealth Serum Laboratories strain (males and females). The dose required to produce neurological deficit caused significant decreases in brain levels of norepinephrine and 5-hydroxyindoleacetic acid but did not affect levels of dopamine or 5-hydroxytryptamine. The value reported by Gluckman (9.3 mg/kg) is essentially the same as that reported by Fennessy and Lee (1972), although strain and sex of mice are not given.

B. DIAZEPAM

1. Maximal Metrazole Seizures

The ED_{50} reported by Robichaud *et al.* (1970), determined in Manor Farms female mice, does not differ significantly from the value reported by Swinyard and Castellion (1966) for CF#1 males. Banziger's (1965) value for CF#1 male mice does differ from those of the other investigators.

It is clear, however, that diazepam is a potent antagonist of maximal electroshock seizures, both in the mouse and in the cat (Table V), more potent than phenobarbital, and less potent than DPH by this test. Accordingly, one would predict that diazepam would have some value in the management of grand mal in man (Woodbury, 1972).

2. Metrazole Seizure Threshold (sc and iv Met) Test

Banziger (1965) and Robichaud *et al.* (1970) reported essentially identical ED_{50} values in CF#1 male and Manor Farms female mice, respectively.

The value reported by Swinyard and Castellion for CF#1 male mice is significantly less than that reported by other investigators (Table V). The difference may possibly be explained by the fact that Swinyard and Castellion's study was conducted at 30 minutes, the previously determined time of peak effect of diazepam, and presumably differs from that employed by the other investigators. Straw (1968) reported that a dose of 0.25 mg/kg of diazepam raised the threshold significantly for intravenously administered pentylene-tetrazole in the cat.

The values recorded for Marcucci *et al.* (1971) are given as a range, since larger amounts of drug are required to protect against pentylenetetrazole seizures, depending on the interval following intravenous injection, and the actual ED_{50} reflects the drug's metabolism to oxazepam. Thus, the ED_{50} after 5 minutes was 0.28 mg/kg, corresponding to a brain level of 0.097 μg/gm of diazepam and only 0.010 μg/gm of oxazepam. After 180 minutes the ED_{50} of diazepam was 0.68 mg/kg, corresponding to 0.86 μg/gm of oxazepam. After 720 minutes the ED_{50} increased to 2.8 mg/kg, corresponding to a brain level of 0.125 μg/gm of oxazepam. Straw (1968) reported significant suppression of pentylenetetrazole siezures in the cat following doses of 1–2 mg/kg of chlordiazepoxide.

A significantly higher value is shown for the rat, based on studies by Banziger (1965) in male Wistar strain rats. This difference may be explained by the finding of Marcucci *et al.* (1968) that active N-demethyl metabolites of diazepam accumulated in mouse brain but were practically undetectable in rat brain. Effective doses for the rabbit (Banziger, 1965) and the monkey (Kopeloff and Chusid, 1967) are extremely low, indicating that the sensitivity of these species for diazepam is very great. Comparison of the values for diazepam and chlordiazepoxide versus sc Met reveals that the former drug is substantially more potent than the latter. The high level of potency against pentylenetetrazole-induced seizures is in line with the expected therapeutic activity shown by both drugs for petit mal in man.

3. Maximal Metrazole Seizures

The value reported by Spehlmann and Colley (1968) (Table V) derives from an experiment in which a dose of 5–10 mg/kg pentylenetetrazole (Metrazole) was injected intramuscularly into cats at intervals until repetitive seizures, referred to as "status," were produced. A single intramuscular 1 mg/kg dose of diazepam terminated this status. Intramuscular 30–60 mg/kg doses of phenobarbital were required for this effect.

4. Minimal Electroshock Seizure Threshold
(60 Hz EST)

In the study by Randall *et al.* (1970) (Table V) a current of 6 mA was used, the end point being a humping of the back in CF#1 mice. The investigation by Banziger (1965) also utilized CF#1 mice, but the ED_{50} he obtained was much lower. In both cases, however, it is apparent that far greater amounts of diazepam are required to elevate 60 Hz seizure threshold than to suppress maximal electroshock seizures.

5. Minimal Electroshock Seizure Threshold (6 Hz EST)

In contrast to the large dosage of diazepam needed to elevate the threshold for high-frequency shock, only one-fourth as much drug sufficed to elevate the threshold when low frequency (lf EST) was used, as shown in Table V. This study, reported by Swinyard and Castellion (1966), was conducted in CF#1 male mice at peak time (30 minutes). It should be noted that, in contrast to diazepam, chlordiazepoxide has a peak time of 120 minutes following oral administration to mice.

6. Audiogenic Seizures

Robichaud *et al.* (1970) employed young (12–18 gm) male mice of the O'Grady strain for determining the ED_{50} (ca. 1.5 mg/kg) shown in Table V. This value is statistically indistinguishable from that for the sc Met test, suggesting a high level of sensitivity for both pentylenetetrazole-induced and audiogenic seizures.

7. Strychnine Seizures

Values reported by Robichaud *et al.* (1970) and by Randall *et al.* (1970), appearing in Table V, are virtually identical. This is somewhat surprising since the former investigators employed adult female albino mice (Manor Farms) and a dose that is probably a multiple of the lethal dose of strychnine sulfate (4 mg/kg ip). Their effective dose is given as a conventional ED_{50} (13.0 mg/kg po). The value of Randall *et al.* (16.0 mg/kg po) was determined in CF#1 mice by means of a different technique. The ED_{50} is the dose required to increase the threshold of intravenously administered strychnine by 50%. Since strychnine is primarily a stimulant that is thought to block postsynaptic inhibition (Vernadakis and Woodbury, 1965), antagonism of this effect by diazepam at low dosage indicates that the latter drug has potent cord-depressant activity, at least in the mouse. Costa *et al.* (1975) suggested a mechanism involving GABA-ergic inhibitory neurons.

8. Bemegride Seizures

The extremely low dose of diazepam recorded in Table V (2 mg/kg sc) for the cat (Van Duijn and Visser, 1972) caused a 232 (87–416%) increase in the threshold for bemegride seizures. Since the site of action of bemegride on the brain is thought to be the same as that of pentylenetetrazole (Hahn, 1960), it is not at all surprising that diazepam would be of value in petit mal.

9. Focal Seizures (Cobalt)

According to Woodbury (1972), the test should have predictive value for compounds capable of suppressing both generalized and clonic seizures. It is surprising, therefore, to find that diazepam not only failed to inhibit cobalt-induced seizures but actually exacerbated them in the experiment by Van Duijn and Visser (1972), as recorded in Table V. The explanation for this unexpected finding remains undetermined.

10. Intermittent Photic Stimulation

Intramuscular doses of 0.5, 1.0, and 2.0 mg/kg of diazepam offset the effect of photic stimulation at 25 Hz in the baboon for a period of 24 hours (Table V). On the basis of the low doses required, one would predict that diazepam would have therapeutic potential in grand mal (Woodbury, 1972).

11. Alumina Cream Seizures

Kopeloff and Chusid (1967) reported that 0.05 mg/kg protected 20% of epileptic monkeys; 0.20 mg/kg protected 100%.

12. Picrotoxin Seizures

Typical spike-and-wave formations were produced in the electrocortico-gram following intravenous injection of 2.5 mg/kg of picrotoxin in the rabbit. Diazepam in low dosage (0.33 mg/kg iv; Table V) antagonized these changes in the ECoG to the extent that they returned almost completely to the pre-treatment pattern within 4–5 minutes. Inhibition of the spike-and-wave pattern is associated with anti-petit-mal activity (Barrada and Oftedal, 1970).

13. Flurothyl Seizures

The value shown in Table V (Boissier *et al.*, 1968) is the intraperitoneal dose required to prevent tonic seizures in mice following an intravenous dose of 0.05 ml 1% flurothyl in polyethyleneglycol (PEG-400). Diazepam antagonized flurothyl at extremely low dosage, suggesting possible therapeutic value in the management of grand mal (Woodbury, 1972).

14. Neurological Deficit

The value shown in Table V (Swinyard and Castellion, 1966) is actually a TD_{50} value, obtained at peak time (30 minutes) for diazepam following oral administration to adult male mice (CF#1 strain). Although comparable values are not shown for other species, it is apparent from the mouse data that the protective index of diazepam is high for all of the tests recorded above, except for the Met Test.

Fennessy and Lee (1972) reported a much smaller TD_{50}. Here, again, presumably the Commonwealth Serum strain of mouse used by these investigators was more sensitive than the CF#1 strain with respect to central nervous system depressant activity. The dose required to cause neurological deficit (7.3 mg/kg po) increased the brain concentration of norepinephrine significantly (from the control value of 0.42 to 0.58 μg/gm) 30 minutes after oral administration of diazepam. Dopamine (DA), 5-hydroxytryptamine (5-HT) and 5-hydroxyindoleacetic acid (5-HIAA) levels were not affected significantly. Another low TD_{50} value was reported by Gluckman (1971), although he did not state the strain and sex of mice employed.

15. Acute Toxicity

Values shown in Table V are LD_{50} values representing CF#1 albino mice (Randall *et al.*, 1970) and female albino Manor Farms mice (Robichaud *et al.*, 1970). It is clear from these large values that diazepam has extremely low acute oral toxicity in the mouse. Corresponding therapeutic indices (LD_{50}/ED_{50}) for the various tests, accordingly, are highly favorable.

C. OXAZEPAM

1. Maximal Electroshock Seizures

The effective dose shown in Table V is an ED_{50} (28 mg/kg) in CF#1 mice. This value is somewhat higher than that shown for diazepam. As one of the metabolites of diazepam (Marcucci *et al.*, 1968), oxazepam possesses strong anticonvulsant activity in mice. One would predict that oxazepam would have therapeutic potential in grand mal (Woodbury, 1972). The marked difference in size of the ED_{50} reported by Gluckman (1971) presumably reflects strain differences.

2. Metrazole Seizure Threshold (sc Met) Test

The value reported by Randall *et al.* (1970) shown in Table V is an ED_{50} determined by antagonism of a large dose of pentylenetetrazole (125 mg/kg sc) in CF#1 mice. The effective dose shown for Marcucci *et al.* (1971) is expressed as a range. These investigators found that the ED_{50} for oxazepam, as was also the case for diazepam, increased with time following intravenous injection of either drug. Peak time for oxazepam under these experimental conditions appears to be 5 minutes, at which time the ED_{50} was 0.342 (0.263–0.445) mg/kg. Tested after 180 minutes, the value had jumped to 4.85 mg/kg. When the ED_{50} corresponding to each of the three time intervals was given intravenously, and brain levels of the drug were determined at the same intervals thereafter, the levels of oxazepam remained unchanged (0.094–0.96 μg/gm). All values are for male albino Swiss mice, and pentylenetetrazole dosage was 120 mg/kg ip.

3. Minimal Electroshock Seizure Threshold (60 Hz EST)

The dose required to elevate seizure threshold was nearly three times that required for diazepam, as shown in Table V. The value recorded for Randall *et al.* (1970) was determined in CF#1 male albino mice.

4. Strychnine Seizures

As shown in Table V, more than five times as much oxazepam as diazepam was required to antagonize strychnine seizures in CF#1 mice. This would appear to indicate that oxazepam has definite, but weak, cord-depressant activity in the mouse.

5. Neurological Deficit

The effective dose (1 mg/kg po) of oxazepam for the cat (Table V) is shown to be five times the dose required to cause neurological deficit following diazepam administration. In each instance the dose shown was the smallest dose required to induce skeletal muscle relaxation, as identified by limpness of the legs when the cat was suspended by the scruff of the neck. Gluckman (1971) reported a TD_{50} of 4.9 mg/kg po for the mouse, but did not specify the strain or sex of the animals.

6. Acute Toxicity

Oxazepam is shown to have extremely low acute toxicity following both oral and intraperitoneal administration to mice. Variations in the actual ED_{50} values reported by Randall *et al.* (1970) and Marcucci *et al.* (1968, 1971) presumably reflect differences in the strains of mice employed.

D. MEDAZEPAM

1. Maximal Electroshock Seizures

The ED_{50} recorded in Table V (36 mg/kg po) was determined in CF#1 male mice using a current strength of 30 mA. Medazepam is therefore in the potency range of oxazepam and chlordiazepoxide but is distinctly less potent than diazepam. One would predict from these findings that medazepam would have potential for the management of grand mal in man.

2. Metrazole Seizure Threshold (sc Met) Test

The value shown in Table V (7 mg/kg po) was determined in CF#1 male mice. Medazepam is thus in the potency range of chlordiazepoxide and is clearly less potent than either oxazepam or diazepam. From these findings one would predict that medazepam might have therapeutic potential in petit mal.

3. Minimal Electroshock Seizure Threshold
   (60 Hz EST)

The ED_{50} shown in Table V (238 mg/kg po), determined in CF#1 male mice, is virtually identical to the value found by the same investigators (Randall *et al.*, 1970) for oxazepam, diazepam, or chlordiazepoxide (Banziger, 1965).

4. Strychnine Seizures

The effective dose recorded in Table V (20 mg/kg po) is in the range of the values for diazepam (16 mg/kg po, Randall *et al.*, 1970; 13.0 mg/kg, Robichaud *et al.*, 1970). Oxazepam and chlordiazepoxide appear to be vastly different since roughly five times as much of these drugs is required to overcome strychnine seizures, as shown in Table V. Medazepam is thus shown to have potent cord-depressant activity, and one would predict that it, like diazepam, would have potential as a centrally acting muscle relaxant, and that oxazepam and chlordiazepoxide, however, would have less therapeutic potential in this area.

5. Neurological Deficit

The dose shown in Table V (15.4 mg/kg) represents a TD_{50} for the mouse which, in this instance, is the amount of drug required to produce motor incoordination as shown by inability to negotiate a rotarod (Dunham and Miya, 1957) 30 minutes following oral administration of the drug. Neurological deficit is associated with a significant increase in the DA concentration in the brain, from 1.27 ± 0.04 to 2.0 ± 0.26 μg/gm wet brain tissue.

This large increase in DA suggests that medazepam may have therapeutic potential in Parkinsonism. It may be noted, however, that chlorpromazine and haloperidol, both of which exacerbate the idiopathic disease and produce Parkinsonian symptoms in others, are capable of increasing brain DA levels, presumably as a compensatory response following postsynaptic receptor blockade. It would be of interest, therefore, to consider the possibility that medazepam may be acting to block dopaminergic receptor sites and that the drug may have utility in the management of schizophrenia. The small changes in the levels of 5-HT and 5-HIAA suggest that an adrenergic rather than a tryptaminergic mechanism may be responsible for the central effects exhibited by medazepam. Other brain amines (norepinephrine, 5-HT, and 5-HIAA) were not altered significantly (Fennessy and Lee, 1972). The latter investigators employed Commonwealth Serum Laboratories strain of mouse, which yielded much lower TD_{50} values than for the more commonly used strains. One hesitates, therefore, to use their figure (15.4 mg/kg po) as the basis for computing protective indices for the tests reported above since different strains of mice were used. One wonders also whether alterations in brain amines shown in the Commonwealth Serum Laboratories strain of mice are necessarily representative of mice as a species.

6. Acute Toxicity

The values shown in Table V are for CF#1 mice, and the LD_{50} values are sufficiently high (1070 mg/kg po and 360 mg/kg ip) (Randall *et al.*, 1970) to guarantee favorable therapeutic indices (LD_{50}/ED_{50}) for each of the tests. It may be concluded that medazepam has low acute oral toxicity for CF#1 mice. It would be of interest to know whether the LD_{50} would be significantly different in the Commonwelath Serum Laboratories strain.

E. PRAZEPAM

1. Maximal Electroshock Seizures

The value shown in Table V is an ED_{50} (24.6 mg/kg po) determined in Manor Farms adult (20–25 gm) female mice (Robichaud *et al.*, 1970). Potency, therefore, is in the range shown by medazepam, oxazepam, and chlordiazepoxide. Prazepam should have the same potential as these drugs for management of grand mal seizures.

2. Metrazole Seizure Threshold (sc Met) Test

The value shown in Table V (3.2 mg/kg po) is low, in the potency range of medazepam and chlordiazepoxide. One would predict, therefore, that prazepam would have therapeutic potential in petit mal.

3. Audiogenic Seizures

The value shown in Table V (1.7 mg/kg po) is an ED_{50} determined in young (12–18 gm) O'Grady strain mice. Potency is clearly in the range of chlordiazepoxide and diazepam. It could be predicted from this test, as well as from the MES test, that prazepam would have therapeutic potential in grand mal (Woodbury, 1972).

4. Strychnine Seizures

The value listed in Table V (36 mg/kg po) is an ED_{50} determined by Robichaud *et al.* (1970) in adult female Manor Farms mice. Here, again, prazepam shows potency in the range of medazepam and far greater than that of chlordiazepoxide, diazepam, and oxazepam. To the extent that the test is a measure of cord-depressant activity, one would predict additional therapeutic potential for prazepam as a centrally acting cord depressant.

5. Acute Toxicity

The value shown in Table V is an LD_{50}. This high value (2000 mg/kg po) may be accepted as representing bona fide acute oral toxicity in the mouse (female, Manor Farms), since significant interference with absorption from the gastrointestinal tract, or enzymatic destruction at this site, would appear to be unlikely in view of the low oral ED_{50} values recorded for anticonvulsant activity. Although the pattern of toxicity is not described, it seems that prazepam differs from the other benzodiazepines in two respects: It does not cause loss of the righting reflex, and it produces convulsions following intravenous injection but not by any other route of administration.

F. LORAZEPAM

1. Maximal Electroshock Seizures

The effective dose (2.0 mg/kg po) shown in Table V represents an ED_{50} in mice of unspecified strain and sex. This low value indicates a high level of potency of lorazepam, in the range of oxazepam, as reported by the same investigator (Gluckman, 1971) but not by Randall *et al.* (1970), who reported an ED_{50} of 0.7 mg/kg for oxazepam. The large discrepancy in ED_{50} values is probably attributable to species differences. In all events, one would predict therapeutic potential in grand mal (Woodbury, 1972).

2. Metrazole Seizure Threshold (sc Met) Test

The extremely low ED_{50} shown in Table V (0.07 mg/kg po) suggests that lorazepam may be the most potent of the benzodiazepines as an antagonist of pentylenetetrazole-induced clonic seizures. This is indeed the case for the series investigated by Gluckman (1971) which included oxazepam (0.6 gm/kg po), chlordiazepoxide (3.7 mg/kg po), and diazepam (0.4 mg/kg po). Since the strain and sex of mice are not specified, it would perhaps be wise to reserve judgment on the potency of lorazepam pending confirmatory studies in other species and strains of experimental animals.

3. Neurological Deficit

The effective dose shown in Table V for the mouse (0.9 mg/kg po) is the TD_{50} based on inability to negotiate a rotating rod (Gluckman, 1971). Lorazepam thus appears to produce neurological deficit at a dosage far below that of any benzodiazepine in his series which includes oxazepam (4.9 mg/kg po), diazepam (1.9 mg/kg po), and chlordiazepoxide (9.3 mg/kg po). Here, again, one would hope to see TD_{50} values in other strains of mice. The value reported for the monkey (5 mg/kg iv) is a dose that produced ataxia for a period of 60 minutes.

4. Acute Toxicity

All of the values shown in Table V (Owen *et al.*, 1971) were determined in species and strains as follows: mice (neonatal and adult, Charles River CD strain); rats (neonatal and adult, male and female Charles River strain) and both male and female dogs. Results indicate an extraordinary sensitivity of the neonatal mouse as compared to the neonatal rat. This difference would appear to reflect differences in the development of the blood–brain barrier in neonates of the two species. Oral LD_{50} values for mice, rats, and dogs are extraordinarily high, as are intraperitoneal doses for the mouse and rat. The findings for the dog are surprising in that the oral lethal dose is at least 80 times the amount required following intramuscular injection. In all events, lorazepam rates as a benzodiazepine of extremely low acute oral toxicity, at least in the adult mouse, rat, and dog.

G. NITRAZEPAM

1. Maximal Electroshock Seizures

The value shown in Table V for the rat (35 mg/kg po) was determined in Sprague-Dawley male albino rats (150–200 gm). Nitrazepam is thus in the potency range of diazepam and oxazepam but is much less potent than chlordiazepoxide. One would predict activity against grand mal seizures (Woodbury, 1972).

2. Metrazole Seizure Threshold (im and iv Met) Test

The value shown in Table V for the monkey (rhesus) was determined in animals made chronically epileptic by the application of alumina cream to the motor cortex. The convulsive threshold for each animal was established by injecting a dose of 25 mg/kg pentylenetetrazole intramuscularly at 15-minute intervals until generalized seizures occurred. Nitrazepam was administered at three dosage levels: 0.77, 1.55, and 2.30 mg/kg. The dose shown in Table V (0.77 mg/kg) was sufficient to raise the threshold for generalized seizures six- to ten-fold (Berman *et al.*, 1968). Somnolence did not occur following any of the above doses of nitrazepam.

The value shown in Table V for the cat (Straw, 1968) (0.125 mg/kg) was determined in adult cats of both sexes that were immobilized with deca-methonium bromide and supplied with respiration by means of a Harvard pump. The threshold for pentylenetetrazole seizures was determined by injecting 5 mg/kg of pentylenetetrazole intravenously every 30 seconds until a sustained seizure pattern appeared in the electrocorticogram. In non-pretreated (control) animals, seizure threshold was recorded as six injections, and seizure duration was 53 ± 7.2 seconds. After injection of 0.125 mg/kg nitrazepam, nearly twice as many injections (11 ± 1.6) were required to evoke a seizure, lasting 44 ± 7.6 seconds. In the acutely paralyzed cat, therefore, a dose of 0.125 mg/kg of nitrazepam significantly raised the threshold for pentylenetetrazole-induced seizures but had no significant effect on seizure duration. The values reported by Christmas and Maxwell (1970) were determined in Charles River S51 male mice and Sprague-Dawley young adult (150–200 gm) male rats. The results show that nitrazepam had more than ten times the potency in the rat than in the mouse against sub-cutaneously administered pentylenetetrazole.

3. Audiogenic Seizures

The value shown in Table V was determined by Collins and Horlington (1969) in the F_1 generation of mice obtained by crossing DBA/1 males with SNR albino female mice. The dose (0.14 mg/kg ip) is the ED_{50} required to prevent the running component of the audiogenic seizure pattern. To the ex-tent that such activity has predictive value for grand mal seizures, one would expect nitrazepam to be among the most potent of the benzodiazepines.

4. Picrotoxin Seizures

The value shown in Table V (0.33 mg/kg iv) was determined by Barrada and Oftedal (1970) in rabbits of unspecified strain and sex. Bilateral electro-corticograms were recorded through a cranial flap made under light urethane anesthesia. A dose of 2.5 mg/kg of picrotoxin was injected intravenously, producing typical spike-and-wave formations occurring after 14–19 minutes. Nitrazepam and diazepam (0.33 mg/kg iv) returned the ECoG pattern to normal within 4–5 minutes. The investigators concluded that nitrazepam was superior to diazepam in that it returned the ECoG and respiratory changes to normal earlier and more completely. One would predict therapeutic potential for petit mal seizures.

5. Neurological Deficit

The value recorded in Table V (23.5 mg/kg po) was determined by Fen-nessy and Lee (1972) in Commonwealth Serum Laboratories strain of mice. Here, again, it would be unwise to assign protective indices to the various tests since different strains of mice were used. It is of interest that the TD_{50} value shown in the table was accompanied by a significant increase in the brain dopamine level, from a control concentration of 1.27 ± 0.04 to 1.42 $\mu g/gm$ wet brain tissue, and an increase in 5-HIAA from a control level of 0.41 ± 0.01 to 0.51 ± 0.05 $\mu g/gm$ wet brain tissue. It should be noted that, although nitrazepam is widely used as a hypnotic agent, motor incoordina-tion and hypnosis appear to be unrelated.

6. Acute Toxicity

The value shown in Table V (275 mg/kg) represents an LD_{50} determined by Collins and Horlington (1969) in a strain of mice bred for audiogenic sensitivity and conceivably may not be representative of the species. It is clear that nitrazepam is a compound of low acute toxicity in this species.

H. CLONAZEPAM

1. Bemegride Seizures

The effective dose shown in Table V, reported by Van Duijn (1973), was determined in the alert cat as follows. Clonazepam was injected subcutaneously at a dose of 0.2 mg/kg. Four minutes later, bemegride was injected intravenously, and the time required for the appearance of tonic seizures was recorded. This time was compared to control time established 2 days earlier with drug. In this instance, 105 ± 18 seconds was the control time, and 653 ± 86 seconds was the threshold time after clonazepam administration, a sixfold increase. The 4-minute pretreatment time selected is not necessarily the peak time, but it was clearly adequate, based on the marked increase in threshold. Since bemegride is thought to act on the same area of the brain (cortex) as does pentylenetetrazole (Hahn, 1960), one would predict that clonazepam would have therapeutic potential in petit mal.

2. Cobalt Seizures

As part of the investigative series reported in the previous section, Van Duijn (1973) included an investigation of the ability of clonazepam to overcome the focal seizure pattern that follows application of 50 mg of cobalt metal powder to the left anterior suprasylvian gyrus of the cat. Clonazepam was injected subcutaneously at a dose of 0.2 mg/kg 2 days following the operative procedure. Forty-five minutes later the ECoG was recorded for 30 minutes and periods containing spikes were counted. Significant reduction in spikes was taken as a measure of anticonvulsant activity. In this instance the mean number of spikes per 10 seconds was 4.5 ± 0.5 before clonazepam administration (control), and 2.4 ± 0.3 per 10 seconds after administration of 0.2 mg/kg of clonazepam. This may be considered additional evidence suggesting the therapeutic potential of clonazepam in petit mal.

3. Neurological Deficit

An oral dose of 2.5 mg/kg of clonazepam induced loss of motor coordination in 50% of mice after 30 minutes, as recorded in Table V. Associated with neurological deficit were significant increases in brain levels of norepinephrine, from 0.41 ± 0.02 to 0.56 ± 0.04; dopamine, from 1.27 ± 0.04 to 2.55 ± 0.19, and 5-hydroxytryptamine, from 0.83 ± 0.03 to 1.03 ± 0.05 μg/gm of wet brain tissue (Fennessy and Lee, 1972). The authors suggested that the large increase in dopamine brain level following clonazepam administration suggests that it may have potential in the management of Parkinsonism. The central behavioral effects may involve both adrenergic and tryptaminergic mechanisms.

If these aminergic changes occurred at the doses used to block seizures, we could make a better appraisal of the possible underlying monoaminergic mechanisms. As things stand, these changes may be secondary, reflecting merely toxic effects of the drug.

VIII. MISCELLANEOUS ANTICONVULSANTS

A. PHENACEMIDE

1. Maximal Electroshock Seizures

The figure reported by Goodman *et al.* (1953a) (108.6 mg/kg; Table VI) was determined in adult CF#1 albino mice of both sexes. For uniformity of reporting, we are expressing dosage in terms of milligrams per kilogram rather than as 0.61 mmol/kg as reported in their paper. Mouse values reported by Chen and Ensor (1950) and Swinyard *et al.* (1952) are not significantly different. The value shown for Everett and Richards (1952), however, is significantly greater, presumably attributable to strain difference. Values for the rat also differ by a wide margin, e.g., 20 mg/kg po (Chen and Ensor, 1950) and 200 mg/kg po (Everett and Richards, 1952). Smaller differences are recorded for the cat: 100–200 mg/kg (Chen and Ensor, 1950) and 400 mg/kg (Everett and Richards, 1952). In suppressing maximal electroshock seizures, one would predict that phenacemide would have therapeutic potential in grand mal. However, the order of potency is considerably lower than that of phenobarbital and DPH, the agents most commonly employed in the management of grand mal. The figures shown in Table VI emphasize that

TABLE VI MISCELLANEOUS ANTICONVULSANTS

Test	Species	Effective dose (mg/kg)	Route of adminis- tration	Reference
		Phenacemide		
MES	Mouse	108.6	po	Goodman *et al.* (1953a)
	Mouse	100	po	Swinyard *et al.* (1952)
	Mouse	150 ± 14	po	Chen and Ensor (1950)
	Mouse	400	po	Everett and Richards (1952)
	Rat	20 ± 1.7	po	Chen and Ensor (1950)
	Rat	200	po	Everett and Richards (1952)
	Cat	100–200	po	Chen and Ensor (1950)
	Cat	400	po	Everett and Richards (1952)

TABLE VI—*Continued*

Test	Species	Effective dose (mg/kg)	Route of adminis-tration	Reference
sc Met	Mouse	250–400	po	Chen and Ensor (1950)
	Mouse	400	po	Everett and Richards (1952)
	Mouse	125	po	Swinyard *et al.* (1952)
	Rat	200	po	Swinyard *et al.* (1952)
MMS	Mouse	58.7	po	Goodman *et al.* (1953a)
	Cat	400	po	Everett and Richards (1952)
MET (60 Hz EST)	Mouse	118	po	Swinyard *et al.* (1952)
	Rat	40	po	Swinyard *et al.* (1952)
HET	Mouse	140	po	Swinyard *et al.* (1952)
	Rat	230	po	Swinyard *et al.* (1952)
Strychnine seizures	Mouse	400	po	Everett and Richards (1952)
Picrotoxin seizures	Mouse	400	po	Everett and Richards (1952)
Intermittent photic stimulation	Rabbit	Inactive	ip	Barnes (1954)
Neurological deficit	Mouse	650	po	Swinyard *et al.* (1952)
	Rat	750	po	Swinyard *et al.* (1952)
Acute toxicity	Mouse	5000	po	Everett and Richards (1952)
	Rat	8000	po	Everett and Richards (1952)
	Cat	2000	po	Everett and Richards (1952)
	Dog	4000	po	Everett and Richards (1952)
		Sulthiame		
MES	Mouse	35	po	Wirth *et al.* (1961)
Strychnine seizures	Mouse	Inactive	po	Wirth *et al.* (1961)
Neurological deficit	Cat	50–100	po	Wirth *et al.* (1961)
	Dog	50–100	po	Wirth *et al.* (1961)
sc Met	Mouse	35	po	Wirth *et al.* (1961)
Acute toxicity	Mouse	> 5000	po	Wirth *et al.* (1961)
	Rat	> 5000	po	Wirth *et al.* (1961)
	Rabbit	> 1000	po	Wirth *et al.* (1961)

ED_{50} values can differ significantly, even by orders of magnitude within a species, depending on the strain of animal and the experimental procedure employed.

2. Metrazole Seizure Threshold (sc Met) Test

Similar but less marked variations occur in the effective doses required to suppress clonic seizures in response to pentylenetetrazole. Swinyard *et al.* (1952) reported a value of 125 mg/kg, determined at peak time in CF#1 mice. Chen and Ensor (1950) reported a much higher figure (250–400 mg/kg), which is close to the value shown for Everett and Richards (1952). Only a single value (200 mg/kg po) was reported for the rat (Swinyard *et al.*, 1952). On the basis of positive antagonism of pentylenetetrazole, one would predict that phenacemide would have therapeutic potential in petit mal. This, of course, has been established for both phenacemide and trimethadione. Since ED_{50} values are high for both drugs, it seems clear that potency, as represented by low ED_{50} values in the experimental animal, serves as a guide in screening drugs for petit mal. However, antagonism of pentylenetetrazole, and not dosage, should be the criterion for screening purposes. Trimethadione, one of the best drugs we have for the management of petit mal, might easily have been eliminated in a pharmacological screen because of its high ED_{50} in this test.

3. Maximal Metrazole Seizures

The values shown in Table VI illustrate how different species respond to a drug. Much larger doses are required to antagonize maximal seizures in the cat than in the mouse. In any case, phenacemide is shown to be effective, and the test provides additional evidence of its potential for suppressing grand mal seizures.

4. Minimal Electroshock Seizure Threshold and Hyponatremic Electroshock Seizure Threshold

The values reported by Swinyard *et al.* (1952) were determined in CF#1 adult male mice and Sprague-Dawley adult male rats. These investigators made a point that has become axiomatic over the years, namely, that mice and rats must have access to food and water, except during the actual experiment. In support of this claim, Swinyard *et al.* (1952) cited a study by Davenport and Davenport (1948), who found that starvation reduces the threshold for MET and, incidentally, prolongs the extensor component of the maximal seizure pattern. The ED_{50} values show that much more phenacemide was required to elevate minimal seizure threshold in the mouse than in the rat (118 and 40 mg/kg, respectively). The reverse appears to be the case in animals rendered hyponatremic (HET). The ED_{50} values determined 2 hours after glucose administration in the mouse and 4 hours in rats were 140 and 230 mg/kg, respectively.

5. Strychnine and Picrotoxin Seizures

As shown in Table VI the same dose of phenacemide was required to antagonize both strychnine and picrotoxin. One would predict, therefore, that the drug might have potential as a centrally acting muscle relaxant, as well as for the management of petit mal.

6. Intermittent Photic Stimulation

Barnes (1954) reported (Table VI) an experiment in which electroencephalographic recordings were made of a seizure in response to a flickering light in the curarized rabbit. Phenacemide was injected at a dose of 150 mg/kg ip daily for 5 days, and flicker was tested 12–14 hours following each injection. Phenacemide failed to abolish the flicker effect.

7. Neurological Deficit

The figures shown in Table VI (Swinyard *et al.*, 1952) represent TD_{50} values determined in CF#1 male mice and Sprague-Dawley male rats. These values are high, indicating that protective indices would generally be favorable. It may be mentioned as a caution that, for protective indices to be meaningful, TD_{50} and ED_{50} values must be determined in animals of the same strain and under the same experimental conditions.

8. Acute Toxicity

Values shown in Table VI (Everett and Richards, 1952) show clearly that the acute oral toxicity of phenacemide is extremely low in the mouse, rat, cat, and dog. A serious limitation to the value of the LD_{50} for predicting toxicity for man is illustrated in the present case, in which toxicity is based on a single administration of phenacemide to the experimental animal. The high LD_{50} values shown have little meaning in view of the toxicity encountered following chronic administration of this drug to man.

B. SULTHIAME

The values shown in Table VI (Wirth *et al.*, 1961) were determined in mice, rats, and rabbits of unspecified strain.

1. Maximal Electroshock Seizures

The value reported (35 mg/kg) is an ED_{50}; a higher dose (50 mg/kg) protected 65% of the animals. Peak time is stated to be 3 hours. A dose of 50 mg/kg po administered daily for 11 consecutive days did not result in any change in the level of protection; i.e., there were no signs of either cumulative activity or tachyphylaxis.

2. Metrazole Seizure Threshold (sc Met) Test

The dose shown in Table VI (35 mg/kg) is an ED_{50} and shows that sulthiame antagonized pentylenetetrazole at the same dose as that required to protect against electroshock. It would appear, therefore, that the drug would have therapeutic potential in both grand mal and petit mal. In addition, the authors (Wirth *et al.*, 1961) claimed clinical effectiveness of sulthiame in psychomotor epilepsy.

3. Strychnine Seizures

Failure of sulthiame to antagonize strychnine seizures suggest that it does not act on the afferent portion of the spinal reflex arc, and hence would not be expected to have potential as a centrally acting cord depressant.

4. Neurological Deficit

Doses of 50–100 mg/kg caused vomiting in both cats and dogs, the former being the more sensitive. Wirth *et al.* (1961) also reported that the drug has mild tranquilizing activity following an oral dose of 80 mg/kg to the golden hamster, but doses as high as 3000 mg/kg were not hypnotic.

5. Acute Toxicity

As shown in Table VI, the LD_{50} exceeds 5000 mg/kg in both mice and rats and 1000 mg/kg in the rabbit. The pattern of toxicity was not disclosed. It is evident that sulthiame has extremely low acute toxicity, at least in the mouse, rat, and rabbit.

REFERENCES

Alexander, G. J., Kopeloff, L. M., and Taylor, R. M. (1969). *Proc. Soc. Exp. Biol. Med.* **130**, 19–23.
Banziger, R. F. (1965). *Arch. Int. Pharmacodyn. Ther.* **154**, 131–136.
Banziger, R. F., and Hane, D. (1967). *Arch. Int. Pharmacodyn. Ther.* **167**, 245–249.
Barnes, C. D., and Eltherington, L. G. (1966). "Drug Dosage in Laboratory Animals— A Handbook." Univ. of California Press, Berkeley.
Barnes, T. C. (1954). *Fed. Proc., Fed. Am. Soc. Exp. Biol.* **26**, 333–334.
Barrada, O., and Oftedal, S. I. (1970). *Electroencephalogr. Clin. Neurophysiol.* **29**, 220–221.
Baumel, I. P., Gallagher, B. B., DiMicco, J., and Goico, H. (1973). *J. Pharmacol. Exp. Ther.* **186**, 305–314.
Berman, A. J., Pomina, A. C., and Nepomuceno, N. R. (1968). *Electroencephalogr. Clin. Neurophysiol.* **24**, 187.
Boissier, J. R., Simon, A., Villeneuve, A., and Larousse, C. (1968). *Can. J. Physiol. Pharmacol.* **46**, 93–100.
Brown, W. C., Schiffman, D. O., Swinyard, E. A., and Goodman, L. S. (1953). *J. Pharmacol. Exp. Ther.* **107**, 273–283.

Chen, G., and Ensor, C. R. (1950). *Arch. Neurol. Psychiatry* **63**, 55–60.

Chen, G., Weston, J. K., and Bratton, A. C. (1963). *Epilepsia* **4**, 66–76.

Christmas, A. J., and Maxwell, D. R. (1970). *Neuropharmacology* **9**, 17–29.

Chusid, J. G., and Kopeloff, L. M. (1961). *Electroencephalogr. Clin. Neurophysiol.* **13**, 825–826.

Collins, A. J., and Horlington, M. (1969). *Br. J. Pharmacol. Chemother.* **37**, 140–150.

Conney, A. H., Davison, C., Gastel, R., and Burns, J. J. (1960). *J. Pharmacol. Exp. Ther.* **130**, 1–8.

Costa, E., Guidotti, A., Mao, C. C., and Suria, A. (1975). *Life Sci.* **17**, 167–186.

Craig, C. R., and Shideman, F. E. (1971). *J. Pharmacol. Exp. Ther.* **176**, 35–41.

Dashputra, P. G., and Kharpe, M. D. (1970). *Indian J. Med. Res.* **58**, 1459–1466.

Davenport, V. D., and Davenport, H. W. (1948). *J. Nutr.* **36**, 139–151.

Davis, W. M., and Webb, O. L. (1963). *Med Exp.* **9**, 263–267.

Dunham, A. W., and Miya, T. S. (1957). *J. Am. Pharm. Assoc.* **46**, 208–209.

Everett, G. M., and Richards, R. K. (1944). *J. Pharmacol. Exp. Ther.* **81**, 402–407.

Everett, G. M., and Richards, R. K. (1952). *J. Pharmacol. Exp. Ther.* **106**, 303–313.

Faeth, W. H., Walker, A. E., Kaplan, A. D., and Warner, W. A. (1955). *Proc. Soc. Exp. Biol. Med.* **88**, 329–331.

Fennessy, M. R., and Lee, J. R. (1972). *Arch. Int. Pharmacodyn. Ther.* **197**, 37–44.

Ferngren, H. (1965). *Acta Pharmacol. Toxicol.* **23**, 27–35.

Ferngren, H. (1968). *Acta Pharmacol. Toxicol.* **26**, 177–188.

Fink, G. B., and Swinyard, E. A. (1959). *J. Pharmacol. Exp. Ther.* **127**, 318–324.

Frey, H. H. (1969). *Acta Pharmacol. Toxicol.* **27**, 295–300.

Frey, H. H., and Hahn, I. (1960). *Arch. Int. Pharmacodyn. Ther.* **128**, 281–289.

Frey, H. H., and Kretschmer, B. H. (1971). *Arch. Int. Pharmacodyn. Ther.* **193**, 181–190.

Gallagher, B. B., Smith, D. B., and Mattson, R. H. (1970). *Epilepsia* **11**, 181–190.

Gellhorn, E., and Ballin, H. M. (1948). *Proc. Soc. Exp. Biol. Med.* **68**, 540–543.

Glazko, A. J., and Dill, W. A. (1972). *In* "Antiepileptic Drugs" (D. M. Woodbury, J. K. Penry, and R. P. Schmidt, eds.), pp. 455–464. Raven, New York.

Gluckman, M. I. (1971). *Arzneim.-Forsch.* **21**, 1049–1055.

Goodman, L. S., and Lih, B. (1941). *J. Pharmacol. Exp. Ther.* **72**, 18.

Goodman, L. S., Toman, J. E. P., and Swinyard, E. A. (1948). *Proc. Soc. Exp. Biol. Med.* **68**, 584–587.

Goodman, L. S., Toman, J. E. P., and Swinyard, E. A. (1949). *Arch. Int. Pharmacodyn. Ther.* **78**, 144–162.

Goodman, L. S., Grewal, M. S., Brown, W. C., and Swinyard, E. A. (1953a). *J. Pharmacol. Exp. Ther.* **108**, 168–176.

Goodman, L. S., Swinyard, E. A., Brown, W. C., Schiffman, D. O., Grewal, M. S., and Bliss, E. L. (1953b). *J. Pharmacol. Exp. Ther.* **108**, 428–436.

Hahn, F. (1960). *Pharmacol. Rev.* **12**, 447–530.

Halberg, F., and Jacobsen, E. (1958). *Science* **128**, 657–658.

Hansen, J. M., Kristensen, M., and Skovsted, L. (1968). *Epilepsia* **9**, 17–22.

Jailer, J. W. (1951). *Endocrinology* **49**, 826–827.

Killam, K. F., Jr. (1969). *Epilepsia* **10**, 229–238.

Killam, K. F., Jr., Killam, E. K., and Naquet, R. (1967). *Electroencephalogr. Clin. Neurophysiol.* **22**, 497–513.

Kopeloff, L. M., and Chusid, J. (1967). *Int. J. Neuropsychiatry* **3**, 469–471.

Kopeloff, L. M., Chusid, J. G., and Kopeloff, N. (1954). *Neurology* **4**, 218–227.

Litchfield, J. T., Jr., and Wilcoxon, F. (1949). *J. Pharmacol. Exp. Ther.* **96**, 99–113.

Mancia, M., and Lucioni, R. (1966). *Epilepsia* **7**, 308–317.

Marcucci, F., Guaitani, A., and Kventina, J. (1968). *Eur. J. Pharmacol.* **4**, 467–470.
Marcucci, F., Fanelli, R., Mussini, E., and Garattini, S. (1970). *Eur. J. Pharmacol.* **11**, 115–116.
Marcucci, F., Mussini, E., Guaitani, A., Fanelli, R., and Garattini, S. (1971). *Eur. J. Pharmacol.* **16**, 311–314.
Marshall, P. G., and Vallance, D. K. (1954). *J. Pharm. Pharmacol.* **6**, 740–746.
McQuarrie, D. G., and Fingl, E. (1958). *J. Pharmacol. Exp. Ther.* **124**, 264–271.
Meyer, H., and Frey, H. H. (1973). *Neuropharmacology* **12**, 939–947.
Millichap, J. G. (1969). *Epilepsia* **10**, 315–328.
Millichap, J. G. (1972). *In* "Antiepileptic Drugs" (D. M. Woodbury, J. K. Penry, and R. P. Schmidt, eds.), pp. 275–281. Raven, New York.
Mitchell, C. L., and Keasling, H. H. (1960). *J. Pharmacol. Exp. Ther.* **128**, 79–84.
Naquet, R., Meldrum, B. S., Balzano, E., and Charrier, J. P. (1970). *Brain Res.* **18**, 503–512.
Nellhaus, G. (1958). *Am. J. Physiol.* **193**, 567–572.
Owen, G., Hatfield, G. K., Pollock, J. J., Steinberg, A. J., Tucker, W. E., and Agersborg, H. P. K., Jr. (1971). *Arzneim.-Forsch.* **21**, 1065–1073.
Petty, W. C., and Karler, R. (1965). *J. Pharmacol. Exp. Ther.* **150**, 443–448.
Plotnikoff, N. P., and Green, D. M. (1957). *J. Pharmacol. Exp. Ther.* **119**, 294–298.
Purpura, D. P., Penry, J. K., Tower, D., Woodbury, D. M., and Walter R., eds. (1972). "Experimental Models of Epilepsy." Raven, New York.
Raines, A., Niner, J. M., and Pace, D. G. (1973). *J. Pharmacol. Exp. Ther.* **186**, 315–322.
Randall, L. O. (1961). *Dis. Nerv. Syst.* **22**, 7–15.
Randall, L. O., Scheckel, C. L., and Pool, W. (1970). *Arch. Int. Pharmacodyn. Ther.* **185**, 135–148.
Rauth, C. E., and Gray, W. D. (1968). *J. Pharmacol. Exp. Ther.* **161**, 329–334.
Reinhard, J. F., and Spector, E. (1970). *Toxicol. Appl. Pharmacol.* **17**, 12–22.
Richards, R. K., and Everett, G. M. (1946). *J. Lab. Clin. Med.* **31**, 1330–1336.
Robichaud, R. C., Gylys, J. A., Sledge, K. L., and Hillyard, I. W. (1970). *Arch. Int. Pharmacodyn. Ther.* **185**, 213–227.
Rümke, C. L. (1967). *Eur. J. Pharmacol.* **1**, 369–377.
Schreiber, R. A., and Schlesinger, K. (1971). *Physiol. Behav.* **6**, 635–640.
Spehlmann, R., and Colley, B. (1968). *Neurology* **18**, 52–59.
Stark, L. G., Killman, K. F., and Killman, E. K. (1970). *J. Pharmacol. Exp. Ther.* **173**, 125–132.
Steinmann, H. W. (1967). *Dtsch. Z. Nervenheilkd.* **192**, 226–229.
Straw, R. (1968). *Arch. Int. Pharmacodyn. Ther.* **175**, 464–469.
Swinyard, E. A. (1949). *J. Am. Pharm. Assoc.* **38**, 201–204.
Swinyard, E. A. (1972). *In* "Experimental Models of Epilepsy" (D. P. Purpura *et al.*, eds.), pp. 433–458. Raven, New York.
Swinyard, E. A., and Castellion, A. W. (1966). *J. Pharmacol. Exp. Ther.* **151**, 369–375.
Swinyard, E. A., and Toman, J. E. P. (1950). *J. Pharmacol. Exp. Ther.* **100**, 151–157.
Swinyard, E. A., Brown, W. C., and Goodman, L. S. (1952). *J. Pharmacol. Exp. Ther.* **106**, 319–330.
Toman, J. E. P., Swinyard, E. A., and Goodman, L. S. (1946). *J. Neurophysiol.* **9**, 231–240.
Torchina, M. L., and Stone, C. A. (1959). *Proc. Soc. Exp. Biol. Med.* **100**, 290–293.
Van Duijn, H. (1973). *Epilepsia* **14**, 195–202.
Van Duijn, H., and Visser, S. L. (1972). *Epilepsia* **13**, 409–420.
Vernadakis, A., and Woodbury, D. M. (1965). *J. Pharmacol. Exp. Ther.* **148**, 144–150.
Vernadakis, A., and Woodbury, D. M. (1969). *Epilepsia* **10**, 163–178.

Vida, J. A., Hooker, M. L., Samour, C. M., and Reinhard, J. F. (1973). *J. Med. Chem.* **16**, 1378–1381.

Vida, J. A., O'Dea, M. H., Samour, C. M., and Reinhard, J. F. (1975). *J. Med. Chem.* **18**, 383–385.

Ward, A. A., Jr. (1972). *In* "Experimental Models of Epilepsy" (D. P. Purpura *et al.*, eds.), pp. 13–35. Raven, New York.

Werner, H. W., and Tatum, A. L. (1939). *J. Pharmacol. Exp. Ther.* **66**, 260–278.

Wirth, W., Hoffmeister, F., Friebel, H., and Sommer, S. (1961). *Ger. Med.* **6**, 309–312.

Withrow, C. D., Stout, R. J., Barton, L. J., Beacham, W. S., and Woodbury, D. M. (1968). *J. Pharmacol. Exp. Ther.* **161**, 335–341.

Woodbury, D. A. (1972). *In* "Experimental Models of Epilepsy" (D. P. Purpura *et al.*, eds.) pp. 557–583. Raven, New York.

Woodbury, D. M., Penry, J. K., and Schmidt, R. P., eds. (1972). "Antiepileptic Drugs." Raven, New York.

Wooley, D. E., Timiras, P. S., Rosenzweig, M. R., Krech, D., and Bennett, E. L. (1961). *Nature (London)* **190**, 515–516.

Worum, I., and Porszasz, J. (1968). *Acta Physiol. Acad. Sci. Hung.* **33**, 383–393.

4

PHYSIOLOGICAL DISPOSITION OF ANTICONVULSANTS

John D. Alvin and Milton T. Bush

I. INTRODUCTION

The physiological disposition of a drug—that is, how a drug is handled by the body: how it is absorbed into the blood stream, how it disperses in body tissues, how it is metabolized and excreted—is one of the principal determinants of the intensity and duration of action. Equally important is the fact that variations in these processes, either natural or pathological, can be directly responsible for anomalous therapeutic results. For instance, very rapid metabolism to an inactive compound can preclude the accumulation of a drug in the target organ and result in the lack of a response. On the other hand, inefficient renal excretion or very slow metabolism can cause an agent

113

to persist unexpectedly in the body and, if therapy is long-term, to accumulate to toxic levels. These possibilities have long been recognized, but in practice, disposition has been considered to be more characteristic of the drug than the patient. It was tacitly assumed that, while certain physiological processes may vary from patient to patient, the multiplicity of events that mediate drug disposition tends to moderate the practical importance of any one process. As a result, drug therapy has been largely empirical. In recent years, however, it has become increasingly apparent that this assumption is not valid: Phenotypic variations in the rates of certain enzymatic conversions have been demonstrated (Kutt, 1971; Evans, 1969) and correlated with anomalous therapeutic responses and potentially dangerous toxic effects. The metabolic formation of chemically reactive metabolites has been implicated in hypersensitivity (Erlanger, 1973), tissue necrosis (Gillette *et al.*, 1974) and carcinogenesis (Miller, 1970) in sensitive subjects. The formation of metabolically and pharmacologically active metabolites has been shown to complicate drug therapy by conventional tactics. Moreover, in certain disease states, gross distortion of the disposition profile can be expected.

The appreciation of the importance of these events in drug response has resulted in attempts to place therapy on a more logical basis—one that reflects the concept that there is a quantitative relationship between the drug concentration at the receptor site and the intensity of pharmacological activity. In recent years, significant advances in this regard have been achieved by designing the administration regimen according to pharmacokinetic parameters that account for the various facets of drug disposition. The approach has generally enhanced the therapeutic effect, greatly reduced the incidence of adverse reactions, and eliminated the use of certain drugs in susceptible individuals. The benefits obtained with the cardiac glycosides and certain anticonvulsants have been the most notable examples (Jelliffe *et al.*, 1972; Ogilvie and Ruedy, 1972; Sherwin *et al.*, 1973). The pharmacokinetic parameters so employed are mathematical descriptions of the drug disposition processes: half-life in blood, renal clearance, hepatic (metabolic) clearance, and volume of distribution. These values reflect the way in which individual patients handle a dose of the drug and, as such, can be used to design or adjust the dosage regimen to achieve effective yet nontoxic blood concentrations. Such advances in therapeutic status have been achieved only after careful quantitative studies of the hepatic, distributive, and renal processes of the drug's disposition. Once these processes are understood, the pharmacokinetic constants are readily determined from the plasma concentrations or, in some cases, from urine levels. The successful application of these principles to therapy with a few important agents has broadened the basis of rational drug therapy to include the tactic of managing drug concentrations in the blood. Many observers feel that this trend will result in the use of fewer but better understood drugs that can be closely controlled for effective blood levels and monitored for patient compliance. Even in an empirical sense, such a status for drug therapy has been a perpetual goal of the allied drug sciences.

The chemicals administered therapeutically to control epilepsy are dispersed in body fluids and tissues according to their physical interactions with aqueous electrolyte solutions, macromolecules, lipoidal membranes, and formed elements of the cell. For the most part, these are rapidly reversible interactions, involving intermolecular forces that leave the drug molecule intact. Embedded in the endoplasmic reticulum membrane of hepatocyte cells, however, are nonspecific enzyme complexes that mediate covalent changes in a wide variety of chemical types (substrates). The products (metabolites) are generally more polar than the substrate and thus have a greater affinity for body fluids than for the lipoidal structures of cells. This conversion not only reduces their ability to interact with the cellular components that mediate pharmacological and toxicological effects but also promotes their excretion in urine. Although the immediate consequence of metabolism is not always inactivation, these enzymes are one of the body's major lines of defense against exogenous substances and, as such, are principal determinants of the inactivation profile of anticonvulsants.

For the commonly used anticonvulsants, the gross distribution pattern and the major metabolic pathways are well defined. This understanding has permitted the application of sound pharmacokinetic principles to the task of predicting, achieving, and monitoring efficacious blood concentrations. The quantitative approach to therapy has led to significant advances in the treatment of the epilepsies with diphenylhydantoin and phenobarbital, and it seems likely that such a status can soon be achieved for primidone and ethosuximide as well. As a result, investigations into this aspect of anticonvulsant disposition have become a prominent feature of epilepsy research. Less well defined than the gross distribution and metabolic profiles are (1) the interactions of the agents with subcellular macromolecules and formed elements and (2) the importance of the metabolic pathways which involve chemically reactive intermediates that may bind covalently (and therefore irreversibly) to endogenous structures. The philosophy prevails that interactions such as these are the qualitative determinants of drug action and toxicity. While these questions are being vigorously pursued, meaningful advances have been restrained by technical limitations in the experimental techniques.

The purpose of this review is to delineate what is known about the physiological disposition of anticonvulsant drugs as it relates to their desired and untoward effects and, wherever possible, to indicate the direction of current investigations. Other observers have dealt with the subject in great detail (Woodbury *et al.*, 1972; International Encyclopedia of Pharmacology and

Therapeutics, 1973), taking account of historical developments, experimental approach, species variations, etc. It is not our intention to duplicate the comprehensive nature of these reviews, but we have attempted to consolidate and update the available information and to give it perspective.

II. DIPHENYLHYDANTOIN AND OTHER HYDANTOINS

Diphenylhydantoin is a very lipid soluble, weak acid (pK 8.6) that is largely undissociated at physiological pH and thus diffuses readily through the lipid–protein complexes that comprise biological barriers. Its absorption from the small intestine following oral administration is limited not by its ability to diffuse through the intestinal lining but by low solubility in the aqueous lumenal fluid. When administered orally, even in solution as the sodium salt, it is virtually insoluble in gastric acid (17 $\mu g/ml$); and, although solubility is enhanced by the duodenal pH (7–8) and the detergent action of bile salts, the accumulation of diphenylhydantoin in blood is directly dependent on the rate of dissolution of the remaining crystalline material. The plasma profile of diphenylhydantoin can thus be materially affected by the dosage form.

An interest in circumventing the complications imparted by the low aqueous solubility of diphenylhydantoin has led some investigators to explore the possibility of administering a water soluble "pro-drug," which is converted to the active drug in the body. The basis for this approach is the observation that esters of hydantoic acids are hydrolyzed and converted to hydantoins, *in vivo* (Stella and Higuchi, 1973). The use of the diethylamino ester of diphenylhydantoic acid was specifically recommended, since this highly water soluble compound was shown to be easily converted to diphenylhydantoin in biological systems (Stella *et al.*, 1975).

Diethylamino ester of   diphenylhydantoin
diphenylhydantoic acid

The compound was found to be well absorbed after intramuscular administration in the rat and dog and after oral administration in the rat (Glazko *et al.*, 1975). The plasma levels of the compound decreased rapidly due to distribution in the tissues and to its conversion to diphenylhydantoin. The decrease in the plasma levels of the compound was accompanied by an increase in the plasma levels of diphenylhydantoin. Additional metabolic studies are required before the approach can be undertaken as a clinical tactic. In rats some of the hydantoic acid ester is excreted unchanged. If this also occurs in humans, the unchanged fraction would constitute a quantity of pro-drug that could be added to the diphenylhydantoin pool in patients who convert the ester to the hydantoin more rapidly than most or under physiologic conditions that stimulate the conversion. This could result in toxic levels of diphenylhydantoin. Further, since it is possible that the diphenylhydantoin generated could reach a saturation point, crystalluria or deposition of crystals in the renal tissue could occur (Glazko *et al.*, 1975). Thus, the feasibility of using the pro-drug clinically remains to be demonstrated.

The need for such a tactic is not acute in any event. Studies have shown that blood levels following oral administration of a microcrystalline suspension of sodium diphenylhydantoin compare favorably with those achieved by intravenous administration (Glazko and Chang, 1972). This suggests that the limitations presented by the low aqueous solubility of diphenylhydantoin can be overcome without resorting to other chemical forms. In a practical sense, perhaps too much attention has been given to the question of rapid absorption, because anticonvulsants are never administered orally for their acute effects. The minimal acceptable requirement is that absorption be a relatively consistent and eventually complete process so that efficacious blood levels can be achieved and reliably maintained.

In the blood, diphenylhydantoin is highly but reversibly bound to albumin and to α-globulin proteins. This increases the capacity of blood to carry diphenylhydantoin well above the aqueous solubility. The binding is believed to occur at sites on the proteins that normally carry free fatty acids and the thyroid hormone thyroxine (Lightfoot and Christian, 1966). Diphenylhydantoin displaces thyroxine from these sites but can itself be displaced by free fatty acids. These are also the sites that bind other commonly used drugs. Phenylbutazone, for instance, can significantly reduce diphenylhydantoin binding by competing for the carrier sites (Lunde *et al.*, 1970). Since only the unbound drug in blood is free to diffuse into tissue and elicit a pharmacological response, interactions of this type can have important consequences. In man, for instance, 10% of the blood diphenylhydantoin is in the unbound state; a factor that reduces binding by 5% (i.e., 90 to 85%) produces a 50% increase in freely diffusable drug. Fortunately, diphenylhydantoin is not readily displaced by other anticonvulsants that might be administered concomitantly. The binding profile may, however, be altered in pathological conditions that comprise changes in the concentration or molecular form of blood proteins. Diphenylhydantoin binding is reduced in hepatic diseases accompanied by hypoalbuminemia (Hooper *et al.*, 1973) and in uremia associated with renal malfunction (Reidenberg *et al.*, 1971). The cause of decreased binding in uremia appears to be twofold: (1) Renal malfunction results in elevated levels of diphenylhydantoin metabolites which then compete with the parent drug for binding site (Letteri *et al.*, 1971); and (2) minor changes in the structure of a portion of the albumin molecules reduce the affinity of carrier sites for the drug (Shoeman and Azarnoff, 1972). The relative quantitative importance of these events has not been established.

The lipoidal nature of undissociated diphenylhydantoin causes it to penetrate cell membranes very rapidly by nonionic diffusion. For this reason it is almost totally reabsorbed from the glomerular filtrate across the lipoidal uriniferous tubule wall, and very little is excreted in the urine. It accumulates significantly in body tissue. Tissue to plasma concentration ratios are greater than 1.0 for every tissue studied, varying, for example, from 1.5 in muscle to about 4 in liver (Noach *et al.*, 1958). The accumulation in tissue is mainly a function of binding to and solubility in subcellular components. Binding is probably the quantitatively more important process. For example, in adipose tissue, the concentration of diphenylhydantoin rises when the mobilization of fats from the cells is stimulated, as in starvation or epinephrine-induced lipolysis. This suggests that the intracellular binding processes are quantitatively more important than fat solubility. The techniques for studying subcellular drug–macromolecule interactions directly are crude and inexact. The evidence that is available by these techniques suggests that the intracellular binding processes for diphenylhydantoin are as avid or more avid than those for plasma proteins. Binding to subcellular proteins is usually in the range of 80–95% (Woodbury and Swinyard, 1972). As a consequence of the high capacity and accessibility of cells for diphenylhydantoin, when it is administered, it accumulates first in highly perfused tissues: liver, kidney, and brain. These organs, along with blood, then provide a source of diphenylhydantoin for less perfused tissues; that is, the drug redistributes to the so-called depot tissues: fat and muscle. During chronic administration, diphenylhydantoin levels must reach a steady state between blood and the depot tissues before brain levels can be maintained.

The qualitative aspects of the intracellular distribution of diphenylhydantoin are under intensive investigation. The outlook of the researchers in this field is that the subcellular drug–macromolecule interaction may be involved in eliciting its pharmacological and toxicological responses. The validity of studies of this type has been questioned on the technical basis that, as the structural integrity of the cell is disrupted during the fractionation process, the macromolecular superstructure is altered and therefore the binding processes change qualitatively. Further, it is suggested that since the physical environment is altered during fractionation the drug may redistribute among the fractions irrespective of possible alterations at the binding sites. For these reasons, it is contended by critics that what is measured in these studies is not reflective of the distribution pattern in the physiological state. Investigators in this field acknowledge these limitations, but they maintain that much of the subcellular structural integrity is preserved and that at least the relative affinity of the cell fractions for the drug can thus be determined. Moreover, they contend that such mechanistically important events as (1) irreversible binding and (2) changes in binding parameters during drug treatment can be determined. Yanagihara and Hamberger (1971) have shown that diphenylhydantoin has a high affinity for nerve cells (for the neuronal fraction relative to the glial fraction), probably because the plasma membranes of neuronal endings, nerve cell bodies, and nucleii bind diphenylhydantoin selectively. Kemp and Woodbury (1971) have proposed that diphenylhydantoin binds rapidly and irreversibly (possibly covalently) to the nuclear fraction of brain cells and that, subsequently, nucleoprotein-bound diphenylhydantoin is transported to and accumulates in the microsomal fraction. These findings clearly have mechanistic implications. Other investigators (Goldberg and Todoroff, 1973; Wilensky and Lowden, 1972), however, have not been able to substantiate these findings. They refute the claim that diphenylhydantoin binds covalently in the brain and suggest that the findings of Kemp and Woodbury may be artifactual consequences of the high affinity of diphenylhydantoin for plasma membranes and of redistribution of the drug during fractionation. This controversy may not be resolved until the technical limitations are overcome.

Diphenylhydantoin is metabolized principally by the hepatic hydroxylase complex in the endoplasmic reticulum of hepatocyte cells. The hydroxy metabolites are converted to very polar glucuronic acid conjugates that are both filtered and secreted into kidney tubules and secreted into the bile. The conjugates are too polar to be reabsorbed by nonionic diffusion out of the tubular lumens, but, in the intestine, the material from bile may be hydrolyzed by the bacterial flora and absorbed to blood as free hydroxyphenylphenylhydantoin. The metabolic hydroxylations occur at one of the 5-phenyl groups, presumably via an arene oxide intermediate, to products analogous to those for benzene: phenols, 5-(3- or 4-hydroxyphenyl)-5-phenylhydantoin (HPPH), and a dihydrodiol, 5-(3,4-dihydroxy-1,5-cyclohexadien-1-yl)-5-phenylhydantoin (Fig. 1). The phenols, HPPH, account for about 90% of an administered dose of diphenylhydantoin. Arene oxide intermediates are thought to be common features of all aromatic hydroxylations. None has been directly demonstrated for diphenylhydantoin, but the evidence is strong that the pathway is typical (Glazko and Chang, 1972). Arene oxides rearrange nonenzymatically in the presence of liver microsomes to phenols (Daly *et al.*, 1969) and are enzymatically hydrated to dihydrodiols by epoxide hydrase, an enzyme coupled to the cytochrome fraction of the liver endoplasmic reticulum.

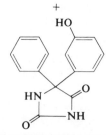

Arene oxide intermediate

5-(4-Hydroxyphenyl)-5-
phenylhydantoin (HPPH)

5-(3,4-Dihydroxy-1,5-cyclohexadien-1-yl)-
5-phenylhydantoin (dihydrodiol)

+

5-(3-Hydroxyphenyl)-5-
phenylhydantoin (HPPH)

Fig. 1. Metabolism of diphenylhydantoin.

The hepatic hydroxylase mechanism has attracted considerable attention recently due to findings that arene oxide intermediates can spontaneously rearrange to free radicals that attack biological macromolecules. Such attacks have been implicated in the toxic effects of environmental chemicals and some drugs. The possibility that diphenylhydantoin toxicities are similarly mediated is currently being studied. The dihydrodiol of diphenylhydantoin can be further oxidized to the corresponding catechol, which is extensively methylated to the 3-*O*-methylcatechol (Chang *et al.*, 1972b). The possibility exists that the free catechol may compete with catecholamine neurotransmitters for 3-*O*-methylation and thereby exert a sparing effect. It has been speculated (Glazko, 1973) that the catechol metabolite may also mediate some of the catecholaminergic actions attributed to diphenylhydantoin: alteration of the uptake and binding of catecholamines by brain synaptosomes (Hadfield, 1972) and inhibition of the oxidative deamination of catecholamines (Azzaro and Gutrecht, 1973).

Diphenylhydantoin can also be converted to a very limited extent to the corresponding open-ring hydantoic acid. The conversion is thought to be enzymatic, but the site of catalysis has not been established. The endogenous enzyme known to be capable of lysing the hydantoin ring has been shown to be specific for 5-monosubstituted hydantoin stereoisomers (Dudley *et al.*, 1974a).

The rate of diphenylhydantoin hydroxylation is dose dependent. At blood concentrations high in the therapeutic range (above 15–20 μg/ml) metabolism is a zero-order process; the rate is independent of concentration. At lower blood levels, metabolism is a first-order process; the rate declines as the concentration declines. These characteristics are consistent with the hypothesis that the capacity limit for diphenylhydantoin hydroxylation is relatively low; that is, the diphenylhydantoin saturation of the enzyme complex occurs at therapeutic blood concentrations (Gerber *et al.*, 1971).

The hydroxylation rate can be markedly reduced by competitors for the catalytic site (Fouts and Kutt, 1972). This is apparently a reflection of a very "loose" binding of diphenylhydantoin to the hepatocyte endoplasmic reticulum. Thus, concomitant administration of other anticonvulsants that are substrates for arylhydroxylase can inhibit diphenylhydantoin metabolism and cause its concentration in blood to rise above the capacity limit. Phenobarbital is especially interesting in this regard because it not only displaces diphenylhydantoin from the catalytic site, but also induces a proliferation of the hydroxylase-containing hepatic endoplasmic reticulum. In the clinical setting, these interactions are further complicated by the time-dependent nature of endoplasmic reticulum proliferation and the relative intensity of the two phenomena. It has been predicted, on the basis of the "loose" binding of diphenylhydantoin to the endoplasmic reticulum, that competition for the catalytic sites would be a quantitatively more important process than endo-plasmic reticulum proliferation (Fouts and Kutt, 1972); and experimental evidence has supported this contention (Kutt, 1972). Diphenylhydantoin can also be displaced from endoplasmic reticulum binding sites by its metabolite, HPPH. If blood HPPH levels are elevated experimentally by inhibiting its glucuronidation, diphenylhydantoin metabolism is reduced (Levy and Ashley, 1973).

The complications that these interactions impose on diphenylhydantoin therapy have been largely surmounted in recent years by designing the administration regimen according to pharmacokinetic parameters. The parameters so employed, half-life in blood, renal clearance, hepatic (metabolic clearance), and volume of distribution, account for the various facets of drug disposition. This approach has generally enhanced the therapeutic effect and markedly reduced the incidence of adverse reactions (Sherwin *et al.*, 1973). The success with diphenylhydantoin, in fact, has made it the model drug for this tactic. The minimum requirement for such a strategy, of course, is the capability for obtaining plasma and urine levels of diphenylhydantoin and, occasionally, HPPH. Several gas chromatographic assays are available. The simplest of these, involving on-column flash-heater methylation with tri-methylanilinium hydroxide, has been evaluated by gas chromatography–mass spectrometry and found to be quite satisfactory (Estas and Dumont, 1973).

The other therapeutic hydantoins have not been nearly so intensively studied as diphenylhydantoin because they are not popular agents. Like diphenylhydantoin, they are lipid-soluble chemicals that readily penetrate brain and other body tissues. They are known to have brain to blood con-centration ratios of 1.0 or greater but the details of their distribution are not known. The 5,5-disubstituted hydantoins are metabolized through aromatic hydroxylase pathways analogous to those for diphenylhydantoin (Butler, 1956). The *N*-methyl analogues are nearly quantitatively dealkylated prior to hydroxylation (Butler, 1952; Butler and Waddell, 1958). Thus mephenytoin (3-methyl-5-ethyl-5-phenylhydantoin) and meteoin (1-methyl-5-ethyl-5-phenylhydantoin) are converted to the active anticonvulsant nirvanol (5-ethyl-5-phenylhydantoin) prior to inactivation by hydroxylation. For these com-pounds, dealkylation is much more rapid than the subsequent hydroxylation; so nirvanol accumulates and is responsible for much of the associated anti-

Mephenytoin   Ethylphenylhydantoin

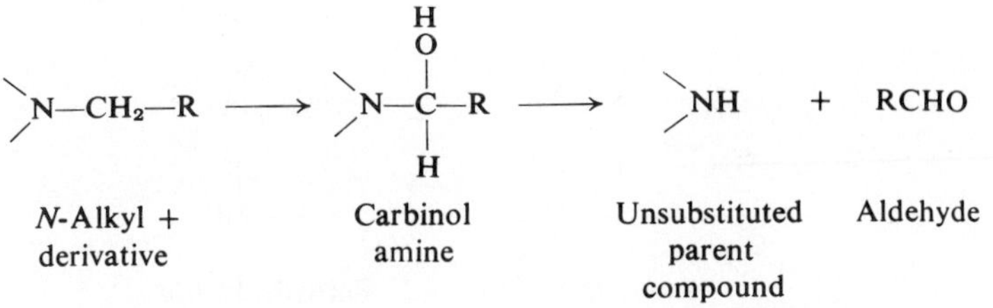

$$\underset{\substack{N\text{-Alkyl } + \\ \text{derivative}}}{\overset{\diagdown}{\underset{\diagup}{N}}-CH_2-R} \longrightarrow \underset{\substack{\text{Carbinol} \\ \text{amine}}}{\overset{\substack{H \\ O \\ |}}{\underset{|}{\overset{\diagdown}{\underset{\diagup}{N}}-\underset{H}{C}-R}}} \longrightarrow \underset{\substack{\text{Unsubstituted} \\ \text{parent} \\ \text{compound}}}{\overset{\diagdown}{\underset{\diagup}{N}}H} \quad + \quad \underset{\text{Aldehyde}}{RCHO}$$

Fig. 2. Proposed pathway for metabolic *N*-dealkylation.

convulsant activity. *N*-Dealkylation has been proposed (Brodie *et al.*, 1958) to proceed via hydroxylation to the corresponding carbinolamine (or -amide), which is not stable and breaks down spontaneously to an aldehyde and the unsubstituted parent compound (Fig. 2). As with the arene oxide intermediate in aromatic hydroxylation, it is suspected that the spontaneous rearrangement of carbinolamines may involve a free radical that reacts with biological macromolecules. The quantitative importance of this possibility is being investigated.

The anticonvulsant activity of mephenytoin in relation to its metabolism to ethylphenylhydantoin has been quantitatively studied in mice (Kupferberg and Yonekawa, 1974, 1975). The ED_{50} values against maximal electroshock seizures for mephenytoin and ethylphenylhydantoin are 42 and 23 mg/kg, respectively, at 30 minutes and 35 and 30 mg/kg, respectively, at 120 minutes after intraperitoneal administration of the drugs. Brain and plasma levels of mephenytoin and ethylphenylhydantoin were determined by gas–liquid chromatography after intraperitoneal administration of 40 mg of mephenytoin per kilogram. At 30 minutes the brain levels of mephenytoin and ethylphenylhydantoin were 9.2 and 8.1 μg/gm, respectively. The brain levels of mephenytoin fell to 5.8 μg/gm and those of ethylphenylhydantoin rose to 18.2 μg/gm at 2 hours. The total molar concentration of mephenytoin and ethylphenylhydantoin, however, did not change more than 10% during the 2-hour period. Although the anticonvulsant activity of mephenytoin did not vary greatly during 2 hours after administration, the early activity is due in major part to mephenytoin and the later activity to ethylphenylhydantoin.

The distribution and metabolism of ethotoin, 3-ethyl-5-phenylhydantoin, has been studied in epileptic patients (Yonekawa *et al.*, 1975). After oral administration of 0.5 or 2.0 gm of ethotoin to epileptic patients, the plasma half-life of ethotoin in different patients was in the range of 5–11 hours. The plasma half-life was the same for the two dose levels in the same patient. Two distinct pathways were established for the metabolism of ethotoin: (1) hydroxylation of the phenyl ring followed by conjugation with glucuronic acid

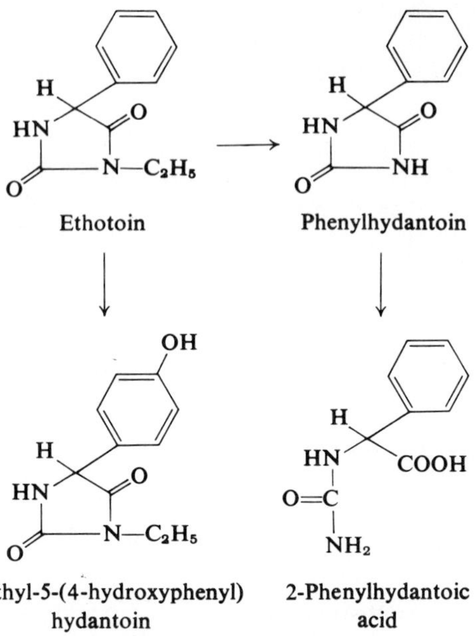

Ethotoin   Phenylhydantoin

3-Ethyl-5-(4-hydroxyphenyl)   2-Phenylhydantoic
hydantoin   acid

Fig. 3. Route of metabolism of ethotoin.

and (2) *N*-deethylation followed by enzymatic ring opening to form 2-phenyl-hydantoic acid (Fig. 3). No ring-hydroxylated metabolites of 5-phenylhydan-toin were found. In separate experiments 2-phenylhydantoic acid was isolated from human urine and shown to have the *R* configuration.

In more detailed studies of the ring-opening pathway, it was found that the racemic forms of 5-phenylhydantoin and its 3-methyl and 3-ethyl derivatives are converted by the dog to *R*(−)-2-phenylhydantoic acid (Dudley *et al.*, 1970) (Fig. 4). The enzyme that converts 5-phenylhydantoin to 2-phenyl-hydantoic acid was subsequently identified as dihydropyrimidinase, which is found in the kidney and liver of the rat, mouse, guinea pig, rabbit, and dog

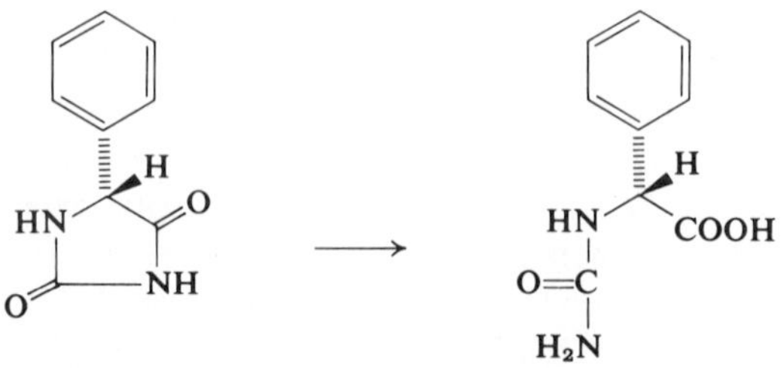

R(−)-5-Phenylhydantoin   *R*(−)-2-Phenylhydantoic acid

Fig. 4. Conversion of *R*(−)-5-phenylhydantoin to *R*(−)-2-phenylhydantoic acid.

(Dudley *et al.*, 1974a). It was noted that 5,5-disubstituted hydantoins and *N*-substituted hydantoins are not substrates for dihydropyrimidinase. Since ethotoin, an *N*-substituted hydantoin, was found to undergo ring cleavage it was postulated that *N*-dealkylation must take place first for the compound to become a substrate for dihydropyrimidinase (Dudley *et al.*, 1974a). Furthermore it was also found that only the $R(-)$ enantiomer of 5-phenylhydantoin is a substrate for the rat liver enzyme, while the $S(+)$ enantiomer must undergo racemization before it is metabolized. The reversible conversion of $R(-)$-2-phenylhydantoic acid to 5-phenylhydantoin by rat liver enzyme is also demonstrable.

III. THE BARBITURATES

The barbiturate type of anticonvulsant differ widely in their biophysical properties. Phenobarbital and barbital are polar compounds that only slowly penetrate the brain and other lipoidal tissues, while the *N*-substituted analogues, mephobarbital and metharbital, are highly lipid soluble and can be expected to behave more like diphenylhydantoin. The *N*-methyl compounds are dealkylated *in vivo* (Butler, 1952), however; and much of their activity is due to the unsubstituted metabolites, which are long acting because they are only slowly metabolized and/or excreted. Recently, there has also been an interest in *N,N'*-dialkyl barbiturates as therapeutic agents. These, too, are dealkylated to long-acting parent barbiturates, with one alkyl group being removed almost instantly, so that the subsequent disposition profile is quite analogous to that of mephobarbital. The disposition of eterobarb, which is representative of this group, is discussed in Chapters 2 and 5.

In a practical sense, the intestinal absorption of the barbiturates, as with diphenylhydantoin, appears to be more dependent on solubility and accessibility to the intestinal mucosa than any other factor. A recent study of phenobarbital in man showed that intestinal absorption is essentially complete in 10 minutes when it is administered by duodenal intubation as a solution buffered at pH 6.8 (Alvin *et al.*, 1975b). The variability observed in previous studies (Lous, 1954; Hogben *et al.*, 1957) can probably be explained on the basis of gastric emptying time, contents of the intestinal lumen, and the dosage form, which affects the rate of dissolution. Metharbital is also well absorbed. The absorption of mephobarbital, on the other hand, is greatly limited by its low aqueous solubility and, in some instances, large portions of the dose have passed into the feces (Butler, 1952; Butler and Waddell, 1958). When solubility is not limiting, as when solutions buffered to keep the drug in the nonionized state are introduced into the intestine, the rate of absorption is dependent on binding to the mucosal protein, not on lipid solubility (Kakemi *et al.*, 1967). This suggests that the drug is held at the site of absorption by its association with proteins in the mucosal lining and that this association process, not the diffusion process, is rate limiting. Thus, phenobarbital, which is more highly bound to mucosal proteins that mephobarbital and metharbital, is the most rapidly absorbed of the three.

The details of the distribution of metharbital and mephobarbital have not been systematically examined, but these compounds must concentrate in fatty tissues because their oil to water partition ratios are high and their volumes of distribution are well above 100% of the body weight (Butler, 1952, 1953). They are not excreted in the urine to a significant extent because, although they are filtered from blood in the glomerulus, they back-diffuse into blood across the lipoidal uriniferous tubule lining. This is a consequence of their high lipid solubility. Phenobarbital achieves nearly equal concentrations in all of the tissues and fluids of the body, except fat. This limited ability of phenobarbital to cross lipoidal barriers is exemplified by its localized distribution pattern in brain. Following intravenous administration, phenobarbital enters the nonmyelinated gray matter much more rapidly than the white matter that is protected by lipoidal myelin sheaths (Roth and Barlow, 1961). The low lipid solubility of phenobarbital also causes it to be partially retained in the glomerular filtrate, and thus large portions of a dose are excreted unchanged in the urine. Some reabsorption does occur, however, and the clearance is considerably less than the glomerular filtration rate (Waddell and Butler, 1957). When the urine is alkaline, the fraction of a phenobarbital dose excreted unchanged increases because the process of backdiffusion (tubular reabsorption) is further retarded by significant ionization of the drug in the tubule. The low pK of phenobarbital (7.4) makes it particularly labile to urine pH changes. In contrast, the higher pK values of diphenylhydantoin, mephobarbital, and metharbital make them refractory to fluctuations in urine pH since it rarely rises above 7.8.

The metabolism of the barbiturates has been extensively studied. Phenobarbital undergoes phenyl hydroxylation, probably by way of an arene oxide intermediate, as suggested for diphenylhydantoin. The predominant metabolite is *p*-hydroxyphenobarbital (Butler, 1954). This compound has weak anticonvulsant activity of its own (Craig *et al.*, 1960), but it does not contribute to the action of phenobarbital because it is rapidly removed from the blood by metabolic conjugation and renal filtration. It appears in the urine as glucuronide and sulfate conjugates (Butler, 1956). The other products of aromatic hydroxylation, the dihydrodiol and the catechol, have also been found in the urine in trace quantities (Harvey *et al.*, 1972). In addition, 1'-hydroxyethylphenobarbital has been identified as a metabolite. The question of whether, or to what extent, ring scission occurs has not been adequately resolved.

Mephobarbital is extensively demethylated to phenobarbital (Butler, 1952).

The relative amounts of these compounds in the blood is dependent on the rate of demethylation. During chronic administration of many anticonvulsants, the rate of drug metabolism is increased by induction of the hepatic microsomal enzyme system. As a result, the rate of dealkylation is nearly as great as the slow absorption of mephobarbital from the intestine. Thus, blood levels of mephobarbital do not rise very rapidly, but phenobarbital does accumulate. It should also be noted that phenyl hydroxylation may be a primary route for a small portion of a mephobarbital dose (Alvin *et al.*, unpublished observations) thus bypassing the phenobarbital pathway.

In order to determine the extent to which the anticonvulsant activity of mephobarbital is dependent on metabolic conversion to phenobarbital, mephobarbital was administered acutely and chronically to rats (Craig and Shideman, 1971). The brain concentration of mephobarbital and phenobarbital was correlated with anticonvulsant activity. The maximal activity against electroshock was observed at 3 hours after administration of a single dose of mephobarbital, when the phenobarbital brain level was too low to account for the activity. At 4 hours after drug administration, when the anticonvulsant activity has passed its peak, the brain level of mephobarbital was low and that of phenobarbital was high.

The routes of metabolism for phenobarbital and mephobarbital are presented in Fig. 5.

Metharbital is quantitatively dealkylated to barbital (Butler, 1953), most of which is excreted in the urine. Chronic administration of metharbital brings about considerable concentrations of both metharbital and barbital.

Analysis of the barbiturates is readily accomplished by gas chromatographic procedures that can be quite specific and sensitive; many procedures have been described. Flash-heater on-column methylation with trimethylphenylammonium hydroxide has become very popular because it eliminates the wet-chemistry derivatization step. Special care should be taken in the use of this procedure, however, because, unlike the hydantoins, barbiturates break down during the flash alkylation (Van Meter and Gillen, 1973). It is even possible to quantitate the breakdown product rather than the derivatized barbiturate. Preinjection derivatization with diazoethane is probably a more reliable procedure. There are hazards associated with the generation and use of this material, but these can be avoided by employing specialized equipment to vent the gas and eliminate the risk of explosion.

IV. PRIMIDONE

Primidone, a 2-deoxybarbiturate, is a polar compound that is well absorbed and distributed. In animals, significant brain levels of primidone are achieved

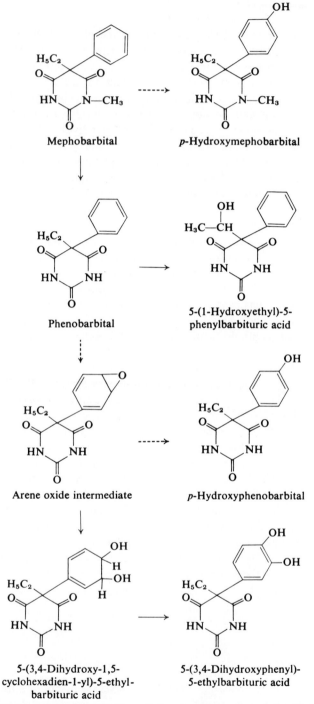

Fig. 5. Route of metabolism of phenobarbital and mephobarbital.

at about one hour after oral administration, but they are always less than that in plasma (Baumel *et al.*, 1973). In man, peak blood levels are achieved within a few hours after administration (Gallagher *et al.*, 1970; Booker *et al.*, 1970). The details of its tissue distribution have not been studied. Because of its low lipid solubility, primidone is cleared rapidly by the kidneys. In the rat, over 50% of the dose appears in the urine unchanged (Alvin and Bush, 1973). Since primidone is a neutral compound, fluctuations in urinary pH do not affect the renal clearance.

Primidone is converted to 2 active metabolites by the enzymatic oxidation of the urea carbon: phenobarbital and phenylethylmalonamide (PEMA) (Fig. 6). The reactions are localized in the microsomal fraction of rat liver homogenates, are TPNH dependent, have a pH optimum of 7.4 and are inhibited by SKF-525A (DiMicco and Gallagher, 1975). These reactions are induced by prior treatment of the animals with diphenylhydantoin, carbamazepine, phenobarbital or primidone (DiMicco and Gallagher, 1975; Alvin *et al.*, 1975a). It has been proposed that 2-hydroxyprimidone is a common intermediate that can spontaneously form PEMA or be further oxidized to phenobarbital (DiMicco and Gallagher, 1975; Alvin *et al.*, 1975a).

The plasma half-life of primidone is about 14 hours in patients not exposed to other anticonvulsants and about 7 hours in patients receiving anticonvulsants chronically. PEMA accounts for about 60% of the primidone metabolized in the former group and about 80% in the latter group. In this latter group of patients, PEMA had an average half-life of 41 hours. In these same subjects, the average half-life of phenobarbital derived from primidone was 83 hours, which is consistent with the frequently observed accumulation of

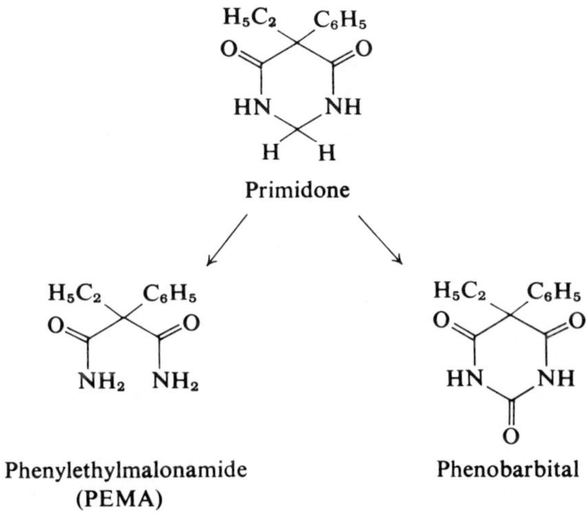

Fig. 6. Route of metabolism of primidone.

phenobarbital during chronic primidone therapy (Zavadil and Gallagher, 1975). Interestingly, while prior administration of other anticonvulsants decreased the primidone half-life, prior administration of primidone itself has been reported to increase the primidone half-life (Gallagher and Baumel, 1972) in some patients.

Primidone, phenobarbital, and PEMA all possess anticonvulsant activity, each with a different potency and spectrum of activity against various experimental models of epilepsy (Baumel *et al.*, 1973). Phenylethylmalonamide has also been shown to potentiate the anticonvulsant and hypnotic activity of barbiturates (Gallagher and Baumel, 1972). Further, the metabolites may have opposing effects on the rate of primidone metabolism, that is, on their own formation. Phenobarbital, of course, is one of the most potent inducers (stimulators) of drug-metabolizing enzymes known. On the other hand, PEMA inhibited primidone metabolism in the perfused rat liver (Alvin *et al.*, 1975a). The inhibitory action of this metabolite may explain the finding that in some, but not all, patients the primidone blood half-life increases (rate of metabolism decreases) up to threefold during chronic administration (Gallagher and Baumel, 1972). Since the intensity of these influences must be graded according to the blood concentrations and duration of therapy, it would not be surprising to find that wide variability occurs in the formation of PEMA and phenobarbital and therefore in the plasma concentrations of all three active compounds. If so, the efficacy of primidone against specific seizure types would depend directly on which compound(s) is favored by the existing status of the disposition process. Likewise, in the instance where phenobarbital and PEMA are both favored, their synergistic sedative effects might produce untoward reactions, such as primidone-induced ataxia and depression. In the clinical setting, predominant concentrations of any of the three active compounds have been reported during chronic primidone administration. A rational pharmacokinetic strategy for the administration of primidone, with the option of administering the metabolites, would clearly enhance its therapeutic efficacy. Other aspects of primidone disposition and their clinical implications are reviewed in detail in Chapter 2.

V. THE SUCCINIMIDES

A. METHSUXIMIDE

Methsuximide is a highly lipophilic compound that concentrates in fat (Butler and Waddell, 1958; Nicholls and Orton, 1972). It is rapidly demethylated, however; and it has been suggested that for most of the duration

Methsuximide (I)

of anticonvulsant activity associated with methsuximide, the desmethyl metabolite (**I**) is the predominant compound (Nicholls and Orton, 1971; Strong *et al.*, 1974). This metabolite has been detected in patients receiving chronic methsuximide therapy (Strong *et al.*, 1974; Muni *et al.*, 1973; Barron *et al.*, 1974). Methsuximide is also extensively hydroxylated to inactive metabolites that appear in the urine and bile as conjugates (Stillwell *et al.*, 1973; Horning *et al.*, 1973b). These studies did not distinguish whether hydroxylation occurred before or after *N*-demethylation. The pathways given below showing the *N*-methyl groups intact are suggested by the investigators, who are in the process of determining the sequence of hydroxylation and *N*-dealkylation. The hydroxylation of methsuximide, like that of diphenyl-hydantoin and phenobarbital, may follow the arene oxide pathway, giving rise to *N*, 2-dimethyl-2-(4-hydroxyphenyl)-succinimide (**II**) the major product, and to *N*,2-dimethyl-2-(3-hydroxyphenyl)-succinimide (**III**) and *N*,2-dimethyl-2-(3,4-dihydroxy-1,5-cyclohexadien-1-yl)-succinimide (**IV**). These metabolites have been isolated from the urine of rat, guinea pig and human; and their structures have been determined by mass spectrometry. Three monohydroxy metabolites not associated with the arene oxide pathway have also been identified: *N*-methyl-2-hydroxymethyl-2-phenylsuccinimide (**V**) and the diastereoisomers of *N*,2-dimethyl-3-hydroxy-2-phenylsuccinimide (**VI** and **VII**). The structure of *N*,2-dimethyl-2-(4-hydroxyphenyl)-3-hydroxysuccin-imide (**VIII**) was assigned to the only dihydroxy metabolite that was detected in the urine of all three species.

The principal metabolites isolated from the urine of the dog after oral administration of methsuximide were 2-methyl-2-(4-hydroxyphenyl)succin-imide (**IX**) and *N*-2-dimethyl-2-(4-hydroxyphenyl)succinimide (**II**) (Dudley *et al.*, 1974b). These metabolites were present in urine largely as glucuronic acid conjugates. The *N*-demethylation reaction was proposed to be primary. There was no evidence for the presence of the potential ring-opened metabolites, 2-methyl-2-phenylsuccinamic acid and 3-methyl-3-phenylsuccinamic acid, in the urine of dogs.

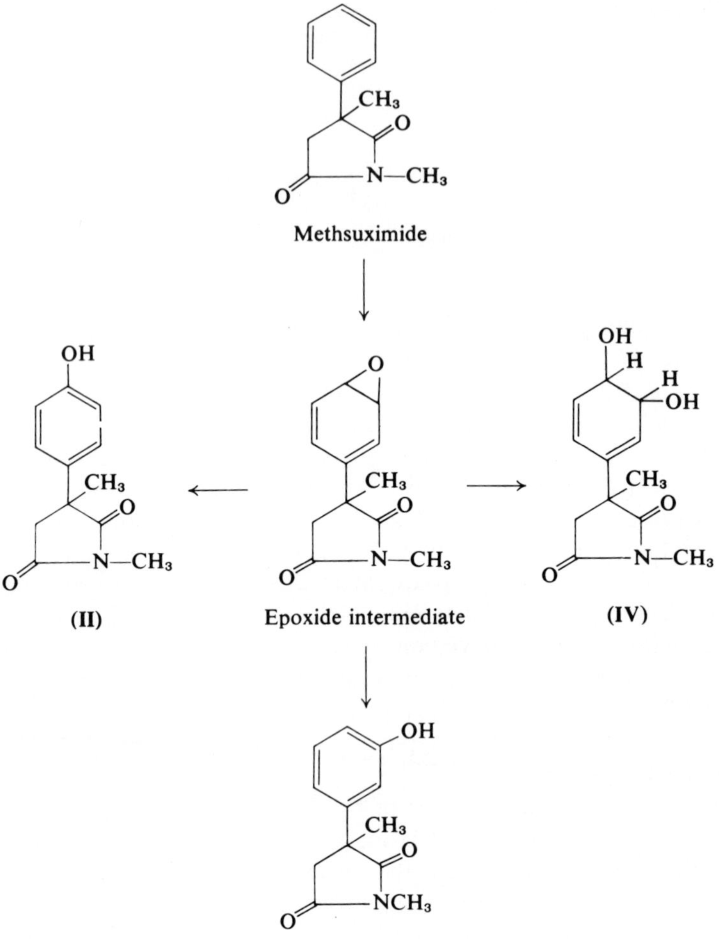

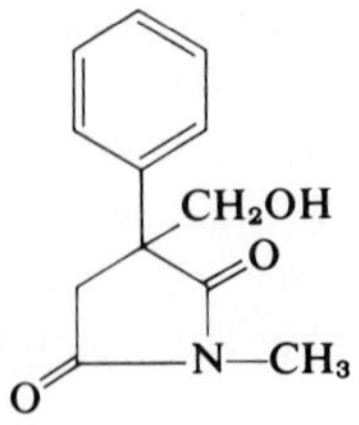

Methsuximide

(II)

Epoxide intermediate

(IV)

(III)

(V)

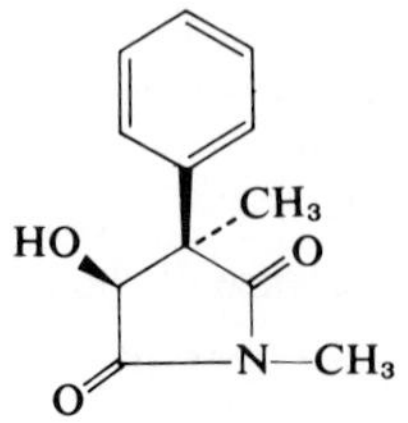

(VI)

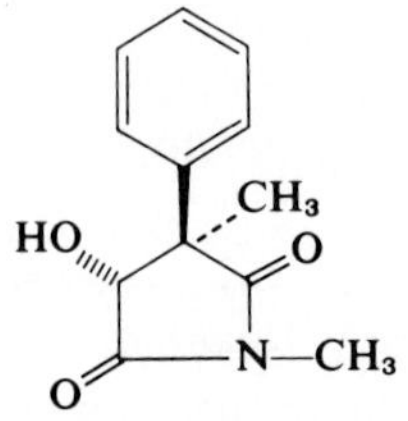

(VII)

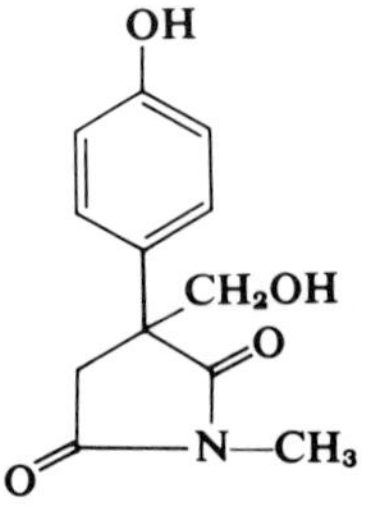

(VIII)

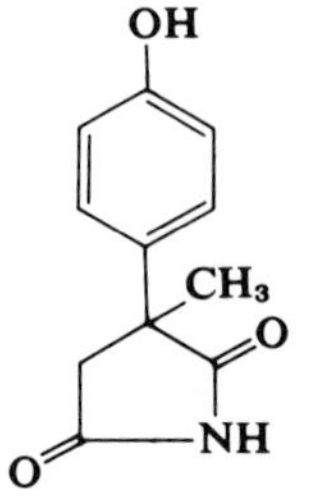

(IX)

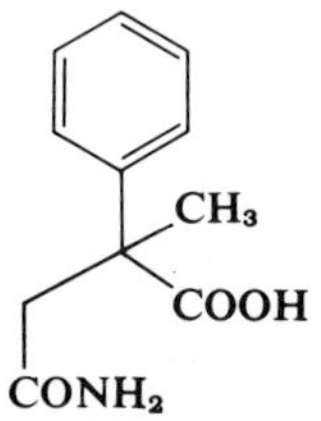

2-Methyl-2-phenylsuccinamic acid

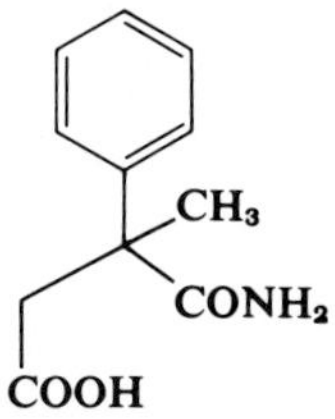

3-Methyl-3-phenylsuccinamic acid

B. PHENSUXIMIDE

Phensuximide (*N*-methyl-*a*-phenylsuccinimide) is evenly dispersed in body tissues (Glazko *et al.*, 1954); and a small quantity is excreted unchanged. Like other drugs containing an aromatic ring, phensuximide is metabolized by the arene oxide pathway. The urine of human subjects has been shown to contain the dihydrodiol, *N*-methyl-2-hydroxy-2-(3,4-dihydroxycyclohexadien-1-yl)-succinimide (**X**), a catechol, *N*-methyl-2-hydroxy-2(3,4-dihydroxy-phenyl)-succinimide (**XI**), and three phenols, *N*-methyl-2-hydroxy-2-(4-hydroxyphenyl)-succinimide (**XII**), *N*-methyl-2-hydroxy-2-(3-hydroxyphenyl)-succinimide (**XIII**), and *N*-methyl-2-(4-hydroxyphenyl)-succinimide (**XIV**). These are excreted as glucuronide conjugates in urine. Two monohydroxy metabolites not associated with the arene oxide pathway have also been

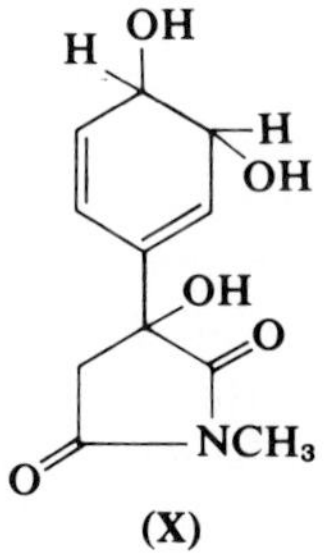

(X)

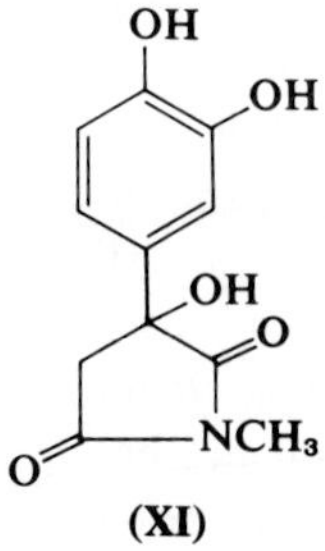

(XI)

(XII)   (XIII)   (XIV)

identified: *N*-methyl-2-hydroxy-2-phenylsuccinimide **(XV)** and 2-hydroxy-2-phenylsuccinimide **(XVI)** (Horning *et al.*, 1974).

(XV)   (XVI)

Phensuximide also undergoes ring scission to 2-phenylsuccinamic acid **(XVII)** and/or *N*-methyl-2-phenylsuccinamic acid **(XVIII)**. In the dog, a

(XVII)   (XVIII)

stereospecific ring opening occurs with 2-phenylsuccinimide but apparently not with *N*-methyl-2-phenylsuccinimide (Dudley *et al.*, 1974a). No *N*-alkylsuccinamic acid was found in the urine of the dog, and other evidence supported the conclusion that *N*-dealkylation was a primary pathway. The result of this study in the dog is in contrast to those in the rat, in which the ring-opened products were thought to contain the *N*-methyl group intact (Glazko *et al.*, 1954). The study with phensuximide (Dudley *et al.*, 1974a) is also in contrast to a study of methsuximide (Dudley *et al.*, 1974b) indicating that potential ring-opened metabolites of methsuximide, i.e., disubstituted succinimides, are not present in dog urine. The enzyme responsible for the metabolic ring cleavage reaction has been identified as dihydropyrimidinase

(Dudley *et al.*, 1974a). Only the $R(-)$ isomer of 2-phenylsuccinimide is subject to the enzymatic ring opening in the dog (Dudley *et al.*, 1972). The $S(+)$ isomer of 2-phenylsuccinimide undergoes the enzymatic ring opening reaction only after racemization to a mixture of $R(-)$ and $S(+)$ isomers has taken place. Racemization may be promoted by general base catalysis.

$R(-)$-2-Phenylsuccinimide $R(-)$-2-Phenylsuccinamic acid

The extent and position of N-demethylation in the metabolic profile of phensuximide have not been satisfactorily determined. (Certainly dealkylation occurs because desmethyl hydroxy and succinamic acid metabolites have been isolated.) Thus, neither has the possible role of desmethyl metabolites in the anticonvulsant activity associated with phensuximide been evaluated. These questions are central to the problem of basing phensuximide therapy on sound pharmacokinetic principles.

C. ETHOSUXIMIDE

Ethosuximide (2-methyl-2-phenylsuccinimide) is a relatively polar compound that has biophysical properties similar to those of phenobarbital. It is well absorbed from the intestine, with peak levels occurring one to four hours after administration (Dill *et al.*, 1965). It is uniformly distributed in all tissues and fluids except fat, where the levels are about one-third those in plasma. Both urinary excretion and metabolism are slow processes. In man, the drug persists for several days (t $\frac{1}{2}$ 60–100 hours). About 20% of a dose is excreted unchanged (Buchanan *et al.*, 1973); the rest is extensively hydroxylated.

Five monohydroxy metabolites of ethosuximide have been identified in the urine of rat and man. These are the diastereoisomers of 2-(1-hydroxyethyl)-2-methylsuccinimide (**XIX** and **XX**), 2-(2-hydroxyethyl)-2-methylsuccinimide (**XXI**), 2-ethyl-2-hydroxy-methylsuccinimide (**XXII**), and 2-ethyl-2-methyl-3-hydroxysuccinimide (**XXIII**) (Horning *et al.*, 1973a; Preste *et al.*, 1974). These metabolites appear in the urine as glucuronides. A dihydroxyethosuximide was present in small quantities in rat urine. Although it was not possible to make a definite structural assignment from the mass spectrum, this metabolite is most likely 2-(1-hydroxyethyl)-2-hydroxymethyl-succinimide (**XXIV**) (Horning *et al.*, 1973a). In addition, a ketonic metabolite of ethosuximide has been identified (Chang *et al.*, 1972a; Burkett *et al.*, 1971) as 2-acetyl-2-methylsuccinimide (**XXV**).

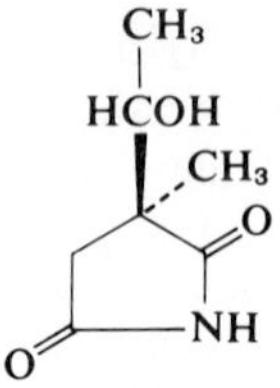

(XIX) 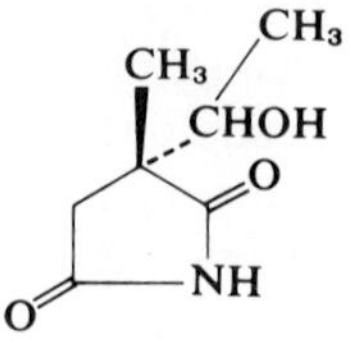   (XX) 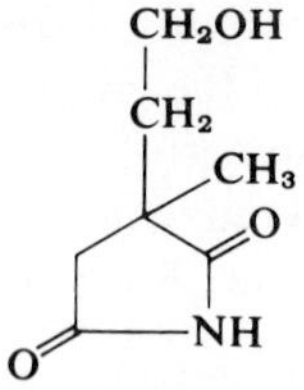   (XXI)

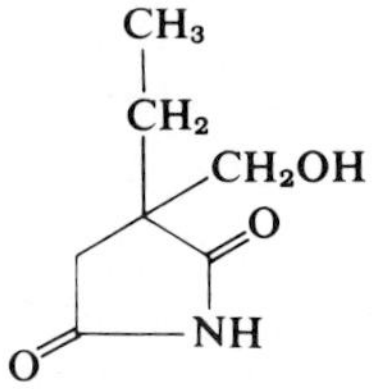

(XXII) 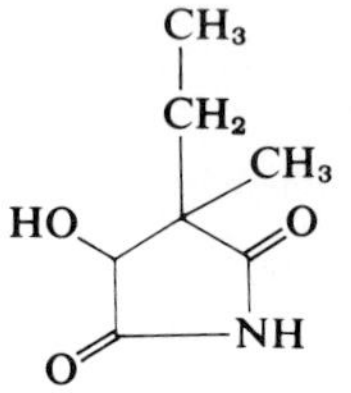   (XXIII)

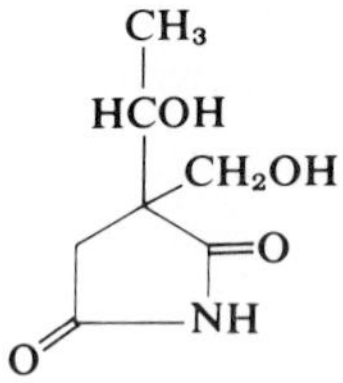

(XXIV) 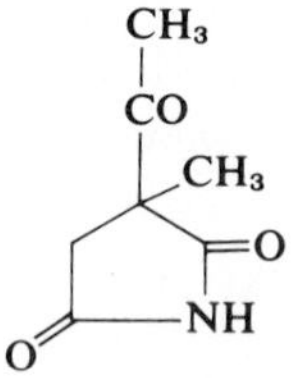   (XXV)

The metabolic profiles obtained from the plasma of the rat and man were different. In the rat plasma, ethosuximide was present in high concentration and only trace amounts of the hydroxyethosuximides (**XIX** and **XX**) were present. In human plasma these hydroxyethosuximides were present in larger quantities than the unchanged drug (Horning *et al.*, 1973a).

These results indicate that the drug is metabolized extensively and that free as well as conjugated metabolites are excreted in the urine. The effect of acute and chronic drug administration on the rate of metabolism and the kinetics of drug disappearance from the blood have not as yet been investigated.

VI. THE OXAZOLIDINEDIONES

Trimethadione and paramethadione are fat-soluble, neutral compounds. Like the other *N*-alkyl anticonvulsants, they are rapidly absorbed; they

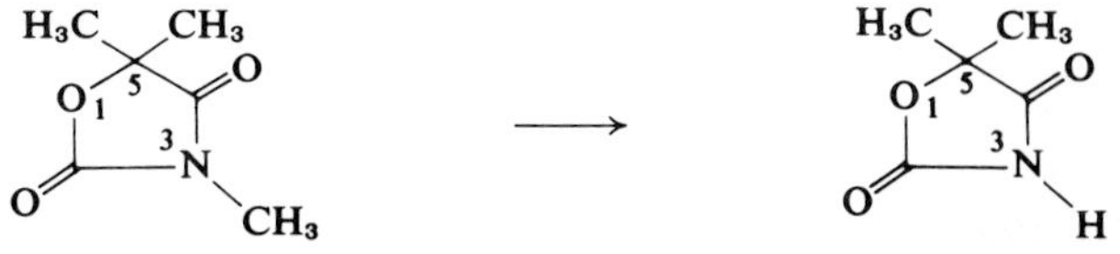

Trimethadione
(3,5,5-trimethyloxazolidine-2,4-dione)

Dimethadione
(5,5-dimethyloxazolidine-2,4-dione)

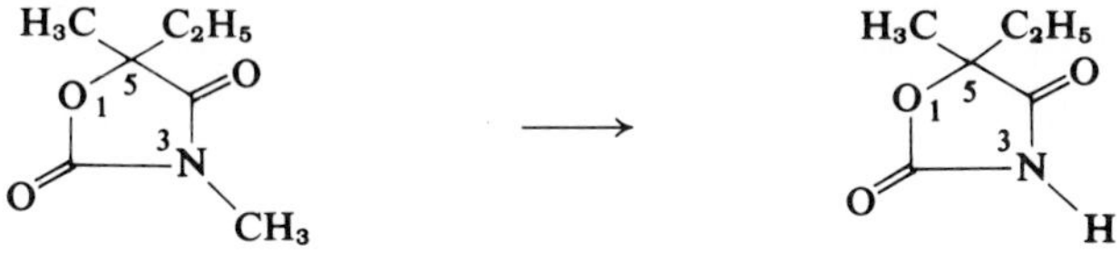

Paramethadione
(3,5-dimethyl-5-ethyloxazolidine-2,4-dione)

N-Demethylparamethadione
(5-methyl-5-ethyloxazolidine-2,4-dione)

Fig. 7. Route of metabolism of oxazolidinediones.

cannot be excreted in the urine unchanged; and they are extensively *N*-dealkylated to active metabolites that persist in the body and accumulate during chronic administration. Unlike the other *N*-alkyl compounds they do not concentrate in tissues; the tissue to blood ratios are less than 1.0 in brain, liver, muscle, and kidney (Taylor and Bertcher, 1952). This may indicate that binding to subcellular structures is not extensive. Trimethadione and paramethadione are potent anticonvulsants (Frey, 1969), but during chronic therapy their blood concentrations are only one-tenth those of the metabolites (Frey and Schulz, 1970).

N-Dealkylation is apparently the only route of metabolism for these drugs (Fig. 7). There is no evidence of ring scission. The metabolites, dimethadione and *N*-demethylparamethadione, are weak acids (p*K* 6.1 and 5.9, respectively). They are not further metabolized so termination of activity is dependent on renal excretion, which is slow. Only about 35% of the body load is excreted in a week (Withrow and Woodbury, 1972). The rate of excretion is increased when the urine is alkaline. The distribution of these compounds is unique. The low p*K* values cause them to be extensively ionized at physiological pH. The volume of distribution is about 40% of the body weight, which is more than the extracellular water volume but less than the total water volume (Waddell and Butler, 1959). The accessibility of neural sites to dimethadione may depend on active transport processes. Dimethadione apparently meets the structural requirements for the transport of weak acids; it is actively transported by the rat intestine (Dietschy and Carter, 1965) and out of the cerebrospinal fluid (Rollins and Reed, 1970). The active transport of dimethadione may also be responsible for trimethadione-associated toxicities.

VII. ACETYLUREAS

Phenylacetylurea is metabolized by aryl hydroxylation and hydrolysis of the ureide group (Fig. 8) (Tatsumi *et al.*, 1967). The 4-hydroxyphenyl, catechol, and 3-*O*-methylcatechol metabolites have been identified as products of hydroxylation. The dihydrodiol is a likely intermediate in the formation of the catechol, but this has not been demonstrated. Ureide hydrolysis yields phenylacetic acid. This is subsequently conjugated with glycine to phenylaceturic acid. The metabolic products of ethylphenylacetylurea have not been identified, but the pathways are probably analogous.

VIII. CARBAMAZEPINE

Carbamazepine is a major anticonvulsant compound with a broad spectrum of activity for partial and generalized seizures except those of the absence type. Typical clinical use of the drug in adults requires doses in the range of 600–1200 mg/day, yet serum concentrations rarely exceed 10–15 μg/ml. Consequently, the metabolism and disposition of the compound must be extensive and rapid. It would also be reasonable to assume that one or more metabolites might contribute to the total anticonvulsant activity.

There has been considerable variation in the reports, to date, of the blood

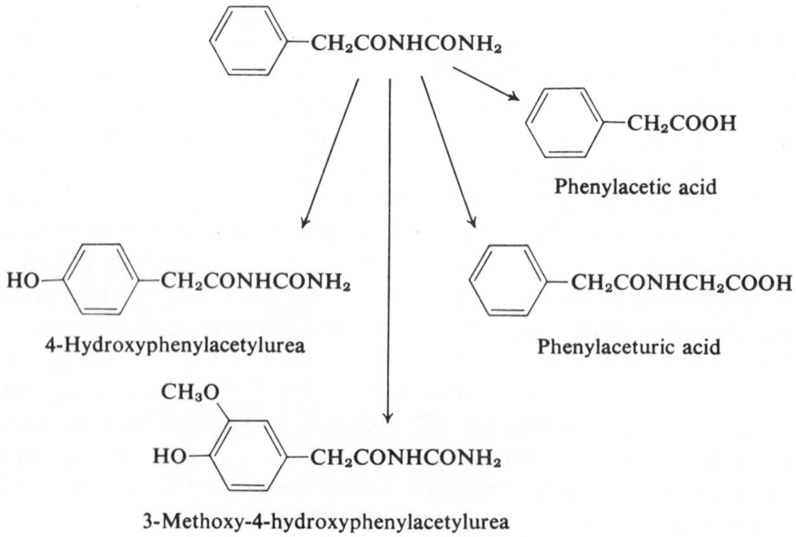

Fig. 8. Metabolic fate of phenylacetylurea.

profile of carbamazepine. In rats, while maximum protection against electro-shock seizure occurs in one hour or less (Theobald and Kunz, 1963) suggesting rapid absorption, a study of plasma and brain concentrations after oral administration indicated that the time to peak levels is up to six hours (Morselli *et al.*, 1971). In humans, time to peak plasma levels has been reported to be $2\frac{1}{2}$ hours in one group of volunteers (Meinardi, 1971), 10 hours in another group of volunteers, and 2–6 hours in a group of patients (Morselli, 1975). Further, there has been significant intra- and inter-patient variations in the blood levels achieved after oral carbamazepine administration (Meinardi, 1971). These discrepancies may be related in part to complexities in the gas chromatographic analysis of carbamazepine. Frigerio *et al.* (1973) reported that carbamazepine breaks down, partially, during analysis to 9-acridine carboxaldehyde. At least one of the metabolites also undergoes rearrangement during analysis (Frigerio, 1972).

The metabolism and distribution of carbamazepine have not yet been completely elucidated. In rats, the greatest tissue concentrations are found in the liver and kidney; and the brain to plasma ratio is greater than one (Morselli *et al.*, 1971). About 80% of blood carbamazepine is bound to plasma proteins (Johannessen and Strandjord, 1973). Carbamazepine is metabolized to a 10,11-epoxide, a 10,11-dihydrodiol and to iminostilbene (Baker *et al.*, 1973). These have been identified in urine along with the parent compound (Fig. 9). Both iminostilbene and the 10,11-dihydrodiol are

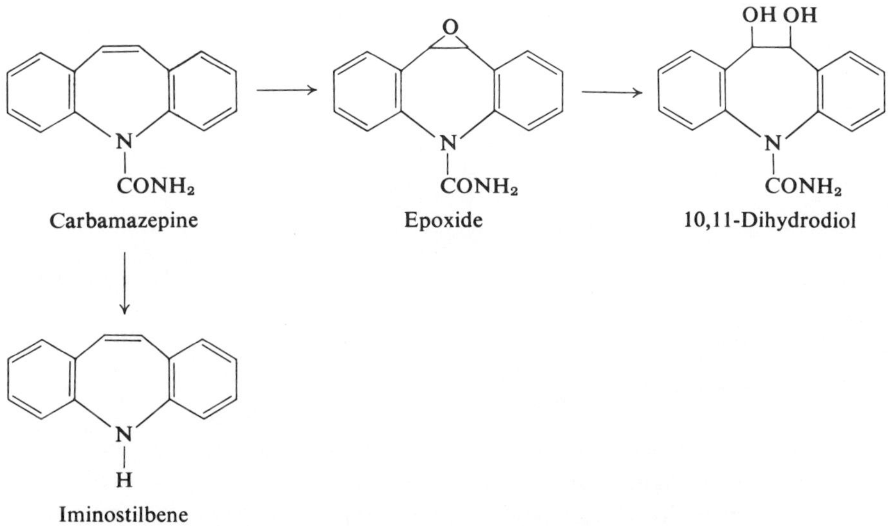

Fig. 9. Route of metabolism of carbamaazepsine.

excreted in urine as such and as conjugates of glucuronic acid. About two-thirds of an intraperitoneal dose of carbamazepine is recovered in urine and stools during a 120-hour interval with 29% of the dose in urine and 38% in stool. Therefore, enterohepatic circulation is possible (Csetenyi *et al.*, 1973). The major urinary metabolite identified thus far is the 10,11-dihydrodiol. In man, the same metabolites have been identified in plasma, urine, and feces. Only 28% of the administered dose was recovered in feces and most of this was unchanged carbamazepine. The major urinary metabolite was the 10,11-dihydrodiol, which accounted for 20% of the administered dose. The remaining identified metabolites accounted for less than 5% of the dose collectively. The metabolism and excretion of carbamazepine have been extensively reviewed by Morselli (1975) and Frigerio and Morselli (1975).

IX. THE BENZODIAZEPINES

The benzodiazepines are lipid-soluble compounds. Once absorbed, they are rapidly distributed and they concentrate in body tissues. The limitation to absorption is their low aqueous solubility and the possibility of chemical degradation in gastric acid. The analogues containing a carbonyl function at the C-2 position, nitrazepam and clonazepam, for example, are particularly susceptible to ring scission in acid solution, forming benzophenones. For nitrazepam, these limitations combined can reduce the availability of an administered dose by 50% (Rieder and Wendt, 1973). The presence of a methylene function at C-2, as in medazepam, stabilizes the ring to acid hydrolysis.

Basic structure of
5-phenyl-1,4-benzodiazepines

The 7-chlorobenzodiazepines generally undergo a series of metabolic conversions through metabolites of similar activity until the pharmacological action is terminated by aromatic hydroxylation, ring scission, or glucuronide conjugation. The 7-nitrobenzodiazepines can undergo the same conversions but are more likely to undergo nitro reduction to an aromatic amine. The sites for metabolic conversion are numerous: (1) Dealkylation at N-1, oxidation at C-2, and hydroxylation at C-3 are pathways to pharmacologically active compounds. These metabolites, being less lipophylic, do not achieve the tissue to plasma ratios or metabolic rates of the unchanged drug, but not being polar enough for efficient urinary excretion, their action is generally more prolonged. Much of the activity associated with the administered drug can be shown to correspond with peak levels of the metabolites, which readily penetrate neural tissue. In man, hydroxylation at C-3 is a slow process, allowing active *N*-1-dealkyl and C-2-one metabolites to accumulate. (2) Aromatic hydroxylation at the 9 or 4′ position of the 5-phenyl ring, conjugation of the 3-hydroxy group, or ring scission to the opened lactam produces highly polar, inactive compounds that are excreted in the bile or urine. The transformation of chlordiazepoxide, demoxepam, medazepam, diazepam, nitrazepam, and clonazepam is reviewed here.

The metabolism of chlordiazepoxide is presented in Fig. 10. For most of the duration of anticonvulsant activity associated with chlordiazepoxide, levels of demethylchlordiazepoxide or the lactam, demoxepam, predominate (Coutinho *et al.*, 1969). The elimination of both of these compounds is slower than that of chlordiazepoxide. The subsequent metabolism of demoxepam is presented in Fig. 11.

The metabolism of medazepam is shown in Fig. 12. *N*-Demethylmedazepam, diazepam, and *N*-demethyldiazepam are, pharmacologically, the most important active metabolites. The metabolic pathways for diazepam are presented in Fig. 13. The *N*-demethyl and 3-hydroxy metabolites have activity similar to that of diazepam and are known to accumulate in man.

The 7-nitro analogues, nitrazepam and clonazepam, are extensively reduced

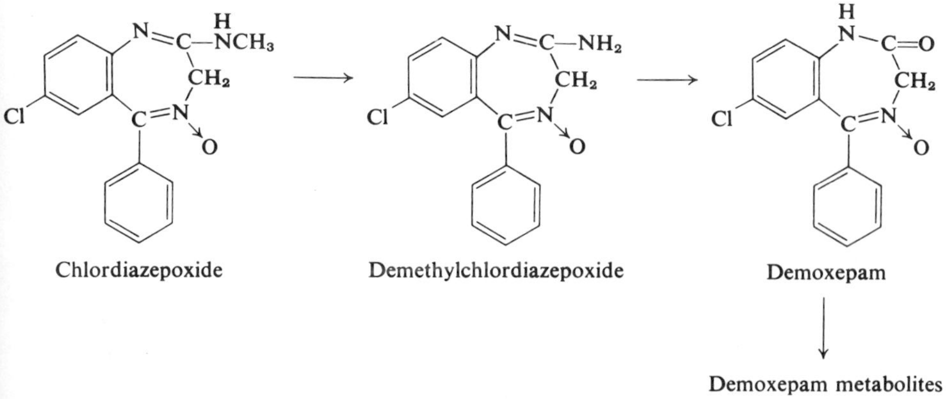

Chlordiazepoxide   Demethylchlordiazepoxide   Demoxepam

Demoxepam metabolites

Fig. 10. Metabolism of chlordiazepoxide.

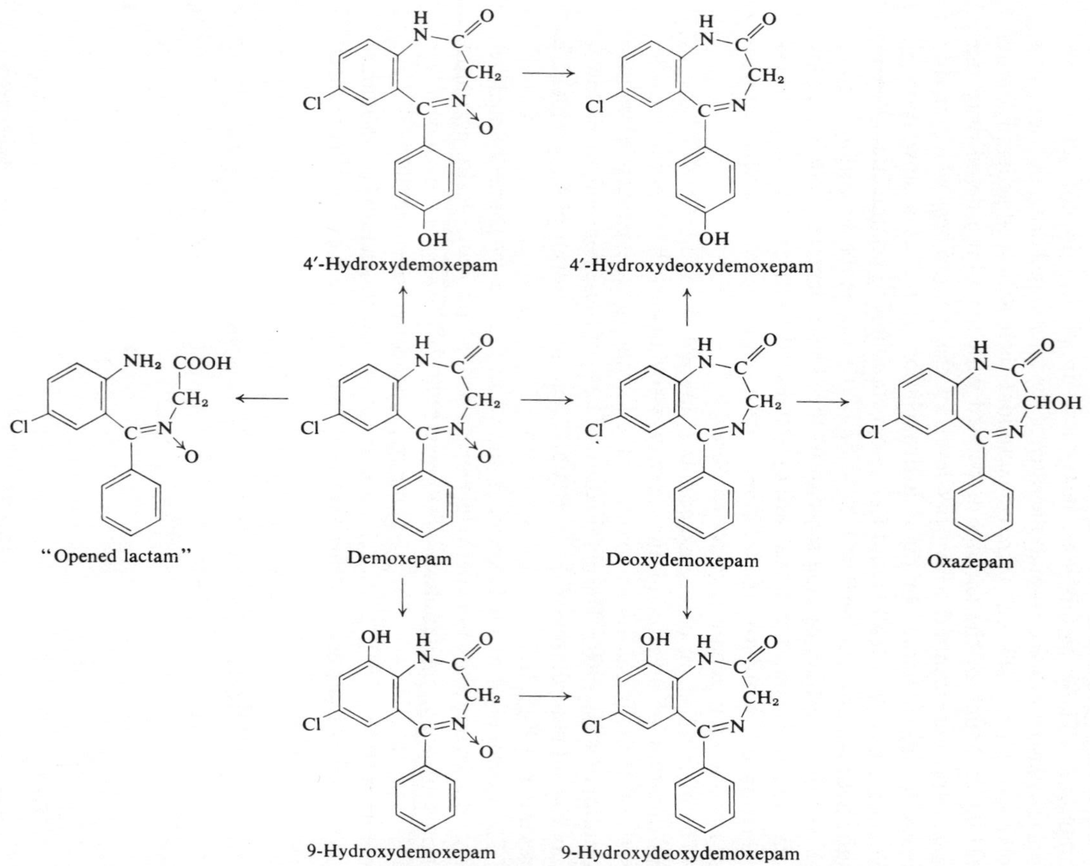

Fig. 11. Metabolism of demoxepam.

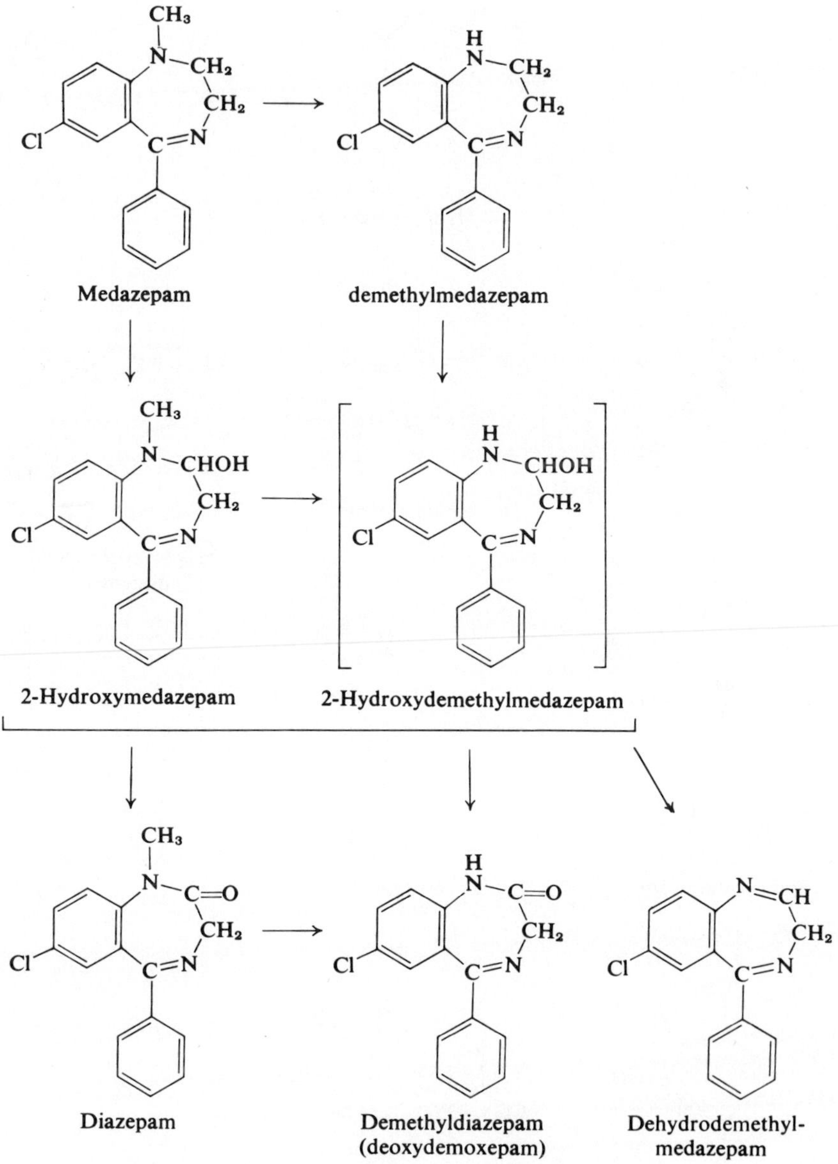

Fig. 12. Metabolism of medazepam.

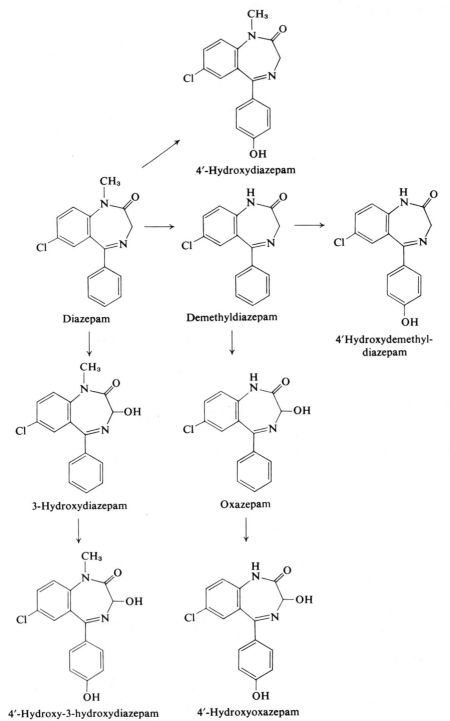

4'-Hydroxydiazepam

Diazepam

Demethyldiazepam

4'Hydroxydemethyl-
diazepam

3-Hydroxydiazepam

Oxazepam

4'-Hydroxy-3-hydroxydiazepam

4'-Hydroxyoxazepam

Fig. 13. Metabolism of diazepam.

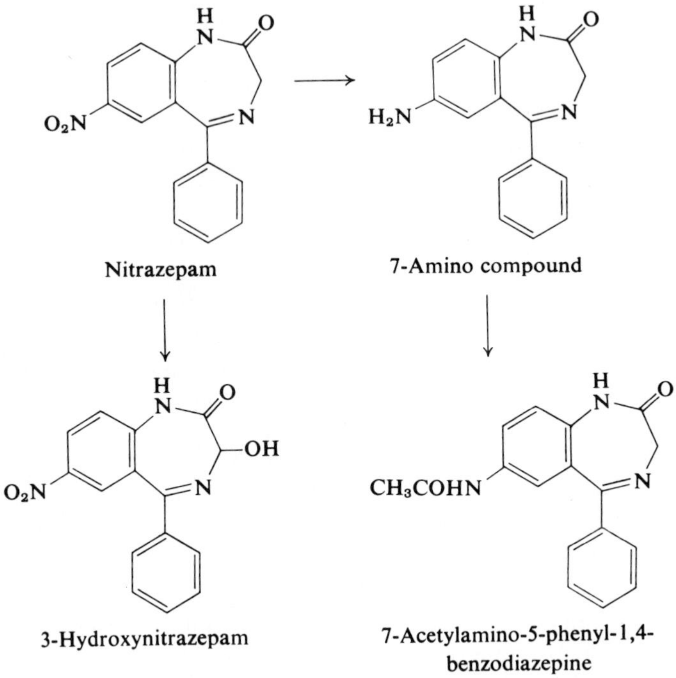

Nitrazepam   7-Amino compound

3-Hydroxynitrazepam   7-Acetylamino-5-phenyl-1,4-
                                 benzodiazepine

Fig. 14. Metabolism of nitrazepam.

to weakly active aromatic amines and then acetylated to inactive acetamides (Rieder and Wendt, 1973). Variable quantities of benzophenones also appear in the urine, but it is not known to what extent these are formed in gastric acid. Hydroxylation at C-3 is a minor metabolic pathway; the product is active. The metabolism of nitrazepam is presented in Fig. 14. Unlike the other benzodiazepines reviewed here, most of the activity following administration of the 7-nitro analogues is due to the parent compound.

Because of the large number of similar compounds in the benzodiazepine class, specific analysis has been difficult. Early gas chromatographic assays were nonspecific, involving degradation of the compounds to benzophenones. Analogues that differ at positions 2 and 3 are not differentiated by these procedures. Marcucci *et al.* (1968) developed a procedure that distinguishes among many of these compounds, but accuracy can still be a problem due to on-column degradation (Frigerio *et al.*, 1973).

X. ACETAZOLAMIDE

Acetazolamide is a rather polar, weak acid. It has a physical affinity for the enzyme carbonic anhdrase, which it inhibits, and for plasma proteins, to which it is extensively bound (95% in man). Its physiological disposition is mainly a reflection of these properties (Maren, 1967). It is well absorbed from the gastrointestinal tract. Because of its hydrophilic character, acetazolamide has rapid access to transcellular fluids and tissue waters. It concentrates in tissues with high carbonic anhydrase levels (renal cortex, erythrocytes, choroid plexus, salivary glands) and in areas that secrete weak acids (liver, as well as the aforementioned tissues). The action of acetazolamide on carbonic anhydrase in the choroid plexus reduces the rate of cerebrospinal fluid production. The concentration in brain is low, about one-half that in plasma, and it is probably localized in the glial cells, which contain carbonic anhydrase. The concentration in tissues that do not contain carbonic anhydrase is similar to that in plasma. Subcellularly, acetazolamide concentrates in the cytoplasm, although some is found in association with mitochondrial carbonic anhydrase (Karler and Woodbury, 1960).

Acetazolamide is not metabolized (Maren, 1967). It is efficiently removed from blood in the kidney by a combination of filtration and the tubular secretory mechanism for weak organic acids. In the minutes immediately after acetazolamide administration, its removal from blood is very rapid due to the high renal clearance. Later, after the drug has equilibrated with tissue carbonic anhydrase, the rate of appearance in urine is slower, reflecting the low dissociation constant for the enzyme–inhibitor complex. The pK_a for acetazolamide, 7.4, makes the rate of renal excretion particularly labile to fluctuations in urinary pH, as discussed for phenobarbital. Acetazolamide is peculiar, however, in that, through its action on carbonic anhydrase, it directly affects the pH gradient across the uriniferous tubule wall. By inhibiting the hydration of carbon dioxide, acetazolamide interrupts the formation of carbonic acid in the tubule cells. Since carbonic acid is the donor for secretion of hydrogen ions into the tubular lumen, alkalinization of the lumenal fluid results. This decreases the proportion of nonionized acetazolamide available for reabsorption into blood and thereby increases the excretion of the drug. However, after sustained inhibition of the mechanism for excretion of hydrogen ion, systemic acidosis develops. This decreases the proportion of blood acetazolamide available in the ionized form for tubular secretion. Thus, the rate of excretion of acetazolamide is closely dependent on the dose, the duration of therapy, and the acid–base balance of the subject.

XI. SULTHIAME

The disposition of sulthiame may also be related to its action as an inhibitor of carbonic anhydrase. It is well absorbed. It concentrates in erythrocytes and accumulates to a lesser extent in liver and kidney. Brain levels are about the same as those in plasma (Duhm *et al.*, 1963). Most of a dose of sulthiame is excreted unchanged; a small amount appears in the urine as an oxidized metabolite (Diamond and Levy, 1963). Much of the clinical interest in sulthiame has centered on its action as an inhibitor of diphenylhydantoin metabolism (Houghten and Richens, 1973). When administered concomitantly with sulthiame, diphenylhydantoin levels rise.

REFERENCES

Alvin, J. D., and Bush, M. T. (1973). *Fed. Proc., Fed. Am. Soc. Exp. Biol.* **32**, 684.
Alvin, J. D., Goh, E., and Bush, M. T. (1975a). *J. Pharmacol. Exp. Ther.* **194**, 117.
Alvin, J. D., McHorse, T., Hoyumpa, A., Bush, M. T., and Schenker, S. (1975b). *J. Pharmacol. Exp. Ther.* **192**, 224.
Azzaro, A. J., and Gutrecht, J. A. (1973). *Neurology* **23**, 431.
Baker, K. M., Csetenyi, J., Frigerio, A., Morselli, P. L., and Parravicini, F. (1973). *J. Med. Chem.* **16**, 703.
Barron, S. A., Darcey, B. A., and Booker, H. A. (1974). *Neurology* **24**, 386.
Baumel, I. P., Gallagher, B. B., DiMicco, J., and Goico, H. (1973). *J. Pharmacol. Exp. Ther.* **186**, 305.
Booker, H. E., Hosokowa, K., Burdette, R. D., and Darcey, B. (1970). *Epilepsia* **11**, 395.
Brodie, B. B., Gillette, J. R., and LaDu, B. (1958). *Annu. Rev. Biochem.* **27**, 427.
Buchanan, R. A., Kinkel, A. W., and Smith, T. C. (1973). *Int. J. Clin. Pharmacol., Ther. Toxicol.* **7**, 213.
Burkett, A. R., Chang, T., and Glazko, A. J. (1971). *Fed. Proc., Fed. Am. Soc. Exp. Biol.* **30**, 391.
Butler, T. C. (1952). *J. Pharmacol. Exp. Ther.* **106**, 235.
Butler, T. C. (1953). *J. Pharmacol. Exp. Ther.* **108**, 474.
Butler, T. C. (1954). *Science* **120**, 494.
Butler, T. C. (1956). *J. Pharmacol. Exp. Ther.* **116**, 326.
Butler, T. C., and Waddell, W. J. (1958). *Neurology* **1**, 106.
Chang, T., Burkett, A. R., and Glazko, A. J. (1972a). *In* "Antiepileptic Drugs" (D. M. Woodbury, J. K. Penry, and R. P. Schmidt, eds.), p. 425. Raven, New York.
Chang, T., Okerholm, R. A., and Glazko, A. J. (1972b). *Res. Commun. Chem. Pathol. Pharmacol.* **4**, 13.
Coutinho, C. B., Cheripko, J. A., and Carbone, J. J. (1969). *Biochem. Pharmacol.* **18**, 303.
Craig, C. R., and Shideman, F. E. (1971). *J. Pharmacol. Exp. Ther.* **176**, 35.
Craig, C. R., Hirano, K., and Shideman, F. E. (1960). *Fed. Proc., Fed. Am. Soc. Exp. Biol.* **19**, 280.
Csetenyi, J., Baker, K. M., Frigerio, A., and Morselli, P. L. (1973). *J. Pharm. Pharmacol.* **25**, 340.
Daly, J., Jorina, D., Witkop, B., Baltzman-Nirenberg, P., and Udenfriend, S. (1969). *Fed. Proc., Fed. Am. Soc. Exp. Biol.* **28**, 546.
Diamond, S., and Levy, L. (1963). *Curr. Ther. Res.* **5**, 325.
Dietschy, J. M., and Carter, N. W. (1965). *Science* **150**, 1294.
Dill, W. A., Peterson, L., Chang, T., and Glazko, A. J. (1965). *Abstr., 149th Natl. Meet., Am. Chem. Soc., Detroit, Mich., 1965*, p. 30N.

DiMicco, J., and Gallagher, B. B. (1975). *Fed. Proc., Fed. Am. Soc. Exp. Biol.* **34**, 726.

Dudley, K. H., Bius, D. L., and Butler, T. C. (1970). *J. Pharmacol. Exp. Ther.* **175**, 27.

Dudley, K. H., Bius, D. L., and Grace, M. E. (1972). *J. Pharmacol. Exp. Ther.* **180**, 167.

Dudley, K. H., Butler, T. C., and Bius, D. L. (1974a). *Drug Metab. Dispos.* **2**, 103.

Dudley, K. H., Bius, D. L., and Waldrop, C. D. (1974b). *Drug Metab. Dispos.* **2**, 113.

Duhm, B., Maul, W., Medenwald, H., Patzchke, K., and Wegner, L. A. (1963). *Z. Naturforsch., Teil B* **18**, 475.

Erlanger, B. F. (1973). *Pharmacol. Rev.* **25**, 271.

Esfås, A., and Dumont, P. A. (1973). *J. Chromatogr.* **83**, 307.

Evans, D. A. P. (1969). *J. Med. Genet.* **6**, 405.

Fouts, J. R., and Kutt, H. (1972). *In* "Antiepileptic Drugs" (D. M. Woodbury, J. K. Penry, and R. P. Schmidt, eds.), Chapter 15. Raven, New York.

Frey, H. H. (1969). *Acta Pharmacol. Toxicol.* **27**, 295.

Frey, H. H., and Schulz, R. (1970). *Naunyn Schmiedebergs Arch. Pharmakol.* **266**, 325.

Frigerio, A. (1972). *J. Pharm. Sci.* **61**, 1144.

Frigerio, A., and Morselli, P. L. (1975). *Adv. Neurol.* (in press).

Frigerio, A., Baker, K. M., and Belvedere, G. (1973). *Anal. Chem.* **45**, 1846.

Gallagher, B. B., and Baumel, I. P. (1972). *In* "Antiepileptic Drugs" (D. M. Woodbury, J. K. Penry, and R. P. Schmidt, eds.), Chapter 38. Raven, New York.

Gallagher, B. B., Smith, D. B., and Mattson, R. H. (1970). *Epilepsia* **11**, 293.

Gerber, N., Weller, W. L., Lynn, R., Rangno, R. E., Sweetman, B. J., and Bush, M. T. (1971). *J. Pharmacol. Exp. Ther.* **178**, 567.

Gillette, J. R., Mitchell, J. R., and Brodie, B. B. (1974). *Annu. Rev. Pharmacol.* **14**, 271.

Glazko, A. J. (1973). *Drug Metab. Dispos.* **1**, 711.

Glazko, A. J., and Chang, T. (1972). *In* "Antiepileptic Drugs" (D. M. Woodbury, J. K. Penry, and R. P. Schmidt, eds.), Chapter 12. Raven, New York.

Glazko, A. J., Dill, W. A., Wolf, L. M., and Miller, C. A. (1954). *J. Pharmacol. Exp. Ther.* **111**, 413.

Glazko, A. J., Dill, W. A., Wheelock, R. H., Young, R. M., Nemanich, A., Croskey, L., Stella, V., and Higuchi, T. (1975). *In* "Prodrugs as Novel Drug Delivery Systems" (T. Higuchi, and V. Stella, eds.), p. 184. Am. Chem. Soc., Washington, D.C.

Goldberg, M. A., and Todoroff, T. (1973). *Biochem. Pharmacol.* **22**, 2973.

Hadfield, M. H. (1972). *Arch. Neurol.* (*Chicago*) **26**, 78.

Harvey, D. J., Glazener, L., Stratton, C., Nowlin, J., Hill, R. M., and Horning, M. G. (1972). *Res. Commun. Chem. Pathol. Pharmacol.* **3**, 557.

Hogben, C. A., Schanker, L. S., Tocco, D. J., and Brodie, B. B. (1957). *J. Pharmacol. Exp. Ther.* **120**, 540.

Hooper, W., Bochner, F., Eadie, M. D., and Yyrer, J. H. (1973). *Clin. Pharmacol. Ther.* **15**, 276.

Horning, M. G., Stratton, C., Nowlin, J., Harvey, D. J., and Hill, R. M. (1973a). *Drug Metab. Dispos.* **1**, 569.

Horning, M. G., Butler, C., Harvey, D. J., Hill, R. M., and Zion, T. E. (1973b). *Res. Commun. Chem. Pathol. Pharmacol.* **6**, 565.

Horning, M. G., Zion, T. E., and Butler, C. M. (1974). *Fed. Proc., Fed. Am. Soc. Exp. Biol.* **33**, 525.

Houghten, G. W., and Richens, A. (1973). *Br. J. Pharmacol.* **49**, 157.

International Encyclopedia of Pharmacology and Therapeutics. (1973). "Anticonvulsant Drugs." Pergamon, Oxford.

Jelliffe, R. W., Buell, J., and Kalaba, R. (1972). *Ann. Intern. Med.* **77**, 891.

Johannessen, S. I., and Strandjord, R. E. (1973). *Epilepsia* **14**, 373.

Kakemi, K., Takaichi, A., Hori, R., and Konishi, R. (1967). *Chem. Pharm. Bull.* 15, 1883.
Karler, R., and Woodbury, D. M. (1960). *Biochem. J.* 75, 538.
Kemp, J. W., and Woodbury, D. M. (1971). *J. Pharmacol. Exp. Ther.* 177, 342.
Kupferberg, H. J., and Yonekawa, W. (1974). *Pharmacologist* 16, 262.
Kupferberg, H. J., and Yonekawa, W. (1975). *Drug Metab. Dispos.* 3, 26.
Kutt, H. (1971). *Ann. N.Y. Acad. Sci.* 179, 704.
Kutt, H. (1972). *In* "Antiepileptic Drugs" (D. M. Woodbury, J. K. Penry, and R. P. Schmidt, eds.), Chapter 16. Raven, New York.
Letteri, J. M., Mellk, H., Louis, S., Durante, P., Kutt, H., and Glaszco, A. (1971). *N. Engl. J. Med.* 285, 648.
Levy, G., and Ashley, J. J. (1973). *J. Pharm. Sci.* 62, 161.
Lightfoot, R. W., and Christian, C. L. (1966). *J. Clin. Endocrinol. Metab.* 26, 305.
Lous, P. (1954). *Acta Pharmacol. Toxicol.* 10, 147.
Lunde, P. K., Anders, R., Yaffe, S. J., Lund, L., and Sjöqvist, F. (1970). *Clin. Pharmacol. Ther.* 11, 846.
Marcucci, F., Fanelli, R., and Mussini, E. (1968). *J. Chromatogr.* 37, 318.
Maren, T. H. (1967). *Physiol. Rev.* 47, 595.
Meinardi, H. (1971). *Psychiatr., Neurol., Neurochir.* 74, 141.
Miller, J. A. (1970). *Cancer Res.* 30, 559.
Morselli, P. L. (1975). *Adv. Neurol.* (in press).
Morselli, P. L., Gerva, M., and Garrattini, S. (1971). *Biochem. Pharmacol.* 20, 2043.
Muni, I. A., Altshuler, C. H., and Neicheril, J. C. (1973). *J. Pharm. Sci.* 62, 1820.
Nicholls, P. J., and Orton, T. C. (1971). *Br. J. Pharmacol.* 43, 459.
Nicholls, P. J., and Orton, T. C. (1972). *Br. J. Pharmacol.* 45, 48.
Noach, E. L., Woodbury, D. M., and Goodman, D. M. (1958). *J. Pharmacol. Exp. Ther.* 122, 301.
Ogilvie, R. I., and Ruedy, J. (1972). *J. Am. Med. Assoc.* 222, 50.
Preste, P. G., Westerman, C. E., Das, N. P., Wilder, B. J., and Duncan, J. H. (1974). *J. Pharm. Sci.* 63, 467.
Reidenberg, M. M., Odar-Cederlof, J., von Bahr, C., Borga, O., and Sjöqvist, F. (1971). *N. Engl. J. Med.* 285, 264.
Rieder, J., and Wendt, G. (1973). *In* "The Benzodiazepines" (S. Garattini, E. Mussini, and L. O. Randall, eds.), p. 99. Raven, New York.
Rollins, D. E., and Reed, D. J. (1970). *Am. J. Physiol.* 219, 1200.
Roth, L. J., and Barlow, C. F. (1961). *Science* 134, 22.
Sherwin, A. L., Robb, J. P., and Lechter, M. (1973). *Arch. Neurol. (Chicago)* 28, 178.
Shoeman, D. W., and Azarnoff, D. L. (1972). *Pharmacology* 7, 169.
Stella, V., and Higuchi, T. (1973). *J. Pharm. Sci.* 62, 962.
Stella, V., Higuchi, T., Hussain, A., and Truelove, J. (1975). *In* "Prodrugs as Novel Drug Delivery Systems" (T. Higuchi, and V. Stella, eds.), p. 154. Am. Chem. Soc., Washington, D.C.
Stillwell, W. G., Stafford, M., and Horning, M. G. (1973). *Res. Commun. Chem. Pathol. Pharmacol.* 6, 565.
Strong, J. M., Abe, T., Gibbs, E. L., and Atkinson, A. J., Jr. (1974). *Neurology* 24, 250.
Tatsumi, K., Yoshimura, H., and Tsukamoto, H. (1967). *Biochem. Pharmacol.* 16, 1941.
Taylor, J. D., and Bertcher, E. L. (1952). *J. Pharmacol. Exp. Ther.* 106, 277.
Theobald, W., and Kunz, H. A. (1963). *Arzneim.-Forsch.* 13, 122.
Van Meter, J. C., and Gillen, H. W. (1973). *Clin. Chem.* 19, 359.
Waddell, W. J., and Butler, T. C. (1957). *J. Clin. Invest.* 36, 1217.
Waddell, W. J., and Butler, T. C. (1959). *J. Clin. Invest.* 38, 720.

Wilensky, A. J., and Lowden, J. A. (1972). *Can. J. Physiol. Pharmacol.* **50**, 346.

Withrow, C. D., and Woodbury, D. M. (1972). *In* "Antiepileptic Drugs" (D. M. Woodbury, J. K. Penry, and R. P. Schmidt, eds.), Chapter 43. Raven, New York.

Woodbury, D. M., and Swinyard, E. A. (1972). *In* "Antiepileptic Drugs" (D. M. Woodbury, J. K. Penry, and R. P. Schmidt, eds.), Chapter 11. Raven, New York.

Woodbury, D. M., Penry, J. K., and Schmidt, R. P., eds. (1972). "Antiepileptic Drugs." Raven, New York.

Yanagihara, T., and Hamberger, A. (1971). *J. Pharmacol. Exp. Ther.* **179**, 611.

Yonekawa, W., Kupferberg, H. J., Cantor, F., and Dudley, K. H. (1975). *Pharmacologist* **17**, 193.

Zavidil, A. P., and Gallagher, B. B. (1975). *Proc. Int. Symp. Epilepsy, 7th, 1975* (in press).

5

CYCLIC UREIDES

Julius A. Vida and Elisabeth H. Gerry

I. THE CYCLIC UREIDE STRUCTURE

Since the year 1912 when phenobarbital reached the market, 19 other antiepileptic drugs have been marketed in the United States up to January 1, 1976. From the total of 20 marketed antiepileptic drugs 3 have since been withdrawn. A close examination of the structures of the remaining 17 anti-convulsant drugs on the market reveals that 14 of them have common structural features; i.e., they contain the ureide structure (Table I).

This chapter describes anticonvulsant drugs containing the ureide structure, i.e., barbiturates, hydantoins, oxazolidine-2,4-diones, and succinimides. In addition two drugs with closely related structures are discussed in detail. These are primidone (5-ethyl-5-phenylhexahydropyrimidine-4,6-dione) and doxenitoine (5,5-diphenylimidazolin-4-one). Glutarimides, which have much less practical significance, are included only in the tables.

Table I contains the anticonvulsant drugs with ureide structure and structurally similar nonureide drugs. The application of the cyclic ureide drugs in various kinds of epilepsies is shown in Fig. 1. This illustration is based on applied clinical therapy.

II. BARBITURATES

A. HISTORY

The discovery of barbituric acid was reported by von Baeyer (1864). He reduced 5,5-dibromobarbituric acid, obtained by bromination from 5,5′-bis(barbituric acid), with sodium amalgam. The structure of barbituric acid was confirmed by Mulder (1873). The first synthesis of barbital (5,5-diethyl-barbituric acid) was accomplished by the alkylation reaction of the silver salt of barbituric acid with ethyl iodide (Conrad and Guthzeit, 1882). Subsequently, Fischer and von Mering (1903) employed a condensation reaction for the synthesis of barbital using diethylmalonic acid and urea in the presence of phosphorous oxychloride. This disclosure not only provided a practical method for the synthesis of barbiturates, but also was coupled with the revolutionary discovery that barbital possesses hypnotic properties.

TABLE I ANTICONVULSANT DRUGS WITH UREIDE AND CLOSELY RELATED STRUCTURE[a]

Class of compounds	Z
Barbiturates	C—N (‖O, H)
Hydantoins	N—H
Succinimides	C H₂
Oxazolidinediones	O
Glutarimides	CH₂—CH₂

Structurally similar drugs (nonureides)

Class of compounds	Z	R_1	R_2	R_3
Primidone (5-ethyl-5-phenylhexahydropyrimi-dine-4,6-dione)	C—N (‖O, H)	C_6H_5	C_2H_5	H
Doxenitoine (5,5-diphenylimidazolidin-4-one)	N—H	C_6H_5	C_6H_5	H

[a] R_1, R_2, and R_3 = H, alkyl, or aryl.

As a result of the discovery, Fischer himself became interested in investigating the properties of other barbiturates. A still better method, i.e., condensation of diethyl dialkylmalonates with urea in the presence of sodium ethoxide, was used for the synthesis of several other barbituric acid derivatives (Fischer and Dilthey, 1904). Soon, a second hypnotic barbiturate drug, phenobarbital (5-ethyl-5-phenylbarbituric acid), was introduced into medical practice

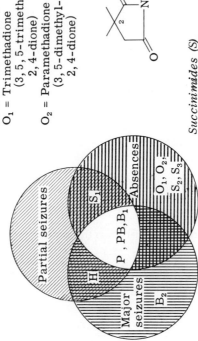

Hydantoins (H)
Diphenylhydantoin (5,5-diphenylhydantoin)
Mephenytoin (3-methyl-5-ethyl-5-phenylhydantoin)
Ethotoin (3-ethyl-5-phenylhydantoin)

Barbiturates (B)
B_2 = Metharbital (1-methyl-5,5-diethyl-barbituric acid)
B_1 = Mephobarbital (1-methyl-5-ethyl-5-phenylbarbituric acid)
PB = Phenobarbital (5-ethyl-5-phenyl-barbituric acid)

Oxazolidinediones (O)
O_1 = Trimethadione (3,5,5-trimethyloxazolidine-2,4-dione)
O_2 = Paramethadione (3,5-dimethyl-5-ethyloxazolidine-2,4-dione)

Succinimides (S)
S_1 = Methsuximide (N-2-dimethyl-2-phenylsuccinimide)
S_2 = Phensuximide (N-methyl-2-phenylsuccinimide)
S_3 = Ethosuximide (2-ethyl-2-methylsuccinimide)

P = Primidone

Fig. 1. Cyclic ureide drug application in various epilepsies.

simultaneously and independently by Loewe (1912), Juliusburger (1912), and Impens (1912). The therapeutic usefulness of phenobarbital in the treatment of epilepsy was disclosed by Hauptmann (1912). In the following years some 3000 barbiturates were synthesized on a trial and error basis. No clear-cut correlation between the chemical structure and hypnotic activity of barbiturates was obtained for many years.

B. ACTIVE CLASSES OF BARBITURATES

In 1951 Sandberg postulated that, in order to possess good hypnotic activity, a barbituric acid must satisfy two criteria: (1) it must be a weak acid, and (2) it must have a lipid/water partition coefficient between certain limits. On the basis of the acidity values, barbituric acid derivatives comprise two classes: hypnotics and inactive compounds (see tabulation below).

Inactive class
 1-Substituted barbituric acids
 5-Substituted barbituric acids
 1,3-Disubstituted barbituric acids
 1,5-Disubstituted barbituric acids
 1,3,5,5-Tetrasubstituted barbituric acids

Potentially active class
 5,5-Disubstituted barbituric acids
 5,5-Disubstituted thiobarbituric acids
 1,5,5-Trisubstituted barbituric acids

In the inactive class, the 1- and 5-substituted as well as the 1,3- and 1,5-disubstituted barbituric acids are strong acids, while the 1,3,5,5-tetra-substituted barbituric acids are not acidic. The metabolism of the last type of compounds gives rise to 1,5,5-trisubstituted barbituric acids, which may be active due to their weakly acidic nature. The other two members of the potentially active class, 5,5-disubstituted barbituric and thiobarbituric acids, are also weak acids.

C. THE ACIDIC NATURE OF BARBITURATES

1. Unsubstituted Barbituric Acids

Due to the acidic nature of the hydrogens, all four hydrogens of the parent compound, barbituric acid, can be exchanged for deuterium. The acidic character of barbituric acid is attributed to lactam–lactim (reaction 1) and keto–enol tautomerism (reaction 2).

$$\underset{\text{Lactam}}{-\overset{\overset{\displaystyle O}{\|}}{C}-NH-} \quad \rightleftharpoons \quad \underset{\text{Lactim}}{-\overset{\overset{\displaystyle OH}{|}}{C}=N-} \tag{1}$$

$$\underset{\text{Keto}}{-\overset{\overset{\displaystyle O}{\|}}{C}-CH_2-} \quad \rightleftharpoons \quad \underset{\text{Enol}}{-\overset{\overset{\displaystyle OH}{|}}{C}=CH-} \tag{2}$$

Barbituric acid contains three groups susceptible to tautomerism. The trioxo form of barbituric acid, therefore, may be in equilibrium with the dioxo, the monooxo, and the trihydroxy tautomeric forms, as shown in reaction (3).

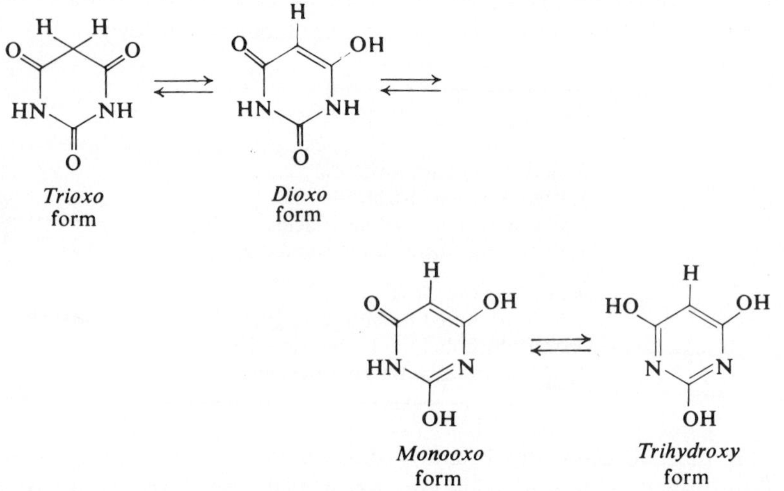

Trioxo
form

Dioxo
form

(3)

Monooxo
form

Trihydroxy
form

X-ray analysis revealed that in the crystalline state barbituric acid exists in the trioxo tautomeric form (Jeffrey *et al.*, 1961; Bolton, 1963). In aqueous solution barbituric acid is in equilibrium among the trioxo, dioxo, and monooxo forms. The relative proportions of the three forms depend on the pH of the solution. In strongly acidic solutions the equilibrium is in favor of the trioxo tautomer, while in strongly basic solutions the monooxo and dioxo tautomers predominate. The occurrence of the trihydroxy tautomer in aqueous solution was ruled out since no ultraviolet bands characteristic of a trihydroxypyrimidine structure were found. The considerable acidity of unsubstituted barbituric acid (pK_a 4.12) accounts for the relative ease of salt formation. Salts of barbituric acid are readily formed by treatment with base, as shown in reaction 4.

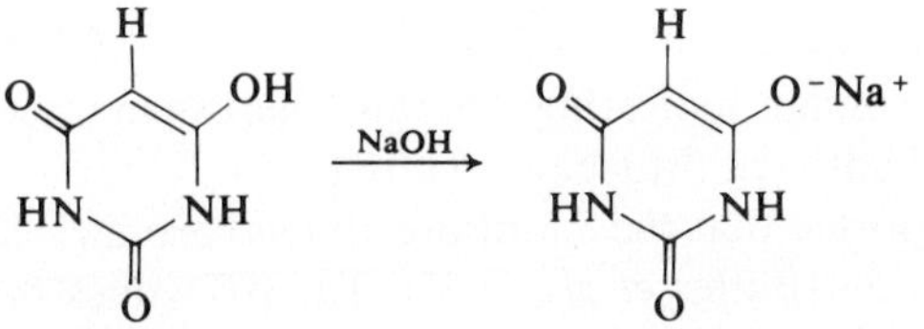

Dioxo tautomeric
form of
barbituric acid

Sodium salt of
barbituric acid

(4)

2. Substituted Barbituric Acids

The number of substituents attached to barbituric acid determines the acidity of barbiturates in aqueous solutions. The strongly acidic mono-substituted (1- or 5-substituted), 1,3-disubstituted, and 1,5-disubstituted barbituric acids in acidic or neutral medium exist predominantly in the dioxo tautomeric form. Salts of these barbituric acids are easily formed by treatment with base, as shown in reaction 5.

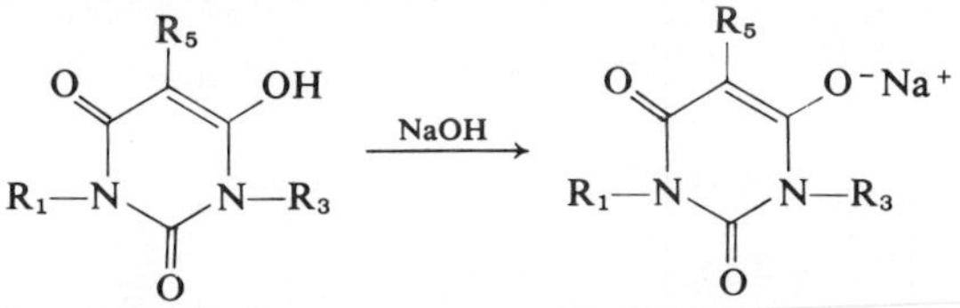

(5)

1-Substituted: R_1 = alkyl or aryl; R_3, R_5 = H
5-Substituted: R_5 = alkyl or aryl; R_1, R_3 = H
1,3-Disubstituted: R_1, R_3 = alkyl or aryl; R_5 = H
1,5-Disubstituted: R_1, R_5 = alkyl or aryl; R_3 = H

On the other hand, the weakly acidic 5,5-disubstituted barbituric acids, 5,5-disubstituted thiobarbituric acids, and 1,5,5-trisubstituted barbituric acids in acidic or neutral medium exist predominantly in the trioxo tautomeric form. The dissociation constants of these compounds (pK_a 7.1–8.1) indicate that they are weaker acids than barbituric acid. Salts of these barbituric acids are, nevertheless, easily formed by treatment with base, as shown in reaction 6.

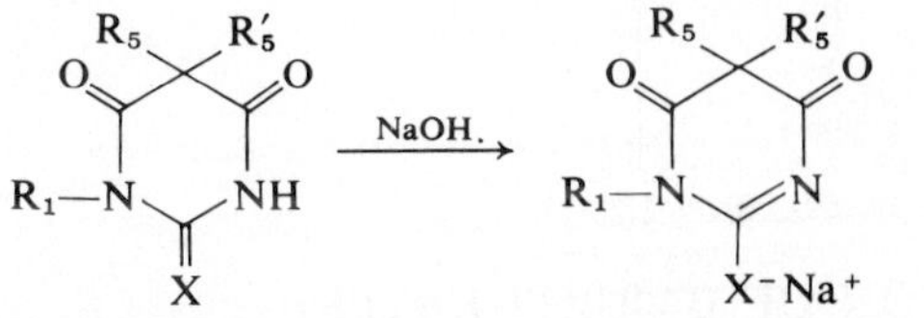

(6)

5,5-Disubstituted barbituric acid: X = O; R_1 = H; R_5, R_5' = alkyl or aryl
5,5-Disubstituted thiobarbituric acid: X = S; R_1 = H; R_5, R_5' = alkyl or aryl
1,5,5-Trisubstituted barbituric acid: X = O; R_1, R_5, R_5' = alkyl or aryl

The ultraviolet spectra of 5,5-disubstituted and 1,5,5-trisubstituted barbituric acids are similar, indicating that tautomerism in these systems involves only one imide hydrogen (Stuckey, 1942).

It has been reported that the 5,5-disubstituted barbituric acids can undergo a second ionization (Butler *et al.*, 1955). The pK values range from 11.7 to 12.7. It is reasonable to assume, therefore, that dialkali metal salts of 5,5-disubstituted barbituric acids could be prepared provided a strong enough base were used. The preparation of a dialkali salt of phenobarbital, as shown in reaction 7, has been reported (Samour *et al.*, 1971).

(7)

D. ALKYLATION OF BARBITURATES AND THIOBARBITURATES

Upon methylation of 5,5-disubstituted barbituric acids, *N*-methylation takes place in preference to *O*-methylation, since in acidic media the ultra-

violet spectra of pure monomethylated and pure dimethylated compounds
are the same as that of the starting material in the lactam tautomeric form.

| Trioxo form (lactam) | *N*-Monomethyl compound | *N,N'*-Dimethyl compound |

If *O*-methylation were to take place the ultraviolet spectra of the pure
monomethylated and pure dimethylated compounds in acidic media would
resemble that of the starting material in the dilactim tautomeric form.

| Monooxo form (dilactim) | *O*-Monomethyl compound | *O,O'*-Dimethyl compound |

On the other hand, alkylation of a 5,5-disubstituted thiobarbituric acid
provides an *N,S*-dialkylated 5,5-disubstituted thiobarbituric aid. Owing to
the greater nucleophilic character of sulfur as compared to that of nitrogen, the
N,S-dialkyl derivative should be formed preferentially over the *N,N*-dialkyl
5,5-disubstituted thiobarbituric acid. Indeed, the dilithium salt of thiophenobarbital, obtained from thiophenobarbital and 2 moles of lithium hydride in
dimethylformamide, was converted to *N,S*-dimethylthiophenobarbital by
treatment with 2 moles of methyl iodide (reaction 8) (Vida, 1973). The

$$\qquad\qquad\qquad\qquad (8)$$

structure of the product was confirmed by its conversion to *N*-methylpheno-
barbital by oxidation, as shown in reaction 9.

$$\qquad\qquad\qquad\qquad (9)$$

As a rule, methylation of the nitrogen leads to weaker acids. The dissociation constants of 1,5,5-trisubstituted barbituric acids (pK_a 8.0–9.0) are slightly higher than those of 5,5-disubstituted barbituric acids.

E. THE EXTENT OF DISSOCIATION

The amounts of barbituric acids in undissociated forms at various pH values can be calculated from the equation

$$\log \frac{[A]}{[HA]} = pH - pK_a$$

where [A] is the concentration of anion and [HA] is the concentration of undissociated acid.

The data in Table II reveal that 1,3,5,5-tetrasubstituted barbituric acids are completely undissociated; 1,5,5-trisubstituted and 5,5-disubstituted barbituric acids are in the undissociated form to a considerable extent; and 5-substituted and unsubstituted barbituric acids are nearly completely dissociated at physiological pH (7.4). All therapeutically useful barbiturates are disubstituted in the 5 position. Other barbiturates, including the 1,5-disubstituted and monosubstituted barbiturates, are dissociated (ionized) almost completely at physiological pH. It has been suggested that these compounds are inactive because they are unable to penetrate the blood–brain barrier (Brodie and Hogben, 1957).

F. STRUCTURE–ACTIVITY RELATIONSHIPS OF BARBITURATES

If a compound satisfies the first requirement for biological activity, i.e., it is a weak acid, it is classified as a member of the potentially active class of barbiturates. In order to elicit biological activity, the compound must also

TABLE II   PERCENTAGE OF BARBITURIC ACIDS IN UNDISSOCIATED FORM AT PHYSIOLOGICAL pH (7.4)

Compound	pK_a	Percentage in undissociated form
Barbituric acid	4.12	0.05
5-Phenylbarbituric acid	3.75	0.02
Phenobarbital	7.29	43.0
Mephobarbital	7.8	61.5
1,3-Dimethyl-5-ethyl-5-phenylbarbituric acid	0	100

satisfy a second requirement; i.e., it must have an appropriate lipid/water partition coefficient. This property, in turn, depends on the structural features of the compound.

Since barbiturates are general central nervous system (CNS) depressants, they can elicit any degree of depression from mild sedation to general anesthesia, depending on the dose and route of administration. Barbituric acid derivatives are often prescribed in low doses as sedatives and hypnotics, while thiobarbituric acid derivatives are frequently used intravenously as anesthetics. In addition, barbiturates may also be employed as anticonvulsants. Conversely, some barbiturates are known to produce convulsions.

A correlation between the chemical structure and hypnotic activity of barbituric acid has emerged. In order to elicit hypnotic activity, a barbituric acid must possess the following structural features:

1. Maximal hypnotic activity is obtained when at carbon 5 the sum of carbon atoms of both substituents is between 6 and 10.

2. The branched-chain isomer has greater hypnotic activity and shorter duration than the corresponding straight-chain isomer.

3. A branched-chain isomer derived from a secondary alcohol is more potent than that derived from a primary alcohol (pentobarbital is a more potent hypnotic than amobarbital).

4. The dextro- and levorotatory stereoisomers have approximately the same hypnotic potencies.

5. The unsaturated allyl, alkenyl, and cycloalkenyl analogues are more potent hypnotics than the corresponding saturated analogues with the same number of carbon atoms.

6. The mixed alicyclic–aliphatic analogues have greater hypnotic potencies than the corresponding dialiphatic analogues with the same number of carbon atoms.

7. The mixed aromatic–aliphatic analogues have greater hypnotic potencies than the corresponding dialiphatic analogues with the same number of carbon atoms.

8. Replacement of the aliphatic group by a second aromatic substituent greatly reduces hypnotic potency (5,5-diphenylbarbituric acid lacks hypnotic activity).

9. Introduction of halogen into the 5-alkyl substituent increases the potency and duration of hypnotic action.

10. Introduction of polar groups (OH, NH_2, RNH, RSO_2, CO, COOH) into the 5-alkyl substituent destroys hypnotic potency.

11. The transition from 5,5-disubstituted barbituric acid to 1,5,5-trisubstituted barbituric acid (methylation of one of the imide hydrogens) does not significantly alter hypnotic activity.

12. Thiobarbiturates, which are obtained by replacement of the carbonyl oxygen by sulfur at carbon 2, produce quick onset and short duration of action.

13. Introduction of more sulfur atoms (2,4-dithio; 2,4,6-trithio) gradually decreases hypnotic potency.

14. Replacement of one or more carbonyl oxygens by imino groups destroys hypnotic activity (2-imino-, 4-imino-, 2,4-diimino-, and 2,4,6-triimino-barbituric acids are inactive).

The following structural features may be responsible for producing a convulsant barbituric acid:

1. Compounds containing at least one aromatic group at carbon 5 are convulsants if the sum of carbon atoms of both substituents at carbon 5 is larger than 10 (5,5-dibenzyl- and 5-ethyl-5-phenylethylbarbituric acids are convulsants).

2. Increasing the size of the alkyl groups attached to nitrogen in 1,5,5-trisubstituted and 1,3,5,5-tetrasubstituted barbituric acids imparts convulsive properties (1,3-diisobutyl-5-ethyl-5-phenylbarbituric acid is a convulsant).

3. Replacement of a saturated secondary pentyl or hexyl group in 5-alkyl-5-ethylbarbituric acid by an unsaturated group having the same carbon skeleton produces a convulsant barbiturate [5-(1-ethylbutenyl)-5-ethyl-barbituric acid is a convulsant].

4. Incorporation of a highly branched aliphatic substituent at carbon 5 into the structure of barbituric acid produces a convulsant even if the sum of carbon atoms of both substituents does not exceed 8 [5-(1,3-dimethylbutyl)-5-ethylbarbituric acid, 5-ethyl-5-(3-methyl-2-butenyl)barbituric acid, and 5,5-di(2-methylallyl)barbituric acids are convulsants].

The two most important methods used in the experimental evaluation of a potential anticonvulsant compound are the maximal electroshock seizures (MES) and metrazole seizure threshold (Met) tests. Protection in experimental animals against electroshock seizures helps to select drugs likely to be effective in grand mal and psychomotor seizures, while protection against a convulsive dose of metrazole indicates that a drug is likely to be active against petit mal. Based on the protective activities obtained in the MES and Met tests, correlations can be made between the chemical structure and anticonvulsant activity of barbiturates.

The following structural features are required for anticonvulsant activity (based on the MES and Met tests):

1. Maximal anticonvulsant activity is obtained when one substituent attached to carbon 5 is a phenyl group.

2. Maximal anticonvulsant activity is obtained when the second substituent attached to carbon 5 is an alkyl group containing two to four carbon atoms (ethyl, propyl, or butyl groups).

3. Replacement of the ethyl group in 5-ethyl-5-phenylbarbituric acid by an alkyl group containing five carbon atoms decreases activity (5-amyl-5-phenylbarbituric acid is less active than 5-ethyl-5-phenylbarbituric acid).

4. Replacement of the ethyl group in 5-ethyl-5-phenylbarbituric acid by an alkyl group containing six or more carbon atoms destroys activity (5-hexyl-5-phenylbarbituric acid is inactive).

5. Replacement of the ethyl group in 5-ethyl-5-phenylbarbituric acid by a phenyl group decreases activity (5,5-diphenylbarbituric acid is less active than 5-ethyl-5-phenylbarbituric acid).

6. Replacement of the phenyl group in 5-ethyl-5-phenylbarbituric acid by an ethyl, butyl, isoamyl, *sec*-pentyl, amyl, or pentenyl group, in order, reduces activity in an increasing manner (5,5-diethylbarbituric acid is more active than 5-ethyl-5-amylbarbituric acid).

7. Replacement of the phenyl group in 5-ethyl-5-phenylbarbituric acid by a methyl or an alkyl group containing more than seven carbons destroys activity (5-ethyl-5-octylbarbituric acid is inactive).

8. Replacement of the phenyl group in 5-ethyl-5-phenylbarbituric acid by a benzyl or phenylethyl group greatly reduces (benzyl group) or destroys (phenylethyl group) anticonvulsant activity.

9. Replacement of both the ethyl and phenyl groups in 5-ethyl-5-phenyl-barbituric acid by methyl groups destroys anticonvulsant activity (5,5-dimethylbarbituric acid is inactive).

10. Replacement of both ethyl and phenyl groups in 5-ethyl-5-phenyl-barbituric acid by methyl groups coupled with methylation of one of the nitrogens retains some of the anticonvulsant activity of the parent compound (1,5,5-trimethylbarbituric acid is active in the Met but inactive in the MES test).

11. Replacement of the phenyl group in 5-ethyl-5-phenylbarbituric acid by an ethyl group coupled with methylation of one of the nitrogens produces a drug with satisfactory properties. Without methylation a less active compound is obtained (1-methyl-5,5-diethylbarbituric acid is more active than 5,5-diethylbarbituric acid).

12. Methylation of one of the nitrogens of 5-ethyl-5-phenylbarbituric acid does not significantly alter anticonvulsant activity.

13. Alkylation of one of the nitrogens in 5-ethyl-5-phenylbarbituric acid with the methoxymethyl group results in a potent anticonvulsant (1-methoxymethyl-5-ethyl-5-phenylbarbituric acid is as potent against MES and more potent against Met than is phenobarbital).

14. Alkylation of both nitrogens in 5-ethyl-5-phenylbarbituric acid with

small groups containing an electronegative atom produces potent anticon-vulsants [e.g., 1,3-bis(methoxymethyl)-, 1,3-bis(acetoxymethyl)-, and 1,3-bis(bromomethyl)-5-ethyl-5-phenylbarbituric acids].

15. Introduction of polar groups (OH, NO_2, hydroxyalkyl, diazoamino, etc.) into the phenyl groups of 5-ethyl-5-phenylbarbituric acid decreases or destroys anticonvulsant activity.

It should also be noted that the structural features responsible for imparting convulsant or sedative–hypnotic properties to a barbiturate should be avoided when the synthesis of a new anticonvulsant barbiturate is being attempted since an ideal anticonvulsant drug should be devoid of neurostimulant or sedative–hypnotic properties.

G. CHEMICAL SYNTHESIS

The barbiturates are usually prepared by the condensation of appropriate malonic acid derivatives with urea or thiourea. These reactions may take place in acidic, neutral, or alkaline medium.

1. Condensation in Alkaline Medium

In an alkaline medium the condensation reactions involve malonic esters or malonic amides, on the one hand, and urea or thiourea on the other (see reaction 10; where $R = OC_2H_5$ or NH_2; $X = O$ or S) (Fischer and Dilthey, 1904).

$$\text{(10)}$$

Alternatively, cyanoacetic esters may be substituted for the malonic acid derivative components (reaction 11) (Bayer Patent, 1915).

$$\text{(11)}$$

In an alkaline medium, cyclization of *N*-substituted ureas also produces barbiturates (reaction 12).

$$\tag{12}$$

In alkaline medium appropriate malonamides undergo a condensation reaction with ethyl carbonate to yield barbiturates (reaction 13) (Shimo and Wakamatsu, 1959).

$$\tag{13}$$

The condensation of malononitrile with urea in alkaline medium produces barbiturates in good yield (reaction 14) (Shimo and Kawasaki, 1964).

$$\tag{14}$$

An improved method for the condensation of a malonate ester with urea uses magnesium methoxide in methanol as the condensing agent (reaction 15) (Lund, 1936).

$$\tag{15}$$

Other variations consist of the use of sodium butoxide in butanol (Halbig and Kaufer, 1934) and the gradual addition of base during the condensation reaction (Phillips, 1948).

2. Condensation in Neutral or Acidic Medium

An appropriate malonic acid can be condensed with urea or thiourea in the presence of phosphorous oxychloride (reaction 16) (Fischer and von Mering, 1903).

$$
\begin{array}{c}
\text{R}' \overset{\displaystyle\text{COOH}}{\underset{\displaystyle\text{COOH}}{\big|}} \text{R}
\end{array}
\quad + \quad
\begin{array}{c}
\text{NH}_2 \\
\text{C}{=}\text{S} \\
\text{NH}_2
\end{array}
\quad \xrightarrow{\text{POCl}_3} \quad
\text{[ring structure]}{=}\text{S}
\qquad (16)
$$

Alternatively, malonyl chloride and urea can be employed (reaction 17) (Einhorn and Diesbach, 1908).

$$
\begin{array}{c}
\text{R}' \overset{\displaystyle\text{COCl}}{\underset{\displaystyle\text{COCl}}{\big|}} \text{R}
\end{array}
\quad + \quad
\begin{array}{c}
\text{NH}_2 \\
\text{CO} \\
\text{NH}_2
\end{array}
\quad \longrightarrow \quad
\text{[ring structure]}{=}\text{O}
\qquad (17)
$$

Another method consists of a condensation reaction between diethyl-malonamide and phosgene (AGFA Patent, 1904) or oxalyl chloride (Einhorn, 1908) (reaction 18; where R = Cl or COCl).

$$
\begin{array}{c}
\text{H}_5\text{C}_2 \overset{\displaystyle\text{CONH}_2}{\underset{\displaystyle\text{CONH}_2}{\big|}} \text{H}_5\text{C}_2
\end{array}
\quad + \quad
\begin{array}{c}
\text{R} \\
\text{C}{=}\text{O} \\
\text{Cl}
\end{array}
\quad \longrightarrow \quad
\text{[ring structure]}{=}\text{O}
\qquad (18)
$$

Malonic acids can be condensed in neutral medium with substituted carbodiimides to produce *N,N*-substituted barbiturates (reaction 19) (Bose *et al.*, 1963).

$$
\begin{array}{c}
\text{R}' \overset{\displaystyle\text{COOH}}{\underset{\displaystyle\text{COOH}}{\big|}} \text{R}
\end{array}
\quad + \quad
\begin{array}{c}
\text{N}{-}\text{R}'' \\
\text{C} \\
\text{N}{-}\text{R}''
\end{array}
\quad \longrightarrow \quad
\text{[ring structure]}{=}\text{O}
\qquad (19)
$$

3. Alkylation of 5-Monosubstituted Barbiturates

Although not practical, it is possible to alkylate a 5-monosubstituted barbituric acid to obtain a 5,5-disubstituted barbituric acid. In fact, one synthesis consists of alkylation, under pressure, of 5-phenylbarbituric acid with ethyl bromide in the presence of 1 equivalent of sodium methoxide (reaction 20).

$$
\text{[ring structure]} \quad \xrightarrow[\text{NaOCH}_3]{\text{C}_2\text{H}_5\text{Br}} \quad \text{[ring structure]}
\qquad (20)
$$

With the discovery of diphenyliodonium chloride (Beringer *et al.*, 1956, 1960), a powerful phenylating agent, it became possible to employ this reagent for the preparation of 5,5-disubstituted barbituric acids starting from a 5-monosubstituted barbituric acid (reaction 21).

$$(21)$$

4. Synthesis of Disubstituted Malonic Ester Precursor

The commercially important diethyl ethylmalonate is obtained from diethyl malonate upon alkylation with ethyl bromide in the presence of sodium ethoxide (reaction 22).

$$(22)$$

Diethyl phenylethylmalonate, the precursor in the synthesis of phenobarbital, is obtained by alkylation of diethyl phenylmalonate, which in turn is obtained from ethyl 1-ethoxyoxalyl-1-phenylacetate by decarbonylation; this compound is obtained by condensation of ethyl phenylacetate with diethyl oxalate in the presence of sodium ethoxide (reaction 23).

$$C_6H_5CH_2COOC_2H_5 + \underset{\underset{COOC_2H_5}{|}}{COOC_2H_5} \xrightarrow{NaOC_2H_5} \underset{\underset{COCOOC_2H_5}{|}}{C_6H_5CHCOOC_2H_5}$$

$$\downarrow \begin{array}{l} 180° \\ -CO \end{array}$$

$$(23)$$

Alternatively, diethyl phenylmalonate can be obtained from ethyl phenylacetate by condensation with ethyl carbonate (reaction 24) (Wallingford *et al.*, 1941).

$$C_6H_5CH_2COOC_2H_5 \xrightarrow{\underset{NaOC_2H_5}{(C_2H_5O)_2CO}} C_6H_5CH(COOC_2H_5)_2 \qquad (24)$$

H. MODE OF ACTION

1. Pharmacological Mechanism

In the normal state the neuronal functions of the brain are at equilibrium between excitatory and inhibitory processes. Energy may be transferred from neuron to neuron by neuronal conduction, an electrical process, or by synaptic transmission, a chemical process. The chemical transmitters responsible for transferring energy across the synaptic space from the terminal branches of the axon of one neuron to another neuron to which the branches are not connected may be excitatory or inhibitory. Convulsions are caused by excessive neuronal activity, which in turn is caused by an increase in the efficiency of excitatory transmission or, alternatively, from a decrease in the efficiency of inhibitory transmission.

Barbiturates are general depressants of the nervous system; they depress both neuronal and muscular activity. By raising the threshold of the postsynaptic nerve cell, the normal action of chemical transmitters does not generate an excitatory postsynaptic potential. The higher threshold required for the stimulation of the postsynaptic nerve cell results from the stabilizing effect of barbiturates on neuronal membranes; they slow down or block active ionic transport across cell membranes.

In experimental animals phenobarbital prevents the spread of electrically or chemically induced seizures. Phenobarbital elevates the threshold for pentylenetetrazole and low-frequency electroshock seizures and abolishes the tonic extensor component of the maximal electroshock seizure.

Electrical stimulation of the brain causes an increased cerebral activity, as observed on the electroencephalogram. Administration of barbiturates brings about a general calming effect, and cerebral activity returns to normal. In general, no real selectivity is observed in the actions of barbiturates. Phenobarbital and other anticonvulsant barbiturates, however, display some selectivity in comparison to the actions of nonanticonvulsant barbiturates. The effect of phenobarbital depends on the dose. In sufficiently large doses it elevates the threshold for electrical or chemical stimulation in the various anatomical areas studied (cortex, subcortex, spinal cord, peripheral nerve, or neuromuscular junction). A paradoxical effect of phenobarbital has also been observed. Small doses cause hyperexcitation and agitation instead of sedation, because the barbiturate concentration is not large enough to depress the excitatory component of synaptic transmission. On the other hand, the concentration of barbiturate is large enough to impede the inhibitory pathways, giving rise to a net excitatory phenomenon

As a rule, depending on the nature of compound, dose, and route of administration, the barbiturates can produce different degrees of depression: sedation, hypnosis, or anesthesia. Anticonvulsant barbiturates display anticonvulsant effects only in doses that usually cause some sedation.

2. Biochemical Mechanism

In general, barbiturates decrease energy production through oxidative metabolism in the brain. Barbiturates also depress synthetic reactions and functional activities in the brain that utilize the extra oxygen produced by excessive cerebral activity. Phenobarbital has a biphasic action. It increases oxygen uptake in cerebral tissues in low concentrations and inhibits it at higher concentrations. The inhibition of oxygen consumption has been ascribed to the uncoupling effect of phenobarbital on oxidative phosphorylation.

Phenobarbital exhibits another biphasic action. In low concentrations it stimulates the synthesis of free acetylcholine and in high concentration it depresses the acetylcholine synthesis. Decreased synthesis of acetylcholine, an excitatory transmitter, may account for the ability of phenobarbital to stabilize membranes and prevent the spread of seizures by decreasing synaptic transmission.

Since barbiturates are lipid soluble, solvation in the cell membrane, which is lipoidal, may alter the permeability of the membrane to xylose, sodium, and potassium ions, which are important in neuronal excitability. This indirect effect on electrolytes may account for the anticonvulsant action of phenobarbital. It has also been suggested that changes in the excitatory and inhibitory processes are caused by a direct effect of phenobarbital: it decreases ATP production, which in turn modifies sodium and potassium fluxes across membranes. The biochemical effects of barbiturates have been the subject of numerous reviews (Aldridge, 1962; Decsi, 1965; Singh and Huot, 1973).

III. ETEROBARB

A. HISTORY

The synthesis of a series of new phenobarbital derivatives has been reported (Samour *et al.*, 1971; Vida *et al.*, 1971, 1973a,b; Vida, 1973). These phenobarbital derivatives are characterized by electronegative substituents attached to the nitrogen of the barbiturate ring. From the several promising candidates, one compound, eterobarb [1,3-bis(methoxymethyl)phenobarbital], has been chosen for drug development. In experimental animals eterobarb displayed marked anticonvulsant activity against both electrically and chemically induced seizures, yet was devoid of hypnotic effects. Therefore, as an anticonvulsant, eterobarb possesses a potential advantage over the parent compound, phenobarbital, a powerful hypnotic drug. The sedative–hypnotic property of phenobarbital often prevents the physician from employing sufficient doses of phenobarbital to fully control seizures. On the other hand, eterobarb, a nonhypnotic anticonvulsant, may provide total seizure control in high enough doses without precipitating undesirable sedative–hypnotic side effects.

B. CHEMICAL SYNTHESIS

Eterobarb is most conveniently obtained by either of the two following procedures:

1. The dilithium salt of phenobarbital, obtained from phenobarbital and 2 moles of lithium hydride in dimethylformamide (DMF), is converted to eterobarb upon treatment with 2 moles of chloromethyl methyl ether (reaction 25) (Vida, 1975a).

$$
\text{(structure: } H_5C_6, C_6H_5, OLi, N, N, OLi) + 2ClCH_2OCH_3 \xrightarrow{\text{DMF}} \text{(structure: } H_5C_6, C_2H_5, O, O, CH_3OCH_2N, NCH_2OCH_3, O) \tag{25}
$$

2. In a two-step reaction 1,3-bis(chloromethyl)phenobarbital is prepared from phenobarbital, formaldehyde, acetyl chloride, and hydrochloric acid in the presence of a Lewis acid (reaction 26) (Vida, 1976).

$$
\text{(structure: } H_5C_6, C_2H_5, O, O, HN, NH, O) + HCHO + HCl \longrightarrow \text{(structure: } H_5C_6, C_2H_5, O, O, ClCH_2N, NCH_2Cl, O) \tag{26}
$$

In the second step 1,3-bis(chloromethyl)phenobarbital (Vida and Wilber, 1972, 1973) is solvolyzed with sodium methoxide in methanol to yield eterobarb (reaction 27).

$$
\text{(structure: } H_5C_6, C_2H_5, O, O, ClCH_2N, NCH_2Cl, O) + NaOCH_3 \longrightarrow \text{(structure: } H_5C_6, C_2H_5, O, O, CH_3OCH_2N, NCH_2OCH_3, O) \tag{27}
$$

C. PHARMACOLOGY AND METABOLISM

The pharmacological data are summarized in Table III.

Eterobarb displayed more potent anticonvulsant activity in the maximal electroshock seizure and hyponatremic electroshock seizure threshold tests than phenobarbital. On the other hand, eterobarb was less active in the minimal electroshock seizure threshold and metrazole seizure threshold tests

TABLE III PHARMACOLOGICAL ACTIVITY OF ETEROBARB COMPARED TO PHENOBARBITAL IN MICE AFTER ORAL ADMINISTRATION OF DRUGS[a]

| Agent | TPE | ED_{50} (mg/kg) | | | | HD_{50} (mg/kg) | LD_{50} (mg/kg) |
		MES	MET[b]	HET[b]	sc Met		
Eterobarb	2	13.5	57	22	47.0	None	470
		(8–22.7)	(33.1–98.0)	(13.8–35.2)	(29.4–75.2)		(376–588)
Phenobarbital	3	20	25	29	9.8	100	270
		(13.8–29.0)	(18.5–34.0)	(22–38)	(6.7–14.2)	(72.5–138)	(216–337.5)

[a] Key to abbreviations: TPE, time of peak effect; MES, maximal electroshock seizure test; MET, minimal electroshock seizure threshold test; HET, hyponatremic electroshock seizure threshold test; sc Met, subcutaneous metrazole threshold test; ED_{50}, effective dose required to induce effect in 50% of the animals; HD_{50}, hypnotic dose required to induce sleep in 50% of the animals; LD_{50}, lethal dose required to kill 50% of the animals.
[b] Unpublished data (J. F. Reinhard, personal communication).

than phenobarbital. Most importantly, eterobarb was less toxic than pheno-barbital, and unlike phenobarbital, which is a powerful hypnotic drug, eterobarb was devoid of hypnotic activity (Samour *et al.*, 1971).

The metabolism and distribution of eterobarb were examined in the rat (Gallagher *et al.*, 1973a). Eterobarb is converted to two major metabolites, 1-methoxymethylphenobarbital (MMP) and phenobarbital. At 10 and 30 minutes after intraperitoneal administration of [^{14}C]eterobarb the plasma contained less than 3% eterobarb, 78% MMP, and 12% phenobarbital. Eterobarb was not detectable in plasma, brain, or liver 60 minutes after drug administration. Peak levels of MMP in plasma, brain, and liver were reached at 30 minutes and maintained through 60 minutes. From 1 to 3 hours, plasma and brain MMP declined linearly with a half-life of 0.8 and 1.7 hours, respec-tively, to 7% of total radioactivity at 4 hours, while phenobarbital increased to a maximum of 93% of total radioactivity (Gallagher *et al.*, 1973a). In rat, approximately 90% of the radioactivity in a dose of [^{14}C]eterobarb is ex-creted in the urine during 96 hours after administration (Alvin and Bush, 1974). Phenobarbital accounted for 5–13%, free *p*-hydroxyphenobarbital for 41–49%, and conjugates of the latter for 24–33% of the dose. It was also found that liver homogenates effectively converted eterobarb to MMP in 8 minutes while, in a separate experiment, in 1 hour only 4% MMP was con-verted to phenobarbital. The rate of microsomal dealkylation of eterobarb *in vitro* is 75 times that of its primary metabolite, MMP (Alvin and Bush, 1974).

An unequivocal synthesis of 1-methoxymethylphenobarbital was accom-plished by oxidation of *N,S*-bis(methoxymethyl)phenobarbital, which in turn was obtained from the dilithium salt of thiophenobarbital and 2 moles of chloromethyl methyl ether (reaction 28) (Vida, 1973).

(28)

In man, two metabolites, MMP and phenobarbital, appeared in plasma within 5 minutes after oral administration of [^{14}C]eterobarb (Matsumoto and

Gallagher, 1975). No eterobarb was found in the plasma at any time. The MMP reached a peak plasma concentration at 30 minutes after administration and subsequently declined at a rate equivalent to a 4- to 6-hour half-life. Although phenobarbital also appeared rapidly in the plasma, a biphasic rise and fall in concentration was observed: The first peak usually appeared within 4 hours and the second within 10 hours after dosing. Phenobarbital was cleared from plasma with a half-life of 4–6 days. The metabolism of eterobarb to MMP and to phenobarbital was considerably accelerated after chronic eterobarb treatment (Matsumoto and Gallagher, 1975).

IV. PRIMIDONE

A. HISTORY

The synthesis of primidone, 5-ethyl-5-phenylhexahydropyrimidine-2,4-dione, was first reported in 1953 by Bogue and Carrington. These researchers noted the considerably toxic properties of hydantoins, especially 5-ethyl-5-phenylhydantoin, and, conversely, the relative lack of toxicity of barbiturates. In an effort to obtain nonhypnotic anticonvulsants in the barbiturate series, primidone was synthesized and tested. Subsequently, primidone was reported to be clinically effective as an anticonvulsant (Handley and Stewart, 1952).

B. CHEMICAL SYNTHESIS

Two syntheses of primidone possess practical significance: electrolytic reduction of phenobarbital (reaction 29) (Boon *et al.*, 1952) and reductive

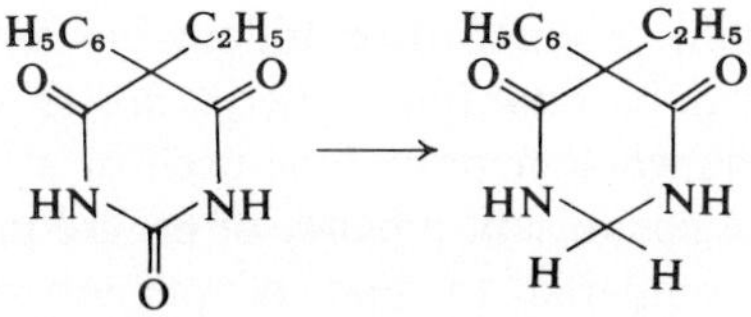

(29)

desulfurization of 2-thiophenobarbital obtained by condensation of diethyl ethylphenylmalonate and thiourea (reaction 30) (Boon *et al.*, 1952).

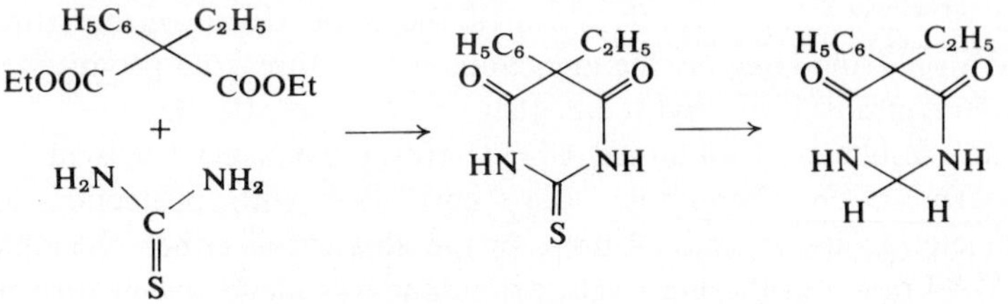

(30)

C. MODE OF ACTION

1. Pharmacological Mechanism

Using a modified MES test (Bogue and Carrington, 1953), primidone was slightly more effective than phenobarbital in abolishing the tonic extensor component of electrically induced seizures in rats. On the other hand, primidone was less effective than phenobarbital against pentylenetetrazole-induced (metrazole-induced) seizures (Met test). More importantly, however, primidone was found to be much less toxic than phenobarbital. A dose of primidone of approximately 20 times that of phenobarbital was required to produce a similar degree of neurotoxicity in laboratory animals. The lack of serious toxicity and the anticonvulsant activity of primidone in grand mal epilepsy were confirmed in man (Handley and Stewart, 1952). The transient side effects (nausea, dizziness, and mild ataxia) observed at the beginning of treatment disappeared in a few days of continuous treatment (Handley and Stewart, 1952).

In mice and dogs, primidone was found to be more effective against pentylenetetrazole-induced seizures than phenobarbital, although phenobarbital blood levels were the same in the two groups of animals (Frey and Hahn, 1960). In rats, the anticonvulsant properties of primidone against fluorothyl-induced seizures were compared to those of phenobarbital. The effect of comparable plasma levels of phenobarbitals obtained as a result of primidone therapy or phenobarbital therapy on the seizure threshold was examined in order to determine if primidone has an anticonvulsant action beyond that attributable to metabolically derived phenobarbital. The results showed that although there is a significant *in vivo* metabolic conversion of primidone to phenobarbital, as evidenced by considerable phenobarbital plasma levels, primidone or a metabolic product of primidone has anticonvulsant properties independent of phenobarbital (Gallagher *et al.*, 1970).

In order to determine whether primidone itself or a metabolite is responsible for the greater anticonvulsant potency of primidone against fluorothyl-induced seizures as compared to that of phenobarbital, the effect of phenylethylmalondiamide (PEMA) was investigated (Gallagher and Baumel, 1972a). Phenylethylmalondiamide has been found in rat urine after the administration of large doses of primidone (Goodman *et al.*, 1953). Administration of PEMA significantly elevated the tonic–clonic seizure threshold and, to a very small degree, the myoclonic seizure threshold produced in rats by the convulsant fluorothyl (Gallagher and Baumel, 1972).

Similar results were obtained when brain and plasma levels of PEMA, phenobarbital, and primidone were correlated with protection against pentylenetetrazole-induced seizures. In the absence of either phenobarbital or PEMA brain and plasma levels, primidone was ineffective against pentylenetetrazole-induced seizures even at brain and plasma levels of primidone fivefold greater than necessary to protect against electroshock seizures in the absence of either metabolite (Gallagher and Baumel, 1971, 1972).

On the other hand, complete protection against maximal electroshock seizures was observed in the absence of phenobarbital (and PEMA). It was concluded that primidone possesses independent anticonvulsant activity and is more potent than phenobarbital in protecting against maximal electroshock seizures (Gallagher and Baumel, 1972).

The aspects of acute and chronic toxicity of primidone were investigated in man (Gallagher *et al.*, 1973). Toxicity associated with first exposure to primidone in epileptic patients was related to plasma levels of primidone itself rather than to those of PEMA or phenobarbital. Both PEMA and phenobarbital are metabolites of primidone possessing anticonvulsant activity of their own. None of these patients had any apparent phenobarbital formed from primidone during the period of toxicity, while half of the patients had measurable but small amounts of PEMA plasma levels. In contrast, subjects on phenobarbital prior to the first exposure to primidone experienced no signs of toxicity in spite of primidone plasma levels that were similar to those in the toxic group. These patients, however, also had detectable plasma levels of PEMA and phenobarbital, but the concentrations varied considerably from one patient to another. This study clearly indicates that primidone itself produced the toxicity rather than either one of its metabolites and that phenobarbital could induce a tolerance to the toxic effects of primidone.

2. Biochemical Mechanism

The biochemical mechanism of action of primidone has not been extensively studied. Like many other anticonvulsant drugs, primidone increases cerebral 5-hydroxytryptamine levels *in vivo* (Bonnycastle *et al.*, 1957). In experimental animals a chronic administration of primidone in daily doses of 100 mg/kg for 37 days increases the oxygen consumption of brain cells by 30% and respiration of liver cells by 20% (Salgarello and Turri, 1957). Folic acid deficiency caused by chronic administration of primidone may lead to megaloblastic anemia (Braun and Kayser, 1954; Fuld and Moorhouse, 1956; Girdwood and Lenman, 1956; Christenson *et al.*, 1957; Stokes and Fortune, 1958; Reynolds *et al.*, 1966). It was proposed that primidone may interfere with folic acid metabolism in the tissue (Chanarin *et al.*, 1958; Baker *et al.*, 1962). The anemia caused by prolonged primidone administration is reversible with the administration of folic acid or vitamin B_{12}. Unlike phenobarbital, which fully protected mice from tremors and convulsions caused by orally administered DDT [1,1,1-trichloro-2,2-bis(4'-chlorophenyl)-ethane] primidone failed to protect the animals from DDT-induced convulsions (Matin and Kar, 1974). The protection provided by phenobarbital was ascribed to the significant increase in the cerebral γ-aminobutyric acid

(GABA) content produced by the drug. The increase counterbalanced the cerebral GABA depletion caused by the administration of DDT. Primidone did not raise the cerebral GABA level depleted in the animals by the DDT dose. Failure to restore cerebral GABA levels to normal may account for the inability of primidone to protect the animals from DDT-induced convulsions. The sodium salt of primidone restored cerebral GABA content previously reduced by isoniazid to normal, but only when depletion was slight (Saad *et al.*, 1972). Consistently with cerebral GABA levels, the protective effect of primidone against isoniazid-produced convulsions was weak.

V. HYDANTOINS

A. HISTORY

The first synthesis of 5,5-diphenylhydantoin was accomplished by Biltz (1908) by the condensation reaction of benzil with a substituted urea. The anticonvulsant action of 5,5-diphenylhydantoin was not discovered, however, until Merritt and Putnam (1938b) disclosed its efficacy against electrically induced seizures in cats. The compound was submitted for testing to Merritt and Putnam because of its low toxicity and lack of sedative activity and its close structural similarity to barbiturates. In the same year, Merritt and Putnam (1938a) reported on the anticonvulsant activity of diphenylhydantoin in man. Since its introduction into clinical practice, diphenylhydantoin has become one of the most extensively used anticonvulsant drugs in the treatment of generalized convulsive and psychomotor seizures.

Although a great number of hydantoin analogues of diphenylhydantoin have been synthesized and tested for anticonvulsant activity in experimental animals, only two were marketed, mephenytoin (3-methyl-5-ethyl-5-phenyl-hydantoin) in 1947 and ethotoin (3-ethyl-5-phenylhydantoin) in 1957. Only one other analogue has since been seriously considered for marketing, albutoin, which is still under evaluation.

B. SALT FORMATION AND ALKYLATION

Diphenylhydantoin is a weak acid as indicated by the value of pK_a 8.3 (Agarwal and Blake, 1968). Under different experimental conditions the value of pK_a 9.2 has been reported (Dill *et al.*, 1956). Diphenylhydantoin is poorly soluble in water. Salts of diphenylhydantoin, which are easily formed by treatment with base, are, however, readily soluble in water. Salt formation of diphenylhydantoin takes place with the involvement of the imidic hydrogen through the occurrence of lactam–lactim tautomerism (reaction 31). Salts of

$$\underset{\text{O}}{\overset{\displaystyle\|}{-\text{C}}}-\text{NH}- \;\rightleftharpoons\; -\underset{}{\overset{\displaystyle\text{OH}}{\text{C}}}=\text{N}- \tag{31}$$

the lactim form are easily formed, as shown in reaction 32.

$$\tag{32}$$

In addition to the imide group, diphenylhydantoin also contains an amide group. Although the imide hydrogen is much more acidic than the amide hydrogen, the latter may also undergo the lactam–lactim tautomerism. Therefore, it is not surprising that alkylation involving the amide hydrogen could be carried out with sodium hydride as a base in nonpolar solvents (benzene) or in DMF (reaction 33) (Orazi *et al.*, 1974).

$$\xrightarrow{\begin{array}{c}\text{1. NaH–DMF}\\\text{2. RX}\end{array}} \tag{33}$$

Using lithium hydride in dimethylformamide, disubstitution of diphenyl-hydantoin could be achieved in one step (reaction 34) (Vida *et al.*, 1975).

$$\xrightarrow{\begin{array}{c}\text{1. LiH–DMF}\\\text{2. ClCH}_2\text{OR}\end{array}} \tag{34}$$

Upon alkylation of 5,5-diphenylhydantoin, *N*-methylation takes place in preference to *O*-methylation (compare with Chapter 4, Section III).

C. STRUCTURE–ACTIVITY RELATIONSHIPS

A large number of hydantoins have been synthesized and evaluated for anticonvulsant activity. The following structural features are important in eliciting anticonvulsant activity based on the MES and Met tests:

1. Significant MES activity is obtained when the hydantoin possesses at least one phenyl substitution at carbon 5.
2. Maximal MES activity is obtained when the hydantoin has a second phenyl group at carbon 5.
3. Replacement of the second phenyl group at carbon 5 of 5,5-diphenyl-hydantoin by an ethyl group imparts moderate Met activity with a slight decrease in the MES activity.
4. Replacement of the second phenyl group of 5,5-diphenylhydantoin

by an ethyl group and, concomitantly, introduction of a methyl group at nitrogen 3 confers marked Met activity without altering MES activity.

5. Introduction of a second methyl group at nitrogen 1 into 3-methyl-5-ethyl-5-phenylhydantoin does not alter Met activity but decreases MES activity.

6. Replacement of the second phenyl group in 5,5-diphenylhydantoin by a thienyl or methyl group decreases MES activity.

7. Replacement of both phenyl groups at carbon 5 in 5,5-diphenyl-hydantoin by isobutyl groups decreases MES activity.

8. Replacement of both phenyl groups in 5,5-diphenylhydantoin by other alkyl groups destroys activity.

9. Introduction of a third phenyl group at nitrogen 3 in 5,5-diphenyl-hydantoin destroys activity.

10. Any substitution on the phenyl group in 5,5-diphenylhydantoin suppresses activity.

11. Replacement of both phenyl groups in 5,5-diphenylhydantoin by benzyl groups destroys activity.

12. Methylation at nitrogen 3 in 5,5-diphenylhydantoin reduces MES activity.

13. Introduction of a *n*-butoxymethyl or benzyloxymethyl group at nitrogen 3 in 5,5-diphenylhydantoin imparts Met activity while decreasing MES activity only slightly.

14. Replacement of oxygen in 5,5-diphenylhydantoin at carbon 2 by sulfur reduces MES and confers small Met activity.

15. Replacement of one phenyl group in 5,5-diphenyl-2-thiohydantoin by an ethyl group increases Met and reduces MES activity.

16. Replacement of both phenyl groups in 5,5-diphenyl-2-thiohydantoin by diethyl, dimethyl, or mixed ethyl–methyl groups greatly increases Met and destroys MES activity.

D. CHEMICAL SYNTHESIS

The hydantoins can be synthesized from aldehydes, ketones, hydroxy acids, or cyanoacetamides by condensation reactions.

1. The Bucherer reaction condenses a ketone (or aldehyde), ammonium carbonate, and potassium cyanide in a mole ratio of $1:3:2$ (reaction 35).

$$(35)$$

2. Aminonitriles, obtained from aldehydes and primary amines, are condensed with cyanates to produce 1-substituted hydantoins (reaction 36).

$$\text{(36)}$$

3. Oxidation of cyanoacetamides with sodium hypobromite yields hydantoins through the intermediate isocyanates (reaction 37).

$$\text{(37)}$$

Isocyanate
intermediate

4. Condensation of hydroxy acids with urea produces hydantoins (reaction 38).

$$\text{(38)}$$

E. MODE OF ACTION

1. Pharmacological Mechanism

In adult animals diphenylhydantoin inhibits maximal seizure activity and reduces spread of seizures from the focus. The effect of diphenylhydantoin is most likely due to its action on normal neurons rather than on pathologically altered neurons or on nonneuronal systems. Diphenylhydantoin exerts its action on normal neurons by preventing their detonation.

Diphenylhydantoin is without effect on two out of four threshold tests. Unlike phenobarbital, diphenylhydantoin does not raise the threshold for seizures induced by 60-cycle alternating current. Diphenylhydantoin, therefore, is unable to prevent all seizure activity after stimulation with a current 20% above the minimal electroshock threshold (EST test). Moreover, diphenylhydantoin, unlike phenobarbital, does not elevate the threshold for seizures induced by a convulsive dose of pentylenetetrazole (Met test).

Diphenylhydantoin is weakly active in the third threshold test; it elevates the low-frequency (six per second) electroshock seizure threshold. Diphenyl-hydantoin, therefore, prevents seizures after stimulation with interrupted (six per second) direct current 100% above psychomotor thresholds (PsM test), although to a much lesser degree than phenobarbital and trimethadione (Woodbury and Esplin, 1959). Diphenylhydantoin is moderately active in the fourth threshold test; it partially restores to normal the alternating current threshold abnormally lowered by acute hyponatremia (HET test) (Swinyard *et al.*, 1946).

The lack of activity of diphenylhydantoin in the EST and Met threshold tests and its poor performance in the PsM threshold and HET tests is attribu-ted to the dual action of the drug. In addition to suppressing the excitatory system, diphenylhydantoin also exerts a moderate blocking action on the inhibitory systems, giving rise to a net excitatory effect. Accordingly, the excitatory effect of diphenylhydantoin predominates over its threshold-elevating effect in the EST and Met tests.

In the MES test diphenylhydantoin modifies the pattern of seizures. It abolishes the tonic phase and slightly exaggerates and prolongs the clonic phase (Raduoco-Thomas *et al.*, 1954). This blocking effect is observed in the cerebrum (Gangloff and Monnier, 1957) and at higher doses in the thala-mus, limbic system (Delgado and Mihailovic, 1956), and spinal cord (Esplin and Freston, 1960) but not in the reticular activating system (Rosati *et al.*, 1967).

Diphenylhydantoin inhibits the spread of seizures by its stabilizing effect on all neuronal membranes (e.g., excitable and nonexcitable) without inter-fering with the normal functions of the excitable neurons (except at toxic doses). Since diphenylhydantoin is ineffective in abolishing the tonic seizure produced by strychnine (Eccles, 1964), an agent known to block postsynaptic inhibition, it was concluded that diphenylhydantoin affects presynaptic rather than postsynaptic events.

The most pronounced effect of diphenylhydantoin, the inhibition of spread of seizures to the entire brain, is also shown by the ability of this drug to inhibit posttetanic potentiation (PTP) (Esplin, 1957). After rapid, repetitive presynaptic stimulation, synaptic transmission may become potentiated (posttetanic potentiation) to include all areas of brain. Posttetanic potentia-tion leads to a rapid and progressive detonation of virtually all neurons in the brain. Diphenylhydantoin prevents the progressive spread of seizure discharge produced by posttetanic potentiation in the brain (Franz and Esplin, 1965).

2. Biochemical Mechanism

Diphenylhydantoin has a marked effect on electrolyte metabolism and ionic transport through membranes. It decreases the total Na content without affecting the total K content in the cortex and other tissues of rats (Woodbury, 1955).

Diphenylhydantoin can also restore abnormal Na–K ratios produced by digitalis (high value) (Helfant *et al.*, 1968) or ouabain (low value) (Watson and Woodbury, 1969) to normal values.

It has been reported that diphenylhydantoin stimulates Na–K-ATPase activity at high Na–K ratio (50:1) but inhibits the activity of enzyme at low Na–K ratio (5:1) (Festoff and Appel, 1968). During seizures the Na content of excitable neurons is increased, which in turn stimulates the activity of Na–K-ATPase enzyme. The enhanced enzyme activity transports Na out of the cell and K into the cell. These changes stabilize the membrane and prevent spread of seizures. The anticonvulsant activity of diphenylhydantoin, therefore, is understandable. The excitatory component of diphenylhydantoin action may also be explained by its influence on the regulatory action of Na–K-ATPase enzyme. Under normal conditions the Na–K ratio is low (Rawson and Pincus, 1968). Under these conditions a small dose of diphenyl-hydantoin inhibits the Na–K-ATPase enzyme activity, which in turn creates an increase in intracellular Na and a decrease in intracellular K concentration. These changes account for the paradoxical excitatory effects of diphenyl-hydantoin in small concentrations (Pincus *et al.*, 1970).

It has also been suggested that diphenylhydantoin may decrease membrane permeability to Ca^{2+} and thereby stabilize membranes against Ca^{2+} fluxes. This mechanism may explain the PTP inhibitory effect of diphenylhydantoin, since posttetanic potentiation is known to involve Ca^{2+} ions (Woodbury and Kemp, 1971).

In large doses, diphenylhydantoin, unlike phenobarbital and trimethadione, does not depress the respiration of cerebral tissue. Diphenylhydantoin decreases xylose concentration (Gilbert *et al.*, 1965) but increases glucose and glycogen concentration in brain (Woodbury, 1954, 1955). Diphenylhydantoin also promotes conversion of glutamic acid via the Krebs cycle to glutamine, GABA, and α-ketoglutarate (Vernadakis and Woodbury, 1960). Experimental evidence indicates that diphenylhydantoin increases protein synthesis, but the claim that it increases the availability of high-energy phosphates is not well documented.

Folic acid treatment of patients suffering from folate deficiency reverses the anticonvulsant effects of diphenylhydantoin, phenobarbital, and primidone. It is possible that the anticonvulsant effect of these drugs is caused by tissue depletion of folic acid or interference with folate reductase enzyme (Smith and Racusen, 1973).

Diphenylhydantoin stimulates acetylcholine release from parasympathetic nerve endings in the wall of gastrointestinal smooth muscle in the heart and in the brain (McLellan and Elliott, 1951). The release of the excitatory transmitter acetylcholine produced by low concentrations of diphenylhydantoin may account for some of its excitatory effects. As mentioned before, diphenylhydantoin also increases the brain levels of the inhibitory transmitter, GABA (Woodbury and Esplin, 1959). This may account for some of the inhibitory effects produced by diphenylhydantoin.

VI. DOXENITOINE

A. HISTORY

Doxenitoine (5,5-diphenylimidazolin-4-one) is a reduced hydantoin having a CH_2 group in place of the CO group at carbon 2. Doxenitoine bears the same structural relationship to 5,5-diphenylhydantoin as primidone does to phenobarbital.

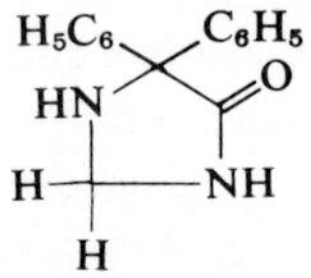

Doxenitoine

Although doxenitoine has been known for many years, the anticonvulsant properties of doxenitoine were revealed only in the 1950's (Goodman *et al.*, 1954). The impetus to test doxenitoine for anticonvulsant properties was provided by the discovery (Handley and Stewart, 1952) that primidone exhibits anticonvulsant properties. It became of interest to find out whether the CO group at carbon 2 is necessary for the anticonvulsant activity of 5,5-diphenylhydantoin. The investigations revealed definite anticonvulsant activity associated with doxenitoine, suggesting that the presence of the CO group at carbon 2 in diphenylhydantoin is not essential for anticonvulsant activity.

B. CHEMICAL SYNTHESIS

The only method of practical significance consists of the reductive desulfurization of 5,5-diphenyl-2-thiohydantoin (reaction 39).

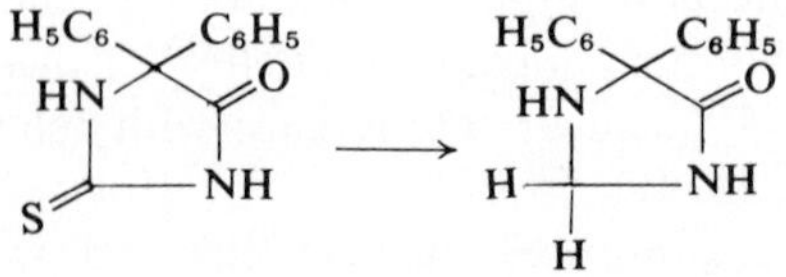

(39)

The reagents used for the reductive desulfurization include sodium in boiling pentyl alcohol (Biltz and Seydel, 1912), Raney nickel in ethyl alcohol (Carrington *et al.*, 1953; Whalley *et al.*, 1955), or zinc in KOH (Cahen, 1962).

C. MODE OF ACTION

It was found that the pharmacological profile of doxenitoine resembles that of diphenylhydantoin and is dissimilar to that of trimethadione (Goodman *et al.*, 1954; Goodman and Cahen, 1959; Cahen and Goodman, 1959).

Doxenitoine was tested in psychiatric patients undergoing electroshock therapy for its anticonvulsant effect. All patients exhibited tonic–clonic generalized (grand mal) seizures as a result of electroshock therapy. Oral doses (0.8–2.4 gm) of doxenitoine prevented the tonic component of the generalized seizure in six out of nine patients. In the remaining three patients the duration of the tonic phase was significantly reduced (Goodman *et al.*, 1954). Continued administration of doxenitoine eliminated first the tonic and eventually the clonic component of generalized seizures. Finally, a "missed shock" resembling a brief psychomotor seizure was the only response to electroshock therapy. In the same test diphenylhydantoin usually converts the tonic–clonic seizures to a completely clonic pattern (Toman and Goodman, 1948). In order to modify the pattern of electrically induced seizures in psychiatric patients, the required doses of other anticonvulsant drugs are usually in the toxic range. Doxenitoine, therefore, is distinguished by its ability to modify therapeutically induced generalized seizures in relatively nontoxic doses (Goodman *et al.*, 1954).

The metabolism of doxenitoine was studied in rats. It was found that doxenitoine was not metabolized oxidatively to diphenylhydantoin (Glasson *et al.*, 1963a).

VII. OXAZOLIDINEDIONES

A. HISTORY

Trimethadione was synthesized in the course of a program aimed at finding new analgesics (Spielman, 1944). A short time later the anticonvulsant properties in experimental animals were discovered (Everett and Richards, 1944; Richards and Everett, 1946). The ability of trimethadione to raise the threshold for both chemically and electrically induced seizures was confirmed (Goodman *et al.*, 1946). Subsequent studies revealed that the outstanding property of trimethadione was its anticonvulsant action against pentylenetetrazole-induced seizures (Toman and Goodman, 1948). Clinical studies showed that trimethadione was effective in the treatment of absences (petit mal) but gave little protection against generalized major seizures (grand mal) or partial convulsive seizures. As a result of the clinical trials, trimethadione was introduced into clinical practice in 1946 specifically for the treatment of absences. The acceptance of trimethadione was complete, since at that time there was no drug available for the effective control of absences. However, the toxic effects of trimethadione soon became apparent. In some cases, it caused acute aplastic anemia, agranulocytosis, and death, even in doses that were not unusually large. A related drug, paramethadione, was introduced in 1949. This drug was claimed to be much less toxic than trimethadione, but it turned out to be much less effective, too (Davis and Lenox, 1949).

The oxazolidinediones, nevertheless, were widely used for the treatment of absences until the introduction of the first of the succinimide drugs in 1953, phensuximide. Today the oxazolidinediones are usually employed only in patients who fail to respond or cannot tolerate a succinimide drug or a combination of other drugs (e.g., acetazolamide and mephobarbital).

B. CHEMICAL SYNTHESIS

Condensation of α-hydroxy esters (glycolic ester) with urea in the presence of sodium ethoxide produces oxazolidine-2,4-diones (reaction 40) (Aspelund,

$$\begin{matrix} R & R' \\ & X \\ HO & COOR'' \end{matrix} + NH_2CONH_2 \longrightarrow \qquad (40)$$

1939; Stoughton, 1941). In the course of the synthesis acylurea intermediates may be formed, which are known to be cyclized by base to oxazolidine-2,4-diones (reaction 41) (Aspelund, 1938).

$$\begin{matrix} R & R' \\ & X \\ HO & C{=}O \\ & | \\ H_2NOC{-}NH \end{matrix} \longrightarrow \qquad (41)$$

Substitution of guanidine for urea in the condensation reaction gives rise to 2-imino-4-oxazolidones, which are hydrolyzed by acids to oxazolidine-2,4-diones (reaction 42) (Traube and Ascher, 1913).

$$\begin{matrix} CH_2OH \\ | \\ COOC_2H_5 \end{matrix} + \begin{matrix} NH_2 \\ | \\ C{=}NH \\ | \\ NH_2 \end{matrix} \longrightarrow \qquad \longrightarrow \qquad (42)$$

The amides of α-hydroxy acids are converted to oxazolidine-2,4-diones with ethyl chloroformate (British Patent 1920) or with alkyl carbonates in the presence of base (reaction 43) (Wallingford *et al.*, 1945).

$$
\underset{\substack{HO \quad CONH_2 \\ R \diagdown \diagup R'}}{} + \underset{\substack{OCH_3 \\ C=O \\ OCH_3}}{} \longrightarrow \underset{\substack{O \diagdown \diagup O \\ R \diagdown \diagup R' \\ O \diagdown NH}}{} \tag{43}
$$

N-substituted oxazolidine-2,4-diones are obtained by condensing α-hydroxy esters with alkyl isocyanates in the presence of sodium (reaction 44) (Rekker and Nauta 1951).

$$
\underset{\substack{CH_2—COOR' \\ OH}}{} + \ OCNR \longrightarrow \underset{\substack{CH_2COOR' \\ OCONHR}}{} \longrightarrow \underset{\substack{O \diagdown \diagup O \\ O \diagdown N—R}}{} \tag{44}
$$

Alkylation of the sodium salt of 5,5-dimethyloxazolidine-2,4-dione with alkyl halides or sulfates in aqueous (Spielman, 1944) or anhydrous (Davies and Hook 1950) medium gives the *N*-alkyl derivatives. Alkylation of the silver salt gives the *O*-alkyl derivative, which on heating rearranges to the *N*-alkyl derivative (reaction 45) (Rekker and Nauta, 1951).

$$\tag{45}$$

C. STRUCTURE–ACTIVITY RELATIONSHIPS

To a limited extent a correlation between the chemical structure and anticonvulsant activity based on the MES and Met tests of oxazolidine-2,4-diones has emerged. The following points are of interest:

1. At least two substituents in the 3,5 or 5,5 positions or three substituents in the 3,5,5 positions are required for anticonvulsant activity.

2. Best anticonvulsant activity in the 3,5,5-trisubstituted, 3,5-disubstituted, or 5,5-disubstituted oxazolidine-2,4-dione series is obtained when the substituents are small alkyl groups.

3. Introduction of two methyl groups at the 3,5 and one ethyl group at the 5 position of unsubstituted oxazolidine-2,4-dione confers maximal anticonvulsant activity (3,5-dimethyl-5-ethyl-oxazolidine-2,4-dione is paramethadione).

4. Replacement of the ethyl group at the 5 position by a methyl group reduces both Met and MES activity.

5. Replacement of the 3-methyl group in 3,5,5-trimethyloxazolidine-2,4-dione by an ethyl group decreases both MES and Met activity.

6. Replacement of both methyl groups in 5,5-disubstituted oxazolidine-2,4-dione by *n*-propyl groups does not substantially alter MES but destroys Met activity.

7. Replacement of the small alkyl groups (methyl or ethyl) in 3,5,5-trisubstituted, 3,5-disubstituted, or 5,5-disubstituted oxazolidine-2,4-diones by larger alkyl groups (butyl, pentyl, hexyl) decreases activity.

8. Replacement of the small alkyl groups (methyl or ethyl) in 3,5,5-trisubstituted, 3,5-disubstituted, or 5,5-disubstituted oxazolidine-2,4-dione by long-chain alkyl groups (heptyl or larger) or amine-containing groups confers convulsant properties.

9. Replacement of both methyl groups in 5,5-disubstituted oxazolidine-2,4-dione by phenyl groups increases MES but destroys Met activity.

10. Replacement of the 3-methyl group in 3,5-dimethyloxazolidine-2,4-dione by an allyl group slightly decreases Met activity. The compound 3-allyl-5-methyloxazolidine-2,4-dione has been marketed in Europe (allomethadione).

11. Replacement of both methyl groups at the 5 position in 3,5,5-trimethyloxazolidine-2,4-dione by a spirocyclohexyl group slightly increases MES but slightly decreases Met activity.

12. Replacement of the oxygen in oxazolidine-2,4-diones in the 1 position (derivatives of thiazolidine-2,4-diones) or 2 position (derivatives of oxazolidine-2-thion-4-ones) by sulfur decreases activity and increases toxicity.

13. Replacement of the oxygen in the 2 position of 5-phenyloxazolidine-2,4-dione by an imino group produces 2-imino-5-phenyloxazolidin-4-one, which retains some anticonvulsant properties and also exhibits CNS-stimulant activity. This compound has been marketed as a psychostimulant (pemoline).

14. Replacement of a methyl group in the 5 position of 3,5,5-trimethyl-oxazolidine-2,4-diones and 3,5-dimethyloxazolidine-2,4-diones by a substituted phenyl group destroys anticonvulsant activity.

15. Replacement of the methyl group in the 3 position of 3,5,5-trimethyloxazolidine-2,4-diones by a carbohydroxymethyl group decreases anticonvulsant activity.

D. MODE OF ACTION

1. Pharmacological Mechanism

Trimethadione exerts an action on both excitatory and inhibitory synaptic transmission, which may account for the specificity of trimethadione for absences. Trimethadione prolongs the recovery period of postsynaptic neurons in the synaptic systems where the repetitive discharges take place to produce absences. This action is particularly effective in the rostral reticular activating system, especially in the thalamus, which possesses reciprocal connections with cortical neurons. There is direct evidence that trimethadione raises the threshold for seizure discharges by electrical stimulation of the medial nucleus of the thalamus of the cat (Schallek and Kuehn, 1963). It was also shown that propagation of seizure activity from cortical focus to the thalamus was blocked by trimethadione, while the local cortical spread of seizures was relatively unaffected (Morrell *et al.* 1958). Since the reticular activating system (thalamocortical projections) is very much involved in the generation of absences, the therapeutic effectiveness of trimethadione in controlling absences may be due to its selective action on the thalamus.

The mode of action of trimethadione is just the opposite of that of diphenyl-hydantoin, which does not affect this region of the thalamus (accounting for its ineffectiveness in absences) but prevents the spread of seizures in the cortex (explaining its usefulness in preventing generalized major seizures). Although phenobarbital is similar in its action in the reticular activating system to that of trimethadione, phenobarbital may exacerbate absences due to the additional central synaptic action that it exerts. It was suggested that phenobarbital potentiates the inhibitory but not the excitatory factors involved in absence discharges by reinforcing central inhibition. On the other hand, trimethadione depresses both inhibitory and excitatory activity in the reticular activating system (Toman, 1970). Trimethadione selectively depresses polysynaptic transmission (Toman, 1970). The fact that trimethadione reduces transmission during repetitive stimulation is in agreement with the finding that it does not affect PTP in the spinal cord or stellate ganglion. In effect, trimethadione, which reduces transmission during repetitive stimulation, does not control self-sustained discharges (e.g., PTP) in a given neuronal system. Trimethadione does not inhibit strychnine-induced seizures, indicating a lack of interference on its part with postsynaptic inhibition.

Trimethadione very effectively inhibits pentylenetetrazole-induced seizures. It was postulated that a competitive antagonism existed between trimethadione and pentylenetetrazole at the excitatory synapses (Toman and Goodman, 1948). Trimethadione could act by preventing the pentylenetetrazole-induced increase in the synthesis or release of acetylcholine in the CNS (Torda and Wolff, 1950).

While trimethadione differs from acetazolamide in that it selectively depresses polysynaptic transmission in the spinal cord of the cat without affecting monosynaptic transmission, the two drugs act similarly in protecting rats against CO_2-induced and CO_2-withdrawal seizures (Withrow *et al.*, 1969; Woodbury *et al.*, 1958). Dimethadione (5,5-dimethyl-2,4-oxazolidinedione), the N-demethylated metabolite of trimethadione, is also effective against CO_2-induced and CO_2-withdrawal seizures.

Trimethadione is only weakly effective in the three electroshock seizure tests (MES, EST, and HET). Dimethadione, which has a similar mechanism of action, is even less potent in these tests (Withrow *et al.*, 1969).

In man only about 4% of chronically administered trimethadione is excreted unchanged (Booker, 1972b). Trimethadione is N-demethylated in the liver (Butler and Waddell, 1954), but no products of ring cleavage have been found *in vivo* (Taylor and Bertcher, 1952). Furthermore, in man, 99% of orally administered dimethadione is excreted unchanged (Waddell and Butler, 1957). These facts suggest that dimethadione is the only important metabolite formed from trimethadione. Since dimethadione is excreted very slowly and does not metabolize to an appreciable degree, administration of trimethadione results in the gradual accumulation of dimethadione in the serum.

Dimethadione possesses anticonvulsant activity on its own (Chamberlin *et al.*, 1965; Withrow *et al.*, 1969). In fact, it was reported that unmetabolized trimethadione contributes no more than 15% to the total anticonvulsant effect of trimethadione therapy. Dimethadione, in large part, is responsible for the observed anticonvulsant effect of trimethadione (Frey and Schulz, 1970).

2. Biochemical Mechanism

Trimethadione and dimethadione have no effect on electrolytes of the brain and plasma. On the other hand, trimethadione has an effect on acid–base metabolism of the brain. At the pH of plasma (7.4) dimethadione with a pK_a value of 6.1 exists predominantly in the dissociated anionic form. Since trimethadione is administered in relatively large doses, large amounts of dimethadione are metabolically formed. Accumulation of dimethadione anion in the plasma causes extracellular acidosis, decreasing the pH and bicarbonate levels. At this point an increase in the nondissociated form takes place. Since the proportion of nondissociated dimethadione to dissociated dimethadione anion increases, more dimethadione enters the brain. This is due to the fact that only nondissociated dimethadione can cross the blood–brain barrier. It appears that the amount of drug given influences the pH of the plasma, which in turn determines the plasma and brain dimethadione concentration. It was found that as a result of trimethadione or dimethadione administration the total CO_2 content of the brain was increased (Withrow *et al.*, 1969). This effect of dimethadione is similar to that of acetazolamide. The changes in pH of brain cells may influence brain metabolic processes including H^+ ion transport, decarboxylation reactions, CO_2 production, and Na, K, or Cl fluxes across brain cells.

Dimethadione *in vitro* accelerates xylose transport into brain cells at low xylose concentrations and decelerates it at high xylose concentrations (Gilbert *et al.*, 1965). This effect is the opposite of that of diphenylhydantoin. In high concentrations trimethadione *in vitro* weakly decreases oxygen uptake of the motor cortex of dogs without significantly affecting uptake of the sensory cortex (Struck *et al.*, 1950). The effects of trimethadione and dimethadione on other biochemical processes have not been studied.

VIII. SUCCINIMIDES

A. HISTORY

Introduction of oxazolidine-2,4-diones (trimethadione, and paramethadione) into clinical therapy in the late 1940's proved that it was possible to market drugs selectively for the treatment of absences. Since oxazolidine-2,4-diones are relatively toxic drugs, a great number of classes of compounds were synthesized and tested. Among others, a series of alkylated and arylated succinimides were synthesized (Miller and Long, 1951, 1953a; Miller *et al.*, 1951) and tested (Chen *et al.*, 1951). Several of the succinimides were found to be effective against pentylenetetrazole and some against electroshock. Since phensuximide (*N*-methyl-2-phenylsuccinimide) was effective against chemically induced seizures in nondepressive doses, it was tried in epileptic patients. Phensuximide was found to be as effective as oxazolidine-2,4-diones against absences but less toxic (Zimmerman, 1951). Although the efficiency was later confirmed, a much higher degree of toxicity was also observed (Millichap, 1952). Methsuximide (*N*-2-dimethyl-2-phenylsuccimide) was tried next. It was found to be effective in absences (Zimmerman, 1956) and in psychomotor seizures (Livingston and Pauli, 1957). The effectiveness of methsuximide in absences and psychomotor seizures was later confirmed, but a number of side effects, including ataxia, nausea, rash, and drowsiness, were also reported (Prichard *et al.*, 1957; Scholl *et al.*, 1959; Rabe, 1960). In laboratory animals ethosuximide (2-ethyl-2-methylsuccinimide) proved to be twice as effective as phensuximide and four times as effective as trimethadione against pentylenetetrazole-induced seizures. Due to its high pharmacological activity, ethosuximide was tested in epileptic subjects. It was found to be effective in controlling absences (Zimmerman and Burgemeister, 1958). It was ineffective in controlling psychomotor seizures (Vossen, 1958; Gordon, 1961). Ethosuximide, however, proved to be the least toxic of the succinimides (Lorentz de Haas *et al.*, 1960) and became the drug of choice in the treatment of absences (Browne *et al.*, 1975). Side effects are occasionally observed in patients taking ethosuximide. Therefore, periodic blood cell counts are required.

B. CHEMICAL SYNTHESIS

Succinimides can be prepared by any of the following reactions.

1. Succinimides are formed when succinic anhydrides are heated in a current of dry ammonia (reaction 46).

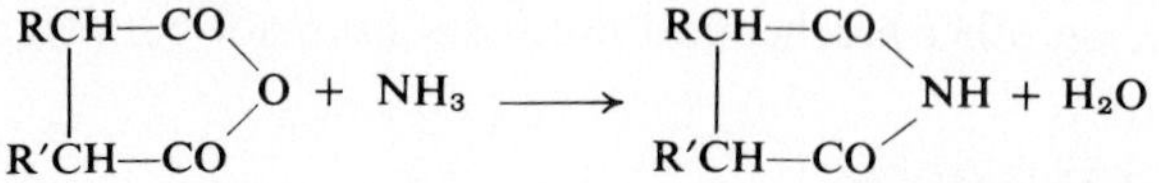

$$\begin{array}{c} RCH-CO \\ | \qquad\qquad O \\ R'CH-CO \end{array} + NH_3 \longrightarrow \begin{array}{c} RCH-CO \\ | \qquad\qquad NH \\ R'CH-CO \end{array} + H_2O \qquad (46)$$

2. Succinamic acid (**I**) and succinamide (**II**) are both readily converted to succinimides when heated (reaction 47).

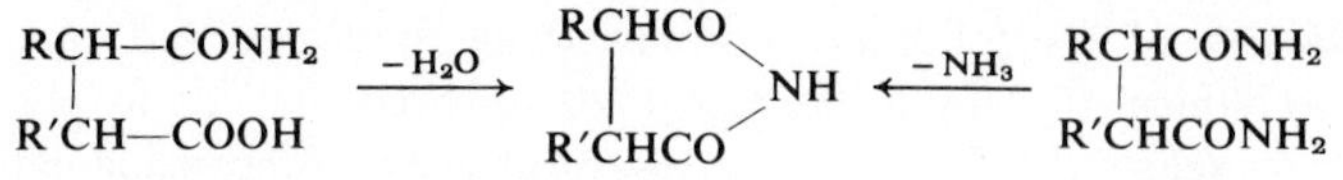

$$\begin{array}{c} RCH-CONH_2 \\ | \\ R'CH-COOH \end{array} \xrightarrow{-H_2O} \begin{array}{c} RCHCO \\ | \qquad\quad NH \\ R'CHCO \end{array} \xleftarrow{-NH_3} \begin{array}{c} RCHCONH_2 \\ | \\ R'CHCONH_2 \end{array} \qquad (47)$$

$$\text{(I)} \qquad\qquad\qquad\qquad\qquad\qquad\qquad\qquad \text{(II)}$$

3. Succinimides are produced from dinitriles by partial hydration (reaction 48).

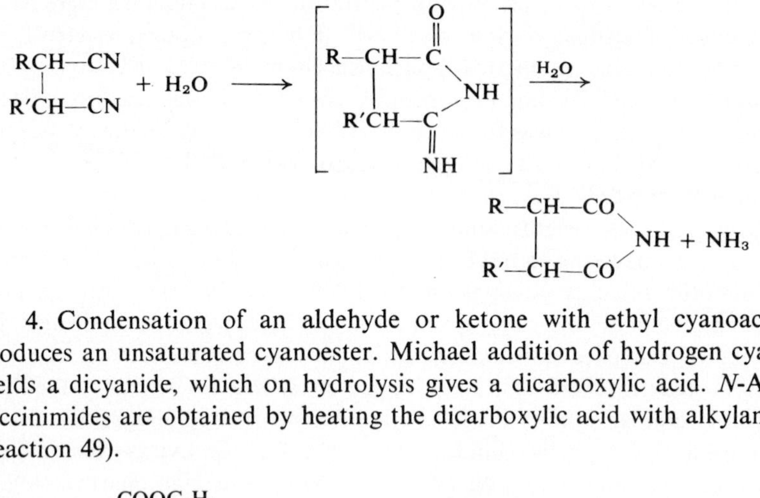

$$\begin{array}{c} RCH-CN \\ | \\ R'CH-CN \end{array} + H_2O \longrightarrow \left[\begin{array}{c} O \\ \| \\ R-CH-C \\ | \qquad\qquad NH \\ R'CH-C \\ \| \\ NH \end{array} \right] \xrightarrow{H_2O}$$

$$\begin{array}{c} R-CH-CO \\ | \qquad\qquad NH + NH_3 \qquad (48) \\ R'-CH-CO \end{array}$$

4. Condensation of an aldehyde or ketone with ethyl cyanoacetate produces an unsaturated cyanoester. Michael addition of hydrogen cyanide yields a dicyanide, which on hydrolysis gives a dicarboxylic acid. *N*-Alkyl-succinimides are obtained by heating the dicarboxylic acid with alkylamines (reaction 49).

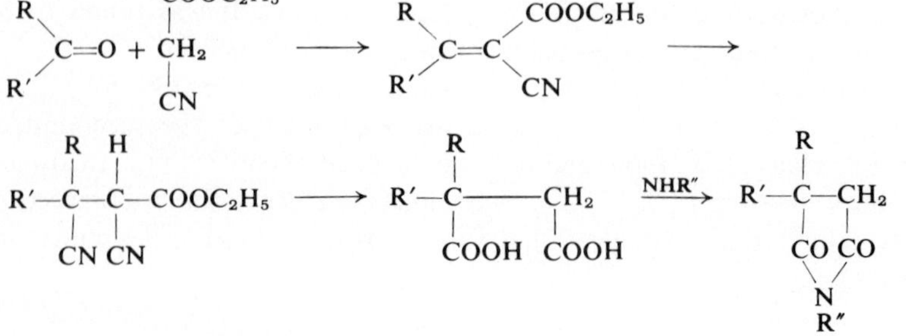

$$\begin{array}{c} R \\ \quad\ \ \diagdown \\ \qquad C=O \\ \quad\ \ \diagup \\ R' \end{array} + \begin{array}{c} COOC_2H_5 \\ | \\ CH_2 \\ | \\ CN \end{array} \longrightarrow \begin{array}{c} R \qquad\quad COOC_2H_5 \\ \diagdown \quad\ \ \diagup \\ \ \ C=C \\ \diagup \quad\ \ \diagdown \\ R' \qquad\quad CN \end{array} \longrightarrow$$

$$\begin{array}{c} R \ \ H \\ | \ \ | \\ R'-C-C-COOC_2H_5 \\ | \ \ | \\ CN \ CN \end{array} \longrightarrow \begin{array}{c} R \\ | \\ R'-C\text{-----}CH_2 \\ | \qquad\quad | \\ COOH \ COOH \end{array} \xrightarrow{NHR''} \begin{array}{c} R \\ | \\ R'-C-CH_2 \\ | \qquad | \\ CO \ CO \\ \diagdown \ \diagup \\ N \\ | \\ R'' \end{array} \qquad (49)$$

5. Alkylation of carbethoxysuccinonitriles and subsequent conversions to the dicarboxylic acid and succinimides provide 2,3-substituted succinimides (reactions 50).

(50)

C. STRUCTURE–ACTIVITY RELATIONSHIPS

The structural features that are important in eliciting biological activity based on the MES and Met tests in succinimides can be summarized.

1. At least two substituents in the 2 position or N-2 positions or three substituents in the N-2,2 positions (one substituent attached to the nitrogen and two substituents attached to the 2 position) are required for anticonvulsant activity.

2. Best anticonvulsant activity in the N-2,2-trisubstituted series is obtained when two of the substituents (one attached to the nitrogen, one attached to the 2 position) are small alkyl groups with the remaining substituent (attached to the 2 position) being a phenyl group.

3. Best anticonvulsant activity in the N-2-disubstituted series is obtained when the N-substituent is a small alkyl group and the 2 substituent is a phenyl group.

4. Best anticonvulsant activity in the 2,2-disubstituted series is obtained when both groups are small alkyl groups.

5. In the N-2,2-trisubstituted series and in the N-2-disubstituted series replacement of the small N-alkyl group by larger alkyl radicals decreases activity (with the exception of the allyl radical in the N-2-disubstituted series, which produces a compound equipotent to the N-methyl analogue in the same series).

6. In the N-2-disubstituted series, replacement of the small N-alkyl group by a hydroxylated alkyl substituent does not alter activity against pentylenetetrazole but strongly reduces the activity against electroshock.

7. In the N-2-disubstituted series, replacement of the small N-alkyl group by a dialkylaminoalkyl group reduces both Met and MES activity.

8. Introduction of a 2-methyl group into *N*-methyl-2-phenylsuccinimide (the conversion of an *N*-2-disubstituted succinimide to a *N*-2,2-trisubstituted succinimide) increases both Met and MES activity without altering toxicity.

9. Replacement of the 2-methyl group in *N*-2-dimethyl-2-phenylsuccinimide by an ethyl group does not significantly alter the activity but increases the toxicity.

10. Introduction of a 3-methyl group into *N*-methyl-2-phenylsuccinimide (the conversion of an *N*-2-disubstituted succinimide to *N*-2,3-trisubstituted succinimide) increases the anticonvulsant activity.

11. Introduction of an *N*-alkyl group into 3-methyl-2-phenylsuccinimide (the conversion of a 2,3-disubstituted succinimide into a *N*-2,3-trisubstituted succinimide) decreases the anticonvulsant activity. The greater the *N*-substituent the greater the reduction in the activity.

12. Introduction of an alkyl group into the 2 position of 3-alkyl-2-phenylsuccinimide or into the 3 position of 2-alkyl-2-phenylsuccinimide (the conversion of a 2,2-disubstituted or 2,3-disubstituted succinimide to a 2,2,3-trisubstituted succinimide) slightly increases antipentylenetetrazole activity.

13. Replacement of the alkyl group in 2-alkyl-2-phenylsuccinimide by a second phenyl group reduces Met activity.

14. Introduction of an *N*-methyl group into 2,2-diphenylsuccinimide decreases MES activity.

15. Transfer of a phenyl group in 2,2-diphenylsuccinimide from the 2 position to the 3 position decreases anticonvulsant activity.

16. Introduction of an *N*-methyl group into 2,3-diphenylsuccinimide increases the Met activity but decreases MES activity.

17. Introduction of an *N*-alkyl group into 2-ethyl-2-phenylsuccinimide or 2-ethyl-2-methylsuccinimide decreases anticonvulsant activity.

D. MODE OF ACTION

The succinimides were not investigated in experimental animals to the extent that oxazolidine-2,4-diones were until after their introduction into clinical therapy. When the tests in laboratory animals were completed it was found that ethosuximide greatly resembled trimethadione. Like trimethadione, ethosuximide was effective against electrically and chemically induced seizures. The degree of protection for the two drugs was similar although at different doses. On the other hand, methsuximide, like phenacemide, was more effective against maximal electroshock seizures than in elevating the threshold for metrazole-induced seizures. Interestingly, methsuximide was effective in experimental animals in the psychomotor electroshock seizure test as well as in patients in the control of psychomotor seizures (Chen *et al.*, 1963). The third succinimide drug, phensuximide, is relatively less potent in chemically induced seizures and is slightly less effective than methsuximide in protecting against maximal electroshock seizures. These observations, along with those obtained for trimethadione, pointed to the usefulness of test methods in predicting activity against various types of epilepsy. Succinimides and oxazolidinediones are particularly effective in providing protection against seizures induced by subcutaneous injection of a convulsive dose of pentylene-tetrazole (metrazole). Since these drugs are effective in the treatment of absences, the assumption is that metrazole threshold tests help to select drugs likely to be active against absences.

To date there is no experimental evidence for the central synaptic actions of succinimides.

The importance of monitoring plasma ethosuximide level to achieve improved control of seizures has been demonstrated (Sherwin *et al.*, 1973). Of 70 patients, 37 had uncontrolled seizures and lower average ethosuximide plasma levels than the control group (33 patients). When the plasma etho-suximide levels were adjusted by increasing the dose of ethosuximide, a reduction of seizures in 18 of previously uncontrolled (37) patients was obtained.

In a comprehensive study 37 patients with previously untreated absence seizures were treated with ethosuximide (Browne *et al.*, 1975). An attempt was made to correlate seizure control with plasma levels of ethosuximide. The therapeutic range of ethosuximide concentration in the plasma was 40–100 μg/ml. The plasma ethosuximide concentration increased with dose. Variability in the plasma concentration produced by a given ethosuximide dose was too great, however, to allow meaningful correlation between the dose and the plasma level of ethosuximide. A 50–100% seizure control was achieved in 35 out of 37 patients (95%), 90–100% control in 18 out of 37 patients (49%), and complete control in 7 out of 37 patients (19%). Etho-suximide produced only minor side effects. The psychometric performance improved in 17 subjects. Impairment of the psychometric performance was not observed in any of the patients.

IX. ADDENDUM: TABLES (1–62)

CONTENTS OF THE TABLES

USE OF THE TABLES

The organization of the tables is patterned after that of the tables in W. J. Close and M. A. Spillman, "Anticonvulsant Drugs," *Medicinal Chemistry Vol. V*, Wiley, 1961, which covered the literature to January 1, 1959. These tables cover the literature from January 1, 1959, to January 1, 1976, and include those compounds tested for anticonvulsant activity in experimental animals and listed in *Chemical Abstracts* under the heading "Antispasmodics" or "Anticonvulsants." The compounds in this chapter fall into the following classes: (I) barbiturates; (II) hydantoins; (III) succinimides; (IV) oxazalidinediones; (V) glutarimides; (VI) deoxybarbiturates. The patent literature is included. Whenever possible the original papers and patents were used to extract the data. When the original publication was not available and only the abstract was used, the reference includes the abstract reference.

The list of abbreviations outlines the designations used in reporting data. Specific data for anticonvulsant activity are listed as ED_{50} mg/kg when the pharmacological methods used were those in common use, essentially as described in Swinyard *et al.* (1952). General designations for anticonvulsant activity, such as MES act., weak act., or inact., are used (1) when methods were not clearly defined, (2) when methods were significantly different from those described in Swinyard *et al.* (1952), or (3) when the results were not expressed in terms of ED_{50}. The designation Act. is used when no data were given, as often occurs in the patent literature, or when only the abstract was available. Generally, LD_{50} for acute toxicity and evaluation of hypnotic and sedative activity are presented just as given in each publication, without any attempt to standardize methods used by different laboratories. The original work should be consulted for further information about data and methods.

The compounds are listed in order from simple R to more complex R, with similar compounds listed together when this was convenient. Compounds are listed as free bases rather than salts, except as noted in the tables. A species belonging in more than one category is placed in the earliest table. For example, a compound containing a heterocyclic and a halide is placed in the table of heterocycles. An examination of the Contents of the Tables will help to explain the organization.

Anticonvulsant activity data for compounds already in clinical use are included when those standard compounds are compared to new compounds. However, not all references to these standard compounds are included.

ABBREVIATIONS USED IN THE TABLES

Abbreviation	Explanation
Act.	No data given; most often a patent or an abstract
^{14}C study	Radioactive compound studied *in vivo* or *in vitro*
ED_{50}	Results determined graphically as by method of Litchfield and Wilcoxon (1949); effective dose in 50% of experimental animals
ES act., inact.	Activity determined by unspecified electroshock method
EST (ED_{50} mg/kg)	No seizure after stimulation with a current 20% above minimal electroshock threshold; results expressed as ED_{50} in milligrams per kilogram
act., weak act., inact.	Results not expressed as ED_{50}
H; not H	Hypnotic; not hypnotic
HD_{50}	Hypnotic activity with results expressed as determined graphically by method of Litchfield and Wilcoxon (1949)

HET (ED_{50} mg/kg)	No seizure after stimulation with a current 50% above hyponatremic electroshock threshold; results expressed as ED_{50} in milligrams per kilogram
act., weak act., inact.	Results not expressed as ED_{50}
LD_{50}	Lethal dose computed graphically; acute toxicity
MES (ED_{50} mg/kg)	Drug administered orally to mice or rats; method essentially according to Swinyard *et al.* (1952) with ED_{50} determined graphically
MES (ip)	Intraperitoneal administration of drug
MES (iv)	Intravenous administration of drug
MES (sc)	Subcutaneous administration of drug
MES act., weak act., inact.	Method significantly different from that of Swinyard *et al.* (1952) or results not expressed as ED_{50}
Met (ED_{50} mg/kg)	No seizure after subcutaneous administration of pentylenetetrazole in mice or rats according to Swinyard *et al.* (1952); drug administered po; ED_{50} determined graphically
Met (ip)	Intraperitoneal administration of drug
Met (iv)	Intravenous administration of drug
Met (sc)	Subcutaneous administration of drug
Met act., weak act., inact.	Method significantly different from that of Swinyard *et al.* (1952) or results not expressed as ED_{50}
MMS (ED_{50} mg/kg)	Prevention of hindleg tonic extensor component of maximal (iv) pentylenetetrazole seizures in rats or mice; ED_{50} mg/kg determined graphically
MMS act., weak act., inact.	Results not expressed as ED_{50}
Other studies	Includes enzyme, tissue, response, or time studies in experimental animals
PsM (ED_{50} mg/kg)	No seizure after stimulation with unidirectional current at intensity twice threshold; results expressed as ED_{50} determined graphically
act., weak act., inact.	Results not expressed as ED_{50}
S; not S	Sedative; not sedative

I. BARBITURATES

A. BARBITURATES WITH ONLY ALIPHATIC HYDROCARBON SUBSTITUENTS

TABLE 1

$$\begin{array}{c} \text{CO}-\text{NH} \\ R-C \qquad \text{CO} \\ R^1 \qquad \text{CO}-\text{N}-R^2 \end{array}$$

R—	R^1—	R^2—	Activity	Reference
C_2H_5—	$CH_3CH_2CH_2CH(CH_3)$—	H—	MES (ip) 10.5, MMS 12.5, H, S, LD_{50} 103 Other studies	Badische Anilin (1971) Weinreich and Clark (1970)
CH_2=CH—	$CH_3CH_2CH_2CH(CH_3)$—	H—	MES (ip) 17, MMS 12, H, S, LD_{50} 188	Badische Anilin (1971)
CH_2=CH—	$CH_3CH_2CH(C_2H_5)$—	H—	MES (ip) 16, MMS 13, H, S, LD_{50} 196	Badische Anilin (1971)
CH_2=CHCH$_2$—	$CH_3CH_2CH_2CH(CH_3)$—	H—	R(+) isomer: Met (ip) 48, LD_{50} 137; S(−) isomer: Met (ip) 46, LD_{50} 72; racemate: Met (ip) 72, LD_{50} 112	Haley and Gidley (1970)
CH_2=CHCH$_2$—	$(CH_3)_3CCH_2$—	H—	Act., S	Brandstrom (1959)
CH≡CCH$_2$—	$CH_3CH_2CH_2CH(CH_3)$—	H—	Met act.	Martin et al. (1959)
C_2H_5—	C_2H_5—	CH_2=CHCH$_2$—	Met act., H	Prastowski and Zak (1966)
CH≡CCH$_2$—	$CH_3CH_2CH_2CH(CH_3)$—	CH_3—	Met act.	Martin et al. (1959)

B. BARBITURATES WITH AROMATIC HYDROCARBON SUBSTITUENTS

TABLE 2

$$\begin{array}{c} R \\ H_5C_6 \end{array}\!\!\!\!\!\!C\!\!\!\!\!\!\begin{array}{c} CO\!-\!N\!-\!R^1 \\ | \\ CO \\ | \\ CO\!-\!N\!-\!R^2 \end{array}$$

R—	R¹—	R²—	Activity	Reference
H—	H—	H—	Inact.	Craig (1964)
C_2H_5—	H—	H—	MES 27.5, Met 24.5, LD_{50} 250	Swinyard et al. (1963)
			MES 24, Met 15, LD_{50} 263	Gesler et al. (1961)
			MES 25, Met 35, HET 25 EST 35, LD_{50} 250	Craig (1964)
			MES 20, Met 9.8, HD_{50} 100, LD_{50} 270	Vida et al. (1973a)
			MES 50, Met 12.5	Raines et al. (1973)
			MES (ip) 0.078 mmole/kg, Met (ip) 0.042 mmole/kg	Witiak et al. (1972)
			MES 31, other studies	Rapport and Kupferberg (1973)
			Met act., other studies	Enebäck and Alberty (1965)
			Other studies	Baumel et al. (1973), Craig and Shideman (1971) Frey and Magnussen (1971) Weinreich and Clark (1970) Dick and Mitchell (1967)
			MES 61 μmoles/kg, Met 65 μmoles/kg, LD_{50} 1180 μmoles/kg	
			MES act., S. LD_{50} 168	Frommel et al. (1961)

(continued)

TABLE 2—*Continued*

R—	R¹—	R²—	Activity	Reference
C_6H_5—	H—	H—	MES (ip) 63, MES (po) 320, Met (ip) 26, Met (po) 57, LD_{50} 550	Raines *et al.* (1973)
C_2H_5—	H—	CH_3—	MES 50, Met 35, EST 10, HET 10, LD_{50} 250	Craig (1964)
C_2H_5—	H—	C_2H_5—	MES 16, Met 24, HD_{50} 180, LD_{50} ca. 300 MES act., S Other studies	Vida *et al.* (1973a,b) Frommel *et al.* (1961) Craig and Shideman (1971)
C_2H_5—	H—	$C_6H_5CH_2$—	MES 30, Met 18, HD_{50} > 200 < 400, LD_{50} ca. 820	Vida *et al.* (1973b)
C_2H_5—	CH_3—	CH_3—	MES ca. 340, Met ca. 120, HD_{50} > 800, LD_{50} > 800	Vida *et al.* (1973b)
C_2H_5—	C_2H_5—	C_2H_5—	MES ca. 21, Met ca. 15, HD_{50} ca. 190, LD_{50} > 250 < 500	Vida *et al.* (1973b)
C_2H_5—	C_2H_5—	$C_6H_5CH_2$—	MES inact., Met inact., LD_{50} > 1000	Vida *et al.* (1973b)
C_2H_5—	$C_6H_5CH_2$—	$C_6H_5CH_2$—	MES > 100 < 500, Met ca. 500, HD_{50} ca. 500, LD_{50} > 500	Vida *et al.* (1973b)

C. BARBITURATES WITH HETEROCYCLIC SUBSTITUENTS

TABLE 3 MISCELLANEOUS HETEROCYCLES

$$R-\underset{H_5C_2}{\overset{CO-N-R^1}{\underset{}{\overset{}{C}}}}\;\;\begin{array}{c}CO\\CO-N-R^2\end{array}$$

R—	R^1—	R^2	Activity	Reference
CH$_2$— (furyl)	H—	H—	Met act., H, LD$_{50}$ 250	Krnjević et al. (1966)
CH(OH)CH$_2$— (pyridyl)	H—	H—	Met inact., H	Prastowski and Zak (1966)
C$_6$H$_5$—	NCH$_2$— (piperidino)	H—	MES < 12.5, MES < 3.12, HD$_{50}$ > 250 < 500, LD$_{50}$ > 250 < 500	Vida et al. (1973a)
C$_6$H$_5$—	NCH$_2$CH$_2$— (piperidino)	H—	Act.	Fujinaga and Negishi (1960)
C$_6$H$_5$—	NCH$_2$CH$_2$CH$_2$— (piperidino)	H—	Act.	Fujinaga and Negishi (1960)
C$_6$H$_5$—	N—CH$_2$— (morpholino)	H—	EtOH salt: MES 12.5, Met ca. 50, HD$_{50}$ 250, LD$_{50}$ > 250 < 500; HCl salt: MES ca. 25, Met 3.12, HD$_{50}$ > 250 < 500, LD$_{50}$ > 250 < 500	Vida et al. (1973a) - Vida (1975b)
C$_6$H$_5$—	NCH$_2$CH$_2$COCH$_2$— (piperidino)	H—	Met inact., LD$_{50}$ 410	Fujinaga et al. (1961)
p-ClC$_6$H$_4$—	NCH$_2$CH$_2$— (piperidino)	H—	Act.	Fujinaga and Negishi (1960)
C$_6$H$_5$—	NCH$_2$CH$_2$COCH$_2$— (piperidino)	NCH$_2$CH$_2$COCH$_2$— (piperidino)	Met inact., LD$_{50}$ 110	Fujinaga et al. (1961)

D. BARBITURATES WITH HETEROATOMS IN NONHETEROCYCLIC SYSTEMS

TABLE 4 ALCOHOLS

$$R{-}C{<}^{CO-NH}_{R^1}{\diagdown}^{CO}_{CO-N-R^2}$$

R—	R¹—	R²—	Activity	Reference
C$_2$H$_5$—	HOCH$_2$CH$_2$—	H—	Met inact., not H	Prastowski and Zak (1966)
C$_2$H$_5$—	CH$_3$CH$_2$C(OH)(CH$_3$)CH$_2$—	H—	Met inact., H	Prastowski and Zak (1966)
C$_2$H$_5$—	CH$_3$CH(CH$_3$)C(OH)(CH$_3$)CH$_2$—	H—	Met inact., not H	Prastowski and Zak (1966)
C$_2$H$_5$—	Cyclo-C$_6$H$_{11}$CH(OH)CH$_2$—	H—	Met inact.,H	Prastowski and Zak (1966)
C$_2$H$_5$—	p-HOC$_6$H$_4$—	H—	MES 380, Met 400, EST 250, HET 150, LD$_{50}$ 2000	Craig (1964)
CH$_2$=CHCH$_2$—	CH$_3$CH(OH)CH$_2$—	H—	Met act.	Hommel (1965)
CH$_3$CH(CH$_3$)CH(CH$_3$)—	CH$_3$CH(OH)CH$_2$—	H—	Met act., not H, S, LD$_{50}$ 2200	Bobrański and Pomorski (1967)
C$_2$H$_5$—	C$_2$H$_5$	CH$_3$CH(OH)CH$_2$—	Met inact., H	Prastowski and Zak (1966)
C$_2$H$_5$—	C$_6$H$_5$—	HOCH$_2$CH$_2$—	Act.	Fujinaga and Negishi (1960)
C$_2$H$_5$—	p-ClC$_6$H$_4$—	HOCH$_2$CH$_2$—	Act.	Fujinaga and Negishi (1960)

TABLE 5 AMINES

$$R-\underset{H_5C_2}{\overset{CO-N-R^1}{\underset{|}{\overset{|}{C}}}}\underset{CO-N-R^2}{\overset{C}{\underset{}{}}}$$

R—	R¹—	R²—	Activity	Reference
C_6H_5—	$(CH_3)_2NCH_2CH_2$—	H—	Act.	Fujinaga and Negishi (1960)
C_6H_5—	$(C_2H_5)_2NCH_2CH_2$—	H—	Act.	Fujinaga and Negishi (1960)
C_6H_5—	$(CH_3)_2NCH_2CH_2CH_2$—	H—	Act.	Fujinaga and Negishi (1960)
C_6H_5—	$(C_2H_5)NCH_2CH_2CH_2$—	H—	Act.	Fujinaga and Negishi (1960)
C_6H_5—	$(CH_3)_2NCH_2CH_2CH(C_6H_5)$—	H—	Met weak act., LD_{50} 1100	Fujinaga et al. (1961)
C_6H_5—	$(CH_3)_2NCH_2CH_2COCH_2$—	H—	Met inact., LD_{50} 420	Fujinaga et al. (1961)
C_6H_5—	$(CH_3)_2NCH_2CH_2OCOCH_2$—	H—	Met inact., LD_{50} 1050	Fujinaga et al. (1961)
$p\text{-}ClC_6H_5$—	$(CH_3)_2NCH_2CH_2$—	H—	Act.	Fujinaga and Negishi (1960)
$p\text{-}ClC_6H_5$—	$(C_2H_5)_2NCH_2CH_2$—	H—	Act.	Fujinaga and Negishi (1960)
$p\text{-}NH_2C_6H_5$—	CH_3—	H—	MES 100, Met 200, EST 60, HET 60, LD_{50} 650	Craig (1964)
C_6H_5—	$(CH_3)_2N(CH_2)_2CH(C_6H_5)$—	$(CH_3)_2N(CH_2)_2CH(C_6H_5)$—	Met act., LD_{50} 680	Fujinaga and Negishi (1960)
C_6H_5—	$(CH_3)_2NCH_2COCH_2$—	$(CH_3)_2NCH_2COCH_2$—	Met inact., LD_{50} 100	Fujinaga et al. (1961)
C_6H_5—	$(CH_3)_2NCH_2CH_2OCOCH_2$—	$(CH_3)_2NCH_2CH_2OCOCH_2$—	Met inact., LD_{50} 1100	Fujinaga et al. (1961)

TABLE 6   CARBAMYL SUBSTITUENTS[a]

$$\begin{array}{c} H_5C_2 \\ \diagdown \\ \diagup \quad \\ H_5C_6 \end{array} C \begin{array}{c} CO{-}N{-}R \\ | \qquad | \\ \quad CO \\ | \qquad | \\ CO{-}N{-}R^1 \end{array}$$

R—	R¹—	Activity
H—	$NH_2CO_2CHCH_2$— CH_2OCH_3	MES act., S, LD_{50} 618
H—	$NH_2CO_2CHCH_2$— $CH_2OC_2H_5$	MES act., S, LD_{50} 590
H—	$NH_2CO_2CHCH_2$— $CH_2OC_3H_7$	MES act., S, LD_{50} 830
H—	$NH_2CO_2CHCH_2$— $CH_2OCH(CH_3)CH_3$	MES act., S, LD_{50} 660
H—	$NH_2CO_2CHCH_2$— $CH_2OCH_2CH{=}CH_2$	MES act., LD_{50} 830
H—	$NH_2CO_2CHCH_2$— $CH_2O(CH_2)_3CH_3$	MES act., LD_{50} 1065
H—	$NH_2CO_2CHCH_2$— $CH_2OCH_2CH(CH_3)_2$	MES act., S, LD_{50} 710
H—	$NH_2CO_2CHCH_2$— $CH_2O(CH_2)_4CH_3$	MES act., S, LD_{50} ca. 1000
H—	$NH_2CO_2CHCH_2$— $CH_2O(CH_2)_2CH(CH_3)_2$	MES act., LD_{50} > 500
H—	$NH_2CO_2CHCH_2$— $CH_2O(CH_2)_3CH_3$	MES act., S, LD_{50} ca. 750
H—	$(C_2H_5)_2NCO_2CHCH_2$— CH_2OCH_3	MES weakly act., not S, LD_{50} > 1000
H—	$(C_2H_5)_2NCO_2CHCH_2$— $CH_2OCH(CH_3)_2$	MES inact., LD_{50} > 2000
H—	$[(CH_3)_2CH]_2NCO_2CHCH_2$— $CH_2OCH_2CH(CH_3)_2$	MES inact., not S, LD_{50} > 750
$NH_2CO_2CH_2$—	$NH_2CO_2CH_2$—	MES ca. 50, not H, LD_{50} > 500[b]

[a] Data from Frommel et al. (1961) except where indicated otherwise.
[b] Data from Vida et al. (1971).

TABLE 7 ETHERS

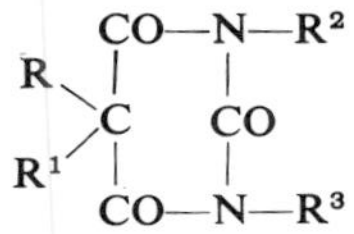

$$\begin{array}{c} R \\ R^1 \end{array} C \begin{array}{c} CO-N-R^2 \\ CO-N-R^3 \end{array}$$

R—	R'—	R²—	R³—	Activity	Reference
CH_3—	$CH_3OCH(CH_3)CH_2$—	H—	H—	Met act., LD_{50} > 3000	Mauvernay and Busch (1968)
CH_3—	$C_2H_5OCH(CH_3)CH_2$—	H—	H—	Met act., LD_{50} 4000	Mauvernay and Busch (1968)
C_2H_5—	$CH_3OCH(CH_3)CH_2$—	H—	H—	Met act., LD_{50} > 3000	Mauvernay and Busch (1968)
C_2H_5—	$C_2H_5OCH(CH_3)CH_2$—	H—	H—	Met act., LD_{50} 1600	Mauvernay and Busch (1968)
$CH_2=CHCH_2$—	$CH_3OCH(CH_3)CH_2$—	H—	H—	H, Met inact.	Prastowski and Zak (1966)
	$C_2H_5OCH(CH_3)CH_2$—		H—	Met act., LD_{50} 2000 H	Mauvernay and Busch (1968)
$CH_2=CHCH_2$—		H—	H—	Met act., LD_{50} 1250	Mauvernay and Busch (1968)
n-C_4H_9—	$CH_3OCH(CH_3)CH_2$—	H—	H—	Met inact., LD_{50} > 3000	Mauvernay and Busch (1968)
n-C_4H_9—	$C_2H_5OCH(CH_3)CH_2$—	H—	H—	Met inact., LD_{50} 3000	Mauvernay and Busch (1968)
$CH_2=C(CH_3)CH_2$—	$CH_3OCH(CH_3)CH_2$—	H—	H—	Met act., LD_{50} > 3000	Mauvernay and Busch (1968)
n-C_5H_{11}—	$CH_3OCH(CH_3)CH_2$—	H—	H—	Met weak act., LD_{50} > 3000	Mauvernay and Busch (1968)
$(CH_3)_2CHCH_2CH_2$—	$C_2H_5OCH(CH_3)CH_2$—	H—	H—	Met inact., LD_{50} > 3000	Mauvernay and Busch (1968)

(continued)

205

TABLE 7—*Continued*

R—	R'—	R^2—	R^3—	Activity	Reference
Cyclo-C_6H_{11}—	$C_2H_5OCH(CH_3)CH_2$—	H—	H—	Met weak act., $LD_{50} > 3000$	Mauvernay and Busch (1968)
C_2H_5—	C_6H_5—	H—	CH_3OCH_2—	MES 22.5, Met 3.9, $HD_{50} > 100 < 250$, $LD_{50} > 250 < 500$	Vida et al. (1973b), Vida (1974)
C_2H_5—	C_6H_5—	H—	$n\text{-}C_4H_9OCH_2$—	MES ca. 125, Met ca. 62.5, HD_{50} ca. 750, LD_{50} ca. 750	Vida et al. (1973b), Vida (1974)
C_2H_5—	C_2H_5—	CH_3—	CH_3OCH_2—	MES > 50 < 100, Met ca. 25, $HD_{50} > 500$,	Vida et al. (1973b), Vida and Samour (1974, 1975a b)
C_2H_5—	C_2H_5—	CH_3—	$n\text{-}C_4H_9OCH_2$—	MES ca. 125, Met > 100, < 250, $HD_{50} > 1000$, $LD_{50} > 1000$	Vida et al. (1973b), Vida and Samour (1974, 1975a,b)
C_2H_5—	C_2H_5—	CH_3OCH_2—	CH_3OCH_2—	MES ca. 50, Met 6.2, not H, $LD_{50} > 1000$	Vida et al. (1971)
C_2H_5—	C_2H_5—	$n\text{-}C_{12}H_{25}OCH_2$—	$n\text{-}C_{12}H_{25}OCH_2$—	Met > 200, not H	Vida et al. (1971)
C_2H_5—	C_6H_5—	CH_3—	CH_3OCH_2—	MES ca. 50, Met 16, $HD_{50} > 500 < 1000$ $LD_{50} > 500 < 1000$	Vida et al. (1973a,b), Vida and Samour (1974, 1975a,b)
C_2H_5—	C_6H_5—	CH_3—	$n\text{-}C_4H_9OCH_2$—	MES ca. 125, Met 32, $HD_{50} > 1000$, $LD_{50} > 1000$	Vida et al. (1973b), Vida and Samour (1974, 1975a,b)

R^1	R^2	R^3	R^4	Pharmacology	Reference
C_2H_5—	C_6H_5—	$C_6H_5CH_2$—	CH_3OCH_2—	MES ca. 100 Met < 100 > 250, HD_{50} > 500, LD_{50} > 500	Vida *et al.* (1973b)
C_2H_5—	C_6H_5—	CH_3OCH_2—	CH_3OCH_2—	MES 13.5, Met 47.0, not H, LD_{50} 470	Vida *et al.* (1971, 1973a)
				MES 42, other studies	Rapport and Kupferberg (1973)
				Other studies	Reinhard *et al.* (1972)
C_2H_5—	C_6H_5—	$C_2H_5OCH_2$—	$C_2H_5OCH_2$—	MES > 12.5 < 25, not H, LD_{50} > 375 < 500	Samour *et al.* (1971)
C_2H_5—	C_6H_5—	$n\text{-}C_4H_9OCH_2$—	$n\text{-}C_4H_9OCH_2$—	MES > 50 < 100, not H, LD_{50} > 500	Samour *et al.* (1971)
C_2H_5—	C_6H_5—	$n\text{-}C_{12}H_{25}OCH_2$—	$n\text{-}C_{12}H_{25}OCH_2$—	MES ca. 50, not H, LD_{50} > 500	Samour *et al.* (1971)
C_2H_5—	C_6H_5—	$C_6H_5CH_2OCH_2$—	$C_6H_5CH_2OCH_2$—	MES ca. 25, Met ca. 50, not H, LD_{50} > 500	Samour *et al.* (1971)
$CH_2{=}CHCH_2$—	$CH_3CH_2CH_2CH(CH_3)$—	CH_3OCH_2—	CH_3OCH_2—	MES < 200, Met ca. 100, not H, LD_{50} > 500 < 1000	Samour *et al.* (1971)
$CH_2{=}CHCH_2$—	$CH_3CH_2CH_2CH(CH_3)$—	$C_6H_5CH_2OCH_2$—	$C_6H_5CH_2OCH_2$—	MES > 200, Met > 200, not H, LD_{50} > 1000	Samour *et al.* (1971)

TABLE 8 HALIDES

$$R-C(R^1)(CO-N-R^2)(CO-N-R^3) \text{ with } CO \text{ bridge}$$

R—	R¹—	R²—	R³—	Activity	Reference
CH_3—	$CH{=}CBrCH_2$—	H—	H—	Met (ip) 82, LD_{50}: 326, other studies	Holck et al. (1961)
C_2H_5—	$CH{=}CBrCH_2$—	H—	H—	Met (ip) 33, H, LD_{50} 140, other studies	Holck et al. (1961)
C_2H_5—	$4\text{-}ClC_6H_4$—	H—	H—	MES 125, Met 60, LD_{50} 290	Swinyard et al. (1963)
C_2H_5—	$3,4\text{-}(Cl)_2C_6H_3$—	H—	H—	MES 26.5, Met 18.4, LD_{50} 190	Swinyard et al. (1963)
$n\text{-}C_3H_7$—	$CH{=}CBrCH_2$—	H—	H—	Met (ip) 44, H, LD_{50} 177, other studies	Holck et al. (1961)
$i\text{-}C_3H_7$—	$CH{=}CBrCH_2$—	H—	H—	Met (ip) 39, H, LD_{50} 97, other studies	Holck et al. (1961)
$CH_2{=}CHCH_2$—	$CH_3CHBrCH_2$—	H—	H—	Met act., H	Prastowski and Zak (1966)
C_2H_5—	C_6H_5—	$BrCH_2CH_2$—	H—	Act.	Fujinaga and Negishi (1960)
C_2H_5—	$p\text{-}ClC_6H_4$—	$BrCH_2CH_2$—	H—	Act.	Fujinaga and Negishi (1960)
C_2H_5—	C_6H_5—	$BrCH_2$—	CH_3—	MES > 500, Met 500, not H, LD_{50} > 1000	Vida et al. (1973a)
C_2H_5—	C_6H_5—	$BrCH_2$—	$BrCH_2$—	MES inact., Met ca. 27, not H, LD_{50} > 1000	Vida et al. (1971, 1973a), Vida and Wilber (1972)
C_2H_5—	C_6H_5—	$ClCH_2$—	$ClCH_2$—	MES inact., Met > 100, not H, LD_{50} > 500 Met 20	Vida et al. (1971) Vida and Wilber (1972, 1973) Vida and Wilber (1972, 1973)
C_2H_5—	C_6H_5—	FCH_2—	FCH_2—	Met > 100, not H	Vida et al. (1971), Vida and Wilber (1972, 1973)

TABLE 9 OTHER FUNCTIONAL GROUPS

$$H_5C_2 - \underset{R}{\overset{CO-N-R^1}{\underset{\displaystyle |}{C}}} {\overset{|}{\underset{CO-N-R^2}{}}}$$

$R-$	R^1-	R^2-	Activity	Reference
C_6H_5-	C_6H_5CO-	$H-$	Act.	Dumennova and Saratikov (1959); Kulev et al. (1960)
C_6H_5-	$CH_3CO_2CH_2-$	$H-$	$LD_{50} > 500$	Vida et al. (1971)
C_2H_5-	$CH_3CO_2CH_2-$	$CH_3CO_2CH_2-$	MES 16.5, not H, LD_{50} 570	Samour and Vida (1970, 1971)
C_6H_5-	$CH_3CO_2CH_2-$	$CH_3CO_2CH_2-$	MES 28, Met 104, not H, LD_{50} 640	Vida et al. (1971)
C_6H_5-	$CH_3CH_2CO_2CH_2-$	$CH_3CH_2CO_2CH_2-$	MES ca. 25, not H, LD_{50} > 500	Vida et al. (1971)
C_6H_5-	CH_3-	NH_2CSCH_2- ($=NH$)	MES > 100 < 250, Met > 100, not H, LD_{50} > 500 < 1000	Vida et al. (1973a)
C_6H_5-	$HBr\cdot H_2NCSCH_2-$ ($=NH$)	$HBr\cdot H_2NCSCH_2-$ ($=NH$)	MES inact., Met inact., HD_{50} > 1000, LD_{50} > 500 < 1000	Vida et al. (1973a), Vida and Hooker (1975)
C_6H_5-	$HBr\cdot C_6H_5NHCSCH_2-$ ($=NH$)	$HBr\cdot C_6H_5NHCSCH_2-$ ($=NH$)	MES > 500, Met 330, not H, LD_{50} > 500	Vida et al. (1973a), Vida and Hooker (1975)
C_6H_5-	$Br^{-\,+}[N_4(CH_2)_6]CH_2-$	$Br^{-\,+}[N_4(CH_2)_6]CH_2-$	MES 42, Met ca. 50, not H, LD_{50} > 1000	Vida et al. (1973a)

209

TABLE 10 OTHER FUNCTIONAL GROUPS: MISCELLANEOUS STRUCTURES

Compound	Activity	Reference
(barbiturate structure: H_5C_2, C_2H_5, O, N, N, O^-)	MES 18, Met 29, H, LD_{50} 424 MES act., Met act., LD_{50} 334 other studies	Dick and Mitchell (1967) Haas (1963)
(cyclohexyl—CH_2—$\overset{+}{C}HNH_2CH_3$—CH_3 ; C_6H_5—N=N— barbituric acid structure with O, HN, NH, O)	Act.	Kulev and Voronova (1961)

MES ca. 25, $LD_{50} > 500$ Vida *et al.* (1971)

MES > 200, $LD_{50} < 1000$ Vida *et al.* (1971)

MES > 200, $LD_{50} > 500$ Vida *et al.* (1971)

E. THIOBARBITURATES

TABLE 11   2-THIOBARBITURIC ACIDS[a]

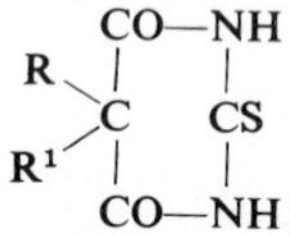

$$
\begin{array}{c}
\text{CO—NH} \\
\text{R} \diagdown \quad | \qquad | \\
\text{C} \quad \text{CS} \\
\text{R}^1 \diagup \quad | \qquad | \\
\text{CO—NH}
\end{array}
$$

R—	R¹—	Activity
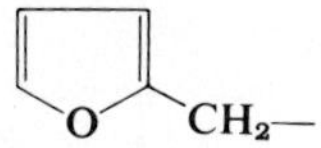 (furan)CH₂—	$CH_3CH(CH_3)$—	Met act., H, LD_{50} 71
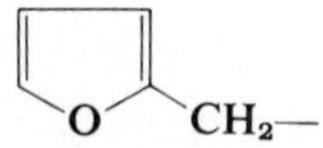 (furan)CH₂—	C_2H_5—	Met act., H, LD_{50} 87
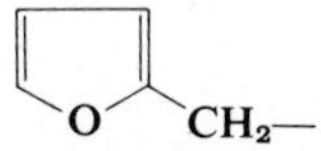 (furan)CH₂—	$CH_2{=}CHCH_2$—	Met act., H, LD_{50} 86

[a] Data from Krnjević *et al.* (1966)

II. HYDANTOINS

A. HYDANTOINS WITH ONLY ALIPHATIC HYDROCARBON SUBSTITUENTS (TABLES 12–13)

TABLE 12

R—	R¹—	R²—	Activity	Reference
CH₃—	Cyclo-C₃H₅—	H—	Act.	Innothera (1962)
CH₃—	(CH₃)₃C—	H—	ES inact., Met weak act., LD₅₀ 2300	Reidel-de Haen Akt-bes (1959)
C₂H₅—	Cyclo-C₃H₅—	H—	Act.	Robba and Moreau (1961)
Cyclo-C₃H₅—	Cyclo-C₃H₅—	H—	Act.	Robba and Moreau (1961)
			Met act., EST inact., LD₅₀ 1200	Innothera (1962)
i-C₃H₇—	Cyclo-C₃H₅—	H—	Act.	Robba and Moreau (1961)
n-C₄H₉—	Cyclo-C₃H₅—	H—	Act.	Robba and Moreau (1961)
CH₃—	CH₃—	CH≡CCH₂—	EST weak act., LD₅₀ > 2300	Danielsson et al. (1965)
Cyclo-C₃H₅—	Cyclo-C₃H₅—	CH₃—	Act.	Robba and Moreau (1961)
			MES act., Met act., EST inact., LD₅₀ 1000	Innothera (1962)

TABLE 13 SPIROHYDANTOINS

$$
\begin{array}{c}
\text{H} \\
\text{N} \\
\text{A} \diagup \diagdown \text{CO} \\
| \qquad | \\
\text{OC} \!\!-\!\!-\!\! \text{NH}
\end{array}
$$

A—	Activity	Reference
H₃C (methyl cycloheptane spiro)	Act.	Brimelow *et al.* (1959b)
H₃C (methyl cycloheptane spiro)	Act.	Brimelow *et al.* (1959b)
(decalin spiro)	Act.	Brimelow *et al.* (1959a)
(CH₂)₁₁	Act.	Chemische Werke (1964)

B. HYDANTOINS WITH AROMATIC HYDROCARBON SUBSTITUENTS (TABLES 14-16)

TABLE 14

$$\begin{array}{c} R \\ R^1 \end{array}\!\!\!>\!\!C\!\!<\!\!\begin{array}{c} \overset{H}{N}\!\!-\!\!CO \\ OC\!\!-\!\!NH \end{array}$$

R—	R¹—	Activity	Reference
CH_3—	C_6H_5—	MES act., LD_{50} 450	Asta Werke A.-G. Chemische Fabrik (1962)
C_2H_5—	C_6H_5—	MES 63, MMS 46, LD_{50} 317	Nakamura et al. (1965)
		^{14}C study	Vigne and Fondarai (1959)
		MES ca. 12.5, Met 16	Vida et al. (1975)
n-C_3H_7—	C_6H_5—	ES act., Met act., LD_{50} 1600	Reidel-de Haen Akt-bes (1959)
Cyclo-C_3H_5—	C_6H_5—	MES act., Met act., EST act., LD_{50} > 2000	Innothera (1962)
$(CH_3)_2CH$—	C_6H_5—	ES act., Met act., LD_{50} 1400	Reidel-de Haen Akt.-bes. (1959)
n-C_4H_9—	C_6H_5—	ES weak act., Met weak act., LD_{50} 5500	Reidel-de Haen Akt.-bes. (1959)
$CH_3CH_2CH(CH_3)$—	C_6H_5—	ES weak act., Met weak act., LD_{50} > 10,000	Reidel-de Haen Akt.-bes. (1959)
$(CH_3)_2CHCHCH_2$—	C_6H_5—	ES act., Met weak act., LD_{50} 1250	Reidel-de Haen Akt.-bes. (1959)
$(CH_3)_3C$—	C_6H_5—	ES act., Met act., LD_{50} 10,000	Reidel-de Haen Akt.-bes. (1959)
C_6H_5—	C_6H_5—	MES 17, MMS 23, LD_{50} 310	Nakamura et al. (1965)
		MES act., Met weak act., LD_{50} 216	Malec (1966)
		ES act., Met inact., LD_{50} 1600	Reidel-de Haen Akt.-bes. (1959)
		MES 16, Met inact, PSM 61	Wolf et al. (1962)
		Met inact., other studies	Enebäck and Alberty (1965)
		MES act., LD_{50} 180	Przegaliński (1969)
		MES 12, LD_{50} 1000	Gesler et al. (1961)
		MES (ip) 0.030 mmole/kg, Met inact.	Witiak et al. (1972)
		MES act., Met inact., EST inact., LD_{50} 360	Carraz and Emin (1967)

(continued)

TABLE 14—*Continued*

R—	R¹—	Activity	Reference
		MES 12.8, Met inact., LD$_{50}$ 1800	Raines *et al.* (1973)
		MES act., LD$_{50}$ 3368	Asta Werke A.-G. Chemische Fabrik (1962)
		Other Studies	Umberkoman and Joseph (1974)
C₆H₅—	C₆H₅—	MES ca. 7.5, Met inact.	Vida *et al.* (1975)
		Other studies	Weinreich and Clark (1970)
		LD$_{50}$ 138	Elkin and Lieberman (1972)
		EST act.	Danielsson *et al.* (1965)
C₆H₅—	C₆H₅CH₂—	MMS inact., other studies	Enebäck and Alberty (1965)
C₆H₅—	C₆H₅CH(CH₃)—	MMS inact., other studies	Enebäck and Alberty (1965)
Cyclo-C₃H₅—	3,4-(CH₃)₂C₆H₃—	Act.	Robba and Moreau (1961)
Cyclo-C₃H₅—	(CH₃)₃CC₆H₄—	Act.	Robba and Moreau (1961)

TABLE 15

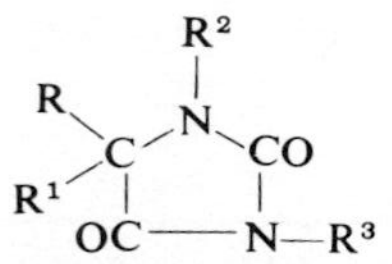

$$\underset{R^1}{\overset{R}{C}}\!\!\begin{array}{c} R^2 \\ | \\ N-CO \\ | \quad\ | \\ OC-N-R^3 \end{array}$$

R—	R¹—	R²—	R³—	Activity	Reference
H—	H—	CH₃—	C₆H₅CH₂—	Met inact.	Natarajan (1971)
H—	H—	C₆H₅—	C₆H₅CH₂—	Met inact.	Natarajan (1971)
H—	C₂H₅—	H—	C₆H₅CH₂—	Met inact.	Natarajan (1971)
CH₃—	CH₃—	CH₃—	C₆H₅CH₂—	Met inact.	Natarajan (1971)

R	R	R	Activity	Reference
C₂H₅—	C₆H₅—	CH₃—	MES 30, LD₅₀ 1460	Schoegl et al. (1961)
C₂H₅—	C₆H₅—	H—	MES 46, Met 40, PsM 65	Wolf et al. (1962)
C₂H₅—	C₆H₅—	H—	Met 75	Natarajan (1971)
C₂H₅—	C₆H₅—	H—	¹⁴C study	Vigne and Fondarai (1959)
C₂H₅—	C₆H₅—	H—	MES 10, Met 30	Achari and Sinha (1967)
C₂H₅—	C₆H₅—	C₂H₅—	MES 230, Met 265, PsM 175	Wolf et al. (1962)
C₂H₅—	C₆H₅—	CH=CCH₂—	EST act., LD₅₀ 1000	Danielsson et al. (1965)
C₂H₅—	C₆H₅—	H—	MES 102, Met 75, PsM 75	Wolf et al. (1962)
C₂H₅—	C₆H₅—	CH₃—	MES (sc) 81, Met (sc) 97	Achari and Sinha (1967)
C₂H₅—	C₆H₅—	CH₃—	MES 110, Met 83, PsM 100	Achari and Sinha (1967)
C₂H₅—	CH=CCH₂—	CH₃—	EST act., LD₅₀ 465	Danielsson et al. (1965)
Cyclo-C₃H₅—	H—	CH₃—	MES act., Met act., EST act., LD₅₀ ca. 1000	Innothera (1962)
C₆H₅—	CH₃—	H—	Act.	Robba and Moreau (1961)
C₆H₅—	H—	H—	MES 58, MMS 31	Nakamura et al. (1965)
C₆H₅—	CH=CCH₂—	CH=CCH₂—	MES > 3.125 < 6.25, Met > 200	Vida et al. (1975)
C₆H₅—	C₆H₅CH₂—	H—	EST act., LD₅₀ 760	Danielsson et al. (1965)
C₆H₅—	CH₃—	H—	MES > 200, Met inact.	Vida et al. (1975)
C₆H₅—	C₆H₅CH₂—	CH₃—	MES 50, Met 25	Vida et al. (1975)
C₆H₅—	CH=CCH₂—	C₆H₅CH₂—	MES > 200, Met 110	Vida et al. (1975)
C₆H₅—	CH=CCH₂—	CH=CCH₂—	EST inact., LD₅₀ > 1000	Vida et al. (1975)

TABLE 16 BISHYDANTOINS [a]

Compound	Activity
(bishydantoin structure) OC—N(H)—CHCH₂CH₂CH(—N(H)—CO ... OC—NC₆H₅) / C₆H₅N—CO	MES inact., S., LD₅₀ > 2500

[a] Data from Przegaliński (1969).

217

C. HYDANTOINS WITH HETEROCYCLIC SUBSTITUENTS (TABLES 17–21)

TABLE 17 THIENYL SUBSTITUENTS

R^a	R^1	R^2	Activity	Reference
2-C_4H_3S—	Cyclo-C_3H_5—	H—	Act.	Robba and Moreau (1961)
			MES act., Met act., EST act., LD_{50} 1000	Innothera (1962)
2-C_4H_3S—	n-C_6H_{13}—	H—	Act.	Robba and Moreau (1961)
2-C_4H_3S—	n-C_7H_{15}—	H—	Act.	Robba and Moreau (1961)
2-C_4H_3S—	C_6H_5—C_6H_4—	H—	Act.	Robba and Moreau (1961)
5-Br, 2-C_4H_2S—	CH_3—	H—	Act.	Robba and Moreau (1961)
5-Br, 2-C_4H_2S—	C_2H_5—	H—	Act.	Robba and Moreau (1961)
5-Br, 2-C_4H_2S—	n-C_3H_7—	H—	Act.	Robba and Moreau (1961)
5-Br, 2-C_4H_2S—	Cyclo-C_6H_{11}—	H—	Act.	Robba and Moreau (1961)
4,5-Br_2, 2-C_4H_1S—	CH_3—	H—	Act.	Robba and Moreau (1961)
4,5-Br_2, 2-C_4H_1S—	C_2H_5	H—	Act.	Robba and Moreau (1961)
2-C_4H_3S—	CH_3—	$HO_2CCH_2CH_2$—	MES inact., Met inact.	Shaffer et al. (1968)
2-C_4H_3S—	Cyclo-C_3H_5—	CH_3—	Act.	Robba and Moreau (1961)
			MES act., Met weak act., EST weak act., LD_{50} 1000	Innothera (1962)
5-Br, 2-C_4H_2S—	CH_3—	CH_3—	Act.	Robba and Moreau (1961)
5-Br, 2-C_4H_2S—	CH_3—	C_2H_5—	Act.	Robba and Moreau (1961)
5-Br, 2-C_4H_2S—	C_2H_5—	C_2H_5—	Act.	Robba and Moreau (1961)
5-Br, 2-C_4H_2S—	n-C_3H_7—	CH_3—	Act.	Robba and Moreau (1961)
5-Br, 2-C_4H_2S—	n-C_3H_7—	C_2H_5—	Act.	Robba and Moreau (1961)
5-Br, 2-C_4H_2S—	Cyclo-C_6H_{11}—	CH_3—	Act.	Robba and Moreau (1961)
5-Br, 2-C_4H_2S—	C_6H_5—	CH_3—	Act.	Robba and Moreau (1961)
4,5-Br_2, 2-C_4H_1S—	CH_3—	CH_3—	Act.	Robba and Moreau (1961)
4,5-Br_2, 2-C_4H_1S—	C_2H_5—	CH_3—	Act.	Robba and Moreau (1961)

[a] C_4H_3S = thienyl.

TABLE 18 OTHER HETEROCYCLIC SUBSTITUENTS

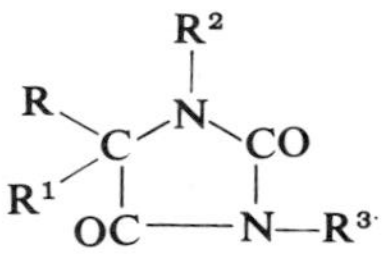

Structure:
$$\begin{array}{c} R^2 \\ R-\!\!\!\underset{R^1}{\overset{}{C}}-N<\!\!\begin{array}{c} CO \\ OC \end{array}\!\!>N-R^3 \end{array}$$

R—	R¹—	R²—	R³—	Activity	Reference
CH_3—	CH_3—	H—	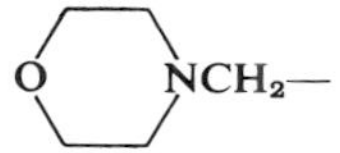 morpholino-NCH_2—	MES inact., Met inact., LD_{50} 830	Malec (1966)
CH_3—	CH_3—	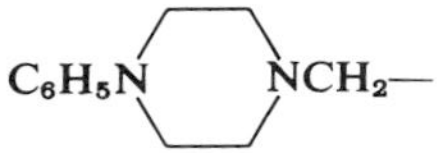 C_6H_5N-piperazinyl-NCH_2—	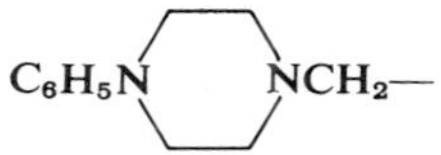 C_6H_5N-piperazinyl-NCH_2—	MES inact., not S, LD_{50} 120	Malec (1970)
CH_3—	CH_3—	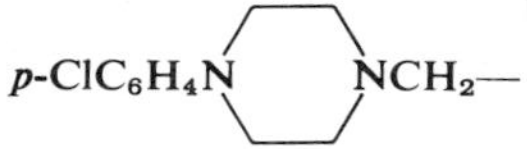 p-ClC_6H_4N-piperazinyl-NCH_2—	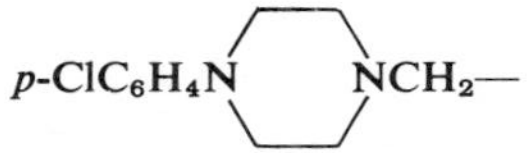 p-ClC_6H_4N-piperazinyl-NCH_2—	MES inact., not S, LD_{50} 1200	Malec (1970)
CH_3—	$C_6H_5CH=CH$—	H—	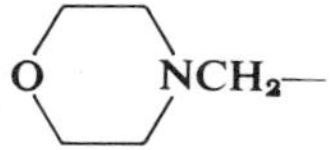 morpholino-NCH_2—	MES inact., not S, LD_{50} 880	Malec (1970)
CH_3—	$C_6H_5CHBrCHBr$—	H—	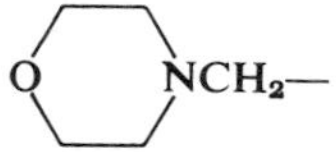 morpholino-NCH_2—	MES inact., not S, LD_{50} 1100	Malec (1970)
C_6H_5—	C_6H_5—	H—	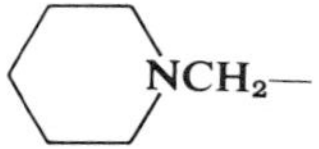 piperidino-NCH_2—	MES inact., Met inact., LD_{50} 193	Malec (1966)
C_6H_5—	C_6H_5—	H—	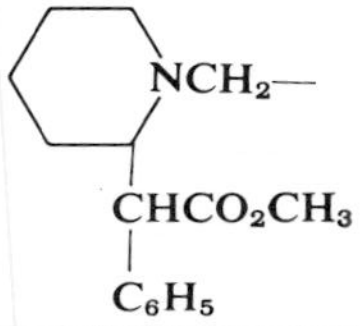 piperidino-NCH_2— $CHCO_2CH_3$ C_6H_5	MES inact., not S, LD_{50} 1000	Malec (1970)

(continued)

219

TABLE 18—*Continued*

R—	R¹—	R²—	R³—	Activity	Reference
C_6H_5—	C_6H_5—	H—	CH_3N piperazine NCH_2—	MES act., Met inact., not S, LD_{50} 125	Malec (1970)
C_6H_5—	C_6H_5—	H—	C_6H_5N piperazine NCH_2—	MES inact., not S, LD_{50} 225	Przegaliński (1969)
C_6H_5—	C_6H_5—	H—	$C_6H_5CH_2N$ piperazine NCH_2—	MES weak act., not S, LD_{50} 250	Przegaliński (1969)
C_6H_5—	C_6H_5—	H—	morpholine NCH_2—	MES act., Met inact., LD_{50} 106	Malec (1966)
C_6H_5—	C_6H_5—	H—	morpholine $NCH_2C\equiv CCH_2$—	EST inact., LD_{50} > 1500	Danielsson *et al.* (1965)
C_6H_5—	C_6H_5—	H—	morpholine (H_3C, C_6H_5) NCH_2—	MES inact not S, LD_{50} 370	Malec (1970)
C_6H_5—	C_6H_5—	H—	$p\text{-}ClC_6H_4N$ piperazine NCH_2—	MES inact., not S, LD_{50} 250	Przegaliński (1969)

TABLE 19 OTHER HETEROCYCLIC SUBSTITUENTS: SPIROBISHYDANTOINS[a]

Compound	Activity
	MES inact., S, LD_{50} 1050

[a] Data from Przegaliński (1969).

TABLE 20 OTHER HETEROCYCLIC SUBSTITUENTS: SPIROHYDANTOINS[a]

A—	R—	Activity
	H—	Act.
	H—	MES act., LD_{50} ca. 2320
	H—	Act.
	H—	MES act., LD_{50} > 2970
	H—	MES act., LD_{50} > 2530
	H—	Act.

(*continued*)

TABLE 20—*Continued*

A—	R—	Activity
H₃C, Cl — benzopyran (chromane) structure	H—	Act.
Cl, CH₃ — chromane structure	H—	Act.
Cl — chromane structure	C₂H₅	Act.
Cl — chromane structure	n-C₄H₉—	Act.
S — thiochromane structure	H—	Act.
O — benzoxepine structure	H—	MES act., LD₅₀ 2111
H₃C — benzoxepine structure	H—	Act.
CH₃ — benzoxepine structure	H—	Act.
H₃C — benzoxepine structure	H—	Act.

TABLE 20—*Continued*

A—	R—	Activity
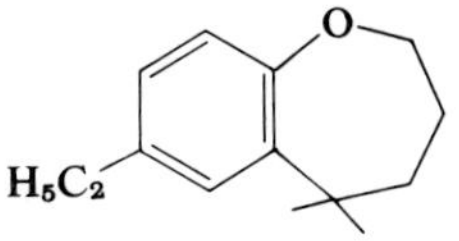	H—	Act.
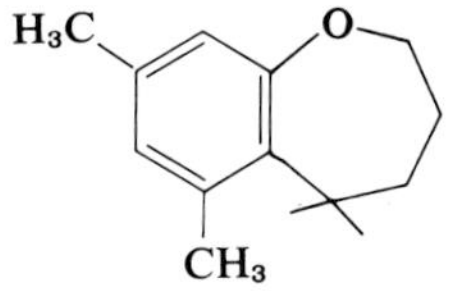	H—	Act.
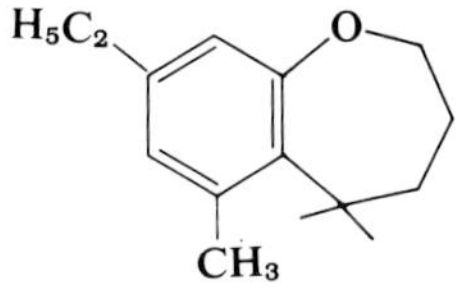	H—	Act.
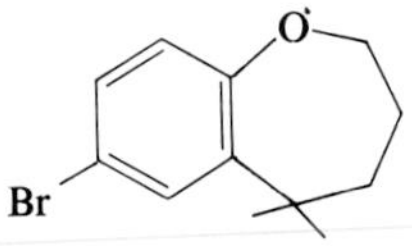	H—	Act
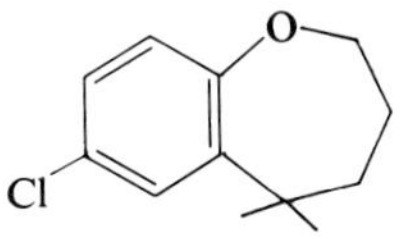	H—	Act.
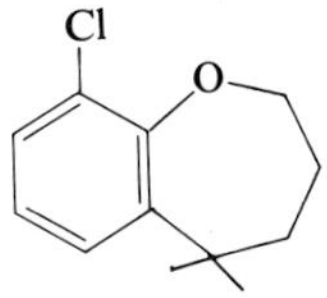	H—	MES act., LD_{50} 3555
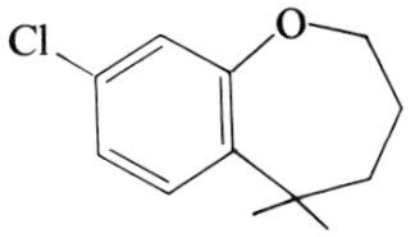	H—	Act.
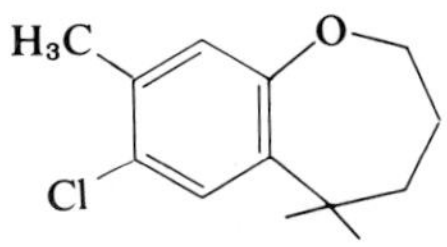	H—	Act.

(*continued*)

TABLE 20—*Continued*

A—	R—	Activity
	H—	Act.
	H	Act.
	H—	Act.
	H—	Act.
	H—	Act.
	H—	Act.
	CH₃—	Act.
	CH₃—	Act.

TABLE 20—*Continued*

A— I	R—	Activity
(bicyclic amine structure)	H—	MMS act., LD_{50} 276[b]
(bicyclic amine structure)	CH_3—	MMS act.[b]
(cyclohexyl structure)	$O\diagdown NCH_2$— (morpholinomethyl)	MES inact., not S, LD_{50} 440[c]
(cyclohexyl structure)	$-CH_2N\diagdown NCH_2$— (benzylpiperazinylmethyl)	MES inact., not S, LD_{50} 320[c]

[a] Data from Asta Werke A.-G. Chemische Fabrik (1962) except where indicated otherwise.

[b] Data from Elkin and Lieberman (1972).

[c] Data from Przegaliński (1969).

TABLE 21 OTHER HETEROCYCLIC SUBSTITUENTS: BISHYDANTOINS

$$\left[\begin{array}{c} R \\ R^1 \end{array} \!\! C \!\! \begin{array}{c} H \\ N-CO \\ | \quad \quad \\ OC-NCH_2 \end{array} \right]_2 B-$$

R—	R¹—	—B—	Activity	Reference
CH₃—	CH₃—	(piperazine)	MES inact., Met weak act., S, LD$_{50}$ 1120	Malec (1966)
			Met inact.	Malec (1967)
CH₃—	C₆H₅CH=CH—	(piperazine)	MES inact., S, LD$_{50}$ > 2000	Malec (1970)
CH₃—	C₆H₅CHBrCHBr—	(piperazine)	MES inact., S, LD$_{50}$ > 2000	Malec (1970)
C₆H₅—	C₆H₅—	(piperazine)	MES inact., Met weak act., S, LD$_{50}$ 1500	Malec (1966)
			Met inact.	Malec (1967)
C₆H₅—	C₆H₅—	(methylpiperazine, CH₃)	MES inact., Met inact., S, LD$_{50}$ > 2000	Malec (1972)
C₆H₅—	C₆H₅—	(dimethylpiperazine, CH₃ / CH₃)	MES inact., Met inact., S, LD$_{50}$ > 2000	Malec (1972)

D. HYDANTOINS WITH HETEROATOMS IN NONHETEROCYCLIC SYSTEMS (TABLES 22–29)

TABLE 22 ALCOHOLS

$$R-\underset{R^1}{\overset{H}{\underset{|}{\underset{C}{\overset{N-CO}{\diagdown}}}}}\quad OC-N-R^2$$

R—	R¹—	R²—	Activity	Reference
H—	C_6H_5—	$HOCH_2CH_2$—	MES 120, LD_{50} 540	Schoegl et al. (1961)
CH_3—	C_6H_5—	$HOCH_2$—	MES 20, LD_{50} 900	Schoegl et al. (1961)
CH_3—	C_6H_5—	$HOCH_2CH_2$—	MES 41, LD_{50} 2200	Schoegl et al. (1961)
CH_3—	p-$HOC_6H_4OCH_2$—	H—	Act.	Blaha and Weichet (1974)
CH_3—	p-BrC_6H_4—	$HOCH_2CH_2$—	MES 76, LD_{50} 3200	Blaha and Weichet (1974)
CH_3—	p-ClC_6H_4	$HOCH_2CH_2$—	MES 142, LD_{50} 2500	Blaha and Weichet (1974)
CH_3—	p-FC_6H_4—	$HOCH_2CH_2$—	MES 290, LD_{50} 2400	Blaha and Weichet (1974)
C_2H_5—	C_6H_5—	$HOCH_2$—	MES 10, LD_{50} 405	Blaha and Weichet (1974)
C_2H_5—	C_6H_5—	$HOCH_2CH_2$—	MES 68, LD_{50} 2000	Blaha and Weichet (1974)
C_2H_5—	p-BrC_6H_4—	$HOCH_2CH_2$—	MES 68, LD_{50} 1300	Blaha and Weichet (1974)
C_2H_5—	p-ClC_6H_4—	$HOCH_2CH_2$—	MES 108, LD_{50} 3000	Blaha and Weichet (1974)
C_2H_5—	p-FC_6H_4—	$HOCH_2CH_2$—	MES 190, LD_{50} 3000	Blaha and Weichet (1974)
C_6H_5—	C_6H_5—	$HOCH_2CH_2$—	MES 48, LD_{50} 530	Blaha and Weichet (1974)
$C_6H_5CH_2$—	o-HOC_6H_4—	H—	MMS inact., other studies	Enebäck and Alberty (1965)
$C_6H_5CH_2$—	2-HO, 4-$CH_3OC_6H_3$—	H—	MMS inact., other studies	Enebäck and Alberty (1965)
o-HOC_6H_4—	p-$CH_3OC_6H_4CH_2$—	H—	MMS inact., other studies	Enebäck and Alberty (1965)
2-HO, 4-$CH_3OC_6H_3$—	p-$CH_3C_6H_4CH_2$—	H—	MMS inact., other studies	Enebäck and Alberty (1965)

TABLE 23 AMINES

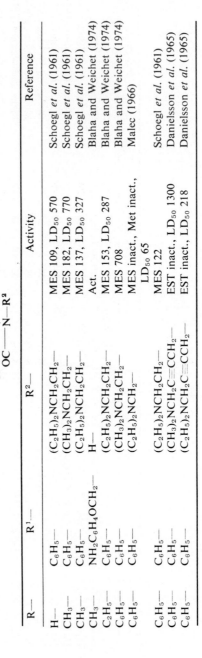

R—	R¹—	R²—	Activity	Reference
H—	C$_6$H$_5$—	(C$_2$H$_5$)$_2$NCH$_2$CH$_2$—	MES 109, LD$_{50}$ 570	Schoegl et al. (1961)
CH$_3$—	C$_6$H$_5$—	(CH$_3$)$_2$NCH$_2$CH$_2$—	MES 182, LD$_{50}$ 770	Schoegl et al. (1961)
CH$_3$—	C$_6$H$_5$—	(C$_2$H$_5$)$_2$NCH$_2$CH$_2$—	MES 137, LD$_{50}$ 327	Schoegl et al. (1961)
CH$_3$—	NH$_2$C$_6$H$_4$OCH$_2$—	H—	Act.	Blaha and Weichet (1974)
C$_2$H$_5$—	C$_6$H$_5$—	(C$_2$H$_5$)$_2$NCH$_2$CH$_2$—	MES 153, LD$_{50}$ 287	Blaha and Weichet (1974)
C$_6$H$_5$—	C$_6$H$_5$—	(CH$_3$)$_2$NCH$_2$CH$_2$—	MES 708	Blaha and Weichet (1974)
C$_6$H$_5$—	C$_6$H$_5$—	(C$_2$H$_5$)$_2$NCH$_2$—	MES inact., Met inact., LD$_{50}$ 65	Malec (1966)
C$_6$H$_5$—	C$_6$H$_5$—	(C$_2$H$_5$)$_2$NCH$_2$CH$_2$—	MES 122	Schoegl et al. (1961)
C$_6$H$_5$—	C$_6$H$_5$—	(CH$_3$)$_2$NCH$_2$C≡CCH$_2$—	EST inact., LD$_{50}$ 1300	Danielsson et al. (1965)
C$_6$H$_5$—	C$_6$H$_5$—	(C$_2$H$_5$)$_2$NCH$_2$C≡CCH$_2$—	EST inact., LD$_{50}$ 218	Danielsson et al. (1965)

TABLE 24 AMINES: BISHYDANTOINS[a]

$$\left[\begin{array}{c} R \\ \\ R^1 \end{array} \begin{array}{c} H \\ N{-}CO \\ C \\ OC{-}NCH_2 \end{array} \right]{-}B{-}$$

R—	R¹—	B—	Activity
—CH₂CH₂CH₂CH₂CH₂—		—N(CH₃)—	MES inact., S, LD_{50} 128
C₆H₅—	C₆H₅—	—N(CH₃)—	MES inact., S, LD_{50} 1440
C₆H₅—	C₆H₅—	—N(C₂H₅)—	MES inact., S, LD_{50} 880
C₆H₅—	C₆H₅—	—N(C₃H₇)—	MES inact., S, LD_{50} 560
C₆H₅—	C₆H₅—	—NHCH₂CH₂NH—	MES inact., not S, LD_{50} 200
C₆H₅—	C₆H₅—	—NCH₂CH₂N— CH₂C₆H₅ CH₂C₆H₅	MES inact., S, LD_{50} 1400[b]

[a] Data from Przegaliński (1969) except where indicated otherwise.
[b] Data from Malec (1970).

TABLE 25 ETHERS

$$\begin{array}{c} R^2 \\ R{-}\underset{R^1{-}OC{-}N{-}R^3}{\overset{}{\underset{}{C}}}\!\!\!\!\diagdown{N}{-}CO \end{array}$$

R—	R¹	R²	R³	Activity	Reference
CH_3-	$CH_3C_6H_4OCH_2-$	H—	H—	Act.	Blaha and Weichet (1974)
CH_3-	$CH_3OC_6H_4OCH_2-$	H—	H—	Act.	Blaha and Weichet (1974)
CH_3-	$ClC_6H_4OCH_2-$	H—	H—	Act.	Blaha and Weichet (1974)
CH_3-	$NO_2C_6H_4OCH_2-$	H—	H—	Act.	Blaha and Weichet (1974)
C_2H_5-	C_6H_5-	H—	CH_3OCH_2-	MES ca. 25, Met ca. 38	Vida et al. (1975)
C_2H_5-	C_6H_5-	H—	$n\text{-}C_4H_9OCH_2-$	MES ca. 200, Met > 200	Vida et al. (1975)
C_2H_5-	C_6H_5-	H—	$C_6H_5CH_2OCH_2-$	MES ca. 100, Met inact.	Vida et al. (1975)
C_2H_5-	C_6H_5-	CH_3OCH_2-	CH_3-	MES 50–80, Met 100	Vida et al. (1975)
Cyclo-C_3H_5-	$p\text{-}CH_3OC_6H_4-$	H—	H—	Act.	Robba and Moreau (1961)
				MES inact., Met inact., EST inact., LD₅₀ 1700	Innothera (1962)
C_6H_5-	C_6H_5-	H—	CH_3OCH_2-	MES ca. 6, Met weak act.	Vida et al. (1971)
C_6H_5-	C_6H_5-	H—	$n\text{-}C_4H_9OCH_2-$	MES < 25, Met ca. 50, LD₅₀ > 500	Samour and Vida (1970) Vida et al. (1971)

R1	R2	R3	Activity	Reference
C_6H_5—	H—	$C_6H_5CH_2OCH_2$—	MES > 25, Met < 50	Vida et al. (1971)
C_6H_5—	H—	$CH_3OCH_2CH_2OCO$—	ES act.	Schaefer (1974a,b)
C_6H_5—	H—	$C_2H_5OCH_2CH_2OCO$—	ES act.	Schaefer (1974a,b)
C_6H_5—	CH_3OCH_2—	CH_3OCH_2—	MES 25, Met 600	Samour and Vida (1970), Vida et al. (1975)
C_6H_5—	CH_3OCH_2—	$C_6H_5CH_2$—	MES > 200, Met > 200	Vida et al. (1975)
C_6H_5—	$n\text{-}C_4H_9OCH_2$—	$n\text{-}C_4H_9OCH_2$—	MES > 200, Met > 1000	Vida et al. (1975)
C_6H_5—	$n\text{-}C_4H_9OCH_2$—	$C_6H_5CH_2$—	MES 200, Met 200	Vida et al. (1975)
C_6H_5—	$p\text{-}CH_3OC_6H_4CH_2$—	H—	MMS weak act., other studies	Enebäck and Alberty (1965)
C_6H_5—	$3,4\text{-}(CH_3O)_2C_6H_3CH_2$—	H—	MMS inact., other studies	Enebäck and Alberty (1965)
$C_6H_5CH_2$	$o\text{-}CH_3OC_6H_4$—	H—	MMS inact., other studies	Enebäck and Alberty (1965)
$C_6H_5CH_2$	$o\text{-}CH_3OCH_2OC_6H_4$—	H—	MMS weak act., other studies	Enebäck and Alberty (1965)
$C_6H_5CH_2$	$2\text{-}CH_3OCH_2O, 4\text{-}CH_3OC_6H_3$—	H—	MMS weak act., other studies	Enebäck and Alberty (1965)
$p\text{-}CH_3OC_6H_4CH_2$	$o\text{-}CH_3OCH_2OC_6H_4$—	H—	MMS weak act., other studies	Enebäck and Alberty (1965)
$p\text{-}CH_3OC_6H_4CH_2$	$3\text{-}CH_3O, 2\text{-}CH_3OCH_2OC_6H_3$	H	MMS inact., other studies	Enebäck and Alberty (1965)
$3,4\text{-}(CH_3O)_2C_6H_3$	$3,4\text{-}(CH_3O)_2C_6H_3CH_2$—	H—	MMS inact., other studies	Enebäck and Alberty (1965)
$3,4,5\text{-}(CH_3O)_3C_6H_2$	$3,4,5\text{-}(CH_3O)_3C_6H_2$	H	Act.	Kapadia et al. (1973)

TABLE 26 HALIDES

R—	R¹—	R²—	Activity	Reference
CH_3—	CF_3—	H—	Act.	Robba and Moreau (1961)
C_2H_5—	p-ClC_6H_4—	H—	Act.	Gerot-Pharmazentika (1966)
C_2H_5—	p-ClC_6H_4—	CH_3—	Act.	Gerot-Pharmazentika (1966)
Cyclo-C_3H_5—	p-BrC_6H_4—	H—	Act.	Robba and Moreau (1961)
			MES act., Met inact., EST inact., $LD_{50} > 2000$	Innothera (1962)
Cyclo-C_3H_5—	p-ClC_6H_4—	H—	Act.	Robba and Moreau (1961)
Cyclo-C_3H_5—	p-FC_6H_4—	H—	Act.	Robba and Moreau (1961)
			MES act., Met act., EST inact., LD_{50} 1000	Innothera (1962)

TABLE 27 SULFIDES: BISHYDANTOINS[a]

—B—	Activity
—CH_2SCH_2—	MES inact., S, LD_{50} 1500
—CH_2SSCH_2—	MES inact., S, LD_{50} 2100
—$CH_2SCH_2SCH_2$—	MES inact., S, LD_{50} 2650

[a] Data from Przegaliński (1969)

TABLE 28 OTHER FUNCTIONAL GROUPS

$R-$	R^1-	R^2-	R^3-	Activity	Reference
CH_3-	C_6H_5-	H—	$HO_2CCH_2CH_2-$	MES inact., Met inact.	Shaffer et al. (1968)
C_2H_5-	C_6H_5-	H—	CH_3CO-	MES 75, MMS 35	Nakamura et al. (1965)
				Act.	Takamatsu et al. (1964)
C_2H_5-	C_6H_5-	H—	C_2H_5OCO-	MES 25, MMS 58	Nakamura et al. (1965)
				Act.	Takamatsu et al. (1964)
C_2H_5-	C_6H_5-	H—	$CH_3CO_2CH_2-$	MES 12.5, Met 100	Vida et al. (1975)
C_2H_5-	C_6H_5-	CH_3CO-	H—	MES > 100, MMS > 100	Nakamura et al. (1965)
C_2H_5-	C_6H_5-	C_2H_5OCO-	H—	MES 100, MMS 100	Nakamura et al. (1965)
C_2H_5-	C_6H_5-	$CH_3CO_2CH_2-$	CH_3-	MES 80, Met 200	Vida et al. (1975)
C_2H_5-	C_6H_5-	$CH_3CO_2CH_2-$	$CH_3CO_2CH_2-$	MES 130, Met > 200	Vida et al. (1975)
C_6H_5-	C_6H_5-	H—	CH_3CO-	MES 19, MMS 25	Nakamura et al. (1965)
				Act.	Takamatsu et al. (1964)
				Act.	Schaefer (1974b)
C_6H_5-	C_6H_5-	H—	CH_3OCO-	MES 15, MMS 12	Nakamura et al. (1965)
				Act.	Takamatsu et al. (1964)
C_6H_5-	C_6H_5-	H—	C_2H_5OCO-	MES < 25	Vida et al. (1971)
C_6H_5-	C_6H_5-	H—	$CH_3CO_2CH_2-$	Act.	Schaefer (1974b)
C_6H_5-	C_6H_5-	H—	$n\text{-}C_4H_9OCO-$	MES 19, MMS 68	Nakamura et al. (1965)
C_6H_5-	C_6H_5-	H—	C_6H_5CO-	Act.	Takamatsu et al. (1964)

(continued)

TABLE 28—*Continued*

R—	R^1—	R^2—	R^3—	Activity	Reference
C_6H_5—	C_6H_5—	H—	$C_6H_5CH_2CO$—	MES 31, MMS 63	Nakamura *et al.* (1965)
C_6H_5—	C_6H_5—	CH_3CO—	H—	MES act, Met act	Takamatsu *et al.* (1964)
C_6H_5—	C_6H_5—	C_2H_5OCO—	H—	MES > 100, MMS > 100	Nakamura *et al.* (1965)
C_6H_5—	C_6H_5—	C_6H_5CO—	H—	MES 58, MMS > 100	Nakamura *et al.* (1965)
C_6H_5—	C_6H_5—	$(C_3H_7)_2CHCO$—	H—	MES > 200, MMS > 200	Nakamura *et al.* (1965)
C_6H_5—	C_6H_5—			MES act., Met (ip) < 50, EST inact., not H, not S, LD_{50} 370	Carraz and Emin (1967)
C_6H_5—	C_6H_5—	CH_3CO—	CH_3CO—	MES > 100, MMS > 100	Nakamura *et al.* (1965)
C_6H_5—	C_6H_5—	CH_3CO—	C_2H_5OCO—	MES > 100, MMS > 100	Nakamura *et al.* (1965)
C_6H_5—	C_6H_5—	C_2H_5OCO—	CH_3CO—	MES > 100, MMS > 100	Nakamura *et al.* (1965)
C_6H_5—	C_6H_5—	C_2H_5OCO—	C_2H_5OCO—	MES 24, MMS 18	Nakamura *et al.* (1965)
C_6H_5—	C_6H_5—	$CH_3CO_2CH_2$—	$CH_3CO_2CH_2$—	MES < 12.5, Met inact., LD_{50} < 500	Vida *et al.*, (1971)
H—	H—	$4\text{-}H_2NSO_2C_6H_4$—	C_6H_5—	Act.	Geistlich (1974)
H—	$CH_3SCH_2CH_2$—	H—	C_6H_5—	MES inact, not S, LD_{50} 1400	Przegaliński (1969)
H—	C_6H_5—	H—	$p\text{-}NH_2SO_2C_6H_4$—	MES 822	Schoegl *et al.* (1961)
CH_3—	C_6H_5—	H—	$NH_2CO_2CH_2CH_2$—	MES 157	Schoegl *et al.* (1961)
C_2H_5—	C_6H_5—	H—	$NH_2CO_2CH_2CH_2$—	MES 203	Schoegl *et al.* (1961)
C_2H_5—	C_6H_5—	H—	$C_2H_5OCONHCH_2$—	MES 327	Schoegl *et al.* (1961)
C_6H_5—	C_6H_5—	H—	$CNCH_2CH_2$—	MES inact., Met inact.	Shaffer *et al* (1968)
C_6H_5—	C_6H_5—	H—	$C_6H_5NHCOCH_2$—	EST inact., LD_{50} > 1000	Danielsson *et al.* (1965)
C_6H_5—	C_6H_5—	H—	$o\text{-}CH_3C_6H_4NHCOCH_2$—	EST inact., LD_{50} > 2000	Danielsson *et al.* (1965)
C_6H_5—	C_6H_5—	H—	$2,6\text{-}(CH_3)_2C_6H_3NHCOCH_2$—	EST inact., LD_{50} > 2000	Danielsson *et al.* (1965)

TABLE 29 SPIROHYDANTOINS

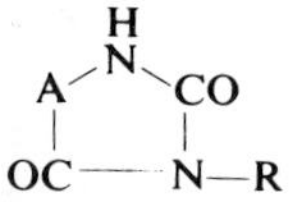

A—	R—	Activity	Reference
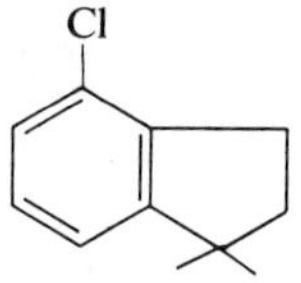	H—	Act.	Waring (1959)
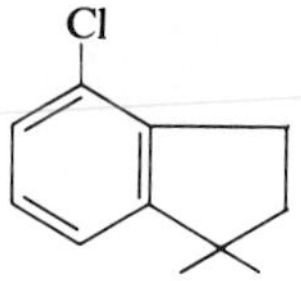	CH_3—	Act.	Waring (1959)
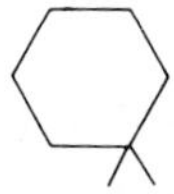	$(C_2H_5)_2NCH_2$—	MES inact., not S, LD_{50} 167	Przegaliński (1969)

E. THIOHYDANTOINS (TABLES 30-34)

TABLE 30 2-THIOHYDANTOINS: BENZILIDENE SUBSTITUENTS

R—	R¹—	R²—	Activity	Reference
H—	H—	C_6H_5—	Act.	Gavrilyuk and Zapadnyuk (1959)
H—	2-CH_3—	C_6H_5—	Met inact.	Musial and Korohoda (1966)
H—	4-CH_3—	C_6H_5—	Met inact.	Musial and Korohoda (1966)
H—	2-CH_3—	4-$CH_3C_6H_4$—	Met inact.	Musial and Korohoda (1966)
H—	4-CH_3—	4-$CH_3C_6H_4$—	Met act.	Musial and Korohoda (1966)
H—	2-CH_3—	4-BrC_6H_4—	MES inact., Met inact., S, LD_{50} 2000	Kleinrok et al. (1972)
H—	4-CH_3—	4-BrC_6H_4—	MES inact., Met inact., S, LD_{50} 2000	Kleinrok et al. (1972)
2-CH_3—	4-CH_3—	C_6H_5—	MES inact., Met inact., LD_{50} 3100	Musial et al. (1972)
3-CH_3—	4-CH_3—	C_6H_5—	MES inact., Met inact., LD_{50} 3700	Musial et al. (1972)
2-CH_3—	4-CH_3—	4-$CH_3C_6H_4$—	MES inact., Met inact., LD_{50} 3300	Musial et al. (1972)
3-CH_3—	4-CH_3—	4-$CH_3C_6H_4$—	MES inact., Met inact., LD_{50} 2600	Musial et al. (1972)
2-CH_3—	4-CH_3—	4-BrC_6H_4—	MES inact., Met inact., S, LD_{50} 2000	Kleinrok et al. (1972)
3-CH_3—	4-CH_3—	4-BrC_6H_4—	MES inact., Met inact., S, LD_{50} 1350	Kleinrok et al. (1972)
H—	2-CH_3O—	C_6H_5—	Met inact.	Musial and Korohoda (1966)
H—	3-CH_3O—	C_6H_5—	Met inact.	Musial and Korohoda (1966)
H—	2-CH_3O—	4-$CH_3C_6H_4$—	Met inact.	Musial and Korohoda (1966)
H—	3-CH_3O—	4-$CH_3C_6H_4$—	Met inact.	Musial and Korohoda (1966)
H—	2-CH_3O—	4-BrC_6H_4—	MES inact., Met inact., S, LD_{50} 1600	Kleinrok et al. (1972)
H—	3-CH_3O—	4-BrC_6H_4—	MES inact., Met inact., S, LD_{50} 2000	Kleinrok et al. (1972)

H—	4-CH$_3$O—	4-BrC$_6$H$_4$—	MES inact., Met weak act., S, LD$_{50}$ 1150	Kleinrok et al. (1972)
2-CH$_3$O—	3-CH$_3$O—	C$_6$H$_5$—	Met inact.	Musial and Korohoda (1967)
2-CH$_3$O—	5-CH$_3$O—	C$_6$H$_5$—	Met inact.	Musial and Korohoda (1967)
3-CH$_3$O—	4-CH$_3$O—	C$_6$H$_5$—	Met inact.	Musial and Korohoda (1967)
2-CH$_3$O—	3-CH$_3$O—	4-CH$_3$C$_6$H$_4$—	Met inact.	Musial and Korohoda (1967)
2-CH$_3$O—	5-CH$_3$O—	4-CH$_3$C$_6$H$_4$—	Met weak act.	Musial and Korohoda (1967)
3-CH$_3$O—	4-CH$_3$O—	4-CH$_3$C$_6$H$_4$—	Met inact.	Musial and Korohoda (1967)
2-CH$_3$O—	3-CH$_3$O—	4-BrC$_6$H$_4$—	MES inact., Met inact., S, LD$_{50}$ 1210	Kleinrok et al. (1972)
2-CH$_3$O—	4-CH$_3$O—	4-BrC$_6$H$_4$—	MES inact., Met inact., S, LD$_{50}$ 1310	Kleinrok et al. (1972)
2-CH$_3$O—	5-CH$_3$O—	4-BrC$_6$H$_4$—	MES inact., Met inact., S, LD$_{50}$ 2000	Kleinrok et al. (1972)
3-CH$_3$O—	4-CH$_3$O—	4-BrC$_6$H$_4$—	MES inact., Met inact., S, LD$_{50}$ 800	Kleinrok et al. (1972)
H—	2-Cl—	C$_6$H$_5$—	Met weak act.	Musial and Korohoda (1967)
H—	4-Cl—	C$_6$H$_5$—	Met inact.	Musial and Korohoda (1967)
H—	3-Cl—	C$_6$H$_5$—	MES (ip) 420, Met (ip) 500, LD$_{50}$ 2370	Musial et al. (1972)
H—	2-Cl—	4-CH$_3$C$_6$H$_4$—	Met act.	Musial and Korohoda (1967)
H—	4-Cl—	4-CH$_3$C$_6$H$_4$—	Met act.	Musial and Korohoda (1967)
H—	3-Cl—	4-CH$_3$C$_6$H$_4$—	MES weak act., Met (ip) 532, LD$_{50}$ 1550	Musial et al. (1972)
H—	2-Cl—	4-BrC$_6$H$_4$—	MES inact., Met weak act., S, LD$_{50}$ 1370	Kleinrok et al. (1972)
H—	3-Cl—	4-BrC$_6$H$_4$—	MES inact., Met weak act., S, LD$_{50}$ 1160	Kleinrok et al. (1972)
H—	4-Cl—	4-BrC$_6$H$_4$—	MES inact., Met inact., S, LD$_{50}$ 1220	Kleinrok et al. (1972)
H—	3-CH$_3$CONH—	C$_6$H$_5$—	MES inact., Met inact., LD$_{50}$ > 4000	Musial et al. (1972)
H—	4-CH$_3$CONH—	C$_6$H$_5$—	MES inact., Met inact., LD$_{50}$ 1760	Musial et al. (1972)
H—	3-CH$_3$CONH—	4-CH$_3$C$_6$H$_4$—	MES weak act., Met inact., LD$_{50}$ > 4000	Musial et al. (1972)
H—	4-CH$_3$CONH—	4-CH$_3$C$_6$H$_4$—	MES weak act., Met inact., LD$_{50}$ > 4000	Musial et al. (1972)

TABLE 31 2-THIOHYDANTOINS: MISCELLANEOUS SUBSTITUENTS

R—	R¹—	R²—	R³—	Activity	Reference
H—	H—	H—	$CH_2{=}CHCH_2{-}$	MES (ip) 141, Met (ip) 60, LD_{50} 600	Gesler et al. (1961)
H—	$CH_3{-}$	H—	$CH_2{=}CHCH_2{-}$	MES (ip) 110, Met (ip) 64, LD_{50} 175	Gesler et al. (1961)
H—	$C_2H_5{-}$	H—	$CH_2{=}CHCH_2{-}$	MES (ip) 125, Met (ip) 44, LD_{50} 350	Gesler et al. (1961)
H—	$n\text{-}C_3H_7{-}$	H—	$CH_2{=}CHCH_2{-}$	MES (ip) 59, Met (ip) 43, LD_{50} 350	Gesler et al. (1961)
H—	$i\text{-}C_3H_7{-}$	H—	$CH_2{=}CHCH_2{-}$	MES (ip) 84, Met (ip) 123, LD_{50} 500	Gesler et al. (1961)
H—	$n\text{-}C_4H_9{-}$	H—	$CH_2{=}CHCH_2{-}$	MES (ip) 60, Met (ip) 37, LD_{50} 500	Gesler et al. (1961)
H—	$sec\text{-}C_4H_9{-}$	H—	$CH_2{=}CHCH_2{-}$	MES (ip) 60, Met (ip) 52, LD_{50} 700	Gesler et al. (1961)
H—	$i\text{-}C_4H_9{-}$	H—	$CH_2{=}CHCH_2{-}$	po: MES 211, Met 40, SD_{50} 139; ip: MES 55, Met 11, SD_{50} 44, LD_{50} 301	Gesler et al. (1961)
H—	$n\text{-}C_6H_{13}{-}$	H—	$CH_2{=}CHCH_2{-}$	MES (ip) 138, Met (ip) 71, LD_{50} 700	Gesler et al. (1961)
H—	$i\text{-}C_4H_9{-}$	H—	H—	MES (ip) 178, Met (ip) 26, LD_{50} 150	Gesler et al. (1961)
H—	$i\text{-}C_4H_9{-}$	H—	$CH_3{-}$	MES (ip) 210, Met (ip) 25, LD_{50} 350	Gesler et al. (1961)

H—	$i\text{-}C_4H_9$—	H—	C_2H_5—	po: MES 190, Met 71; ip: MES 94, Met 12.5, LD_{50} 210	Gesler et al. (1961)
H—	$i\text{-}C_4H_9$—	H—	$n\text{-}C_3H_7$—	po: MES 358, Met 100; ip: MES 50, Met 20, LD_{50} 700	Gesler et al. (1961)
H—	$i\text{-}C_4H_9$—	H—	$n\text{-}C_4H_9$—	MES (ip) 110, Met (ip) 34, LD_{50} 600	Gesler et al. (1961)
H—	$i\text{-}C_4H_9$—	H—	$i\text{-}C_4H_9$—	MES (ip) ca. 300, Met (ip) ca. 75	Gesler et al. (1961)
H—	$i\text{-}C_4H_9$—	H—	$n\text{-}C_6H_{13}$—	MES (ip) 330, Met (ip) 92, $LD_{50} > 1600$	Gesler et al. (1961)
H—	$HO_2CCH_2CH_2$—	C_6H_5—	H—	Act.	Gavrilyuk and Zapadnyuk (1959)
H—	$CH_3SCH_2CH_2$—	C_6H_5—	H—	MES inact., not S, LD_{50} 450	Przegaliński (1969)
CH_3—	CH_3—	C_6H_5—	H—	Act.	Imperial Chemical Industries Limited (1959)
CH_3—	CH_3—	$p\text{-}CH_3C_6H_5$—	H—	Act.	Imperial Chemical Industries Limited (1959)
CH_3—	CH_3—	$m\text{-}ClC_6H_4$—	H—	Act.	Imperial Chemical Industries Limited (1959)
CH_3—	CH_3—	$p\text{-}ClC_6H_4$—	H—	Act.	Imperial Chemical Industries Limited (1959)
CH_3—	C_2H_5—	C_6H_5—	H—	Act.	Imperial Chemical Industries Limited (1959)

(continued)

TABLE 31—*Continued*

R—ᵃ	R¹—ᵃ	R²—	R³—	Activity	Reference
CH_3-	$i\text{-}C_4H_9-$	C_6H_5-	$H-$	Act.	Imperial Chemical Industries Limited (1959)
C_2H_5-	C_2H_5-	C_6H_5-	$H-$	Act.	Imperial Chemical Industries Limited (1959)
C_6H_5-	C_6H_5-	$H-$	$H-$	MES 25, Met weak act.	Sohn et al. (1970)
C_6H_5-	$C_6H_5CH_2-$	$H-$	$H-$	MMS inact., other studies	Enebäck and Alberty (1965)
C_6H_5-	C_6H_5-	$H-$	(morpholin-4-yl)$-CH_2-$	MES inact., Met weak act., S; LD_{50} 265	Malec (1966)
C_6H_5-	C_6H_5-	$H-$	CH_3N(piperazine)$N-CH_2-$	MES weak act., not S, LD_{50} 300	Malec (1970)
$3,4,5\text{-}(CH_3O)_3C_6H_2-$	$3,4,5\text{-}(CH_3O)_3C_6H_2-$	$H-$	$H-$	Act.	Kapadia et al. (1973)
ᵃ		$H-$	C_6H_5-	Act.	Gavrilyuk and Zapadnyuk (1959)

ᵃ R and R', (furan-2-yl)$-CH=$

TABLE 32   SPIRO-2-THIOHYDANTOINS: MISCELLANEOUS STRUCTURES

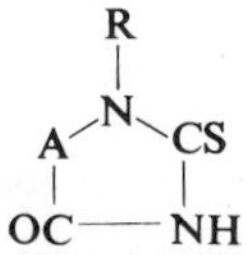

A—	R—	Activity	Reference
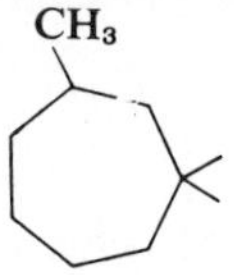 (CH₃)	H—	Act.	Brimelow *et al.* (1959b)
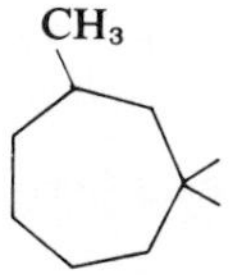 (CH₃)	H—	Act.	Brimelow *et al.* (1959b)
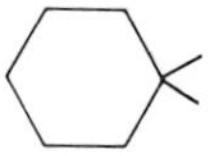	C_6H_5—	Act.	Imperial Chemical Industries Limited (1959)

TABLE 33   BIS-2-THIOHYDANTOINS AND MISCELLANEOUS 2-THIOHYDANTOINS

Compound	Activity	Reference
	MES inact., Met inact, S, LD_{50} 2000	Malec (1966)
	Met inact., S	Malec (1967)
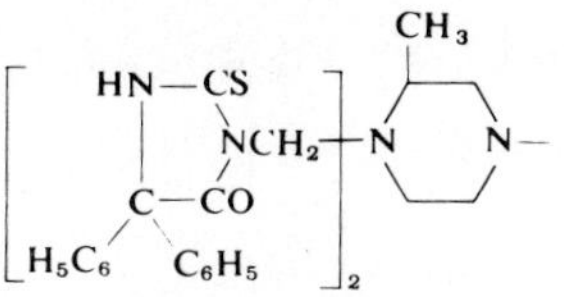	MES inact., Met inact., S, $LD_{50} > 2000$	Malec (1972)
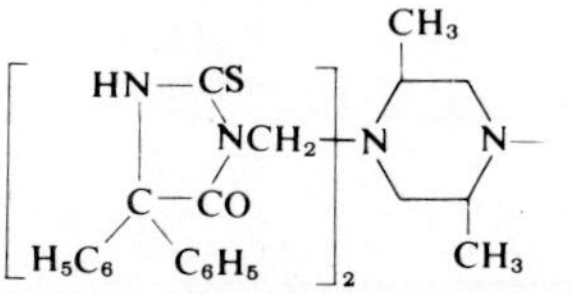	MES inact., Met inact., S, $LD_{50} > 2000$	Malec (1972)

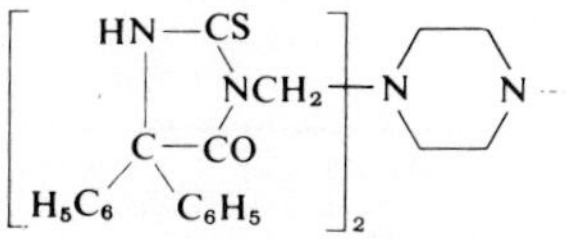

(*continued*)

241

TABLE 33—*Continued*

Compound	Activity	Reference
(structure: C_6H_5, SC–N–CO, HN–CHCH$_2$, $[\ ]_2$–S–)	MES inact., S, $LD_{50} > 2500$	Przegaliński (1969)
(structure: C_6H_5, SC–N–CO, HN–CH–CH$_2$, $[\ ]_2$–S–S–)	MES inact., S, $LD_{50} > 2500$	Przegaliński (1969)
(structure: C_6H_5, SC–N–CO, HN–CHCH$_2$S, $[\ ]_2$–CH$_2$–)	MES inact., S, LD_{50} 395	Przegaliński (1969)
(structure: C_6H_5, SC–N–CO, HN–CHCH$_2$, $[\ ]_2$)	MES inact., S, $LD_{50} > 2500$	Przegaliński (1969)
(structure: H_5C_6, H_5C_6, C, N=, CSCH$_3$, OC–NCH$_2$N, morpholine–O)	MES inact., not S, LD_{50} 620	Malec (1970)
(structure: H_5C_6, H_5C_6, C, N=, CSCH$_3$, OC–NCH$_2$, $[\ ]_2$, piperazine)	MES inact., S, LD_{50} 1620	Malec (1970)

TABLE 34 2,4-DITHIOHYDANTOINS[a]

Compound	Activity
(structure: H_5C_6, H_5C_6, C, N–H, CS, SC–NCH$_2$N, morpholine–O)	MES inact., not S, LD_{50} 980
(structure: H_5C_6, H_5C_6, C, N–H, CS, SC–NCH$_2$, $[\ ]_2$, piperazine)	MES inact., S, LD_{50} 2000

[a] Data from Malec, (1970).

III. SUCCINIMIDES

A. SUCCINIMIDES WITH ONLY ALIPHATIC HYDROCARBON SUBSTITUENTS (TABLES 35–36)

TABLE 35

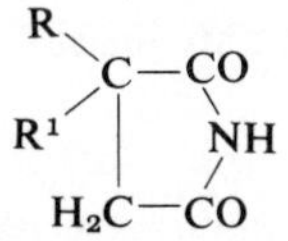

$$R{\diagdown} \atop {R^1} \quad C{-}CO \atop {|} \quad NH \atop H_2C{-}CO$$

R—	R¹—	Activity	Reference
CH_3—	C_2H_5—	MES (po) 1150, (ip) 1400, Met (po) 115, (ip) 125, EST (ip) 660, LD_{50} 1750	Najer *et al.* (1966)
		MES inact., Met act., LD_{50} 930	Fijalkowska *et al.* (1971)
		MES (ip) 4.33 mmoles/kg, Met (ip) 0.52 mmole/kg, MMS (ip) 2.21 mmoles/kg	Witiak *et al.* (1972)
		EST 340 (Carbowax), 600 (gum arabic), LD_{50} 1600	Laboratoires Dausse S. A. and Société B.M.C. (1969)
		LD_{50} 1225	Malec (1972)

TABLE 36   CYCLIC SUBSTITUENTS

Compound	Activity	Reference
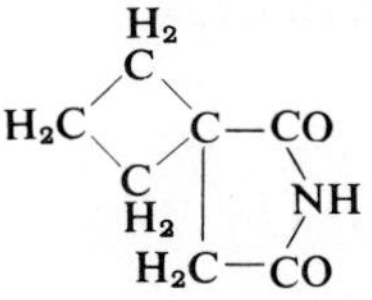	MES (po) 1030, (ip) 840, Met (po) 220, (ip) 200, EST (ip) 340, LD_{50} 1750	Najer *et al.* (1966)
	MES (ip) 840, Met (ip) 200, EST 160 (Carbowax) 340 (gum arabic), LD_{50} 1600	Laboratoires Dausse S. A. and Société B.M.C. (1969)
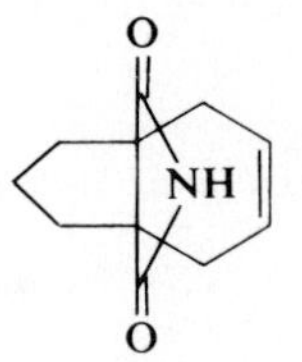	MES inact., Met act.	Wagner and Rudzik (1967)
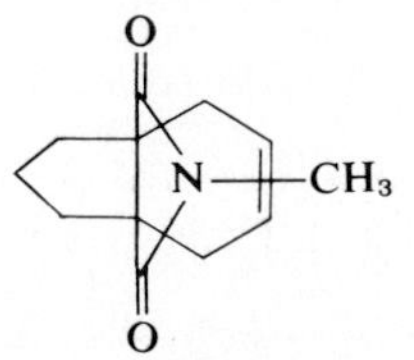	MES inact., Met weak act.	Wagner and Rudzik (1967)

(continued)

TABLE 36—*Continued*

Compound	Activity	Reference
	MES inact., Met inact.	Wagner and Rudzik (1967)
	MES inact., Met inact.	Wagner and Rudzik (1967)
	MES inact., Met inact.	Wagner and Rudzik (1967)
	MES inact., Met (ip) 22, LD_{50} 620	Wagner and Rudzik (1967, 1969)
	Met weak act.	Wagner and Rudzik (1967, 1969)
	Met act.	Wagner and Rudzik (1967, 1969)

TABLE 36—*Continued*

Compound	Activity	Reference
	Act.	Wagner and Rudzik (1967)
	Act.	Wagner and Rudzik (1967)
	MES inact., Met weak act.	Wagner and Rudzik (1967, 1969)
	Act.	Wagner and Rudzik (1969)
	Act.	Wagner and Rudzik (1969)
	MES inact., Met inact., S	Wagner and Rudzik (1969)

(continued)

TABLE 36—*Continued*

Compound	Activity	Reference
	MES inact., Met (ip) 42, S	Wagner and Rudzik (1967, 1969)
	MES inact., Met inact.	Wagner and Rudzik (1967, 1969)
	Act.	Wagner and Rudzik (1969)
	Act.	Wagner and Rudzik (1969)

B. SUCCINIMIDES WITH AROMATIC HYDROCARBON SUBSTITUENTS (TABLES 37–40)

TABLE 37

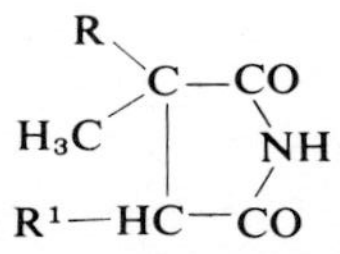

R—C(CH₃)—CO
                | \
                | NH
                | /
          R¹—HC—CO

R—	R¹—	Activity	Reference
C_6H_5-	H—	Met act., ^{14}C study	Nicholls and Orton (1972)
C_6H_5-	C_2H_5-	MES 50–100, Met act.	Hauck et al. (1967)
		MES act., Met act., S	Chen and Bass (1964)
C_6H_5-	$n\text{-}C_3H_7-$	MES weak act., Met act.	Hauck et al. (1967)
C_6H_5-	$i\text{-}C_3H_7-$	MES weak act., Met act.	Hauck et al. (1967)
C_6H_5-	$CH_2=CHCH_2-$	MES weak act., Met act.	Hauck et al. (1967)
C_6H_5-	$CH_3CH=CHCH_2-$	MES inact., Met weak act.	Hauck et al. (1967)
C_6H_5-	$(CH_3)_2C=CHCH_2-$	MES inact., Met weak act.	Hauck et al. (1967)
C_6H_5-	$CH_2=C(CH_3)CH_2-$	MES inact., Met inact.	Hauck et al. (1967)
C_6H_5-	$C_6H_5CH_2-$	MES inact., Met weak act.	Hauck et al. (1967)
C_6H_5-	$C_6H_5CH=CHCH_2-$	MES inact., Met inact.	Hauck et al. (1967)
$o\text{-}CH_3C_6H_4-$	C_2H_5-	MES act., Met weak act.	Hauck et al. (1967)
$p\text{-}CH_3C_6H_4-$	C_2H_5-	MES inact., Met weak act.	Hauck et al. (1967)

TABLE 38

$$R-\underset{R^1}{\overset{}{C}}\!\!-\!\!\underset{H_2C-CO}{\overset{CO}{\diagdown}}NR^2$$

R—	R¹—	R²—	Activity	Reference
H—	$C_6H_5CH_2$—	H—	MES 62, Met 36, LD_{50} 420	Matsuda and Matsuda (1957)
H—	$p\text{-}CH_3C_6H_4CH_2$—	H—	MES 70, Met 68, LD_{50} 1441	Matsuda and Matsuda (1957)
H—	C_6H_5—	CH_3—	MES 70, Met 38, LD_{50} 1580	Matsuda and Matsuda (1957)
			MES 64, Met 87, LD_{50} 950	Akopyan and Gerasimayn (1971b)
			MES 115, Met 134, not H	Clemson et al. (1970)
			MES (ip) 0.39 mmole/kg, Met (ip) 0.43 mmole/kg, MMS (ip) 2.69 mmole/kg	Witiak et al. (1972)
			MES weak act.	Clemson et al. (1968)
			Met act.	Magarian et al. (1973)
			MES act., Met act., LD_{50} 500	Magyar and Walsa (1966)
H—	$p\text{-}CH_3C_6H_4$—	CH_3—	Act.	Akopyan and Gerasimyan (1971a)
H—	$p\text{-}CH_3CH(CH_3)C_6H_4$—	CH_3—	Act.	Akopyan and Gerasimyan (1971a)
H—	$C_6H_5CH_2$—	CH_3—	MES 75, Met 100, LD_{50} 420	Matsuda and Matsuda (1957)
H—	$C_6H_5CH_2$—	C_2H_5—	MES 120, Met 135, LD_{50} 580	Matsuda and Matsuda (1957)
H—	$C_6H_5CH_2$—	$n\text{-}C_4H_9$—	Met inact., LD_{50} 580	Matsuda and Matsuda (1957)
H—	$C_6H_5CH_2$—	$n\text{-}C_{12}H_{25}$—	Met inact., LD_{50} > 2000	Matsuda and Matsuda (1957)
H—	$C_6H_5CH_2$—	C_6H_5—	Met inact., LD_{50} 1650	Matsuda and Matsuda (1957)
H—	$C_6H_5CH_2$—	$C_{10}H_7$—[a]	Met inact., LD_{50} 3850	Matsuda and Matsuda (1957)
CH_3—	C_6H_5—	CH_3—	MES (ip) 0.21 mmole/kg, Met (ip) 0.17 mmole/kg, MMS (ip) 2.03 mmoles/kg	Witiak et al. (1972)
			Met act., ^{14}C study	Nicholls and Orton (1972)
C_6H_5—	$C_6H_5CH_2$—	CH_3—	MES inact., Met inact., not H	Clemson et al. (1970)

[a] Naphthyl.

TABLE 39 SPIROSUCCINIMIDES

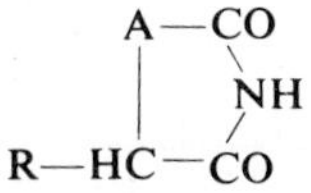

$$A—CO$$
$$| \quad NH$$
$$R—HC—CO$$

A— |	R—	Activity	Reference
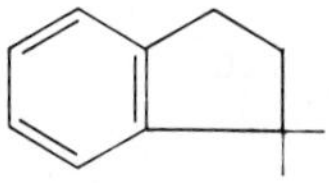	C_2H_5—	MES weak act., Met. act.	Hauck *et al.* (1967)
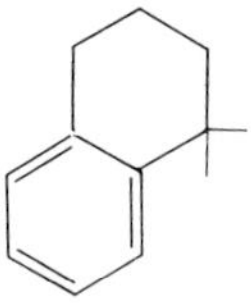	C_2H_5—	MES inact., Met inact	Hauck *et al.* (1967)
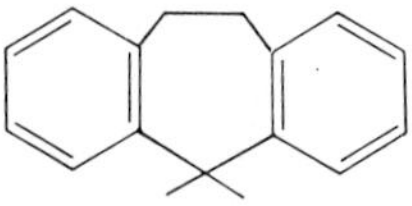	H—	Act.	Davis (1964)

TABLE 40 CYCLIC SUBSTITUENTS[a]

Compound	Activity
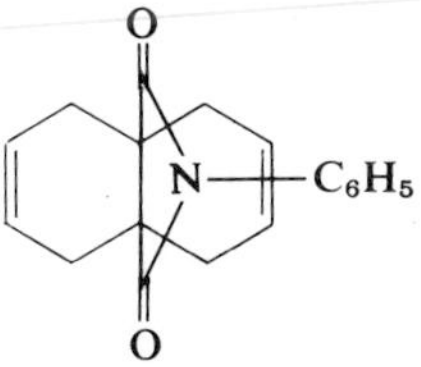 $-C_6H_5$	MES inact., Met inact., S
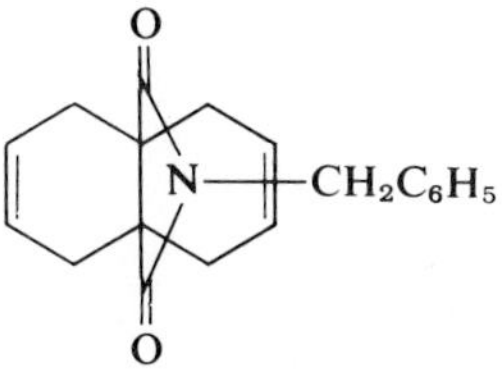 $-CH_2C_6H_5$	MES inact., Met weak act.
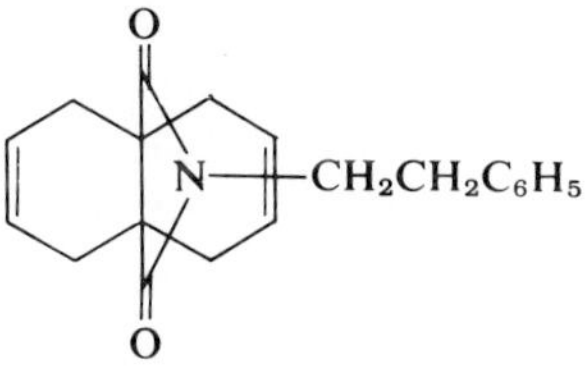 $-CH_2CH_2C_6H_5$	MES inact., Met inact.

[a] Data from Wagner and Rudzik (1967).

C. SUCCINIMIDES WITH HETEROCYCLIC SUBSTITUENTS (TABLES 41–45)

TABLE 41 BOTH CYCLIC AND HETEROCYCLIC SUBSTITUENTS[a]

Compound	Activity
	MES inact., Met inact.[b]
	MES inact., Met inact.[b]
	Act.
	Act.
	Act.
	Act.

TABLE 41—*Continued*

Compound	Activity

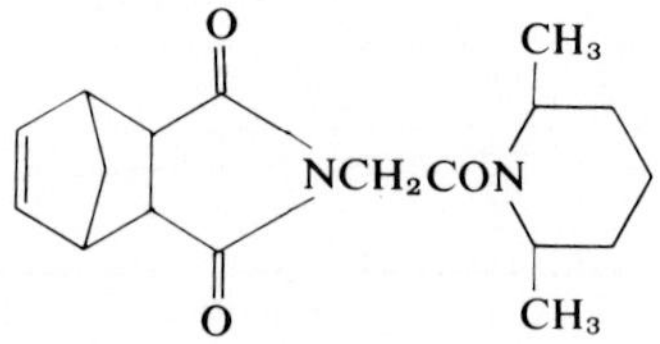

Act.

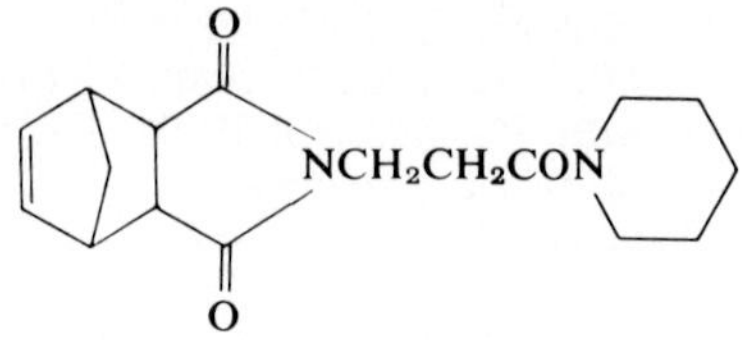

Act.

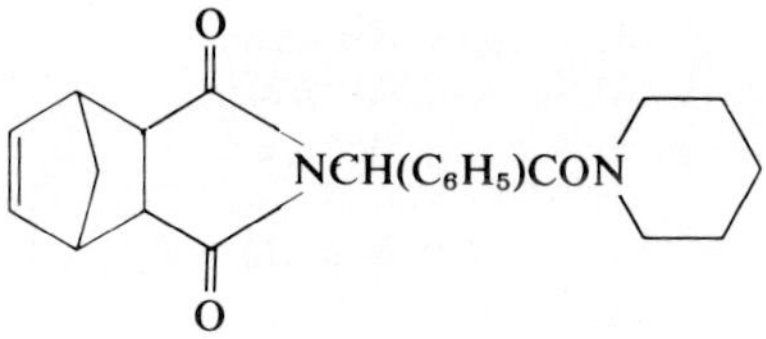

Act.

[a] Data from Serino *et al.* (1970) except where indicated otherwise.

[b] Data from Wagner and Rudzik (1967).

TABLE 42 7-OXABICYCLO[2.2.1]HEPTANE-2,3-DICARBOXIMIDES[b]

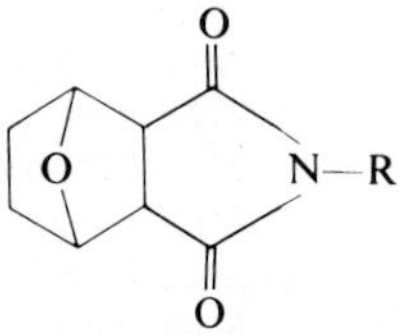

R—	Activity
$(CH_3)_3C$—	MES inact., Met inact.
Cyclo-C_6H_{11}—	MES inact., Met inact.
C_6H_5—	MES 400, Met > 400, LD_{50} 1165
2-$CH_3C_6H_4$—	MES 260, Met > 800, LD_{50} 270
3-$CH_3C_6H_4$—	MES inact., Met inact.
4-$CH_3C_6H_4$—	MES inact., Met inact.
2-$C_2H_5C_6H_4$—	MES inact., Met inact.
2,4-$(CH_3)_2C_6H_3$—	MES inact., Met inact.
2,6-$(CH_3)_2C_6H_3$—	MES 310, Met > 400, LD_{50} > 1000

(*continued*)

251

TABLE 42—*Continued*

R—	Activity
3,4-(CH$_3$)$_2$C$_6$H$_3$—	MES inact., Met inact.
C$_6$H$_5$CH$_2$—	MES 171, Met 285, MMS 51, LD$_{50}$ 1240
C$_6$H$_5$CH$_2$CH$_2$—	MES 154, Met 168, MMS 36, LD$_{50}$ > 1600
C$_6$H$_5$(CH$_2$)$_4$—	MES inact., Met inact.
C$_6$H$_5$CH(CH$_3$)—	MES 340, Met > 400, LD$_{50}$ > 1600
C$_6$H$_5$CH$_2$CH(CH$_3$)—	MES inact., Met inact.
C$_6$H$_5$CH(CH$_3$)CH—	MES 132, Met > 200, LD$_{50}$ > 1600
C$_6$H$_5$CH(C$_2$H$_5$)CH$_2$—	MES inact., Met inact.
(C$_6$H$_5$)$_2$CH—	MES inact., Met inact.
(C$_6$H$_5$)$_2$CHCH$_2$—	MES inact., Met inact.
C$_6$H$_5$CH=CHCH$_2$—	MES 220, Met > 400, LD$_{50}$ > 1600
2-BrC$_6$H$_4$—	MES < 400, Met 315, LD$_{50}$ > 1600
4-BrC$_6$H$_4$—	MES inact., Met inact.
2,4,6-Br$_3$C$_6$H$_2$—	MES inact., Met inact.
2-ClC$_6$H$_4$—	MES 112, Met 185, MMS 19, LD$_{50}$ 1690
3-ClC$_6$H$_4$—	MES 260, Met 280, LD$_{50}$ > 1200
4-ClC$_6$H$_4$—	MES 240, Met > 800, LD$_{50}$ 1450
2,3-Cl$_2$C$_6$H$_3$—	MES 27, Met 52, LD$_{50}$ > 1600
2,4-Cl$_2$C$_6$H$_3$—	MES 43.5, Met 195, MMS 7.6, LD$_{50}$ 1000
2,5-Cl$_2$C$_6$H$_3$—	MES < 200, Met 94, LD$_{50}$ > 1600
2,6-Cl$_2$C$_6$H$_3$—	MES 280, Met > 400, LD$_{50}$ > 1000
3,4-Cl$_2$C$_6$H$_3$—	MES inact., Met inact.
3,5-Cl$_2$C$_6$H$_3$—	MES 49, Met 259, LD$_{50}$ > 800
2,4,5-Cl$_3$C$_6$H$_2$—	MES inact., Met inact.
2,4,6-Cl$_3$C$_6$H$_2$—	MES 175, Met > 400, LD$_{50}$ > 800
2-Cl, 4-CH$_3$C$_6$H$_3$—	MES inact., Met inact.
2-Cl, 5-CH$_3$C$_6$H$_3$—	MES inact., Met inact.
2-Cl, 6-CH$_3$C$_6$H$_3$—[a]	MES inact., Met inact.
3-Cl, 2-CH$_3$C$_6$H$_3$—	MES 24.5, Met 200, LD$_{50}$ > 1600
3-Cl, 4-CH$_3$C$_6$H$_3$—	MES inact., Met inact.
4-Cl, 2-CH$_3$C$_6$H$_3$—	MES 105, Met 90, LD$_{50}$ > 1000

TABLE 42—*Continued*

R—	Activity
5-Cl, 2-CH$_3$C$_6$H$_3$—	MES inact., Met inact.
2-ClC$_6$H$_4$CH$_2$—	MES 225, Met > 400, LD$_{50}$ 1350
4-ClC$_6$H$_4$CH$_2$—	MES 251, Met 870, LD$_{50}$ 600
2,4-Cl$_2$C$_6$H$_3$CH$_2$—	MES inact., Met inact.
3,4-Cl$_2$C$_6$H$_3$CH$_2$—	MES 165, Met > 400, LD$_{50}$ > 2000
2-ClC$_6$H$_4$CH$_2$CH$_2$—	MES 98, Met 125, LD$_{50}$ > 1600
4-ClC$_6$H$_4$CH$_2$CH$_2$—	MES inact., Met inact.
2,4-Cl$_2$C$_6$H$_3$CH$_2$CH$_2$—	MES inact., Met inact.
3-CF$_3$C$_6$H$_4$—	MES 335, Met > 400, LD$_{50}$ > 1600
2-Cl, 5-CF$_3$C$_6$H$_3$—	MES 50, Met > 200, LD$_{50}$ < 400
CH$_3$CHOHCH$_2$—	MES inact., Met inact.
2-HOC$_6$H$_4$—	MES inact., Met inact.
4-HOC$_6$H$_4$—	MES inact., Met inact.
2-CH$_3$OC$_6$H$_4$—	MES 505, Met > 800, LD$_{50}$ 595
4-CH$_3$OC$_6$H$_4$CH$_2$—	MES inact., Met inact.
2-C$_2$H$_5$OC$_6$H$_4$—	MES 296, Met > 800, MMS 200, LD$_{50}$ 410
4-C$_2$H$_5$OC$_6$H$_4$—	MES inact., Met inact.
4-C$_2$H$_5$OC$_6$H$_4$CH$_2$—	MES inact. Met inact.
4-C$_4$H$_9$OC$_6$H$_4$CH$_2$—	MES inact., Met inact.
C$_6$H$_5$OCH$_2$CH$_2$—	MES inact., Met inact.
CH$_3$COC$_6$H$_4$—	MES 290, Met > 400, LD$_{50}$ > 1600
4-(CH$_3$)$_2$NC$_6$H$_4$—	MES inact., Met inact.
C$_6$H$_5$N(CH$_3$)—	MES inact., Met inact.
3-Pyridyl-	MES inact., Met inact.
5-Cl, 2-pyridyl-	MES inact., Met inact.
2-Thiazolyl-	MES inact., Met inact.
2-Benzothiazolyl-	MES inact., Met inact.

[a] Two isomers.
[b] Bockstahler *et al.* (1968).

TABLE 43 MISCELLANEOUS HETEROCYCLES

R—	R¹—	Activity	Reference
H—	(NCH₂—)	Act.	Eckstein et al. (1967)
H—	(NCH₂—)	MES inact., Met weak act. Act.	Magarian et al. (1973) Eckstein et al. (1967)
H—	(NCH₂—)	MES act.(?), Met act.	Magarian et al. (1973)
H—	(NCH₂—)	MES inact., Met inact.	Magarian et al. (1973)
H—	C₆H₅(CH₂)₃— (NCH₂—)	MES weak act., Met weak act.	Magarian et al. (1973)
H—	CH₃N (NCH₂—)	MES weak act., Met act.	Magarian et al. (1973)
H—	(O, NCH₂—)	MES weak act., Met act. Act. MES act., Met act., LD₅₀ 2000	Magarian et al. (1973) Eckstein et al. (1967) Magyar and Walsa (1966)

Structure		Activity	Reference
CH_3-	(morpholine)NCH_2-	Review	Lunsford (1968), Reidl and Kertesi (1968)
		Act.	Eckstein et al. (1967)
(pyrrolidine)NCH_2-	CH_3-	MES inact., Met inact.	Clemson et al. (1968)
(pyrrolidine)NCH_2CH_2-	CH_3-	MES act., Met. Inact.	Clemson et al. (1968)
(piperidine)NCH_2-	CH_3-	MES act., Met. inact.	Clemson et al. (1968)
(piperidine)NCH_2CH_2-	CH_3-	MES act., Met inact.	Clemson et al. (1968)
(bicyclic)NCH_2-	CH_3-	MES act., Met inact.	Clemson et al. (1968)
(bicyclic)NCH_2CH_2-	CH_3-	MES weak act., Met inact.	Clemson et al. (1968)
CH_3N(piperazine)NCH_2-	CH_3-	MES inact., Met inact.	Clemson et al. (1968)
CH_3N(piperazine)NCH_2CH_2-	CH_3-	MES act., Met inact.	Clemson et al. (1968)
(morpholine)NCH_2-	CH_3-	MES inact., Met inact.	Clemson et al. (1968)

(continued)

TABLE 43—*Continued*

R—	R¹—	Activity	Reference
(morpholine)NCH₂CH₂—	CH₃—	MES act., Met inact.	Clemson *et al.* (1968)
(piperidine)NCH₂—	(piperidine)NCH₂—	MES weak act., Met inact.	Magarian *et al.* (1973)
(tetrahydropyridine)NCH₂—	(tetrahydropyridine)NCH₂—	MES inact., Met inact.	Magarian *et al.* (1973)
(bicyclic)NCH₂—	(bicyclic)NCH₂—	MES inact., Met weak act.	Magarian *et al.* (1973)
C₆H₅(CH₂)₃(piperidine)NCH₂—	C₆H₅(CH₂)₃(piperidine)NCH₂—	MES inact., Met inact.	Magarian *et al.* (1973)
CH₃N(piperazine)NCH₂—	CH₃N(piperazine)NCH₂—	MES weak act., Met inact.	Magarian *et al.* (1973)
O(morpholine)NCH₂—	O(morpholine)NCH₂—	MES weak act., Met inact.	Magarian *et al.* (1973)

TABLE 44 MISCELLANEOUS HETEROCYCLES

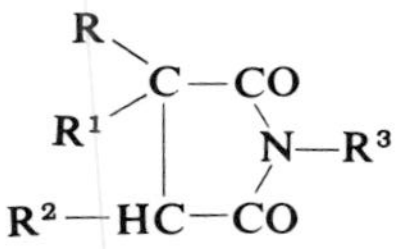

$$R-C-CO$$
$$R^1 \quad N-R^3$$
$$R^2-HC-CO$$

R—	R¹—	R²—	R³—	Activity	Reference
H—	H—	H—	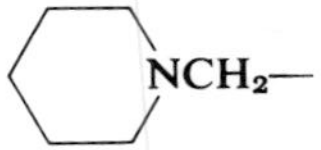 (piperidin-1-yl)CH₂—	MES inact., Met inact.	Das et al. (1975)
H—	H—	H—	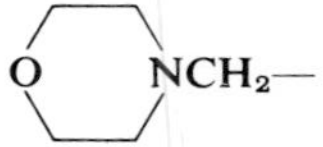 (morpholin-4-yl)CH₂—	MES inact., Met inact.	Das et al. (1975)
H—	H—	H—	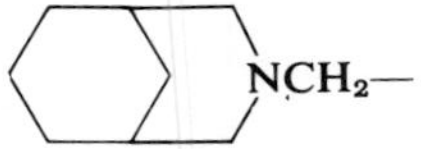 (bicyclic amine)CH₂—	MES inact., Met inact.	Das et al. (1975)
H—	H—	H—	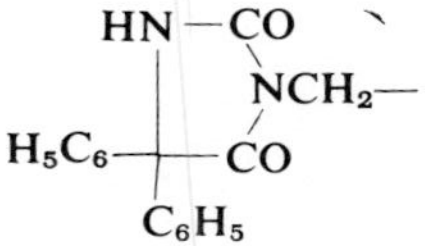 HN—CO, C_6H_5, H_5C_6, NCH₂—CO	MES inact., Met inact.	Das et al. (1975)
H—	$p\text{-}ClC_6H_4$—	H—	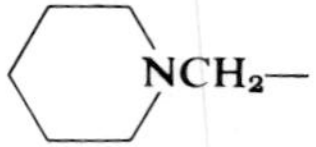 (piperidin-1-yl)CH₂—	Act.	Eckstein et al. (1967)
H—	$p\text{-}ClC_6H_4$—	H—	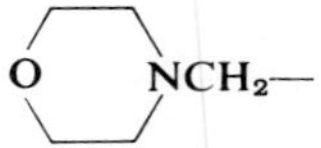 (morpholin-4-yl)CH₂—	Act.	Eckstein et al. (1967)

(Continued)

TABLE 44—Continued

R—	R¹—	R²—	R³—	Activity	Reference
(furan ring)	CH_3—	C_2H_5—	H—	MES weak act., Met weak act.	Hauck et al. (1967)
(thiophene ring)	CH_3—	C_2H_5—	H—	MES weak act., Met weak act.	Hauck et al. (1967)
(imidazole ring)	H—	H—	H—	Act.	Hasegawa and Kotani (1974)
(imidazole ring)	H—	H—	$n\text{-}C_4H_9$—	Act.	Hasegawa and Kotani (1974)
(imidazole ring)	H—	H—	Cyclo-$C_{12}H_{25}$—	Act.	Hasegawa and Kotani (1974)
(imidazole ring)	H—	H—	C_6H_5—	Act.	Hasegawa and Kotani (1974)
H_5C_6 (imidazole ring)	H—	H—	$p\text{-}C_2H_5OC_6H_4$—	Act.	Hasegawa and Kotani (1974)
(indole ring)	H—	H—	H—	MMS act.	Julia and Bagot (1964)

(indole, N–CH₃)	H—	H—	CH₃—	MMS weak act.	Julia and Bagot (1964)
(5-CH₃O-indole, N–CH₃)	H—	H—	C₂H₅—	MMS act.	Julia and Bagot (1964)
(5-CH₃O-indole, N–H)	H—	H—	n-C₃H₇—	MMS act.	Julia and Bagot (1964)

259

TABLE 45 MISCELLANEOUS BISSUCCINIMIDES

R—	R¹—	—B—	Activity	Reference
H—	H—	$-CH_2N$ piperazine NCH_2-	MES inact., Met inact.	Das et al. (1975)
H—	H—	$-CH_2NCH_2-$ cyclohexyl with CH_3	MES act., Met inact.	Das et al. (1975)
H—	H—	$-CH_2NCH_2-$ cyclohexyl with CH_3	MES act., Met inact.	Das et al. (1975)
CH_3-	C_2H_5-	$-CH_2N$ piperazine NCH_2-	Act.	Lucka-Sobstel and Zejc (1971)

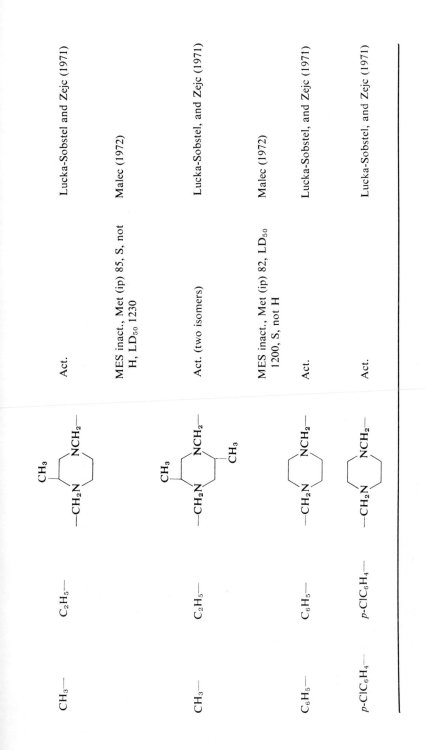

CH$_3$—		Act.	Lucka-Sobstel and Zejc (1971)
C$_2$H$_5$—		MES inact., Met (ip) 85, S, not H, LD$_{50}$ 1230	Malec (1972)
CH$_3$—		Act. (two isomers)	Lucka-Sobstel, and Zejc (1971)
C$_2$H$_5$—		MES inact., Met (ip) 82, LD$_{50}$ 1200, S, not H	Malec (1972)
C$_6$H$_5$—		Act.	Lucka-Sobstel, and Zejc (1971)
p-ClC$_6$H$_4$—		Act.	Lucka-Sobstel, and Zejc (1971)

D. SUCCINIMIDES WITH HETEROATOMS IN NONHETEROCYCLIC SYSTEMS (TABLES 46–51)

TABLE 46 CYCLIC SUBSTITUENTS

Compound	Activity	Reference
	MES 35, MMS 100, $LD_{50} > 3000$	Campaigne et al. (1968)
	Met inact.	Wagner and Rudzik (1967)
	MES inact., Met inact.	Wagner and Rudzik (1967)

Structure	Activity	Reference
NCH_2CONH_2 (imide)	Act.	Serino et al. (1970)
$NCH(CH_3)CONH_2$ (imide)	Act.	Serino et al. (1970)
$NCH_2CON(C_2H_5)_2$ (imide)	Act.	Serino et al. (1970)
$NCH_2CON(C_2H_5)_2$ (imide)	Act.	Serino et al. (1970)
$NCH_2CONHC_6H_4$ (imide)	Act.	Serino et al. (1970)

TABLE 47 HALIDES

X—	R—	R¹—	R²—	Activity	Reference
m-Br—	H—	H—	H—	MES 15, Met act., LD_{50} 600	Fijalkowska et al. (1971)
p-Br—	H—	H—	H—	ES inact., Met act.	Lange et al. (1962)
p-Cl—	H—	H—	H—	Met act.(?)	Lange et al. (1962)
p-F—	H—	H—	H—	ES inact., Met act.	Lange et al. (1962)
p-I—	H—	H—	H—	ES inact., Met act.	Lange et al. (1962)
p-Br—	H—	H—	CH_3—	ES inact., Met act.	Lange et al. (1962)
p-Br—	H—	H—	C_2H_5—	ES weak act., Met act.	Lange et al. (1962)
p-Br—	H—	H—	C_3H_7—	ES weak act., Met inact.	Lange et al. (1962)
p-Br—	H—	H—	CH_2=$CHCH_2$—	ES inact., Met inact.	Lange et al. (1962)
p-Br—	H—	H—	C_4H_9—	ES inact., Met inact.	Lange et al. (1962)
p-Br—	H—	H—	$CH_3CH_2CH(CH_3)$—	ES weak act., Met inact.	Lange et al. (1962)
p-Br—	H—	H—	C_5H_{11}—	ES inact., Met inact.	Lange et al. (1962)
p-Br—	H—	H—	i-C_5H_{11}—	ES inact., Met inact.,	Lange et al. (1962)
p-Br—	H—	H—	C_6H_{13}—	ES inact., Met act.	Lange et al. (1962)
p-Br—	H—	H—	i-C_6H_{13}—	ES inact., Met inact.	Lange et al. (1962)
p-Cl—	H—	H—	CH_3—	Met act.(?)	Lange et al. (1962)
p-Cl—	H—	H—	C_2H_5—	Met inact.	Lange et al. (1962)
p-Cl—	H—	H—	CH_2=$CHCH_2$—	Met inact.	Lange et al. (1962)
p-Cl—	H—	H—	C_4H_9—	ES inact., Met act.	Lange et al. (1962)

Position	R1	R2	Activity	Reference
p-Cl—	H—	i-C_5H_{11}—	ES inact., Met inact.	Lange et al. (1962)
p-Cl—	H—	C_6H_{13}—	ES inact., Met inact.	Lange et al. (1962)
p-Cl—	H—	i-C_6H_{13}—	ES weak act., Met weak act.	Lange et al. (1962)
p-F—	H—	CH_3—	ES inact., Met act.	Lange et al. (1962)
p-F—	H—	C_2H_5—	ES weak act., Met inact.	Lange et al. (1962)
p-F—	H—	C_3H_7—	ES inact., Met inact.	Lange et al. (1962)
p-F—	H—	C_4H_9—	ES inact., Met inact.	Lange et al. (1962)
p-F—	H—	C_5H_{11}—	ES inact., Met inact.	Lange et al. (1962)
p-I—	H—	CH_3—	ES weak act., Met inact.	Lange et al. (1962)
p-I—	H—	C_2H_5—	ES weak act., Met inact.	Lange et al. (1962)
p-I—	H—	C_3H_7—	ES inact., Met weak act.	Lange et al. (1962)
p-I—	H—	C_4H_9—	ES inact., Met inact.	Lange et al. (1962)
p-I—	H—	C_5H_{11}—	ES inact., Met inact.	Lange et al. (1962)
p-I—	H—	i-C_5H_{11}—	ES inact., Met inact.	Lange et al. (1962)
p-I—	H—	C_6H_{13}—	ES inact., Met inact.	Lange et al. (1962)
p-I—	H—	i-C_6H_{13}—	ES inact., Met inact.	Lange et al. (1962)
p-Br—	C_2H_5—	CH_3—	MES weak act., Met act.	Hauck et al. (1967)
p-Cl—	CH_3—	CH_3—	MES weak act., Met weak act.	Hauck et al. (1967)
o-Cl—	C_2H_5—	CH_3—	MES act., Met inact.	Hauck et al. (1967)
m-Cl—	C_2H_5—	CH_3—	MES weak act., Met act.	Hauck et al. (1967)
p-Cl—	C_2H_5—	CH_3—	MES weak act., Met act.	Hauck et al. (1967)
p-Cl—	C_2H_5—	C_2H_5—	MES lethal/200, Met act.	Hauck et al. (1967)
p-Cl—	CH_3—	$CH_2{=}CHCH_2$—	MES weak act., Met weak act.	Hauck et al. (1967)
p-Cl—	CH_3—	n-C_3H_7—	MES inact., Met weak act.	Hauck et al. (1967)
p-Cl—	C_2H_5—	$CH_2{=}CHCH_2$—	MES inact., Met weak act.	Hauck et al. (1967)
p-Cl—	C_2H_5—	CH_3OCH_2—	MES weak act., Met weak act.	Hauck et al. (1967)
o-F—	C_2H_5—	CH_3—	MES act., Met weak act.	Hauck et al. (1967)
m-F—	C_2H_5—	CH_3—	MES weak act., Met act.	Hauck et al. (1967)
p-F—	C_2H_5—	CH_3—	MES weak act., Met act.	Hauck et al. (1967)
p-F—	C_2H_5—	C_2H_5—	MES weak act., Met act.	Hauck et al. (1967)

TABLE 48 HALIDES

R—	R¹—	R²—	R³—	Activity	Reference
H—	C₆H₅CH₂—	Br—	CH₃—	MES inact., Met inact., not H (two isomers)	Clemson et al. (1970)
H—	Br—	H—	CH₃—	MES inact., Met 400(?), not H	Clemson et al. (1970)
H—	2,6-Cl₂C₆H₃—	H—	H—	MES > 10 < 25	Bream and Read (1973)
H—	2,6-Cl₂C₆H₃—	H—	CH₃—	MES act.	Bream and Read (1973)
H—	2,6-Cl₂C₆H₃—	H—	CH₃OCH₂—	MES act.	Bream and Read (1973)
H—	2,6-Cl₂C₆H₃—	H—	HOCH₂—	MES act.	Bream and Read (1973)
H—	CH₃CONH—	H—	p-ClC₆H₄—	D(R) isomer: MES (ip) 1.54 mmoles/kg, Met (ip) 0.77 mmole, (ip) 1.28 mmoles/kg; L(S) isomer: MES (ip) inact., Met (ip) inact., MMS (ip) 0.84 mmoles/kg	Witiak et al. (1972)
CH₃—	C₆H₅—	CH₂=CClCH₂—	H—	MES inact. Met inact.	Hauck et al. (1967)
CH₃—	2,4-Cl₂C₆H₃—	C₂H₅—	H—	MES weak act., Met weak act.	Hauck et al. (1967)
CH₃—	3,4-Cl₂C₆H₃—	C₂H₅—	H—	MES inact., Met inact.	Hauck et al. (1967)
CH₃—	m-CF₃C₆H₄—	C₂H₅—	H—	MES weak act., Met weak act.	Hauck et al. (1967)

TABLE 49 HALOGEN SULFONAMIDES[a]

Structure:

$$\underset{R^1}{\overset{R}{>}}C - CO - \underset{H_2C - CO}{\overset{X}{\underset{N}{|}}} \text{—} \langle \text{—} \rangle \text{—} SO_2NHR^2$$

R—	R¹—	X—	Sulfamoyl position	R²—	Activity
H—	CH₃—	2-Br—	4	H—	MES 25–50, Met 200
H—	C₆H₅—	2-Br—	4	H—	MES 10, Met 200
CH₃—	C₂H₅—	2-Br—	4	H—	Act.
CH₃—	C₂H₅—	2-Br—	5	H—	Act.
CH₃—	C₆H₅—	2-Br—	4	H—	Act.
H—	CH₃—	2-Cl—	4	H—	Act.
H—	CH₃—	2-Cl—	5	H—	Act.
H—	CH₃—	5-Cl—	2	H—	Act.
H—	CH₂=CHCH₂—	2-Cl—	4	H—	MES 25, Met 200
H—	n-C₅H₁₁—	2-Cl—	4	H—	Act.
H—	Cyclo-C₅H₉—	2-Cl—	4	H—	Act.
H—	(cyclopentenyl)	2-Cl—	4	H—	MES 10, Met 200
H—	n-C₆H₁₃—	2-Cl—	4	H—	Met 200
H—	Cyclo-C₆H₁₁—	2-Cl—	4	H—	MES 2.5–5, Met 200
H—	(cyclohexenyl)	2-Cl—	4	H—	Act.
H—	(cyclohexenyl)	2-Cl—	4	H—	MES 25–50, Met 20–100

(continued)

TABLE 49—*Continued*

R—	R¹—	X—	Sulfamoyl position	R²—	Activity
H—	(cyclohexylidene structure)	2-Cl—	4	H—	Act.
H—	n-C_7H_{15}—	2-Cl—	4	H—	Act.
H—	C_6H_5—	2-Cl—	5	H—	Act.
H—	C_6H_5—	2-Cl—	4	H—	MES 5, Met 100, LD_{50} > 7000
H—	C_6H_5—	2-Cl—	4	CH_3CO—	Act.
H—	C_6H_5—	2-Cl—	4	C_2H_5OCO—	Act.
H—	C_6H_5—	3-Cl—	4	H—	MES 50, Met 200
H—	C_6H_5—	3,5-Cl_2—	4	H—	Act.
CH_3—	C_2H_5—	2-Cl—	4	H—	Act.
CH_3—	C_2H_5—	5-Cl—	2	H—	Act.
CH_3—	C_2H_5—	3-Cl—	4	H—	MES 10, Met 200
CH_3—	C_6H_5—	2-Cl—	4	H—	MES 7.5–10, Met 200, LD_{50} 3800
CH_3—	C_6H_5—	3-Cl—	4	H—	Act.
CH_3—	C_6H_5—	2-Cl—	5	H—	Act.
H—	CH_3—	2-F—	4	H—	MES 2.5–10(?)
H—	C_6H_5—	2-F—	4	H—	MES 5, Met 50, LD_{50} 7000
H—	C_6H_5—	3-F—	4	H—	Act.
H—	C_6H_5—	2-F—	4	C_2H_5—	Act.
CH_3—	C_2H_5—	2-F—	5	H—	Act.
CH_3—	C_2H_5—	2-F—	4	H—	MES 15, Met 200–300, LD_{50} 3500
CH_3—	C_2H_5—	2-F—	4	C_2H_5—	MES 25–50, Met 200
CH_3—	C_2H_5—	3-F—	4	H—	MES 25, Met 200
CH_3—	C_6H_5—	2-F—	4	H—	MES 4–5, Met 100, LD_{50} 5500
CH_3—	C_6H_5—	3-F—	4	H—	Act.
CH_3—	C_6H_5—	2-F—	4	C_2H_5—	MES 5–10, Met 200, LD_{50} 7000
CH_3—	C_6H_5—	2-F—	4	CH_3CO—	Act.

[a] Data from Pfirrmann (1970).

TABLE 50 MISCELLANEOUS FUNCTIONAL GROUPS

$$\begin{array}{c} R \\ \diagdown \\ C-CO \\ \diagup \diagdown \\ R^1 \quad NH \\ | \\ R^2-HC-CO \end{array}$$

R—	R¹—	R²—	Activity	Reference
H—	$p\text{-}CH_3OC_6H_4$—	H—	MES 122, Met, 218, LD_{50} 1350	Akopyan and Gerasimyan (1971b)
H—	$p\text{-}C_2H_5OC_6H_4$—	H—	MES 135, Met 175, LD_{50} 1220	Akopyan and Gerasimyan (1971b)
H—	$p\text{-}C_2H_5OC_6H_4CH_2$—	H—	Act.	Akopyan et al. (1974)
H—	$p\text{-}C_3H_7OC_6H_4$—	H—	MES 70, Met 145, LD_{50} 940	Akopyan and Gerasimyan (1971b)
H—	$p\text{-}CH_3CH(CH_3)OC_6H_4$—	H—	MES 77, Met 86, LD_{50} 2150	Akopyan and Gerasimyan (1971b)
H—	$p\text{-}n\text{-}C_4H_9OC_6H_4$—	H—	MES 87, Met 142, LD_{50} 950	Akopyan and Gerasimyan (1971b)
H—	$p\text{-}i\text{-}C_4H_9OC_6H_4$—	H—	MES 54.2, Met 170, LD_{50} 1200	Akopyan and Gerasimyan (1971b)
H—	$p\text{-}n\text{-}C_5H_{11}OC_6H_4$—	H—	MES 61, Met 220, LD_{50} 895	Akopyan and Gerasimyan (1971b)
H—	$p\text{-}i\text{-}C_5H_{11}OC_6H_4$—	H—	MES 45, Met 123, LD_{50} 660	Akopyan and Gerasimyan (1971b)
H—	$p\text{-}n\text{-}C_6H_{13}OC_6H_4$—	H—	MES 65, Met 215, LD_{50} 1390	Akopyan and Gerasimyan (1971b)
H—	$p\text{-}n\text{-}C_7H_{15}OC_6H_5$—	H—	MES 61, Met 280, LD_{50} 1200	Akopyan and Gerasimyan (1971b)
H—	$p\text{-}n\text{-}C_8H_{17}\text{-}OC_6H_4$—	H—	MES inact., Met inact.	Akopyan and Gerasimyan (1971b)
CH_3—	$p\text{-}C_4H_9OC_6H_4$—	H—	Act.	Akopyan et al. (1974)
CH_3—	C_6H_5—	$(C_2H_5)_2NCH_2CH_2$—	MES inact., Met inact.	Hauck et al. (1967)
CH_3—	C_6H_5—	$(CH_3)_2NCH(CH_3)CH_2$—	MES inact., Met inact.	Hauck et al. (1967)
CH_3—	C_6H_5—	$CH_3CH_3OCH_2CH_2$—	MES inact., Met weak act.	Hauck et al. (1967)
CH_3—	C_6H_5—	$CH_3OCH_2CH_2CH=CHCH_2$—	MES weak act., Met inact.	Hauck et al. (1967)
CH_3—	C_6H_5—	$C_6H_5OCH_2CH_2$—	MES inact., Met weak act.	Hauck et al. (1967)
CH_3—	C_6H_5—	$o\text{-}C_2H_5OC_6H_4OCH_2CH_2$—	MES inact., Met inact.	Hauck et al. (1967)
CH_3—	$p\text{-}HOC_6H_4$—	C_2H_5—	MES weak act., Met weak act.	Hauck et al. (1967)
CH_3—	$o\text{-}CH_3OC_6H_4$—	C_2H_5—	MES inact., Met act.	Hauck et al. (1967)
CH_3—	$m\text{-}CH_3OC_6H_4$—	C_2H_5—	MES inact., Met weak act.	Hauck et al. (1967)
CH_3—	$p\text{-}CH_3OC_6H_4$—	C_2H_5—	MES inact., Met inact.	Hauck et al. (1967)
CH_3—	$p\text{-}C_6H_5CH_2OC_6H_4$—	C_2H_5—	MES weak act., Met inact.	Hauck et al. (1967)
CH_3—	$p\text{-}NO_2C_6H_4$—	C_2H_5—	MES weak act., Met inact.	Hauck et al. (1967)
CH_3—	$p\text{-}NH_2C_6H_4$—	C_2H_5—	MES weak act., Met inact.	Hauck et al. (1967)
C_6H_5—	CH_3OCH_2—	C_2H_5—	MES weak act., Met inact.	Hauck et al. (1967)

TABLE 51 MISCELLANEOUS FUNCTIONAL GROUPS

$$\begin{array}{c} R \\ \diagdown \\ R^1 - C - CO \\ | \quad \diagdown \\ H_2C - CO \end{array} N - R^2$$

R—	R¹—	R²—	Activity	Reference
H—	H—	$(C_4H_9)_2NCH_2$—	MES inact., Met weak act.	Das *et al.* (1975)
H—	H—	$[(CH_3)_2CHCH_2]_2NCH_2$—	MES act., Met inact.	Das *et al.* (1975)
H—	H—	$(Cyclo\text{-}C_6H_{11})_2NCH_2$—	MES weak act., Met inact.	Das *et al.* (1975)
H—	H—	$(C_6H_5CH_2)_2NCH_2$—	MES act., Met inact.	Das *et al.* (1975)
H—	H—	$C_2H_5N(C_6H_5)CH_2$—	MES inact., Met inact.	Das *et al.* (1975)
H—	H—	$C_6H_5CH_2CONHCH_2$—	MES act., Met inact.	Das *et al.* (1975)
H—	H—	$C_2H_5OCOC(C_6H_5)_2CH_2$—	MES act., Met weak act., S	Das *et al.* (1975)
H—	H—	$C_2H_5OCOCHC_6H_4NO_2$ $|$ CH_2—	MES act., Met act.	Das *et al.* (1975)
H—	H—	$NH_2CSNHCH_2$—	MES inact., Met inact.	Das *et al.* (1975)
H—	C_6H_5—	$(n\text{-}C_4H_9)_2NCH_2$—	Act.	Eckstein *et al.* (1967)
H—	$p\text{-}ClC_6H_4$—	$(C_2H_5)_2NCH_2$—	Act.	Eckstein *et al.* (1967)
H—	$p\text{-}ClC_6H_4$—	$(C_6H_5CH_2)_2NCH_2$—	Act.	Eckstein *et al.* (1967)

H—	CH₃CONH—	C₆H₅—	D(R) isomer: MES (ip) 3.79 mmoles/kg, Met (ip) 1.42 mmoles/kg, MMS (ip) 2.07 mmoles/kg; L(S) isomer: MES (ip) 5.39 mmoles/kg, Met inact., MMS (ip) 1.20 mmoles/kg	Witiak et al. (1972)
H—	CH₃CONH—	p-CH₃C₆H₅—	D(R) isomer: MES (ip) inact., Met inact., MMS (ip) 0.91 mmole/kg; L(S) isomer: MES (ip) inact., Met inact., MMS (ip) 0.71 mmole/kg	Witiak et al. (1972)
H—	CH₃CONH—	p-CH₃OC₆H₄—	D(R) isomer: MES (ip) inact., Met inact., MMS (ip) 1.17 mmoles/kg; L(R) isomer: MES (ip) inact., MMS (ip) 1.08 mmoles/kg	Witiak et al. (1972)
C₆H₅—	(CH₃)₂NCH₂—	CH₃—	MES act., Met inact.	Clemson et al. (1968)
C₆H₅—	(C₂H₅)₂NCH₂—	CH₃—	MES act., Met inact.	Clemson et al. (1968)
C₆H₅—	(CH₃)₂NCH₂CH₂—	CH₃—	MES weak act., Met inact.	Clemson et al. (1968)
C₆H₅—	(C₂H₅)₂NCH₂CH₂—	CH₃—	MES act., Met inact.	Clemson et al. (1968)
C₆H₅—	CH₃CO—	CH₃—	MES 96, Met 86, not H	Clemson et al. (1970)
C₆H₅—	C₆H₅CO—	CH₃—	MES inact., Met ca. 610, not H	Clemson et al. (1970)

H

IV. 2,4-OXAZOLIDINEDIONES

A. 2,4-OXAZOLIDINEDIONES WITH ONLY ALIPHATIC HYDROCARBONS

TABLE 52

$$\begin{array}{c} R \\ \diagdown \\ R^1 \diagup \end{array} C \underset{OC-N-R^2}{\overset{O-CO}{<}}$$

R—	R¹—	R²—	Activity	Reference
H—	H—	CH₂=CHCH₂—	Met inact.	Shapiro et al. (1959b)
H—	CH₃—	CH₂=CHCH₂—	Met inact., S	Shapiro et al. (1959b)
H—	CH₃—	i-C₄H₉—	Met act., LD₅₀ 250	Shapiro et al. (1959b)
H—	CH₃—	Cyclo-C₆H₁₁—	Met inact.	Shapiro et al. (1959b)
H—	CH₃—	CH₃CH₂CH₂CH₂CH₂CH(C₂H₅)CH₂—	Met inact.	Shapiro et al. (1959b)
CH₃—	CH₃—	H—	MES act., Met act., LD₅₀ 850	Malec (1966)
			MES (ip) 610 rats, 2100 mice, MMS act., EST weak act.	Withrow et al. (1968)
				Frey (1969)
			MET (iv) 360, other studies	Frey and Kretschmer (1971)
			Other studies	Brink and Freeman (1972)
CH₃—	CH₃—	CH₃—	MES > 400, Met 225, LD₅₀ 3450	Gesler et al. (1961)
			MES (ip) 4.92 mmoles/kg, Met (ip) 1.75 mmoles/kg	Witiak et al. (1972)
			Met (iv) 335, other studies	Frey (1969)
			MMS (ip) 62, other studies	Brink and Freeman (1972)
			Met 470, other studies	Frey and Kretschmer (1971)
			MMS act., other studies	Enebäck and Alberty (1965)
			Other studies	Tapia et al. (1965)
CH₃—	CH₃—	Cyclo-C₆H₁₁—	MES act., Met act., S, LD₅₀ 2000	Malec (1966)
			Met inact.	Shapiro et al. (1959b)
CH₃—	C₂H₅—	CH₃—	MES (ip) 1.24 mmoles/kg, Met (ip) 0.42 mmole/kg	Witiak et al. (1972)

B. 2,4-OXAZOLIDINEDIONES WITH AROMATIC HYDROCARBON SUBSTITUENTS

TABLE 53[a]

$$R-O-O-CO$$
$$R^1-O-OC---N-R^2$$

R—	R¹—	R²—	Activity
H—	H—	C_6H_5—	Met inact.
H—	H—	$2\text{-}CH_3C_6H_4$—	Met inact.
H—	H—	$4\text{-}CH_3C_6H_4$—	Met inact.
H—	H—	$C_6H_5CH_2$—	Met act., LD$_{50}$ 450
H—	H—	$C_6H_5CH_2CH_2$—	Met act., LD$_{50}$ 125
H—	H—	$C_6H_5CH(CH_3)$—	Met act., not S, LD$_{50}$ 450
H—	H—	$(C_6H_5)_2CH$—	Met inact.
H—	CH_3—	C_6H_5—	Met inact.
H—	CH_3—	$2\text{-}CH_3C_6H_4$—	Met inact.
H—	CH_3—	$4\text{-}CH_3C_6H_4$—	Met inact.
H—	CH_3—	$2,4\text{-}(CH_3)_2C_6H_3$—	Met inact.
H—	CH_3—	$C_6H_5CH_2$—	Met inact.
H—	CH_3—	$C_6H_5CH_2CH_2$—	Met inact.
H—	CH_3—	$C_6H_5CH(CH_3)$—	Met act., S, LD$_{50}$ 1000
H—	CH_3—	$(C_6H_5)_2CH$—	Met inact.
H—	C_6H_5—	H—	MMS (ip) 375, ^{14}C Studies, LD$_{50}$ 872[b]
H—	C_6H_5—	$i\text{-}C_3H_7$—	Met inact.
H—	C_6H_5—	$i\text{-}C_4H_9$—	Met inact.
H—	C_6H_5—	C_6H_5—	Met inact.
H—	C_6H_5—	$C_6H_5CH_2$—	Met inact.
H—	C_6H_5—	$C_6H_5CH_2CH_2$—	Met inact.
CH_3—	CH_3—	C_6H_5—	Met inact.
CH_3—	CH_3—	$2\text{-}CH_3C_6H_4$—	Met act., LD$_{50}$ 200
CH_3—	CH_3—	$4\text{-}CH_3C_6H_4$—	Met inact.
CH_3—	CH_3—	$C_6H_5CH_2$—	Met act., LD$_{50}$ 1000
CH_3—	CH_3—	$C_6H_5CH_2CH_2$—	Met Act., LD$_{50}$ 450
CH_3—	CH_3—	$C_6H_5CH(CH_3)$—	Met act., LD$_{50}$ 450

[a] Data from Shapiro *et al.* (1959b) except when indicated otherwise.
[b] Data from Brink and Freeman (1972).

C. 2,4-OXAZOLIDINEDIONES WITH HETEROCYCLIC SUBSTITUENTS (TABLES 54–56)

TABLE 54 PYRIDYL SUBSTITUENTS

R—	R¹—	R²—	Position of pyridyl attachment	Activity	Reference
H—	H—	H—	2	Act.	Shapiro et al. (1958a,b)
H—	H—	H—	4	Act.	Shapiro et al. (1958a,b)
H—	H—	$5\text{-}C_2H_5$—	2	Act.	Shapiro et al. (1958a,b)
H—	CH_3—	H—	2	Act.	Shapiro et al. (1958a,b)
H—	CH_3—	H—	4	Act.	Shapiro et al. (1958a,b)
H—	CH_3—	$5\text{-}C_2H_5$—	2	Act.	Shapiro et al. (1958a,b)
H—	C_2H_5—	H—	2	Act.	Shapiro et al. (1958a,b)
H—	C_2H_5—	H—	4	Act.	Shapiro et al. (1958a,b)
H—	C_2H_5—	$5\text{-}C_2H_5$—	2	Act.	Shapiro et al. (1958a,b)
H—	$i\text{-}C_3H_7$—	H—	2	Act.	Shapiro et al. (1958a,b)
H—	$i\text{-}C_3H_7$—	H—	4	Act.	Shapiro et al. (1958a,b)
H—	$i\text{-}C_3H_7$—	$5\text{-}C_2H_5$—	2	Act.	Shapiro et al. (1958a,b)
H—	$n\text{-}C_4H_9CH(C_2H_5)$—	H—	2	Act.	Shapiro et al. (1958a,b)
H—	$n\text{-}C_4H_9CH(C_2H_5)$—	H—	4	Act.	Shapiro et al. (1958a,b)
H—	$n\text{-}C_4H_9CH(C_2H_5)$—	$5\text{-}C_2H_5$—	2	Act.	Shapiro et al. (1958a,b)
H—	$(CH_3)_2C(CH_2OH)$—	H—	2	Act.	Shapiro et al. (1958a,b)
H—	$(CH_3)_2C(CH_2OH)$—	H—	4	Act.	Shapiro et al. (1958a,b)
H—	$(CH_3)_2C(CH_2OH)$—	$5\text{-}C_2H_5$—	2	Act.	Shapiro et al. (1958a,b)
H—	C_6H_5—	H—	2	Act.	Shapiro et al. (1958a,b)

H—	C_6H_5—	H—	4	Act.	Shapiro *et al.* (1958a,b)
H—	C_6H_5—	5-C_2H_5—	2	Act.	Shapiro *et al.* (1958a,b)
CH_3—	CH_3—	H—	2	Act.	Shapiro *et al.* (1958a,b)
CH_3—	CH_3—	H—	4	Act.	Shapiro *et al.* (1958a,b)
CH_3—	CH_3—	5-C_2H_5—	2	Act.	Shapiro *et al.* (1958a,b)
CH_3—	C_2H_5—	H—	2	Act.	Shapiro *et al.* (1958a,b)
CH_3—	C_2H_5—	H—	4	Act.	Shapiro *et al.* (1958a,b)
CH_3—	C_2H_5—	5-C_2H_5—	2	Act.	Shapiro *et al.* (1958a,b)
CH_3—	*i*-C_3H_7—	H—	2	Met inact.	Shapiro *et al.* (1958a,b, 1959a)
CH_3—	*i*-C_3H_7—	H—	4	Met inact.	Shapiro *et al.* (1958a,b, 1959a)
CH_3—	*i*-C_3H_7—	5-C_2H_5—	2	Met inact.	Shapiro *et al.* (1958a,b, 1959a)
CH_3—	Cyclo-C_3H_5—	H—	2	Met act.	Shapiro *et al.* (1958a,b, 1959a)
CH_3—	Cyclo-C_3H_5—	H—	4	Met inact., S	Shapiro *et al.* (1958a,b, 1959a)
CH_3—	Cyclo-C_3H_5—	5-C_2H_5—	2	Met inact.	Shapiro *et al.* (1958a,b, 1959a)
CH_3—	Cyclo-C_6H_{11}—	H—	2	Met inact.	Shapiro *et al.* (1958a,b, 1959a)
CH_3—	Cyclo-C_6H_{11}—	H—	4	Act.	Shapiro *et al.* (1958a,b)
CH_3—	Cyclo-C_6H_{11}—	5-C_2H_5—	2	Met inact.	Shapiro *et al.* (1958a,b, 1959a)
CH_3—	$C_6H_5CH_2CH_2$—	H—	2	Met inact., S	Shapiro *et al.* (1958a,b, 1959a)
CH_3—	$C_6H_5CH_2CH_2$—	H—	4	Met inact., S	Shapiro *et al.* (1958a,b, 1959a)
CH_3—	$C_6H_5CH_2CH_2$—	5-C_2H_5—	2	Met inact.	Shapiro *et al.* (1958a,b, 1959a)
CH_3—	$C_6H_5CH{=}CH$—	H—	2	Met inact.	Shapiro *et al.* (1959a)

(*continued*)

TABLE 54—*Continued*

R—	R¹—	R²—	Position of pyridyl attachment	Activity	Reference
CH₃—	C₆H₅CH=CH—	H—	4	Met inact.	Shapiro et al. (1959a)
CH₃—	C₆H₅CH=CH—	5-C₂H₅—	2	Met inact.	Shapiro et al. (1959a)
CH₃—	4-ClC₆H₄—	H—	2	Met inact.	Shapiro et al. (1958a,b, 1959a)
CH₃—	4-ClC₆H₄—	H—	4	Met inact.	Shapiro et al. (1958a,b, 1959a)
CH₃—	4-ClC₆H₄—	5-C₂H₅—	2	Met inact.	Shapiro et al. (1958a,b, 1959a)
C₂H₅—	C₆H₅—	H—	2	Met inact.	Shapiro et al. (1958a,b, 1959a)
C₂H₅—	C₆H₅—	H—	4	Met inact., S	Shapiro et al. (1958a,b, 1959a)
C₂H₅—	C₆H₅—	5-C₂H₅—	2	Met inact.	Shapiro et al. (1958a,b, 1959a)
C₆H₅—	C₆H₅—	H—	2	Act.	Shapiro et al. (1958a,b)
C₆H₅—	C₆H₅—	H—	4	Act.	Shapiro et al. (1958a,b)
C₆H₅—	C₆H₅—	5-C₂H₅—	2	Act.	Shapiro et al. (1958a,b)

TABLE 55 PYRIDYL SUBSTITUENTS: SPIROOXAZOLIDINEDIONES

A—C(—O—CO / OC—N—CH₂CH₂—)—[pyridine ring with R and N]

$$A-\!\!\!\underset{}{C}\!\!<\genfrac{}{}{0pt}{}{O-CO}{OC-N-CH_2CH_2-}\!\!\!\text{—pyridyl}(R)$$

—A—	R—	Position of pyridyl attachment	Activity	Reference
—(CH₂)₄—	H—	2	Act.	Shapiro et al. (1958a,b, 1959b)
—(CH₂)₄—	H—	4	Act.	Shapiro et al. (1958a,b, 1959b)
—(CH₂)₄—	5-C₂H₅—	2	Act.	Shapiro et al. (1958a,b, 1959b)
—(CH₂)₅	H—	2	Act.	Shapiro et al. (1958a,b, 1959b)
—(CH₂)₅	H—	4	Act.	Shapiro et al. (1958a,b, 1959b)
—(CH₂)₅	5-C₂H₅—	2	Act.	Shapiro et al. (1958a,b, 1959b)
—(CH₂)₂CH(CH₃)CH₂—	H—	2	Met inact.	Shapiro et al. (1958a,b, 1959b)
—(CH₂)₂CH(CH₃)CH₂—	H—	4	Met act.	Shapiro et al. (1958a,b, 1959b)
—(CH₂)₂CH(CH₃)CH₂—	5-C₂H₅—	2	Met act., not S	Shapiro et al. (1959b)
			Act.	Shapiro et al. (1958a,b)
—(CH₂)₄CH(CH₃)—	H—	2	Met inact.	Shapiro et al. (1958a,b, 1959b)
—(CH₂)₄CH(CH₃)—	H—	4	Met inact.	Shapiro et al. (1958a,b, 1959b)
—(CH₂)₄CH(CH₃)—	5-C₂H₅—	2	Met inact.	Shapiro et al. (1958a,b, 1959b)
—(CH₂)₃CH(CH₃)CH₂—[a]	H—	2	Met inact., S	Shapiro et al. (1959b)
			Act.	Shapiro et al. (1958a,b)
—(CH₂)₃CH(CH₃)CH₂—[a]	H—	2	Met act.	Shapiro et al. (1958a,b, 1959b)
—(CH₂)₃CH(CH₃)CH₂—[a]	H—	4	Met inact.	Shapiro et al. (1958a,b, 1959b)
—(CH₂)₃CH(CH₃)CH—[a]	5-C₂H₅—	2	Met inact.	Shapiro et al. (1958a,b, 1959b)
—(CH₂)₃CH(CH₃)CH₂—[a]	5-C₂H₅—	2	Met inact.	Shapiro et al. (1958a,b, 1959b)
—(CH₂)₂CH(CH₃)(CH₂)₂—[a]	H—	2	Act.	Shapiro et al. (1958a,b)
—(CH₂)₂CH(CH₃)(CH₂)₂—[a]	H—	4	Act.	Shapiro et al. (1958a,b)
—(CH₂)₂CH(CH₃)(CH₂)₂—[a]	5-C₂H₅—	2	Act.	Shapiro et al. (1958a,b)

[a] Isomer not specified.

TABLE 56   OTHER HETEROCYCLIC SUBSTITUENTS

$$R-\overset{R}{\underset{R^1}{C}}\begin{matrix} O-CO \\ | \quad | \\ OC-N-R^2 \end{matrix}$$

R—	R¹—	R²—	Activity	Reference
H—	H—		Met act., LD_{50} 200	Shapiro et al. (1959b)
CH_3—	CH_3—		MES act., Met inact., LD_{50} 490	Malec (1966)
CH_3—	CH_3—		MES inact., Met inact., LD_{50} 488	Malec (1966)
CH_3—	CH_3—		MES inact., Met act., S, LD_{50} 1110	Malec (1966)

D. 2,4-OXAZOLIDINEDIONES WITH HETEROATOMS IN NONHETEROCYCLIC SYSTEMS (TABLES 57–59)

TABLE 57 ETHERS

$$\begin{array}{c} R \\ \diagdown \\ R^1 \diagup C \diagup O \diagdown CO \\ \mid \qquad \mid \\ OC \!-\!-\! N\!-\!R^2 \end{array}$$

R—	R¹—	R²—	Activity
H—	H—	$2\text{-}CH_3OC_6H_4\text{—}$	Met inact.
H—	H—	$4\text{-}CH_3OC_6H_4\text{—}$	Met inact.
H—	H—	$2\text{-}C_2H_5OC_6H_4\text{—}$	Met inact.
H—	H—	$3,4\text{-}(CH_3O)_2C_6H_3CH_2CH_2\text{—}$	Met inact.
H—	$CH_3\text{—}$	$2\text{-}CH_3OC_6H_4\text{—}$	Met inact.
H—	$CH_3\text{—}$	$4\text{-}CH_3OC_6H_4\text{—}$	Met inact.
H—	$CH_3\text{—}$	$2\text{-}C_2H_5OC_6H_4\text{—}$	Met inact.
H—	$CH_3\text{—}$	$3\text{-}C_2H_5OC_6H_4\text{—}$	Met inact.
H—	$CH_3\text{—}$	$4\text{-}C_2H_5OC_6H_4\text{—}$	Met inact.
H—	$CH_3\text{—}$	$3,4\text{-}(CH_3O)_2C_6H_3CH_2CH_2\text{—}$	Met inact.
$CH_3\text{—}$	$CH_3\text{—}$	$2\text{-}CH_3OC_6H_4\text{—}$	Met inact.
$CH_3\text{—}$	$CH_3\text{—}$	$4\text{-}CH_3OC_6H_4\text{—}$	Met inact.
$CH_3\text{—}$	$CH_3\text{—}$	$2\text{-}C_2H_5OC_6H_4\text{—}$	Met act., LD_{50} 700
$CH_3\text{—}$	$CH_3\text{—}$	$3\text{-}C_2H_5OC_6H_4\text{—}$	Met act., LD_{50} 1000
$CH_3\text{—}$	$CH_3\text{—}$	$3,4\text{-}(CH_3O)_2C_6H_3CH_2CH_2\text{—}$	Met inact.
$CH_3\text{—}$	$CH_3\text{—}$	$2,5\text{-}(CH_3O)_2C_6H_3\text{—}$	Met inact.

[a] Data from Shapiro *et al.* (1959b).

TABLE 58 HALIDES

$$\begin{array}{c} R \\ \diagdown \\ R^1 \diagup C \diagup O \diagdown CO \\ \mid \qquad \mid \\ OC \!-\!-\! N\!-\!R^2 \end{array}$$

R—	R¹—	R²—	Activity
H—	H—	$2\text{-}ClC_6H_4\text{—}$	Met inact.
H—	H—	$4\text{-}ClC_6H_4\text{—}$	Met inact., S
H—	H—	$4\text{-}FC_6H_4\text{—}$	Met inact.
H—	H—	$2\text{-}CH_3, 4\text{-}ClC_6H_3\text{—}$	Met act., not S, LD_{50} 1000
H—	H—	$4\text{-}ClC_6H_4CH_2\text{—}$	Met inact.
H—	$CH_3\text{—}$	$4\text{-}BrC_6H_4\text{—}$	Met inact.
H—	$CH_3\text{—}$	$2\text{-}ClC_6H_4\text{—}$	Met inact.
H—	$CH_3\text{—}$	$4\text{-}ClC_6H_4\text{—}$	Met inact.
H—	$CH_3\text{—}$	$4\text{-}FC_6H_4\text{—}$	Met inact.
H—	$CH_3\text{—}$	$4\text{-}ClC_6H_4CH_2\text{—}$	Met inact.
H—	$C_6H_5\text{—}$	$4\text{-}ClC_6H_4\text{—}$	Met inact.
H—	$C_6H_5\text{—}$	$4\text{-}ClC_6H_4CH_2\text{—}$	Met inact.
$CH_3\text{—}$	$CH_3\text{—}$	$4\text{-}ClC_6H_4\text{—}$	Met inact.
$CH_3\text{—}$	$CH_3\text{—}$	$4\text{-}ClC_6H_4CH_2\text{—}$	Met inact.

[a] Data from Shapiro *et al.* (1959b).

TABLE 59 OTHER FUNCTIONAL GROUPS

$$\begin{array}{c} R \\ R^1 \end{array}\!\!\!> C\!\!\!<\!\!\!\begin{array}{c} O \\ OC \end{array}\!\!\!\!-\!\!\!\!\begin{array}{c} CO \\ N\!\!-\!\!R^2 \end{array}$$

R—	R¹—	R²—	Activity	Reference
H—	H—	4-HO$_2$CC$_6$H$_4$—	Met inact.	Shapiro *et al.* (1959b)
H—	CH$_3$—	4-NO$_2$C$_6$H$_4$—	Met inact.	Shapiro *et al.* (1959b)
CH$_3$—	CH$_3$—	4-HO$_2$CC$_6$H$_4$—	Met inact.	Shapiro *et al.* (1959b)
CH$_3$—	CH$_3$—	(C$_6$H$_5$CH$_2$)$_2$NCH$_2$—	MES weak act., Met inact., LD$_{50}$ 660	Malec (1966)

V. GLUTARIMIDES (TABLES 60–61)

TABLE 60

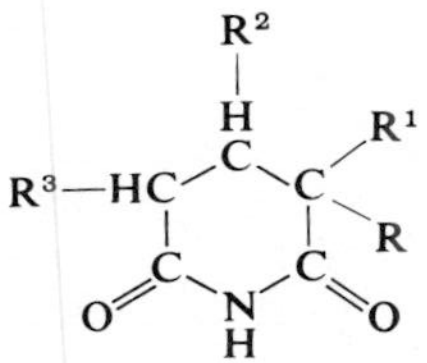

R—	R¹—	R²	R³—	Activity	Reference
H—	H—	p-CH₃OC₆H₄—	H—	Act.	Mndzhoyan et al. (1971)
H—	H—	p-C₂H₅OC₆H₄—	H—	Act.	Mndzhoyan et al. (1971)
H—	H—	p-C₃H₇OC₆H₄—	H—	Act.	Mndzhoyan et al. (1971)
H—	H—	p-i-C₃H₇OC₆H₄—	H—	Act.	Mndzhoyan et al. (1971)
H—	H—	p-C₄H₉OC₆H₄—	H—	Act.	Mndzhoyan et al. (1971)
H—	H—	p-i-C₄H₉OC₆H₄—	H—	Act.	Mndzhoyan et al. (1971)
H—	H—	p-C₅H₁₁OC₆H₄—	H—	Act.	Mndzhoyan et al. (1971)
C₂H₅—	C₆H₅—	H—	H—	Act.	Pakleppa (1959)
C₂H₅—	C₆H₅—	H—	H—	MES (ip) 21.2, H, LD₅₀ 400	Aboul-Enein et al. (1975)
C₂H₅—	C₆H₅—	CH₃—	H—	Act.	Pakleppa (1959)
C₂H₅—	C₆H₅—	H—	H—	Act.	Pakleppa (1959)
C₂H₅—	C₆H₅—	H—	CH₃—	MES (ip) 97.9, H, LD₅₀ > 2000	Aboul-Enein et al. (1975)
C₂H₅—	C₆H₅—	H—	Br—	MES (ip) 16.1, H, LD₅₀ 340	Aboul-Enein et al. (1975)
C₂H₅—	C₆H₅—	H—	OH—	MES (ip) 20.5, H, LD₅₀ 600	Aboul-Enein et al. (1975)
C₂H₅—	C₆H₅—	H—	NH₂	Act.	Pakleppa (1959)
C₂H₅—	p-BrC₆H₅—	H—	H—	ES act.	Ciba Ltd. (1959)
C₂H₅—	p-NH₂C₆H₄—	H—	H—	MES (ip) 14.0, H, LD₅₀ 625	Aboul-Enein et al. (1975)
C₂H₅—	C₆H₄CONHC₆H₄—	H—	H—	ES weak act.	Ciba Ltd. (1959)
n-C₃H₇—	C₆H₅—	H—	H—	Act.	Pakleppa (1959)
3-ClC₃H₆—	C₆H₅—	H—	H—	Act.	Pakleppa (1959)

TABLE 61

R—	R¹—	R²—	R³—	R⁴—	Activity	Reference
NH_2—	H—	H—	CH_3—	C_6H_5—	Act.	Taub (1962)
NH_2—	H—	H—	C_2H_5—	C_6H_5—	Act.	Taub (1962)
NH_2—	H—	H—	C_2H_5—	$p\text{-}CH_3OC_6H_4$—	Act.	Taub (1962)
NH_2—	CH_3—	C_6H_5—	H—	N—	Act.	Taub (1962)
NH_2—	CH_3—	$C_6H_5CH_2$—	H—	H—	Act.	Taub (1962)
NH_2—	C_2H_5—	C_6H_5—	H—	H—	Act.	Taub (1962)
NH_2—	C_2H_5—	C_6H_5—	CH_3—	H—	Act.	Taub (1962)
NH_2—	C_2H_5—	$3,4\text{-}(CH_3)_2C_6H_3$—	H—	CH_3—	Act.	Taub (1962)
NH_2—	C_2H_5—	$3\text{-}CH_3OC_6H_4$—	H—	H—	Act.	Taub (1962)
NH_2—	C_2H_5—	$p\text{-}ClC_6H_4$—	H—	H—	Act.	Taub (1962)
NH_2—	C_2H_5—	$3,4\text{-}Cl_2C_6H_3$—	H—	H—	Act.	Taub (1962)
NH_2—	$n\text{-}C_3H_7$—	C_6H_5—	H—	H—	Act.	Taub (1962)
NH_2—	$CH_2{=}CHCH_2$—	C_6H_5—	H—	H—	Act.	Taub (1962)
NH_2—	$n\text{-}C_4H_9$—	C_6H_5—	H—	H—	Act.	Taub (1962)
C_6H_5—	CH_3CONH—	H—	H—	H—	D(R) isomer (mmoles/kg): MES (ip) 0.50, Met (ip) 0.71, MMS (ip) 1.66; L(S) isomer (mmoles/kg): MES (ip) 0.58, Met (ip) 0.77, MMS (ip) 1.61	Witiak et al. (1972)

$p\text{-}CH_3C_6H_4-$	CH_3CONH-	$H-$	H—	D(R) isomer (mmoles/kg): MES (ip) 1.23, Met (ip) 1.83, MMS (ip) 1.16; L(S) isomer mmoles/kg): MES (ip) 1.62, Met (ip) 1.69, MMS (ip) 2.21	Witiak et al. (1972)
$p\text{-}CH_3OC_6H_4-$	CH_3CONH-	$H-$	H—	D(R) isomer (mmoles/kg): MES (ip) 2.63, Met (ip) 2.23, MMS (ip) 1.17; L(S) isomer (mmoles/kg): MES (ip) 3.39, Met (ip) 3.41, MMS (ip) 1.41	Witiak et al. (1972)
$p\text{-}NO_2\text{-}C_6H_4-$	CH_3CONH-	$H-$	H—	D(R) isomer (mmoles/kg): MES (ip) 1.36, Met (ip) 1.51, MMS (ip) 1.49; L(S) isomer (mmoles/kg): MES (ip) 2.47, Met (ip) 5.50, MMS (ip) 1.38	Witiak et al. (1972)
$p\text{-}ClC_6H_4-$	CH_3CONH-	$H-$	H—	D(R) isomer (mmole/kg): MES (ip) 0.26, Met (ip) 0.77, MMS (ip) 0.994; L(S) isomer (mmoles/kg): MES (ip) 0.56, Met (ip) 0.60, MMS (ip) 1.19	Witiak et al. (1972)

VI. DEOXYBARBITURATES

TABLE 62   DIHYDRO-4,6-PYRIMIDINEDIONES

R—	R¹—	R²—	Activity	Reference
C_2H_5—	C_6H_5—	H—	Other studies	Baumel *et al.* (1973)
C_2H_5—	C_6H_5—	HO_2C—	Act.	Waring (1960)
C_2H_5—	m-ClC_6H_4—	HO_2C—	Act.	Waring (1960)

REFERENCES

Aboul-Enein, H. Y., Schauberger, C. W., Hansen, A. R., and Fischer, L. J. (1975). *J. Med. Chem.* **18**, 736.
Achari, G., and Sinha, S. P. (1967). *J. Indian Med. Assoc.* **49**, 115.
Agawal, S. P., and Blake, M. I. (1968). *J. Pharm. Sci.* **57**, 1434.
AGFA Patent. (1904). German Patent 167,332; *Chem. Zentralbl.* **I**, 881 (1906).
Akopyan, N. E., and Gerasimyan, D. A. (1971a). *Biol. Zh. Arm.* **24**, 88; *Chem. Abstr.* **76**, 107836y (1972).
Akopyan, N. E., and Gerasimyan, D. A. (1971b). *Biol. Zh. Arm.* **24**, 91.
Akopyan, N. E., Gerasimyan, D. A., and Melkonyan, D. (1974). *Biol. Zh. Arm.* **27**, 52.
Aldridge, W. N. (1962). *Enzymes Drug Action, Ciba Found. Symp.*, *1962* p. 155.
Alvin, J., and Bush, M. T. (1974). *J. Pharmacol. Exp. Ther.* **188**, 8.
Aspelund, H. (1938). *Acta Acad. Abo.*, *Ser B* **11**, 7.
Aspelund, H. (1939). *Acta Acad. Abo.*, *Ser. B* **11**, 14.
Asta Werke A.-G. Chem. Fabrik. (1962). *German Patent* 1,135,915 (by H. Arnold, E. Kuehas, and N. Brock).
Badische Anilin-und Soda Fabrik A. G. (1971). French Patent 2,047,864.
Baker, H., Frank, O., Juter, S. H., Aaronson, S., Ziffer, H., and Sobotka, H. (1962). *Experientia* **18**, 224.
Baumel, I. P., Gallagher, B. B., DiMicco, J., and Goico, H. (1973). *J. Pharmacol. Exp. Ther.* **186**, 305.
Bayer Patent. (1915). German Patent 293163; *Chem. Zentralbl.* **2**, 531 (1916).
Beringer, F. M., Geering, E. J., Kuntz, I., and Mausner, M. (1956). *J. Phys. Chem.* **60**, 141.
Beringer, F. M., Forgione, P. S., and Yudis, M. D. (1960). *Tetrahedron* **8**, 49.
Biltz, H. (1908). *Ber. Dtsch. Chem. Ges.* **41**, 1379.
Biltz, H., and Seydel, K. (1912). *Justus Liebigs Ann.* 391, 215, *Chem. Abstr.* **6**, 3277 (1900).
Blaha, L., and Weichet, J. (1974). Czech Patent 151,744; 15 Jan. 1974; *Chem. Abstr.* **81**, 63633b (1974).
Bobranski, B., and Pomorski, J. (1967). *Arch. Immunol. Ther. Exp.* **15**, 751.

Bockstahler, E. R., Weaver, L. C., and Wright, D. L. (1968). *J. Med. Chem.* 11, 603.

Bogue, J. Y., and Carrington, H. C. (1953). *Br. J. Pharmacol. Chemother.* 8, 230.

Bolton, W. (1963). *Acta Crystallogr.* 16, 166.

Bonnycastle, D. D., Giarman, N. J., and Paasonen, M. K. (1957). *Br. J. Pharmacol. Chemother.* 12, 228.

Boon, W. R., Carrington, H. C., and Vasey, C. H. (1952). British Patent 666,027 (I.C.I.).

Bose, A. K., Garrett, S., and Pelosi, J. J. (1963). *J. Org. Chem.* 28, 730.

Brändström, A. (1959). *Acta Chem. Scand.* 13, 613.

Braun, F., and Kayser, W. (1954). *Schweiz. Med. Wochenschr.* 84, 446.

Bream, J. B., and Read, D. M. (1973). German Patent. 2,300,220. 12 Jul 1973.

Brimelow, H. C., Vasey, C. H., and Imperial Chemical Industries Limited (1959a). British Patent 807,676. 21 Jan. 1959.

Brimelow, H. C., Vasey, C. H., and Imperial Chemical Industries Limited (1959b). British Patent 807,678. 21 Jan. 1959.

Brink, J. J., and Freeman, E. (1972). *J. Neurochem.* 19, 1783.

British Patent. (1920). No. 159,153.

Brodie, B. B., and Hogben, A. M. (1957). *J. Pharm. Pharmacol.* 9, 345.

Browne, T. R., Dreifuss, F. E., Dyken, P. R., Goode, D. J., Penry, J. K., Porter, R. J., White, B. G., and White, P. T. (1975). *Neurology* 25, 515.

Butler, T. C., and Waddell, W. J. (1954). *J. Pharmacol. Exp. Ther.* 110, 241.

Butler, T. C., Ruth, J. M., and Tucker, G. F. (1955). *J. Am. Chem. Soc.* 77, 1488.

Cahen, R. (1962). British Patent 904,105.

Cahen, R., and Goodman, L. S. (1959). *Therapie* 14, 117.

Campaigne, E., Roelofs, W. L., and Weddleton, R. J. (1968), *J. Med. Chem.* 11, 395.

Carraz, G., and Emin, N. (1967). *Therapie* 22, 641.

Carrington, H. C., Vasey, C. H., and Waring, W. S. (1953). *J. Chem. Soc.* p. 3105.

Chamberlin, H. R., Waddell, W. J., and Butler, T. C. (1965). *Neurology* 15, 449.

Chanarin, I., Elmes, P. C., and Mollin, D. L. (1958). *Br. Med. J.* 3, 80.

Chemische Werke Huels A. G. German Patent 1,173,102 (W. Stumpf, and K. Rombusch) 2 Jul 1964.

Chen, G., and Bass, P. (1964). *Arch. Int. Pharmacodyn. Ther.* 152, 115.

Chen, G., Portman, R., Ensor, C. R., and Bratton, A. C. (1951). *J. Pharmacol. Exp. Ther.* 103, 54.

Chen, G., Weston, J. K., and Bratton, A. C. (1963). *Epilepsia* 4, 66.

Christenson, W. N., Ultmann, J. E., and Roseman, D. M. (1957). *J. Am. Med. Assoc.* 163, 940.

Ciba Ltd. (1959). Swiss Patent 342,220 (K. Hoffmann, and E. Urech) 31 Dec 1959.

Clemson, H. C., Magarian, E. O., Fuller, C., and Langner, R. L. (1968). *J. Pharm. Sci.* 57, 384.

Clemson, H. C., Magarian, E. O., and Reinhard, J. F. (1970). *J. Pharm. Sci.* 59, 1137.

Conrad, M., and Guthzeit, M. (1882). *Ber. Dtsch. Chem. Ges.* 15, 2844.

Craig, C. R. (1964). "Anticonvulsant Metabolism of Some Barbituric Properties and Acid Derivatives" Order No. 64–3917. University Wisconsin. Madison. (Univ. Microfilms, Ann Arbor, Michigan.)

Craig, C. R., and Shideman, F. E. (1971). *J. Pharmacol. Exp. Ther.* 176, 35.

Danielson, B., Johansson, S., and Paalzow, L. (1965), *Acta. Pharm. Suec.* 2, 155.

Das, P. K., Singh, G. B., Debnath, P. K., Acharya, S. B., and Dube, S. N. (1975). *Indian J. Med. Res.* 63, 286.

Davies, J. S. H., and Hook, W. H. (1950). *J. Chem. Soc.* p. 30.

Davis, M. A. (1964), U.S. Patent 3,153,050 (Am. Home Prod.).

Davis, J. P., and Lennox, W. G. (1949). *J. Pediatr.* **34**, 273.
Davis, J. P., and Schwade, E. D. (1959). *Fed. Proc., Fed. Am. Soc. Exp. Biol.* **18**, 380.
Decsi, L. (1965) *Prog. Drug Res.* **8**, 53.
Delgado, J. M. R., and Mihailovic, L. (1956). *Ann. N. Y. Acad. Sci.* **64**, 644.
Dick, R. W., and Mitchell, C. L. (1967) *Arch. Int. Pharmacodyn. Ther.* **170**, 333.
Dill, W. A., Kazenko, A., Wolf, L. M., and Glazko, A. J. (1956). *J. Pharmacol. Exp. Ther.* **118**, 270.
Dumennova, E. M., and Saratikov, A. S. (1959) *Nov. Lek. Rast. Sib. Ikh Lech. Prep. Primen.* **5**, 165; *Chem. Abstr.* **55**, 20212i (1961).
Eccles, J. C. (1964). "The Physiology of Synapses." Academic Press, New York.
Eckstein, M., Zeje, A., and Klusek, A. (1967) *Diss. Pharm. Pharmacol.* **19**, 263; *Chem. Abstr.* **68**, 59511z (1968).
Einhorn, A. (1909). German Patent 225,457; *Chem. Zentralbl.* **2**, 931 (1910).
Einhorn, A., and Diesbach, H. (1908). *Justus Liebigs Ann. Chem.* **359**, 158.
Elkin, S., and Lieberman, H. (1972) U.S. Patent 3,681,363.
Enebäck, C., and Alberty, J. E. (1965). *Arnzneim.-Forsch.* **15**, 1231.
Esplin, D. W. (1957). *J. Pharmacol. Exp. Ther.* **120**, 301.
Esplin, D. W., and Freston, J. W. (1960). *J. Pharmacol. Exp. Ther.* **121**, 301.
Everett, G. M., and Richards, R. K. (1944). *J. Pharmacol. Exp. Ther.* **81**, 402.
Festoff, B. W., and Appel, S. H. (1968). *J. Clin. Invest.* **47**, 2752.
Fijalowska, M., Kleinrok, Z., and Przegaliński, E. (1971) *Farm. Pol.* **27**, 405.
Fischer, E., and Dilthey, A. (1904). *Justus Liebigs Ann. Chem.* **335**, 334.
Fischer, E., and Von Mering, J. (1903). *Ther. Gegw.* **44**, 97.
Franz, D. N., and Esplin, D. W. (1965). *Pharmacologist* **7**, 174.
Frey, H. H. (1969) *Acta Pharmacol. Toxicol.* **27**, 295.
Frey, H. H., and Hahn, I. (1960). *Arch. Int. Pharmacodyn. Ther.* **128**, 281.
Frey, H. H., and Kretschmer, B. H. (1971) *Arch. Int. Pharmacodyn. Ther.* **193**, 181.
Frey, H. H., and Magnussen, M. P. (1971) *Pharmacology* **5**, 1.
Frey, H. H., and Schulz, R. (1970). *Acta Pharmacol. Toxicol.* **28**, 477.
Frommel, E., Gold-Aubert, P., Fleury, C., Schmidt-Ginskey, J., and Beguin, M. (1961). *Helv. Physiol. Pharmacol. Acta* **19**, 241.
Fujinaga, Z., and Negishi, B. (1960), *Yakugaku Zasshi* **80**, 919.
Fujinaga, Z., Negishi, B., and Ohmoto, M. (1961), *Yakugaku Zasshi* **81**, 851.
Fuld, H., and Moorhouse, E. H. (1956). *Br. Med. J.* **2**, 102.
Gallagher, B. B., and Baumel, I. P. (1971). *Neurology* **21**, 394.
Gallagher, B. B., and Baumel, I. P. (1972). *In* "Antiepileptic Drugs" (D. M. Woodbury, J. K. Penry, and R. P. Schmidt, eds.), pp. 367–371. Raven, New York.
Gallagher, B. B., Smith, D. B., and Mattson, R. H. (1970). *Epilepsia* **11**, 293.
Gallagher, B. B., Baumel, I. P., DiMicco, J. A., and Vida, J. A. (1973a). *Fed. Proc. Fed. Am. Soc. Exp. Biol.* **32**, 684.
Gallagher, B. B., Baumel, I. P., Mattson, R. H., and Woodbury, S. G. (1973b). *Neurology* **23**, 145.
Gangloff, H., and Monnier, M. (1957). *Electroencephalogr. Clin. Neurophysiol.* **9**, 43.
Gavrilyuk, A. A., and Zapadnyuk, V. G. (1959), *Farm. Zh. (Kiev)* **3**, 24; *Chem. Abstr.* **55**, 4779e (1961).
Geistlich, E. (1974), German Patent 2,357,591 (Soehne A.-G. fuer Chem. Ind.); 22 May 1974; *Chem. Abstr.* **81**, 63631z (1974).
Gerot-Pharmazeutika (1966). Austrian Patent 250,383. 10 Nov. 1966.
Gesler, R. M. Lints, C. E., and Swinyard, E. A. (1961) *Toxicol. Appl. Pharmacol.* **3**, 107.
Gilbert, J. C., Ortiz, W. R., and Millichap, J. G. (1965). *Proc. Int. Med. Chicago* **25**, 258.

Girdwood, R. H., and Lenman, J. A. R. (1956). *Br. Med. J.* **1**, 146 (1956).
Glasson, B., Benakis, A., and Ernst, C. (1963a). *Helv. Physiol. Pharmacol. Acta* **21**, 114.
Glasson, B., Benakis, A., and Ernst, C. (1963b). *Therapie* **18**, 1483.
Goodman, L. S., and Cahen, R. (1959). *Therapie* **14**, 109.
Goodman, L. S., Toman, J. E. P., and Swinyard, E. A. (1946). *Am. J. Med.* **1**, 213.
Goodman, L. S., Swinyard, E. A., Brown, W. C., Schiffman, D. O., Grewal, M. S., and Bliss, E. L. (1953). *J. Pharmacol. Exp. Ther.* **108**, 428.
Goodman, L. S., Swinyard, E. A., Brown, W. C., and Schiffman, D. O. (1954). *J. Pharmacol. Exp. Ther.* **110**, 403.
Gordon, N. (1961). *Neurology* **11**, 266.
Haas, V. H. (1963). *Arzneim.-Forsch.* **13**, 613.
Halbig, P., and Kaufler, F. (1934). German Patent 593,673; *Chem. Abstr.* **28**, 3423 (1934).
Haley, T. J., and Gidley, J. T. (1970). *Eur. J. Pharmacol.* **9**, 358.
Handley, R., and Stewart, A. S. R. (1952). *Lancet* **1**, 742.
Hasegawa, G., and Kotani, A. (1974). Japan Kohai 74 49,959; 15 May 1974; *Chem. Abstr.* **81**, 77923h (1974).
Hauck, F., Jr., Demick, J., and Fan, J. (1967). *J. Med. Chem.* **10**, 611.
Hauptmann, A. (1912). *Muench. Med. Wochenschr.* **59**, 1907.
Helfant, R. H., Ricciutti, M. A., Scherlag, B. J., and Damato, A. N. (1968). *Am. J. Physiol.* **214**, 880.
Holck, H. G. O., Malone, M. H., and Kaji, H. K. (1961). *J. Pharm. Sci.* **50**, 747.
Hommel A.-G. (1965). Swiss Patent 385,212 (by Heusser, J.).
Impens, E. (1912). *Dtsch. Med. Nochensch.* **38**, 945.
Imperial Chemical Industries Limited (1959). British Patent 817,745 (by H. C. Carrington and W. S. Waring).
Innothera (1962). French Patent 1,067M (by A. Pons, M. Robba, and P. Laurent).
Jeffrey, G. A., Ghose, A., and Warwicker, J. O. (1961). *Acta Crystallogr. (Copenhagen)* **14**, 88.
Julia, M., and Bagot, J. (1964). *Bull. Soc. Chim. Fr.* p. 1924.
Juliusburger, T. (1912). *Ber. Klin. Wochenschr.* **49**, 940.
Kapadia, B., Shah, M. H., and Deliwala, C. V. (1973). *Bull. Haffkine Inst.* **1**, 48; *Chem. Abstr.* **81**, 3832f (1974).
Kleinrok, Z., Malec, D., and Kruszewska, A. (1972). *Diss. Pharm. Pharmacol.* **24**, 467.
Krnjević, H., Kolačny, L., Tomljanović, D., Glunčić, B., and Hahn, V. (1966). *Farm. Glas.* **22**, 183.
Kulev, L. P., and Voronova, K. R. (1961). *Izv. Tomsk. Politekh. Inst.* **111**, 30; *Chem. Abstr.* **58**, 1832d (1963).
Kulev, L. P., Stepnova, G. M., Stolyarchuk, V. G., and Nechaeva, O. N. (1960). *Zh. Obshch. Khim.* **30**, 1385; *Chem. Abstr.* **55**, 553e (1961).
Laboratoires Dausse S. A., and Société B.M.C. (1969). French Patent 1,559,568.
Lange, J., Urbanski, T., and Venulet, J. (1962). *Rocz. Chem.* **36**, 1631.
Litchfield, J. T., and Wilcoxon, F. (1949). *J. Pharmacol.* **96**, 99 (1949).
Livingston, S., and Pauli, L. (1957). *Pediatrics* **19**, 614.
Livingston, S., and Peterson, D. (1956). *N. Engl. J. Med.* **254**, 327.
Loewe, S. (1912). *Dtsch. Med. Wochenschr.* **38**, 947. *Chem. Abstr.* **6**, 2110 (1912).
Lorentz de Haas, A. M., and Stoel, L. M. K., (1960). *Epilepsia* **1**, 501.
Lucka-Sobstel, B., and Zejc, A. (1971). *Diss. Pharm. Pharmacol.* **23**, 135.
Lund, H. (1936). *Ber. Dtsch. Chem. Ges. B* **69**, 1621.
Lunsford, C. D. (1968). *Annu. Rep. Med. Chem.* p. 28. (A. H. Robins Co., Inc.).
McLennan, H., and Elliott, K. A. C. (1951). *J. Pharmacol. Exp. Ther.* **103**, 35.

Magarian, E. O., Becker, G. W., and Diamond, L. (1973). *J. Pharm. Sci.* **62**, 325.
Magyar, I., and Walsa, R. (1966). *Ther. Hung.* **14**, 97.
Malec, D. (1966). *Diss. Pharm. Pharmacol.* **18**, 337.
Malec, D. (1967). *Diss. Pharm. Pharmacol.* **19**, 479.
Malec, D. (1970). *Diss. Pharm. Pharmacol.* **22**, 209.
Malec, D. (1972). *Diss. Pharm. Pharmacol.* **24**, 1.
Martin, G., Avakian, S., and Gal, A. E. (1959). U.S. Patent 2,868,690.
Matin, M. A., and Kar, P. O. (1974). *Pharmacol. Res. Commun.* **6**, 357.
Matsuda, S., and Matsuda, H. (1957). *Nippon Kagaku Zasshi* **78**, 814.
Matsumoto, H., and Gallagher, B. B. (1975). *Int. Symp. Epilepsy, Int. League Against Epilepsy, 7th,* 1975.
Mattson, R. H. Williamson, P. D., and Hanahan, E. (1975). *Neurology* **25**, 377.
Mauvernay, R. Y., and Busch, N. (1968). French Patent 5,866M. 16 Apr 1968.
Merritt, H. H., and Putnam, T. J. (1938a). *J. Am. Med. Assoc.* **111**, 1068.
Merritt, H. H., and Putnam, T. J. (1938b). *Arch. Neurol. Psychiatry* **39**, 1003.
Miller, C. A., and Long, L. M. (1951). *J. Am. Chem. Soc.* **73**, 4895.
Miller, C. A., and Long, L. M. (1953a). *J. Am. Chem. Soc.* **75**, 373.
Miller, C. A., and Long, L. M. (1953b). *J. Am. Chem. Soc.* **75**, 6256.
Miller, C. A., Scholl, H. I., and Long, L. M. (1951). *J. Am. Chem. Soc.* **73**, 5608.
Millichap, J. G. (1952). *Lancet* **2**, 907.
Mndzhoyan, O. L., Petrasyan, L. M., and Akopyan, N. E. (1971). *Arm. Khim. Zh.* **24**, p. 492; *Chem. Abstr.* **75**, 129485q (1971).
Morrell, F., Bradley, W., and Ptashne, M. (1958). *Neurology* **8**, 140.
Mulder, E. (1873). *Ber. Dtsch. Chem. Ges.* **6**, 1223.
Musial, L., and Korohoda, M. J. (1966). *Rocz. Chem.* **40**, 997.
Musial, L., and Korohoda, M. J. (1967). *Rocz. Chem.* **41**, 1491.
Musial, L., Korohoda, M., Szadowska, A., and Szmigielska, H. (1972). *Acta Pol. Pharm.* **3**, 573.
Najer, H., Giudicelli, R., and Sette, J. (1966). *Bull. Soc. Chim. Fr.* 1966, 1119.
Nakamura, K., O'Hashi, K., Nakatsuji, K., Hirooka, T., Fujimoto, F., and Ose, S. (1965). *Arch. Intern. Pharmacodyn. Ther.* **156**, 261.
Natarajan, P. N. (1971). *Acta Pharm. Sueci.* **8**, 537.
Nicholls, P. J., and Orton, T. C. (1972). *Br. J. Pharmacol.* **45**, 48.
Orazi, O. O., Corral, R. A., and Schurtenberg, H. (1974). *J. Chem. Soc., Perkin Trans. I* p. 219.
Pakleppa, G. (1959). German (East) Patent 16,295; *Chem. Abstr.* **55**, 575f (1961).
Pfirrmann, R. W. (1970). *German Patent* 2,029,821. 23 Dec. 1970.
Phillips, M. A. (1948). British Patent 590,714; *Chem. Abstr.* **42**, 2987 (1948).
Pincus, J. H., Grove, I., Marino, B. B., and Glaser, G. H. (1970). *Arch. Neurol. (Chicago)* **22**, 566.
Prastowski, W., and Zak, A. (1966). *Arch. Immunol. Ther. Exp.* **14**, 662.
Prichard, J. S., Murphy, E. G., and Escardo, F. E. (1957). *Can. Med. Assoc. J.* **76**, 770.
Przegaliński, E. (1969). *Diss. Pharm. Pharmacol.* **21**, 113–123.
Rabe, F. (1960). *Nervenartzt* **31**, 306.
Raduoco-Thomas, C., Gold, P. H., and Raduoco-Thomas, S. (1954). *Boll. Soc. Ital. Biol. Sper.* **30**, 765.
Raines, A., Niner, J., and Pace, D. (1973). *J. Pharmacol. Exp. Ther.* **186**, 315.
Rapport, R. L., and Kupferberg, H. J. (1973). *J. Med. Chem.* **16**, 599.
Rawson, M. D., and Pincus, J. H. (1968). *Biochem. Pharmacol.* **17**, 573.
Reidl, L., and Kertesi, K. (1968). *Gygogyszereszet* **12**, 184.
Reidl-de Haën Akt-Ges. (1959). British Patent 823, 517 (by A. Heymors and W. Persch).

Reinhard, J. F., Samour, C. M., and Vida, J. A. (1972). U.S. Patent 3,663,669.

Rekker, R. F., and Nauta, W. Th. (1951). *Rec. Trav. Chim. Pays-Bas* **70**, 313.

Reynolds, E. H., Millner, G., Matthews, D. M., and Chanarin, I. (1966). *Q. J. Med.* **35**, 521.

Richards, R. K., and Everett, G. M. (1946). *J. Lab. Clin. Med.* **31**, 1330.

Robba, M., and Moreau, R. (1961). *Bull. Soc. Chim. Fr*, p. 2161.

Rosati, R. A., Alexander, J. A., Schaals, S. F., and Wallace, A. G. (1967). *Circ. Res.* **21**, 757.

Saad, S. F., ElMasry, A. M., and Scott, P. M. (1972). *Eur. J. Pharmacol.* **17**, 386.

Salgarello, G., and Turri, E. (1957). *Boll. Soc. Ital. Biol. Sper.* **34**, 628.

Samour, C. M., and Vida, J. A. (1970). German Patent 1,939,787, (Kendall Co.). *Chem. Abstr.* **72**, 132771y (1970).

Samour, C. M., Reinhard, J. F., and Vida, J. A. (1971). *J. Med. Chem.* **14**, 187.

Sandberg, F., *Acta Physiol Scand.* **24** (1951).

Schaefer, H. (1974a). German Patent 1,966,802 (Destin-Werke Carl Klinke GmbH).

Schaefer, H. (1974b). German Patent 1,963,925 (Desitin-Werke Carl Klinke GmbH).

Schallek, W.. and Kuehn, A. (1963). *Proc. Soc. Exp. Biol. Med.* **112**, 813.

Schoegl, K. Wessely, F., Kraupp, O., and Stormann, H. (1961). *J. Med. Pharm. Chem.* **4**, 231.

Scholl, M. L., Abbott, J. A., and Schwab, R. S. (1959). *Epilepsia* **1**, 105.

Serino, E , Antoniu, D., Gamzina, F., and Magi, M. (1970). German Patent 1,933,598 (S.I.R. Labs. Chimico Biologici); 15 Jan 1970; *Chem. Abstr.* **72**, 100163k (1970).

Shaffer, J. W., Steinberg, E., Krimsley, V., and Winstead, M. B. (1968). *J. Med. Chem.* **11**, 462.

Shapiro, S. L., Freedman, L., and Rose, I. M. (1958a). U.S. Patent 2,866,734.

Shapiro, S. L., Rose, I. M., Roskin, E., and Freedman, L. (1958b). *J. Am. Chem. Soc.* **80**, 1648.

Shapiro, S. L., Rose, I. M., Roskin, E., and Freedman, L. (1959a). *J. Am. Chem. Soc.* **81**, 386.

Shapiro, S. L., Rose, I. M., Testa, F. C., Roskin, E., and Freedman, L. (1959b). *J. Am. Chem. Soc.* **81**, 6498.

Sherwin, A. L., Robb, J. P., and Lechter, M. (1973). *Arch. Neurol.* (*Chicago*) **28**, 178.

Shimo, K., and Kawasaki, T. (1964). Kogyo Kagaku Zasshi **67**, 574; *Chem. Abstr.* **61**, 9494 (1964).

Shimo, K., and Wakamatsu, S. (1959). *J. Org. Chem.* **24**, 19.

Singh, P., and Huot, J. (1973). *In* "Anticonvulsant Drugs" (C. Raduoco-Thomas, ed.), Vol. 2, pp. 427–504. Pergamon, Oxford.

Smith, D. B., and Racusen, L. C. (1973). *Arch. Neurol.* (*Chicago*) **28**, 18.

Smith, D. B., Goldstein, S. G., and Roomet, A. (1974). *Am. Epilepsy Soc. Annu. Meet., Program* p. 16.

Smith, D. B., Roomet, A., Goldstein, S., and Pippinger, C. (1975). *Neurology* **25**, 395.

Sohn, Y. J., Levitt, B., and Raines, A. (1970). *Arch. Int. Pharmacodyn.* **188**, 284.

Spielman, M. A. (1944). *J. Am. Chem. Soc.* **66**, 1244.

Stella, V., Higuchi, T., Hussain, A., and Truelove, J. (1975). In "Pro-Drugs as Novel Drug Delivery Systems" (T. Higuchi and V. Stella, eds.), pp. 154–183. *Am. Chem. Soc.* Washington, D.C.

Stokes, J. B., and Fortune, C. (1958). *Australas. Ann. Med.* **7**, 118.

Stroughton, R. W. (1941) *J. Am. Chem. Soc.* **63**, 2376.

Struck, H. C., Strumpff, D. L., and Caffrey, R. J. (1950). *Fed. Proc. Fed. Am. Soc. Exp. Biol.* **9**, 123.

Stuckey, R. E. (1942). *Q. J. Pharm. Pharmacol.* **15**, 377.

Swinyard, E. A., Toman, J. E. P., and Goodman, L. S. (1946). *J. Neurophysiol.* **9**, 47.
Swinyard, E. A., Brown, W. C., Goodman, L. S. (1952). *J. Pharmacol. Exp. Ther.* **106**, 319.
Swinyard, E. A., Miyahara, J. T., and Goodman, L. S. (1963). *J. Pharm. Sci.* **52**, 463.
Takamatsu, H., Umemoto, S., Fujimoto, K., and Nakamura, K. (1964). U.S. Patent 3,161,652.
Tapia, R., Pasantes, H., de la Mora, M. P., Ortega, B. G., and Massieu, G. (1965). *An. Inst. Biol., Univ. Nac. Auton. Mex.* **36**, 9.
Taub, W. (1962). U.S. Patent 3,057,867 (Calanda-Stiftung, Inst. f. Wissenschaft und Tech. Forsch.).
Taylor, J. D., and Bertcher, E. L. (1952). *J. Pharmacol. Exp. Ther.* **106**, 277.
Toman, J. E. P. (1970). *In* "The Pharmacological Basis of Therapeutics" (L. S. Goodman and A. Gilman, eds.), 4th ed., p. 204. Macmillan, New York.
Toman, J. E. P., and Goodman, L. S. (1948). *Physiol. Rev.* **28**, 409.
Torda, C., and Wolff, H. G. (1950). *Proc. Soc. Exp. Biol. Med.* **74**, 744.
Traube, W., and Ascher, R. (1913). *Ber.* **46**, 2077.
Umberkoman, B., and Joseph, T. (1974). *Indian J. Physiol. Pharmacol.* **18**, 29; *Chem. Abstr.* **81**, 86,198c (1974).
Vernadakis, A., and Woodbury, D. M. (1960). *In* "Inhibition in the Nervous System and Gamma-Aminobutyric Acid" (E. Roberts, ed.), p. 242. Pergamon, Oxford.
Vida, J. A. (1973). *Synth. Commun.* **3**, 105.
Vida, J. A. (1974). German Patent 2,405,778 (Kendall Co.) 29 Aug 1974; *Chem. Abstr.* **81**, 169559x (1974).
Vida, J. A. (1975a). U.S. Patent 3,920,656, (Kendall Co.).
Vida, J. A. (1975b). U.S. Patent 3,865,941, (Kendall Co.).
Vida, J. A. (1976). U.S. Patent 3,947,443, (Kendall Co.).
Vida, J. A., and Hooker, M. L. (1975). U.S. Patent 3,900,475 (Kendall Co.). *Chem. Abstr.* **84**, 31112 (1976).
Vida, J. A., and Samour, C. M. (1974). British Patent 1,369,770 (Kendall Co.); *Chem. Abstr.* **83**, 58886y (1975).
Vida, J. A., and Samour, C. M. (1975a). German Patent 2,340,976 (Kendall Co.); *Chem. Abstr.* **83**, 43368g (1975).
Vida, J. A., and Samour, C. M. (1975b). Canadian Patent 961,041 (Kendall Co.); *Chem. Abstr.* **83**, 28268f (1975).
Vida, J. A., Wilber, W. (1972), U.S. Patent 3,635,980 (Kendall Co.).
Vida, J. A., Wilber, W. (1973), U.S. Patent 3,711,607 (Kendall Co.).
Vida, J. A., Wilber, W. R., Reinhard, J. F. (1971). *J. Med. Chem.* **14**, 190.
Vida, J. A., Hooker, M. L., and Reinhard, J. F. (1973a). *J. Med. Chem.* **16**, 602.
Vida, J. A., Hooker, M. L., Samour, C. M., and Reinhard, J. F. (1973b). *J. Med. Chem.* **16**, 1378.
Vida, J. A., O'Dea, M. H., Samour, C. M., and Reinhard, J. F. (1975). *J. Med. Chem.* **18**, 383.
Vigne, J. P., and Fondarai, J. A. (1959). *Pathol. Biol.* **7**, 1219.
von Baeyer, A. (1864). *Ann. Chem. Pharm.* **130**, 129.
Vossen, R. (1958). *Dtsch. Med. Wocheschr.* **83**, 1227.
Waddell, W. J., and Butler, T. C. (1957). *Proc. Soc. Exp. Biol. Med.* **96**, 563.
Wagner, E., and Rudzik, A. D. (1967). *J. Med. Chem.* **10**, 607.
Wagner, E., and Rudzik, A. D. (1969). U.S. Patent 3,463,857.
Wallingford, V. H., Homeyer, A. H., and Jones, D. M. (1941). *J. Am. Chem. Soc.* **63**, 2056.

Wallingford, V. H. Thorpe, M. A., and Stoughton, R. W. (1945). *J. Am. Chem. Soc.* **67**, 522.

Waring, W. S. (1959). U.S. Patent 2,872,454. (Imperial Chemical Industries Limited).

Waring, W. S. (1960). British Patent 845,235. (Imperial Chemical Industries Limited).

Watson, E. L., and Woodbury, D. M. (1969). *In* "Basic Mechanisms of the Epilepsies" (H. H. Jasper, A. A. Ward, and A. Pope, eds.), p. 681, Ref. No. 126. Little, Brown, Boston, Massachusetts.

Weinreich, D., and Clark, L. (1970). *Arch. Int. Pharmacodyn. Ther.* **185**, 269.

Whalley, W. B., Anderson, E. L., Du Gan, F., Wilson, J. W., and Ullyot, G. E. (1955). *J. Am. Chem. Soc.* **77**, 745.

Withrow, C. D., Stout, R. J., Barton, L. J., Beacham, W. S., and Woodbury, D. M. (1968). *J. Pharmacol. Exp. Ther.* **161**, 335.

Withrow, C. D., Barton, L. J., and Woodbury, D. M. (1969). In "Basic Mechanisms of the Epilepsies (H. H. Jasper, A. A. Ward, and A. Pope, eds.), p. 681. Ref. No. 127. Little, Brown, Boston, Massachusetts.

Witiak, D. T., Seth, S. K., Baizman, E. R., Weibel, S. L., and Wolf, B. H. (1972). *J. Med. Chem.* **15**, 1117.

Wolf, H. H., Swinyard, E. A., and Goodman, L. S. (1962). *J. Pharm. Sci.* **51**, 74.

Woodbury, D. M. (1954). *Recent Prog. Horm. Res.* **10**, 65.

Woodbury, D. M. (1955). *J. Pharmacol. Exp. Ther.* **115**, 74.

Woodbury, D. M., and Esplin, D. W. (1959). *Res. Publ., Assoc. Res. Nerv. Ment. Dis.* **37**, 24.

Woodbury, D. M., and Kemp, J. W. (1971). *Psychiat. Neurol. Neurochem.* **74**, 91.

Woodbury, D. M., Rollins, L. T., Gardner, M. D., Hirschi, W. C., Hogan, J. R., Rallison, M. L., Tanner, G. S., and Brodie, D. A. (1958). *Am. J. Physiol.* **192**, 79.

Zimmerman, F. T. (1951). *Arch. Neurol. (Chicago)* **66**, 156.

Zimmerman, F. T. (1956). *N. Y. State J. Med.* **56**, 1460.

Zimmerman, F. T., and Burgemeister, B. B. (1958). *Neurology* **8**, 769.

6

BENZOPYRANS

Nicholas P. Plotnikoff and Harold E. Zaugg

I. INTRODUCTION

An interest in the benzopyrans as anticonvulsants stemmed from the pioneer animal studies of Loewe and Goodman (1947) and clinical studies of Davis and Ramsey (1949) on dimethylheptylpyran (DMHP). Earlier, O'Shaughnessy (1838) had introduced marihuana to Europe to treat various central nervous system (CNS) disorders including epilepsy. Thus, it became of great interest to several investigators to study the anticonvulsant activity of the constituents of marihuana, e.g., Δ^9-tetrahydrocannabinol (THC), Δ^8-THC, cannabidiol, and cannabinol (Garriott *et al.*, 1968; Sofia *et al.*, 1971; Man and Consroe, 1973; Boggan *et al.*, 1973; Corcoran *et al.*, 1973; Wada *et al.*, 1973; Karler, 1973; Karler *et al.*, 1973, 1974a,b; Carlini *et al.*, 1973; Consroe and Man, 1973; Chesher and Jackson, 1974).

In addition to the natural and synthetic C-ring carbocyclic cannabinoids, a wide variety of new analogues including nitrogen- and sulfur-containing compounds as well as water-soluble derivatives have become available for study as anticonvulsants. The syntheses, pharmacological profiles, and structure–activity relationships of these new analogues were described by Pars *et al.* (1976), Razdan *et al.* (1976b), and Winn *et al.* (1976). Preliminary reports on their anticonvulsant action have also appeared (Plotnikoff *et al.*, 1975; Razdan *et al.*, 1976b). The purpose of this review is to detail the specific anticonvulsation action of these new analogues.

II. CHEMISTRY

A. BENZOPYRAN SYNTHESIS

1. Δ^8- and Δ^9-Tetrahydrocannabinols

Methods of synthesis of these naturally occurring cannabinols have been reviewed by Mechoulam (1973). A more recently reported one-step synthesis of Δ^9-THC, however, deserves special mention. Razdan *et al.* (1974) found that *cis/trans*-(+)-*p*-mentha-2,8-dien-1-ol (**I**) and olivetol (**II**) in the presence of 1% boron trifluoride etherate in *dry* methylene chloride at 0°C gave optically pure (−)-Δ^9-THC (**III**) in a 31% yield by a single chromatographic separation.

Because of the relative ease of this synthesis, it was further stated by these workers that the method of choice for the preparation of pure Δ^8-THC (**IV**) has now become isomerization of **III** with *p*-toluenesulfonic acid in refluxing-benzene. Although **IV** can be prepared directly from **I** and **II** with *p*-toluene sulfonic acid (*p*-TSA) (Petrzilka *et al.*, 1969), multiple chromatographies are required for its purification.

2. Δ^{10a}-Tetrahydrocannabinols

The method of synthesis of these analogues was described by Anker and Cook (1946) and more recently by Pars *et al.*, (1976). For example, the preparation of analogues containing a nitrogen atom at the 9 position of ring C (see structure **III**) is illustrated as follows: Von Pechmann condensation of 1-benzyl-4-carbethoxy-3-piperidone (**V**) with a 5-alkylresorcinol (**VI**) gave the tricyclic benzopyrone (**VII**), which with excess methyl Grignard provided the benzopyran (**VIII**). Catalytic debenzylation of **VIII** to **IX** followed by alkylation led to the final product **X** (see Table IV, for example). Overall yields of 10–30% were generally attainable (Pars *et al.*, 1976). In like manner,

using the appropriate cyclic thia-β-ketoester, the corresponding C-ring sulfur heterocyclic analogues (see Table III, compounds 13 and 14) were obtained in 20–50% overall yield (Razdan *et al.*, 1976a).

Among the cannabinoids discussed in this review, the most commonly occurring side chain, R, is the 1,2-dimethylheptyl (DMH) group. The requisite resorcinol (**VI**) was prepared originally by Adams *et al.* (1948), from which they derived the potent synthetic cannabinoid, dimethylheptylpyran (see Table II, compound 5). Their process, necessarily involving the introduction of two chiral centers into the side chain, leads to a mixture of *dl-threo*- and *dl-erythro*-DMH-resorcinols in a ratio of 65:35. Most of the DMH-cannabinoids of this review were prepared from this mixture of resorcinols. Because there was no indication of any isomer separation occurring during purification of the final products of their intermediates, it is concluded that the same isomer ratio pertains to the final products as well. Aaron and Ferguson (1968) and Pars *et al.* (1976) synthesized all of the optically active isomers of DMHP and of the nitrogen analogue **X** (R' = $CH_2C{\equiv}CH$, R = DMH), and H. D. Dalzell (unpublished work) prepared the DL-*threo* and DL-*erythro* isomers of a cyclopenteno analogue. The anticonvulsant properties of these three pairs of *threo* and *erythro* isomers are shown in Table V.

Another commonly occurring side chain discussed in this review is the 1-methyl-4-(*p*-fluorophenyl)butyl group. These derivatives were described by Winn *et al.* (1976). The intermediate resorcinol (**XV**) is prepared from readily available 3,5-dimethoxybenzoic acid. Treatment of its lithium salt (**XI**) with methyl lithium produced the methyl ketone (**XII**). Further treatment with Grignard reagent derived from 3-(*p*-fluorophenyl)propyl bromide gave the carbinol (**XIII**), which, without purification, was hydrogenated in the presence of acid to **XIV**. Hydrobromic acid cleavage of the ether groups produced the resorcinol (**XV**). Overall yields of 60–65% were readily obtainable (Winn *et al.*, 1976).

Other intermediate resorcinols were prepared by published procedures (Adams *et al.*, 1948; Loev *et al.*, 1973; Suter and Weston, 1939).

B. BENZOPYRAN DERIVATIVES

1. Derivatives of the 1-Hydroxy Group

Razdan *et al.* (1976b) prepared many phenolic ester derivatives of the cannabinoids which were studied in the course of the present work. Simple esters (e.g., acetates) were readily prepared by conventional means. However, the basic ester derivatives were made by treating the cannabinoid with an amino acid in the presence of dicyclohexylcarbodiimide in methylene chloride at room temperature by the method of Zitko *et al.* (1972). Yields of 80% or better were usually obtained.

Analogous basic carbamates were also made for comparison with the corresponding basic esters. These were prepared by treatment of the parent cannabinoids in benzene solution with phosgene in the presence of N,N-dimethylaniline. Further treatment of the resulting chlorocarbonates (**XVI**) with the requisite diamines led to the carbamates (**XVII**) in moderate yields (40–80%) (C. M. Lee, unpublished work).

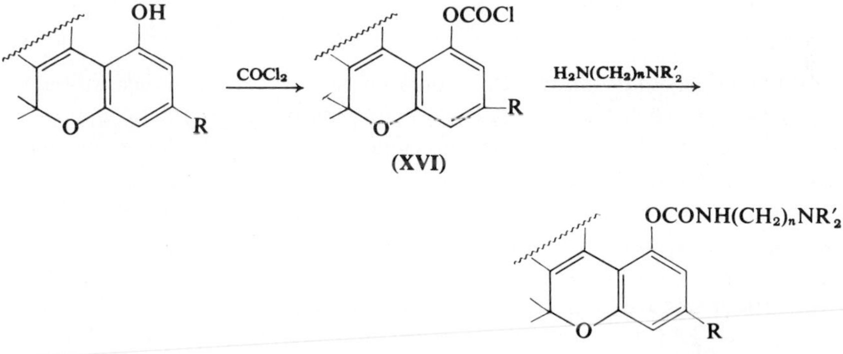

(XVI)

(XVII)

Both simple and basic phenolic ethers were made by alkylation of the corresponding sodium salts (**XVIII**) formed using sodium hydride in dimethylformamide (DMF) or hexamethylphosphoramide solution. Overnight stirring with the alkyl or aminoalkyl halide at room temperature gave good yields (60–90%) of the corresponding ethers (**XIX**) (C. M. Lee, unpublished work).

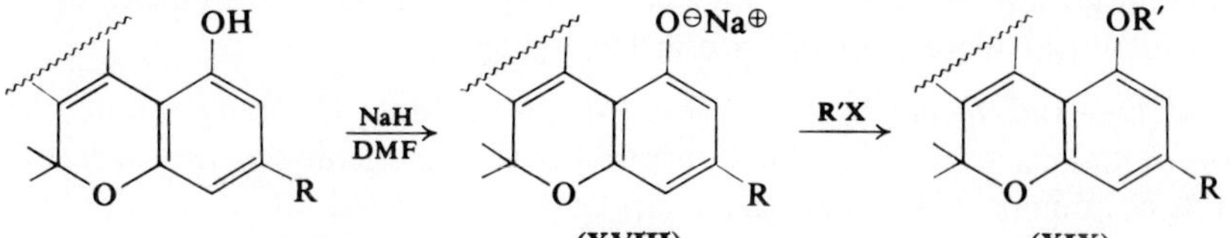

(XVIII)   (XIX)

R' = alkyl or —$(CH_2)_n NR_2''$

2. Dihydro Derivatives

Several dihydro derivatives of the Δ^{10a}-cannabinoids were prepared in either of two ways. The Δ^{10a}-cannabinoid (e.g., structure **IX**) dissolved in a

90:5:5 mixture of ethanol, acetic acid, and water was hydrogenated at 40–50 lb pressure in the presence of 50% (by weight) of 5% palladium-on-charcoal catalyst. Those compounds with a carbocyclic C ring were reduced in 2–3 hours. However, the C-ring nitrogen analogue required 5–7 days (D. A. Dunnigan, unpublished work; also compare Loev *et al.*, 1973; Pars *et al.*, 1976). In the second method, the pyrone intermediate (e.g., compound 94, Table XII) was hydrogenated by the foregoing procedure and then treated with excess methyl Grignard to give the reduced benzopyran.

III. ANTICONVULSANT PROPERTIES

A. TABULAR SURVEY

1. Structure

In the tables that follow, the cannabinoids are grouped according to structural type. The naturally occurring cannabinoids and synthetic analogues with carbocyclic C rings are listed in Table II. Heterocyclic analogues with nitrogen and sulfur in the C ring are in Tables III and IV. Table V summarizes the effect of isomerism in the dimethylheptyl side chain on the activities of three C-ring variants. Derivatives of the parent cannabinoids obtained by esterification of the phenolic hydroxyl are listed in Tables VI–IX. Phenolic basic carbamates are entered in Table X and corresponding ethers in Table XI. Intermediate benzopyrones are recorded in Table XII, and four dihydro-benzopyrans appear finally in Table XIII.

2. Activity

a. Methods. The test procedures were conducted with white male ARS/Sprague-Dawley strain mice, 18–24 gm, and male Long-Evans rats, 170–190 gm. The test compounds were administered orally as a suspension in 10% olive oil and 90% Methocel (0.5%) to ten animals per dose. All drugs were tested for activity at 1, 4, and 24 hours post drug administration in different groups of animals. Statistical analyses were carried out using simultaneous linear regression and probit techniques.

i. AUD—Audiogenic Seizures Test (Mouse). Male O'Grady strain mice (14–16 gm) especially bred for susceptibility to audiogenic seizures were used as test animals. The audiogenic apparatus consisted of a wooden box enclosing a metal container with two doorbells attached to the upper section. After drug administration the animals were placed in the audiogenic chamber and the bells activated for 1 minute and the animals were observed for convulsions (Plotnikoff and Green, 1957).

ii. MES—Supramaximal Electroshock Test (Mouse and Rat). After drug administration each animal received an electroshock (mice received 100 Hz, pulse duration 1.0 msec, at 140 V for 0.3 second; rats received 150 MA at 0.2 second) through corneal electrodes to initiate a hindlimb tonic extension convulsion; anticonvulsant activity was present when the above convulsion was blocked (Swinyard *et al.*, 1952; Toman and Everett, 1964).

iii. PsM—Psychomotor Electroshock Test (Mouse). After receiving drug, each animal was given an electroshock (6 Hz, pulse duration 1.0 msec, at 70 V for 3 seconds) through corneal electrodes to initiate a pyschomotor seizure. Protection from convulsions occurred when either the clonic forepaw activity or facial clonus was blocked (Toman and Everett, 1964).

iv. Maximal Metrazole Seizures Test (Mouse). After drug administration, each animal received pentylenetetrazole (metrazole) at 120 mg/kg subcutaneously to cause a tonic extension convulsion; anticonvulsant activity occurred when this convulsion was blocked (Toman and Everett, 1964).

b. Explanation of Tables. The first line of data in a column refers to the activity expressed in ED_{50} obtained 1 hour after drug administration; the second line refers to that obtained 4 hours after drug administration; and the third line refers to that obtained 24 hours after drug administration. When only two lines of data are given, reference is to 1-hour and 4-hour pretreatment times, respectively. When only one line appears, reference is to a 1-hour pretreatment time, unless otherwise indicated. The first figure in each line is the ED_{50} value for protecting the animals from the tonic extensor component with 95% confidence limits in parentheses. All other figures are the doses employed in milligrams per kilogram followed by the percentage of animals protected from the tonic extensor component.

c. Standards. Comparative data on known agents are listed in Table I. It is apparent that diphenylhydantoin as well as phenacemide exhibited highly significant activity in the audiogenic seizure, supramaximal electroshock, and maximal metrazole test. Considerably less potent activity was seen in the psychomotor test. In contrast, trimethadione as well as phenobarbital were more potent in the audiogenic seizure, psychomotor, and metrazole tests than in the supramaximal electroshock test.

In comparison, most of the benzopyrans are more active in the audiogenic seizure test than in the metrazole, electroshock, or psychomotor test.

B. STRUCTURE–ACTIVITY RELATIONSHIPS

Because relatively few of the compounds listed in the tables were tested for anything but their effects against audiogenic seizures and supramaximal electroshock in mice, the following conclusions regarding structure–activity relationships are based mainly on these two tests, with emphasis on the former.

TABLE I REFERENCE COMPOUNDS

Compounds	AUD (mice)	MES (mice)	MES (rats)	PsM (mice)	MMS (mice)
Phenacemide	14.8 (10–22)	60 (51–70)	30 (21–47)	151 (93–276)	33 (17–165)
	15.2 (19–23)	196 (144–264)	9 (3–20)	155 (91–318)	73 (58–93)
	>200	>800			
Trimethadione	168 (148–182)	680 (594–755)		110 (59–211)	181 (131–233)
	414 (345–478)	1125 (1115–1142)		157 (74–416)	336 (163–168)
	1000	>2000			
Diphenylhydantoin	1.7 (1.3–2.5)	8.1 (5.2–11)	23 (12–51)	102 (32–1107)	2.7 (1.7–5.9)
	3.3 (2.7–4.4)	7.6 (7.0–8.3)	62 (57–67)	86 (29–524)	2.2 (1.8–2.7)
	11.0 (6.5–21.6)	28.3 (22–36)	>200		
Phenobarbital	1.9 (0.8–3.8)	22 (19–25)	4.0 (2.0–6.7)	23 (10–283)	6.6 (4.0–10.0)
	0.3 (0.1–0.9)	18 (14–21)	4.5 (3.0–6.5)	6 (4–11)	4.8 (3.2–7.2)
	6.0 (4.2–8.4)				

1. Natural Cannabinoids and Close Analogues

Inspection of the data of Table II reveals that in the Δ-THC series high potency, among the analogues with a side chain (R) containing six carbons or less, is confined to Δ^9-THC itself (compound 1). Moving the double bond to the Δ^8 (compound 2) or Δ^{10a} position (compounds 3 and 4) markedly reduces activity. However, with certain larger side chains (compounds 5–7), not only is potency restored in the Δ^{10a} series, but also duration of action is strikingly increased over that observed for Δ^9-THC.

Noteworthy is the fact that the potency of DMHP (compound 5) is maintained in its 11-nor homologue (compound 7A). Clearly, metabolism to an 11-hydroxy derivative is not necessary for anticonvulsant activity in this series as appears to be the case for the analgesic action of Δ^8- and Δ^9-THC, e.g., **XX** → **XXI** (Wilson and May, 1975).

(XX)   (XXI)

The virtual absence of activity in the three analogues with five-membered C rings (8–10) clearly demonstrates the need for at least a six-membered C ring in the carbocyclic Δ^{10a} series.

2. C-Ring Heterocyclics

The first two examples of Table III demonstrate that the presence of nitrogen in the C ring can preserve anticonvulsant activity albeit at a somewhat lower level of potency than in DMHP. The last two compounds (13 and 14) clearly suggest that incorporation of divalent sulfur in the C ring is not a promising direction for further structural modification.

3. *N*-Substituted C-Ring Heterocyclics

The 13 variations of *N* substituent (R') and side chain (R) listed in Table IV reveal that the only combinations leading to significant anticonvulsant activity are the *N*-propargyl group with either the dimethylheptyl (C_9H_{19}) or arylalkyl ($C_{11}H_{14}F$) side chains in the 3 position (compounds 11 and 22). As expected, quaternization of the nitrogen, even with a propargyl group (compound 27), destroys activity.

TABLE II NATURAL CANNABINOIDS AND CLOSE ANALOGUES

No.	C Ring	R	AUD (mice)	MES (mice)	MES (rats)	PsM (mice)	MMS (mice)
1		n-C_5H_{11} (Δ^9-THC)	5.0 (2.4–7.7) 39 (29–49) >100	32 (29–35) 102 (96–107)	53 (36–81) 41 (24–143) >200	300 = 20% 300 = 40%	300 = 10% 300 = 0%
2		n-C_5H_{11} (Δ^8-THC)	180 (est.)	600 = 10% 600 = 0%		300 = 20% 300 = 30%	>300 320 (167–2060)
3		—$CH(CH_3)_2$	300 = 0%	100 = 0% 100 = 0%	20 = 80% (4 hours)	1100 (est.) 300 = 30%	500 = 0% 500 = 0%
4		n-C_6H_{13} (synhexyl)	100 = 30%	100 = 0%		64 (38–143) 45 (23–96)	300 = 40% 30 (14–63)

No.	Structure			
5	—CH(CH₃)CH(CH₃)-n-C₅H₁₁ (DMHP)	6.7 (2.1–11) 2.9 (1.8–4.9) 15 (8.2–26)	310 (230–590) 57 (35–80) > 300	7.5 (3.4–11) (4 hours)	5000 (est.) 190 (est.)	9.5 (3.5–22) 10 (5.3–22)
6	—CH₂C(CH₃)₂-n-C₅H₁₁	100 = 80%	100 = 20%		300 = 20% 300 = 30%	67 (est.) 62 (est.)
7	—CH(CH₃)CH₂CH₂CH₂—⟨C₆H₄⟩—F	2.3 (1.3–4.0) 1.4 (0.7–2.7) 30 (est.)	230 (140–1200)	15 (8.5–33) 4 hours	960 (est.) 640 (est.)	40 (17–220) 330 (est.)
7A	—CH(CH₃)CH(CH₃)-n-C₅H₁₁	21 (9.1–305) 7.1 (4.1–13.2)				
8	CH₃	30 = 0%	100 = 0%			
9	n-C₅H₁₁	100 = 0%	100 = 0%			
10	—CH(CH₃)CH(CH₃)-n-C₅H₁₁	35 (16–115) 100 = 40%	100 = 0% 100 = 0%		300 = 30% 300 = 20%	100 = 30% 100 = 30%

TABLE III C-RING HETEROCYCLICS

structure: C ring (with X substituent), B ring, A ring with OH; H$_3$C, H$_3$C–, O; side chain –CH(CH$_3$)CH(CH$_3$)-n-C$_5$H$_{11}$

No.	C Ring	AUD (mice)	MES (mice)	PsM (mice)	MMS (mice)
11	CH$_2$C≡CH, N ring	17 (9.0–35)	300 = 0%[a]	500 = 30%	600 = 30%
		11 (6.4–20)	300 = 40%	500 = 50%	600 = 40%
		>100			
12	N ring	100 = 100%	100 = 0%	260 (est.)	300 = 20%
			100 = 0%	300 = 30%	180 (88–1500)
13	S ring	300 = 10%	300 = 0%	300 = 20%	100 = 10%
			300 = 10%	530 (est.)	100 = 20%
14	S ring	26 (est.)	100 = 0%	300 = 20%	190 (est.)
		100 = 60%	100 = 0%	1400 (est.)	100 = 10%

[a] MES (rats): 150 (est., 1 hour), 52 (21–100, 4 hours).

4. Isomerism in the Dimethylheptyl Side Chain

Without exception, the entire anticonvulsant activity of the three pairs of isomers of Table V resides in the *dl-threo* form (constituting only 35% of the isomeric mixture of all other DMH-cannabinoids listed in the tables). With the exception of a mouse primary screen (Pars *et al.*, 1976), in all other CNS tests to which these isomeric pairs have been subjected, the potency of the *dl-threo* form has invariably exceeded that of the *dl-erythro* isomer. However, in no test system has the separation of activity been so pronounced as it is in the audiogenic seizure test.

5. Esters

In general, the esters listed in Table VI have activity profiles in the audiogenic seizure test rather similar to their parent compounds 5 and 7 (Table II).

Most of them, like their parents, have peak activities at the 4-hour pretreatment time. Even the "hindered" esters 32 and 35 (and presumably also 40) develop respectable potencies after 4 hours even though their 1-hour potencies are much lower than that of compound 5. This strongly suggests that the basic esters must hydrolyze to the phenolic precursor before they can exhibit anticonvulsant activity. This is further borne out by the fact that no basic ester has a peak potency appreciably greater than its parent. The apparent absence of activity in the basic ester 41 is puzzling. A priori, there is no obvious reason why this ester should not hydrolyze as readily as the others.

The action of the simple acetate 28 appears to be exceptional. Although its 4-hour potency is the same as its precursor 5, its activity after only 1 hour is ten times that of 5, suggesting that, unlike the basic esters, the acetate undergoes an enhanced rate of absorption as compared to compound 5.

The results summarized in Table VII are consistent with those of Table VI. In no instance does esterification of an inactive compound produce a significantly active substance (compare compounds 42, 45, and 47 with compound 9, Table II). Nor does esterification of a moderately active cannabinoid produce a derivative with potency any greater than that of the parent (compare compounds 43, 44, 46, 48, and 49 with compound 10, Table II).

Again, in the C-ring *N*-heterocyclic series (Table VIII), a basic ester (compound 55) of an inactive parent (compound 19, Table IV) is itself inactive. Furthermore, in this series, basic ester formation appears to attenuate the activity of the parent. In less than half of those tested (compounds 56, 57, 62–66) does the activity approach that of the parent (e.g., compounds 56, 62, 63, and 65 versus compound 11, Table IV, and compounds 57, 64, and 66 versus compound 22, Table IV). Oddly, the 1-hour potencies of three "hindered" esters (compounds 62, 65, and 66) are not greatly reduced, as was the case in the carbocyclic series (Table VI). Conversely, simple acetylation in this series does not appear to enhance absorption rates (e.g., compounds 50 and 51 versus compounds 11 and 22, respectively).

Activities of the miscellaneous basic esters in Table IX again are in line with previous results. Esterification of Δ^9-THC (compound 67 versus compound 1, Table II) and the active compound 12 (12, Table III, versus compound 71) severely reduces anticonvulsant action. On the other hand, esterification (compound 69) of the moderately active 14 (Table III) merely retards the attainment of peak activity.

6. Basic Carbamates

All of the basic carbamates listed in Table X are either completely inactive or much less active than their parent cannabinoids. Since the carbamate linkage is more resistant to hydrolytic cleavage than the ester group, these

TABLE IV N-SUBSTITUTED C-RING HETEROCYCLICS

$R = C_9H_{19} = CH(CH_3)CH(CH_3)\text{-}n\text{-}C_5H_{11}$

$R = C_{11}H_{14}F = CH(CH_3)CH_2CH_2CH_2\text{-}[\text{4-F-}C_6H_4]$

No.	R	R'	AUD (mice)	MES (mice)	PsM (mice)	MMS (mice)
15	—CH(CH$_3$)$_2$	H	100 = 20%	100 = 0%		
16	n-C$_5$H$_{11}$	H · HCl	100 = 40%	100 = 0%		
17	C$_9$H$_{19}$	H · HCl	30 = 0%			
18	C$_{11}$H$_{14}$F	H	100 = 10% 100 = 20%	100 = 0% 100 = 0%		
19	n-C$_5$H$_{11}$	—CH$_2$C≡CH	30 = 0%	100 = 0%	100 = 0%	100 = 10%
20	n-C$_7$H$_{15}$	—CH$_2$C≡CH	100 = 60%	100 = 0%	100 = 50%	100 = 0%

No.	R	R′				
21	$-CH(CH_3)$-n-C_7H_{15}	$-CH_2C{\equiv}CH$	$100 = 20\%$	$100 = 20\%$	$300 = 0\%$	$30 = 10\%$ $30 = 30\%$
11	C_9H_{19}	$-CH_2C{\equiv}CH$	$17\ (9.0\text{–}35)$ $11\ (6.4\text{–}20)$ >100	$300 = 0\%$ $300 = 40\%$	$300 = 10\%$ $500 = 30\%$ $500 = 50\%$	$600 = 30\%$ $600 = 40\%$
22	$C_{11}H_{14}F$	$-CH_2C{\equiv}CH$	0.3 (est.)	$100 = 0\%$ $100 = 0\%$	1100 (est.)	$300 = 30$ $300 = 70\%$
23	C_9H_{19}	$-CH_2CH_2CH_3$	$300 = 20\%$	$300 = 0\%$	$300 = 30\%$	$100 = 10\%$ $100 = 20\%$
24	C_9H_{19}	$-CH_2CH{=}C(CH_3)_2$	$300 = 40\%$	$300 = 0\%$	$300 = 40\%$ $300 = 30\%$	$100 = 20\%$ $300 = 30\%$
25	C_9H_{19}	$-CH_2CH{=}CHCl$ (cis)	$100 = 30\%$ $100 = 50\%$	$600 = 0\%$ $100 = 0\%$	$300 = 20\%$ $300 = 20\%$	$300 = 0\%$ $300 = 10\%$
26	$-CH(CH_3)_2$	$-CH_2C_6H_5$	$270\ (180\text{–}430)$[a]	$300 = 0\%$ $300 = 0\%$	$300 = 30\%$ $300 = 30\%$	$100 = 10\%$ $100 = 10\%$
27	C_9H_{19}	$CH_3-\overset{\oplus}{N}-CH_2C{\equiv}CH \cdot Br^{\ominus}$ (ring)	$100 = 20\%$	$600 = 0\%$ $600 = 0\%$	$100 = 30\%$ $100 = 20\%$	$300 = 10\%$ $300 = 0\%$

[a] ED_{50} value at 1 hour with 95% confidence limits.

TABLE V DIMETHYLHEPTYL SIDE CHAIN ISOMERS

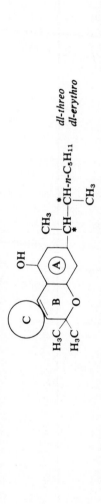

No.	C Ring	Isomer	AUD (mice)	MES (mice)	PsM (mice)	MMS (mice)
5a		dl-threo	30 = 80%			
5b		dl-erythro	100 = 60%	100 = 0%		
10a		dl-threo	30 = 60%	100 = 10%	100 = 60%	
				100 = 20%	100 = 80%	

10b	(cyclopentene–CH₂C≡CH structure)	*dl-erythro*	100 = 0%	100 = 0%	30 = 30% 30 = 70%
11a	(tetrahydropyridine–CH₂C≡CH structure)	*dl-threo*	4.2 5.0 = 30%	100 = 20% 100 = 50%	300 = 50% 300 = 40%	88 (22–180) 100 (47–190)
11b	(tetrahydropyridine structure)	*dl-erythro*	340	100 = 0%	300 = 10% 300 = 20%	100 = 0% 100 = 10%

TABLE VI ESTERS OF DMHP-TYPE COMPOUNDS 5 AND 7

$R = C_9H_{19} = CH(CH_3)CH(CH_3)\text{-}n\text{-}C_5H_{11}$

$R = C_{11}H_{14}F = CH(CH_3)CH_2CH_2\text{-}$ (4-fluorophenyl)

No.	R	R'	AUD (mice)	MES (mice)	MES (rats)	PsM (mice)	MMS (mice)
28	C_9H_{19}	CH_3	0.6 (0.1–2.5)	>100	10 = 100%		52 (est.)
			3.3 (1.9–14)	102 (45–470)			35 (15–110)
29	C_9H_{19}	$-(CH_2)_3N(C_2H_5)_2 \cdot HCl$	7.7 (1.4–20)	100 = 0%			100 = 40%
				100 = 20%			100 = 80%
30	C_9H_{19}	$-(CH_2)_3N$ [piperidinyl] $\cdot HCl$	8.5 (5.1–14)	300 = 0%	>100	200 = 20%	20 (10–41)
			2.8 (1.4–6.8)	59 (42–81)	4.6 (2.8–7.2)	200 = 10%	55 (29–110)
			32 (20–49)	300 = 0%			
31	$C_{11}H_{14}F$	$-(CH_2)_3N$ [piperidinyl] $\cdot HCl$	7.1 (3.5–16)	100 = 40%			140 (est.)
			9.2 (3.2–45)	100 = 0%			460 (est.)
32	C_9H_{19}	$-CH(CH_3)CH_2CH_2N$ [piperidinyl] $\cdot HCl$	26 (6.1–53)	110 (est.)	12 (8.0–22) (4 hours)		
			1.6 (0.7–3.5)	71 (35–270)			
33	C_9H_{19}	$-(CH_2)_3N$ [3-methylpiperidinyl, H_3C] $\cdot HCl$	28 (15–43)	100 = 0%			
			60 = 100%	84 (63–120)			

No.		Structure					
34	C_9H_{19}	$-(CH_2)_3N\!\bigcirc\!(CH_2)_6$	9.3 (6.1–16) 1.1 (0.5–2.4) 66 (28–2100)	68 (62–79) 74 (60–95) 300 = 0%	61 (38–98) 7.4 (4.2–13) >150	200 = 30% 200 = 20%	42 (22–91) 38 (16–90)
35	C_9H_{19}	$-CH(CH_3)CH_2CH_2N\!\bigcirc\!(CH_2)_6$	91 (est.) 12 (est.)				
36	C_9H_{19}	$-(CH_2)_3N\!\bigcirc\!(CH_2)_7$	7.0 (3.0–13) 1.0 (0.3–4.4)	100 = 0% 100 = 0%		13 (2.5–25) 11 (4.8–24)	300 = 50% 23 (3.3–52)
37	C_9H_{19}	$-(CH_2)_3N\!\bigcirc\!(CH_2)_8$	60 (est.) 4.5 (2.4–9.5)	100 = 0% 100 = 20%	20 = 0% (4 hours)		
38	C_9H_{19}	$-(CH_2)_3N\!\bigcirc\!O \cdot HBr$	4.2 (2.1–8.0) 2.4 (1.2–5.5) 19 (13–27)	300 = 40% 68 (41–150) 300 = 0%	>200 25 (5.3–52)	400 = 20% 400 = 80%	31 (16–63) 52 (35–75)
39	$C_{11}H_{14}F$	$-(CH_2)_3N\!\bigcirc\!O \cdot HCl$	8.0 (4.7–14) 2.2 (est.) 30 = 60%	93 (50–1200) 100 = 20%	10 = 60% 20 = 40%	100 = 30% 900 (est.)	66 (19–240) 200–600 = 50–70%
40	C_9H_{19}	$-CH(CH_3)CH_2CH_2N\!\bigcirc\!O \cdot HCl$	100 = 80%	100 = 0% 100 = 30%			
41	C_9H_{19}	$-(CH_2)_3N\!\bigcirc\!S \cdot HCl$	100 = 20%	100 = 0%			

TABLE VII ESTERS OF COMPOUNDS 9 AND 10

$$R = C_9H_{19} = CH(CH_3)CH(CH_3)\text{-}n\text{-}C_5H_{11}$$

No.	R	R'	AUD (mice)	MES (mice)	PSM (mice)	MMS (mice)
42	$n\text{-}C_5H_{11}$	$-(CH_2)_3N$ [pyrrolidine] $\cdot$ HCl	100 = 0%	100 = 0%		
43	C_9H_{19}	$-(CH_2)_3N$ [pyrrolidine] $\cdot$ HCl	51 (est.) 35 (22–59)	100 = 20% 100 = 40%	300 = 20% 300 = 20%	100 = 10% 100 = 20%
44	C_9H_{19}	$-(CH_2)_3N$ [piperidine] $\cdot$ HCl	180 (est.)	100 = 0%		
45	$n\text{-}C_5H_{11}$	$-(CH_2)_3N$ $(CH_2)_6 \cdot$ HCl	100 = 0% 100 = 0%			
46	C_9H_{19}	$-(CH_2)_3N$ $(CH_2)_6 \cdot$ HCl	30 = 0%			
47	$n\text{-}C_5H_{11}$	$-(CH_2)_3N$ [O] $\cdot$ HCl	100 = 50%	100 = 0%		
48	C_9H_{19}	$-(CH_2)_3N$ [O] $\cdot$ HCl	100 = 60%			
49	C_9H_{19}	$-(CH_2)_3N$ [S] $\cdot$ HCl	55 (21–237)	100 = 0%	300 = 20% 300 = 20%	300 = 20% 650 (est.)

TABLE VIII ESTERS OF COMPOUNDS 11, 19, AND 22

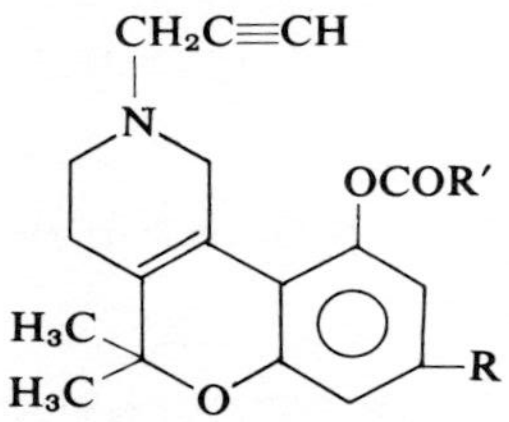

$R = C_9H_{19} = CH(CH_3)CH(CH_3)\text{-}n\text{-}C_5H_{11}$

$R = C_{11}H_{14}F = CH(CH_3)CH_2CH_2\text{-}(4\text{-}FC_6H_4)$

No.	R	R'	AUD (mice)	MES (mice)	PsM (mice)	MMS (mice)
50	C_9H_{19}	CH_3	100 = 30%	100 = 10%	100 = 40%	100 = 20%
51	$C_{11}H_{14}F$	CH_3	3.5 (1.5–7.0)	100 = 0%	300 = 30%	100 = 60%
52	C_9H_{19}	$C(CH_3)_3$	100 = 60%			
53	C_9H_{19}	$-(CH_2)_3N(C_2H_5)_2 \cdot HCl$	30 = 20%			
54	C_9H_{19}	$-(CH_2)_3N\text{(pyrrolidine)} \cdot 2HCl$ 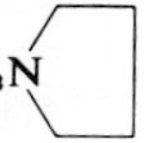	59 (33–220)	100 = 0%	300 = 20% 300 = 30%	100 = 40% 100 = 20%
55	$n\text{-}C_5H_{11}$	$-(CH_2)_3N\text{(piperidine)} \cdot HCl$ 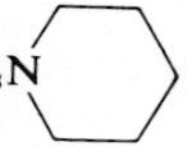	30 = 0%			
56	C_9H_{19}	$-(CH_2)_3N\text{(piperidine)} \cdot HCl$ 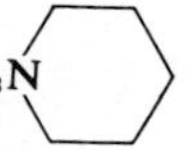	22 (14–37)	100 = 0%	100 = 20% 100 = 60%	100 = 20% 100 = 30%
57	$C_{11}H_{14}F$	$-(CH_2)_3N\text{(piperidine)} \cdot HCl$ 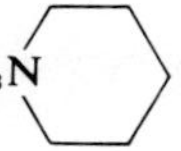	0.45 (est.)	100 = 0% 100 = 0%	100 = 20% 100 = 30%	400 = 40% 230 (est.)
58	C_9H_{19}	$-CH(CH_3)CH_2CH_2N\text{(piperidine)} \cdot 2HCl$ 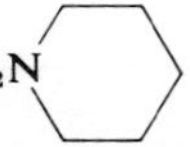	100 = 60%	100 = 0%	300 = 30% 300 = 30%	100 = 10% 100 = 40%

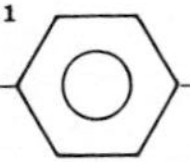

(continued)

313

TABLE VIII—Continued

No.	R	R'	AUD (mice)	MES (mice)	PsM (mice)	MMS (mice)
59	C_9H_{19}	—C(CH$_3$)$_2$CH$_2$CH$_2$N⟨piperidine⟩ · 2HCl	100 = 0%	100 = 0% 100 = 10%	100 = 20% 100 = 60%	100 = 20% 100 = 30%
60	C_9H_{19}	—(CH$_2$)$_4$N⟨piperidine⟩ · HCl	100 = 60%	100 = 40%	300 = 20% 300 = 10%	100 = 50% 100 = 30%
61	C_9H_{19}	—(CH$_2$)$_3$N⟨2-methylpiperidine (CH$_3$)⟩ · HCl	31 (5.7–160)	100 = 0% 100 = 0%	300 = 20% 300 = 20%	300 = 10% 300 = 30%
62	C_9H_{19}	—CH(CH$_3$)CH$_2$CH$_2$N⟨2-methylpiperidine (CH$_3$)⟩ · 2HCl	11 (4.4–23) 33 (est.)	300 = 0% 300 = 70%	300 = 20% 300 = 20%	190 (110–590) 94 (30–2800)
63	C_9H_{19}	—(CH$_2$)$_3$N⟨morpholine O⟩ · HCl	37 (est.) 10 (0.6–17)	100 = 0%	300 = 30% 300 = 20%	6.8 (5.0–17) 6.1 (4.7–12)
64	$C_{11}H_{14}F$	—(CH$_2$)$_3$N⟨morpholine O⟩ · 2HCl	3.9 (est.)	100 = 20% 100 = 0%		
65	C_9H_{19}	—CH(CH$_3$)CH$_2$CH$_2$N⟨morpholine O⟩ · 2HCl	12 (6.1–20)	100 = 0%	300 = 20% 300 = 20%	480 (est.) 74 (3.8–170)
66	$C_{11}H_{14}F$	—CH(CH$_3$)CH$_2$CH$_2$N⟨morpholine O⟩ · 2HCl	4.6 (2.3–9.3)	100 = 30% 100 = 0%	300 = 10% 300 = 20%	350 (est.) 110 (40–1800)

TABLE IX MISCELLANEOUS BASIC ESTERS

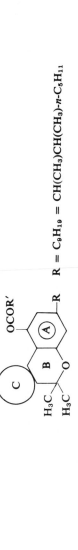

$R = C_9H_{19} = CH(CH_3)CH(CH_3)\text{-}n\text{-}C_5H_{11}$

No.	C Ring	R	R'	AUD (mice)	MES (mice)	PsM (mice)	MMS (mice)
67		$n\text{-}C_5H_{11}$	$-(CH_2)_3N{\bigcirc}O \cdot HCl$	$30 = 20\%$			
68		C_9H_{19}	$-(CH_2)_3N{\bigcirc}O \cdot HCl$	$30 = 80\%$			
69		C_9H_{19}	$-(CH_2)_3N{\bigcirc}O \cdot HCl$	120 (est.) 29 (16–53)	$100 = 0\%$	$300 = 10\%$ $300 = 20\%$	$100 = 30\%$ $100 = 10\%$
70		C_9H_{19}	$-(CH_2)_3N{\bigcirc} \cdot HCl$	$100 = 20\%$	$100 = 0\%$	$300 = 20\%$ $300 = 20\%$	$100 = 20\%$ $100 = 20\%$
71		C_9H_{19}	$-(CH_2)_3N{\bigcirc}O \cdot 2HCl$	$100 = 60\%$	$100 = 60\%$	$300 = 20\%$ $300 = 10\%$	$100 = 50\%$ (4 hours)

315

TABLE X BASIC CARBAMATES

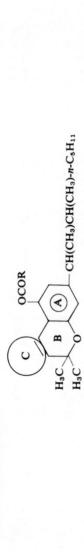

No.	C Ring	R	AUD (mice)	MES (mice)	PsM (mice)	MMS (mice)
72		—NH(CH₂)₃N(CH₃)₂	120 (est.)	300 = 10% 300 = 0%	300 = 20% 180 (55–3000)	100 = 10% 100 = 10%
73		—NH(CH₂)₃N⟨morpholine⟩	100 = 20%	100 = 0%	300 = 20% 300 = 20%	100 = 0% 100 = 30%
74		—N(CH₃)CH₂CH₂N(CH₃)₂	100 = 40%	100 = 0%	300 = 40%	300 = 10%

No.	Structure	Substituent			
75	cyclohexenyl	—N(CH₃)CH₂CH₂CH₂N(CH₃)₂	100 = 20%	100 = 0%	
76	cyclopentenyl	—NH(CH₂)₃N(CH₃)₂	85 (est.)	100 = 0%	300 = 20% 300 = 30%	100 = 40% 100 = 20%
77	cyclopentenyl	—NH(CH₂)₃N$\bigcirc$O	100 = 40%	600 = 0% 600 = 0%	300 = 20% 300 = 20%	100 = 0% 100 = 20%
78	cyclopentenyl	—NH(CH₂)₃N$\bigcirc$NCH₃	100 = 20%	100 = 0%		
79	cyclopentenyl	—N(CH₃)CH₂CH₂CH₂N(CH₃)₂	100 = 20%	100 = 60%		
80	CH₂C≡CH —N$\bigcirc$	—N(CH₃)CH₂CH₂N$\bigcirc$O · 2HCl	100 = 0%	600 = 0% 600 = 0%	300 = 20% 300 = 20%	200 = 10% (est.) 220 = (est.)

TABLE XI ETHERS

$R = C_9H_{19} = CH(CH_3)CH(CH_3)\text{-}n\text{-}C_5H_{11}$

$R = C_{11}H_{14}F = CH(CH_3)CH_2CH_2CH_2$—[4-fluorophenyl]

No.	C Ring	R	R'	AUD (mice)	MES (mice)	PsM (mice)	MMS (mice)
81		C_9H_{19}	CH_3	3.6 (.08–26) (4 hours)	300 = 0% 300 = 0%		
82		$C_{11}H_{14}F$	CH_3	100 = 70% 300 = 50%	100 = 0% 100 = 0%		100 = 30% 100 = 20%
83		C_9H_{19}	—CH_2CH_2N(CH$_2$)$_6$·HCl				200 = 10% 200 = 0%

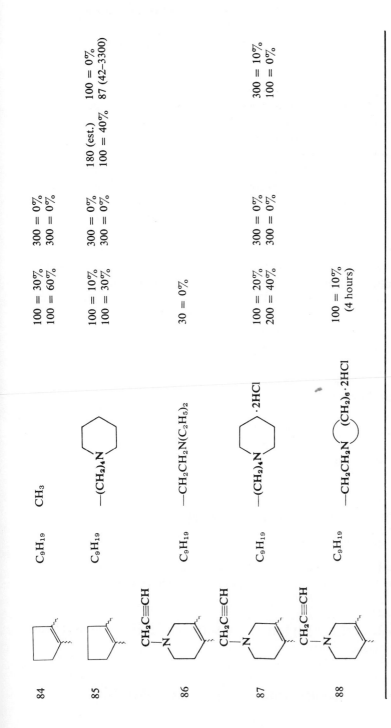

#		Substituent	Data		
84	C₉H₁₉	CH₃	100 = 30% 100 = 60%	300 = 0% 300 = 0%	
85	C₉H₁₉	—(CH₂)₄N (piperidine)	100 = 10% 100 = 30%	300 = 0% 300 = 0%	180 (est.) 100 = 40% 100 = 0% 87 (42–3300)
86	C₉H₁₉	—CH₂CH₂N(C₂H₅)₂	30 = 0%		
87	C₉H₁₉	—(CH₂)₄N · 2HCl	100 = 20% 200 = 40%	300 = 0% 300 = 0%	300 = 10% 100 = 0%
88	C₉H₁₉	—CH₂CH₂N (CH₂)₆ · 2HCl	100 = 10% (4 hours)		

observations are consistent with the view that the phenolic cannabinoid is the active form of the drug.

7. Ethers

Chemically, the ether function is even more resistant to cleavage than the carbamate group. It is not surprising, therefore, that most of the ethers in Table XI are relatively inactive. However the borderline activity exhibited by two methyl ethers (compounds 82 and 84) and the significant 4-hour activity of another (compound 81) strongly suggests that these simple ethers may be undergoing slow biochemical rupture. In fact, 1-hour tests of compound 81 gave highly erratic results. Only at the 4-hour pretreatment time was a dose-response observed that was adequate for the calculation of an ED_{50}.

8. Benzopyrones

It is clear from Table XII that these intermediates are uniformly inactive as anticonvulsants. Neither are any of them active in any of a half-dozen other tests for CNS effects (DOPA potentiation in mice, amphetamine antagonism in rats, reduction of shock-induced mouse fighting behavior, reduction in spontaneous rat motor activity, reduction of acetic acid-induced writhing in mice, and increased threshold for tail flick in the rat).

9. Dihydro Derivatives

Of the four dihydro derivatives in Table XIII, three are no more active or much less active than their Δ^{10a} precursors. However, compound 102, in preliminary tests, appears to be much more potent than its parent (compound 10, Table II). If confirmed by further work, this would be a significant, albeit puzzling, development.

C. COMPOUNDS OF SPECIAL INTEREST

Table II

Compound 7 was found to have outstanding activity in the mouse audiogenic seizure test and the rat supramaximal electroshock test.

Table IV

Compounds 11 (Table III) and 22 (Table IV) were both potent in activity against audiogenic seizures in mice.

Table V

Compound 11a was quite active in the audiogenic seizure test.

TABLE XII BENZOPYRONES

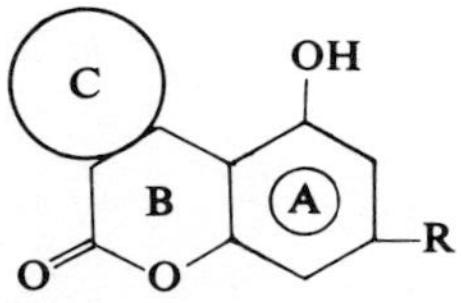

$R = C_9H_{18} = CH(CH_3)CH(CH_3)\text{-}n\text{-}C_5H_{11}$

No.	C Ring	R	AUD (mice)	MES (mice)	PsM (mice)	MMS (mice)
89	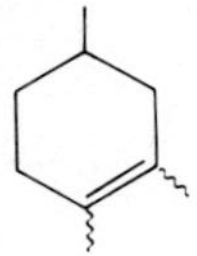	CH_3	100 = 30%		300 = 20% 300 = 20%	
90	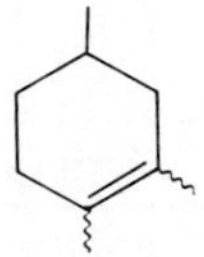	$-CH(CH_3)_2$	100 = 0%	100 = 20% 100 = 0%		100 = 0% 86 (est.)
91	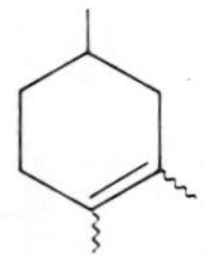	C_9H_{19}	300 = 10% 300 = 20%	300 = 0% 300 = 0%	300 = 10% 300 = 30%	100 = 20% 100 = 30%
92	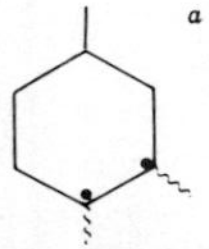	C_9H_{19}	100 = 0%	100 = 0% 100 = 30%	100 = 20% 100 = 90%	100 = 20% 100 = 40%

(continued)

321

TABLE XII—Continued

No.	C Ring	R	AUD (mice)	MMS (mice)	PsM (mice)	MMS (mice)
93	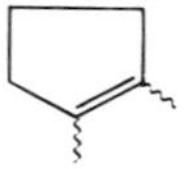	CH$_3$	300 = 10% 300 = 10%	300 = 0% 300 = 0%	300 = 20% 300 = 20%	280 (156–4000) 420 (est.)
94	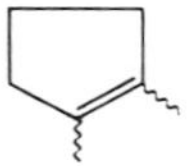	C$_9$H$_{19}$	300 = 10% 300 = 20%	300 = 0% 300 = 0%	300 = 10% 300 = 20%	100 = 20% 410 (est.)
95	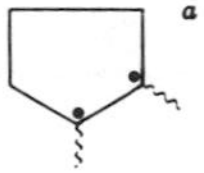	C$_9$H$_{19}$	100 = 0%	100 = 0%		
96	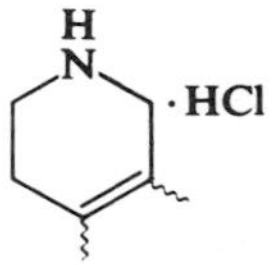	C$_9$H$_{19}$	100 = 20%	100 = 0%		

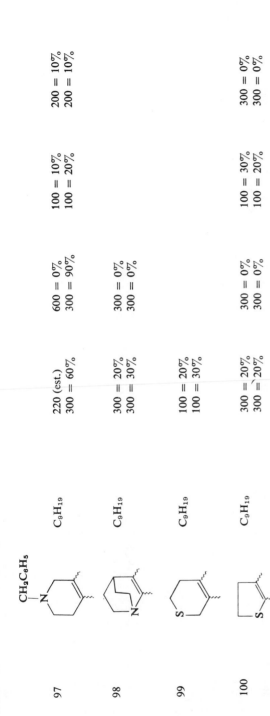

97	CH₂C₆H₅ structure · C₉H₁₉	220 (est.) 300 = 60%	600 = 0% 300 = 90%	100 = 10% 100 = 20%	200 = 10% 200 = 10%
98	C₉H₁₉	300 = 20% 300 = 30%	300 = 0% 300 = 0%		
99	C₉H₁₉	100 = 20% 100 = 30%			
100	C₉H₁₉	300 = 20% 300 = 20%	300 = 0% 300 = 0%	100 = 30% 100 = 20%	300 = 0% 300 = 0%

CH₂C₆H₅

[a] Single Bond with *cis*-fused B–C ring junction.

TABLE XIII DIHYDRO DERIVATIVES

No.	C Ring	AUD (mice)	MES (mice)	PsM (mice)	MMS (mice)
101	(cyclohexyl ring)	$100 = 20\%$	$100 = 0\%$	$300 = 20\%$ $300 = 20\%$	$100 = 20\%$ $100 = 80\%$
102	(cyclopentyl ring)	$30 = 100\%$ $100 = 90\%$	$100 = 0\%$[a] $100 = 40\%$	$100 = 70\%$ $100 = 80\%$	$100 = 40\%$ $100 = 30\%$
103	H—N (piperidine) · HCl	$100 = 40\%$ $100 = 40\%$	$600 = 0\%$ $600 = 0\%$	$300 = 20\%$ $300 = 20\%$	47 (est.) $100 = 20\%$
104	$CH_2CH=CHCl$ (cis) N (piperidine)	$30 = 40\%$			

[a] MES (rat): $5 = 100\%$.

Table VI

The largest number of active compounds were esters of DMHP-type compounds 5 and 7 in the audiogenic seizure test. They include compounds 28, 30, 32, 34, 36, 38, and 39.

Of great interest was the high level of anticonvulsant activity seen in the rat supramaximal electroshock test with compounds 30, 32, and 34 (at 4 hours).

Table VIII

Additional esters of compounds 11, 19, and 22 exhibiting outstanding activity in the mouse audiogenic seizure test include compounds 51, 57, 64, and 66.

Table XI

Only one compound, 81, exhibited significant activity in the mouse audiogenic seizure test.

Table XIII

Of interest is compound 102, which exhibited anticonvulsant activity against both mouse audiogenic seizures and rat supramaximal electroshock seizures.

IV. DISCUSSION

The compounds to date have exhibited remarkable specificity in terms of potential anticonvulsant activity. The singularly most sensitive anticonvulsant test was the audiogenic seizure test in mice. By this criterion, in Table II on natural cannabinoids and close analogues, it is apparent that only Δ^9-THC (compound 1), DMHP (compound 5), and compound 7 exhibit significant activity in the audiogenic seizure test. In addition, the compounds were active in the rat supramaximal electroshock test. Surprisingly, the C-ring heterocyclic compounds were considerably less active, resulting in activity only in the N-substituted analogues (compounds 11 and 22). The most active derivatives found were esters of DMHP-type compounds and esters of compounds 11, 19, and 22. In contrast, ethers of the phenol in ring A, as well as the basic carbamates, benzopyrones, and dihydro derivatives (between rings B and C), were generally inactive. Thus, it would appear that formation of the ester derivatives is ideal for anticonvulsant activity.

The profiles of anticonvulsant activities of the ester derivatives appear to resemble that of diphenylhydantoin. That is, the compounds protect mice from audiogenic seizures, electroconvulsive seizures, and maximal metrazole seizures, but *not* against psychomotor seizures. It is interesting that the new analogues have a longer duration of action than Δ^9-THC against audiogenic seizures in mice. Probably, the most significant finding was that the new analogues (compounds 30, 32, and 34) are considerably more active than diphenylhydantoin against electroconvulsive seizures in rats. This finding alone makes the benzopyrans highly promising in terms of clinical development. It is quite probable that some of the benzopyrans will be found effective in the treatment of major (grand mal) seizure states, as was suggested by an early clinical study in children (Davis and Ramsey, 1949). The long duration of action of these compounds will make them of special interest in the clinic. Finally, DMHP and Δ^9-THC are known to produce significant subjective and cardiovascular effects in man. In view of the different pharmacological profiles previously reported for the new analogues (Pars *et al.*, 1976; Razdan *et al.*, 1976; Winn *et al.*, 1976), it is our belief from our present studies that they will have therapeutic advantages as anticonvulsants.

In conclusion, it is our hope that these new analogues will be evaluated clinically both alone and in combination with other known anticonvulsant agents.

ACKNOWLEDGMENTS

We would like to express our appreciation to Dr. Harvey Kupferberg and the Anticonvulsant Advisory Committee of the National Institute of Neurological Diseases and Stroke for their encouragement of this study (supported in part by contract NO1-NS-3-2314).

The authors are indebted to A. C. Petersen, D. L. Arendsen, and R. F. Anderson for their technical assistance.

REFERENCES

Aaron, H. S., and Ferguson, C. P. (1968). *J. Org. Chem.* 33, 684.
Adams, R., MacKenzie, S., Jr., and Loewe, S. (1948). *J. Am. Chem. Soc.* 70, 664.
Anker, R. M., and Cook, A. H. (1946). *J. Chem. Soc.* 58.
Boggan, W. O., Steele, R. A., and Freedman, D. X. (1973). *Psychopharmacologia* 29, 101–106.
Carlini, E. A., Leite, J. R., Tannhauser, M., and Bernardi, A. C. (1973). *J. Pharm. Pharmacol.* 25, 664–665.
Chesher, G. B., and Jackson, D. M. (1974). *Psychopharmacologia* 37, 255–264.
Consroe, P. F., and Man, D. P. (1973). *Life Sci.* 13, 429–439.
Corcoran, M. E., McCaughran, J. A., Jr., and Wada, J. A. (1973). *Exp. Neurol.* 40, 471–483.
Davis, J. P., and Ramsey, H. H. (1949). *Fed. Proc., Fed. Am. Soc. Exp. Biol.* 8, 284–285.

Garriott, J. C., Forney, R. B., Hughes, F. W., and Richards, A. B. (1968). *Arch. Int. Pharmacodyn. Ther.* **171**, 425–434.

Karler, R. (1973). *Fed. Proc., Fed. Am. Soc. Exp. Biol.* **32**, 756.

Karler, R., Cely, W., and Turkanis, S. A. (1973). *Life Sci.* **13**, 1527–1531.

Karler, R., Cely, W., and Turkanis, S. A. (1974a). *Res. Commun. Chem. Pathol. Pharmacol.* **7**, 353–358.

Karler, R., Cely, W., and Turkanis S. A. (1974b). *Life Sci.* **15**, 931–947.

Loev, B., Bender, P. E., Dowalo, F., Macko, E., and Fowler, P. J. (1973). *J. Med. Chem.* **16**, 1200.

Loewe, S., and Goodman, L. S. (1947). *Fed. Proc., Fed. Am. Soc. Exp. Biol.* **6**, 352.

Man, D. P., and Consroe, P. F. (1973). *J. Int. Res. Commun.* **1**, 12.

Mechoulam, R. (1973). *In* "Marijuana" (R. Mechoulam, ed.), pp. 31–50. Academic Press, New York.

O'Shaughnessy, W. B. (1838). Translations of Medicine, Physiology, and Sociology, Bengal; 1838–1840, pp. 71–102.

Pars, H. G., Granchelli, F. E., Razdan, R. K., Rosenberg, F., Teiger, D., and Harris, L. S. (1976). *J. Med. Chem.* **19**, 445.

Petrzilka, T., Haefliger, W., and Sikemeier, C. (1969). *Helv. Chim. Acta* **52**, 1102.

Plotnikoff, N. P., and Green, D. J. (1957). *J. Pharmacol. Exp. Ther.* **119**, 234.

Plotnikoff, N. P., Zaugg, H. E., Petersen, A. C., Arendsen, D. L., and Anderson, R. F. (1975). *Life Sci.* **17**, 97–104.

Razdan, R. K., Dalzell, H. C., and Handrick, G. R., (1974). *J. Am. Chem. Soc.* **96**, 5860.

Razdan, R. K., Zitko Terris, B., Handrick, G. R., Dalzell, H. C., Pars, H. G., Howes, J., Plotnikoff, N. P., Dodge, P. W., Dren, A. T., Kyncl, J., Shoer, L., and Thompson, W. R. (1976a). *J. Med. Chem.* **19**, 549.

Razdan, R. K., Zitko Terris, B., Pars, H. G., Plotnikoff, N. P., Dodge, P. W., Dren, A. T., Kyncl, J., and Somani, P. (1976b). *J. Med. Chem.* **19**, 454.

Sofia, R. D., Solomon, T. A., and Barry, M., III. (1971). *Pharmacologist* **13**, 246.

Suter, C. M., and Weston, A. W. (1939). *J. Am. Chem. Soc.* **61**, 232.

Swinyard, E. A., Brown, W. C., and Goodman, L. S., (1952). *J. Pharmacol. Exp. Ther.* **106**, 319–330.

Toman, E. P., and Everett, G. M. (1964). *In* "Evaluation of Drug Activities: Pharmacometrics" (D. R. Laurence and A. L. Bacharach, eds.), Vol. I, pp. 287–301. Academic Press, New York.

Wada, J. A., Sato, M., and Corcoran, M. E. (1973). *Exp. Neurol.* **39**, 157–165.

Wilson, R. S., and May, E. L. (1975). *J. Med. Chem.* **18**, 700.

Winn, M., Arendsen, D., Dodge, P. W. Dren, A. T., Dunnigan, D., Hallas, R., Hwang, K., Kyncl, J., Lee, Y.-H., Plotnikoff, N., Young, P., Zaugg, H., Dalzell, H., and Razdan, R. (1976). *J. Med. Chem.* **19**, 461.

Zitko, B. A., Howes, J. F., Razdan, R. K., Dalzell, B. C., Dalzell, H. C., Sheehan, J. C., Pars, H. G., Dewey, W. L., and Harris, L. S. (1972). *Science* **177**, 444.

7

OTHER HETEROCYCLIC DRUGS

Frank D. Popp

ABBREVIATIONS USED IN THE TABLES

ES	Electroshock
MES	Maximal electroshock seizures test; method essentially according to Swinyard *et al.* (1952) with ED_{50} (when given) determined graphically
LD_{50}	Lethal dose computed graphically; acute toxicity in 50% of experimental animals
ED_{50}	Results determined graphically as by method of Litchfield and Wilcoxon; effective dose in 50% of experimental animals
Met	No seizure after subcutaneous administration of pentylene-tetrazole in mice or rats according to Swinyard *et al.* (1952); drug administered po; ED_{50} determined graphically
inact.	Inactive
act.	Active
mod. act.	Moderately active
v. act.	Very active
sl. act.	Slightly active

protn.	Protection
40% protn. at 100	40% protection at 100 mg/kg dose
100 less act. 10 Pb	100 mg/kg dose of compound less active than a 10 mg/kg dose of phenobarbital
100% protn. 0.2 LD_{50}	100% protection at a 0.2 LD_{50} dose
ip	Intraperitoneal administration
iv	Intravenous administration
po	Oral administration
sc	Subcutaneous administration
thresh. raised 15–20 mA	Elevation of theshold by 15–20 mA

This chapter includes all of those heterocyclic compounds screened for anticonvulsant activity that are not included in Chapters 5 and 6. The literature has been surveyed as far as possible from the time of the appearance of the book by Close and Spielman (1961), which covered the literature up to January 1959, until the end of 1975. In a number of cases heterocyclic amines have simply been used as amine substituents on other classes of compounds. Thus, for example, heterocyclic together with nonheterocyclic amines have been used as substituents on 1,1-diaryl-*tert*-aminopropanols (Barron *et al.*, 1965), acetophenone oxime ethers (Buzas *et al.*, 1972a), 1-aryl-2-phenyl-3-aminopropanones (Moffett and Hester, 1972), derivatives of diphenylmethane (Delschlager *et al.*, 1973), phenyl ketones (Sasajima *et al.*, 1974, 1975), 2-benzyl-3-dialkylaminoalkylindenes (Ganellin *et al.*, 1967), *N*-substituted benzenedisulfonamides (Holland *et al.*, 1963), diphenylaminopropanols (Keasling and Moffett, 1971), *N*-substituted amides (Union Chimique, 1966), and tetrafluorobenzenesulfonamides (Young, 1966) and are not included in the tables of this chapter.

In a number of cases anticonvulsant activity has been reported for crude natural product extracts, alkaloid extracts, or natural products of unspecified structure (Azimov *et al.*, 1966; Ghosal *et al.*, 1972; Hashimoto, 1967; Kovaleva and Lazebnik, 1966; Kretzschmar and Meyer, 1969; Roussinov, 1966; K. Rusinov, 1966; K. S. Rusinov, 1968; Tashbaev and Sultanov, 1965; Tursunova *et al.*, 1968; K. Watanabe *et al.*, 1973; Zakirov and Kamilov, 1967). These are not included in the tables in this chapter.

Compounds are listed in the tables starting with small-ring compounds and proceeding to large-ring compounds. In each ring size those compounds with a single heteroatom are listed first followed by the more complicated systems. When a compound contains more than one heteroring, it is generally listed in the table that appears first. An exception to this generalization are the cases in which it is obvious from the author's comments that he is studying the activity of the more complex ring system. With the exception of the compounds included in the section on the benzodiazepines, relatively few really outstanding compounds are included in this chapter. It is for this reason that we have not, in the text, discussed structure–activity relationships for the hundreds of active, but not outstanding, compounds reported. The reader is referred to the tables to draw his own conclusions. Unfortunately, this is not always possible because of the diversity of screening methods and methods of reporting results that are used by various authors.

I. SMALL-RING COMPOUNDS

Relatively little work has appeared on the use of three- and four-membered ring compounds as potential anticonvulsants. A variety of 2-arylglycidamides (**I**) were prepared, but results were presented only for **I** (R = Cl, Ar = 2,4-$Cl_2C_6H_3$), which had an ED_{50} of 24.7 mg/kg in an electroshock screen (Quick, 1973). The aziridine **II** has been reported (Pala *et al.*, 1971) to be active as an anticonvulsant.

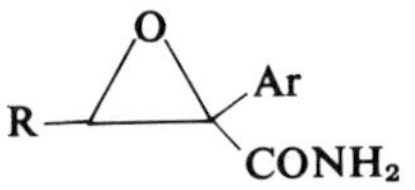

(**I**) 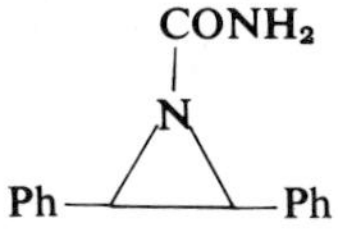　　　　(**II**) 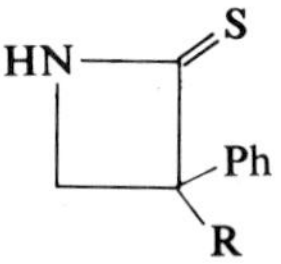　　　　(**III**)

A number of azetidines and azetidinones have shown activity and are listed in Table I. A large number of these were compared to luminol and were less effective (Maffii, 1959). A variety of related 1-substituted 2-azetidinones have also been reported to be active (Calenda-Stiftung, 1963; Testa and Fontanella, 1957) as have the 2-azetidinthiones (**III**) (Testa *et al.*, 1968).

TABLE I FOUR-MEMBERED RING COMPOUNDS

A. Azetidines

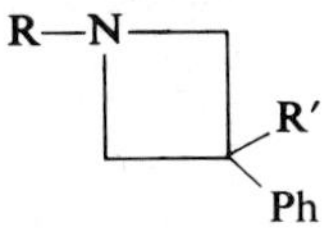

R	R′	Activity	Reference
$CONH_2$	*n*-Pr	Met ED_{50} < 20	Testa *et al.* (1963)
$CONH_2$	*i*-Pr	Met ED_{50} < 20	Testa *et al.* (1963)
$CONH_2$	Me	Met ED_{50} < 20	Testa *et al.* (1963)
COEt	Et	ES ED_{50} 20	Testa *et al.* (1961, 1962)
COBu-*n*	Et	ES ED_{50} 15	Testa *et al.* (1961, 1962)
CO*Et*	$PhCH_2$	ES ED_{50} 10	Testa *et al.* (1961, 1962)

(*continued*)

TABLE I—*Continued*

B. Azetidinones

R	R'	R''	Activity	Reference
2-ArCOC$_6$H$_2$RR		H	MES ED$_{50}$ 400; Met ED$_{50}$ 200–400	Wei and Bell (1972, 1973)
H	Ph	H	MES ED$_{50}$ 0.455[a]; Met ED$_{50}$ 1.358[a]	Maffii (1959)
H	Ph	Me	MES ED$_{50}$ 0.173[a]; Met ED$_{50}$ 0.465[a]	Maffii (1959)
H	Ph	Et (±)	MES ED$_{50}$ 0.182[a]; Met ED$_{50}$ 0.570[a]	Maffii (1959)
H	Ph	Et (+)	MES ED$_{50}$ 0.159[a]; Met ED$_{50}$ —	Maffii (1959)
H	Ph	Et (−)	MES ED$_{50}$ 0.188[a]; Met ED$_{50}$ —	Maffii (1959)
Me	Ph	Et	MES ED$_{50}$ 0.412[a]; Met ED$_{50}$ 0.792[a]	Maffii (1959)
Et	PhCH$_2$	Et	MES ED$_{50}$ 0.368[a]; Met ED$_{50}$ ≥ 0.398[a]	Maffii (1959)
H	cyclohexyl	Et	MES ED$_{50}$ 0.237[a]; Met ED$_{50}$ 0.317[a]	Maffii (1959)
H	4-NO$_2$C$_6$H$_4$	Et	MES ED$_{50}$ 0.717[a]; Met ED$_{50}$ > 1.103[a]	Maffii (1959)
H	4-NH$_2$C$_6$H$_4$	Et	MES ED$_{50}$ 0.295[a]; Met ED$_{50}$ > 0.454[a]	Maffii (1959)
H	Et	Et	MES ED$_{50}$ 0.226[a]; Met ED$_{50}$ ≥ 0.526	Maffii (1959)
H	Ph	n-Pr	MES ED$_{50}$ 1.470; Met ED$_{50}$ 0.471[a]	Maffii (1959)
H	Ph	i-Pr	MES ED$_{50}$ 0.391;[a] Met ED$_{50}$ 0.396[a]	Maffii (1959)
H	Ph	n-Bu	MES ED$_{50}$ 0.132;[a] Met ED$_{50}$ 0.211[a]	Maffii (1959)
H	Ph	i-Bu	MES ED$_{50}$ 0.152;[a] Met ED$_{50}$ 0.368[a]	Maffii (1959)
H	Ph	cyclohexyl	MES ED$_{50}$ 0.201;[a] Met ED$_{50}$ 0.245[a]	Maffii (1959)
H	Ph	cyclohexyl	MES ED$_{50}$ > 0.872;[a] Met ED$_{50}$ > 0.872[a]	Maffii (1959)
H	Ph	PhCH$_2$	MES ED$_{50}$ 0.674;[a] Met ED$_{50}$ 0.716[a]	Maffii (1959)
H	Ph	Ph	MES ED$_{50}$ 0.358;[a] Met ED$_{50}$ 1.119[a]	Maffii (1959)

[a] Dose given in moles per kilogram.

II. FIVE-MEMBERED RINGS

A. WITH ONE NITROGEN

Various pyrroles, pyrrolidines, indoles, and related compounds containing a five-membered nitrogen heterocyclic ring are included in Table II. By far the largest group of compounds studied in this area consists of the various derivatives of indole. It has been observed that no relationship exists between anticonvulsant activity and monoamine oxidase (MAO) inhibitory effectiveness (Rastogi *et al.*, 1974; Whittle and Young, 1963) or tryptophan decarboxylase activity (Whittle and Young, 1963) or the ability to inhibit NAD-dependent oxidations (Agarwal *et al.*, 1974) in a number of types of indoles. The pyrrolidine derivative **IV** (procyclidine) has been reported (Millichap *et al.*, 1968) to reduce the incidence of seizures in 10 of 16 children resistant to other anticonvulsants

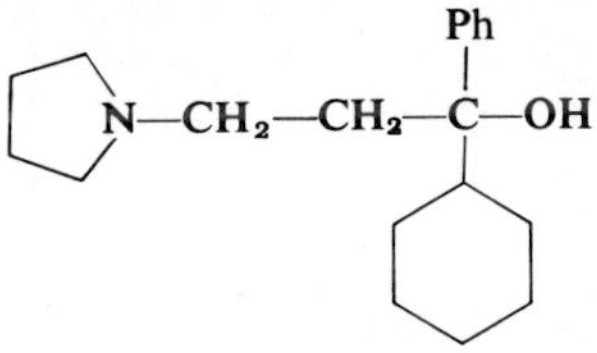

$$\text{N—CH}_2\text{—CH}_2\text{—C—OH}$$

with Ph above the C and a cyclohexyl ring below.

(IV)

B. WITH ONE HETEROATOM

The relatively few furan and thiophene derivatives that have been screened and found to have any degree of activity are included in Tables III and IV, respectively.

TABLE II PYRROLE DERIVATIVES

A. Pyrroles

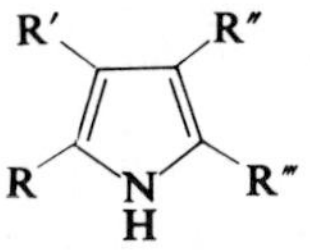

R	R'	R"	R'''	Activity	Reference
Me	Et	Me	H	MES ED_{50} 25 (ip)	Moffett (1968b)
Me	COMe	Me	H	MES ED_{50} 25 (ip)	Moffett (1968b)
Me	COMe	H	Me	MES ED_{50} 20 (ip)	Moffett (1968b)
COMe	Me	Et	Me	MES ED_{50} 50 (ip)	Moffett (1968b)

(*continued*)

TABLE II—*Continued*

B. Pyrrolines

R	Activity	Reference
Me, Et, Ph,	Met, weak activity in doses of at least 60 mg/kg (Me, Et, Ph); MES, inactive at 100 mg/kg (Ph)	van Proosdij-Hartzema et al. (1958)

C. Pyrrolidines

R	R'	R"	Activity	Reference
Various	Ph	OCOAr	Active	Hirata et al. (1974)
Various	Ar	H	ES, active	Helsley et al. (1970)
MeNHCO	PhO	H	MES ED_{50} 50 (ip); Met, 100% protn. at 150	Boswell et al. (1974)
H_2NCO	OC_6H_4Cl-3	H	MES ED_{50} 66 (ip); Met ED_{50} 111 (ip)	Boswell et al. (1974)
MeNHCO	OC_6H_4Cl-3	H	MES ED_{50} 54 (ip); Met ED_{50} 88 (ip)	Boswell et al. (1974)
H_2NCO	OC_6H_4Cl-4	H	MES ED_{50} 35 (ip); Met, 67% protn. at 100	Boswell et al. (1974)
H_2NCO	OC_6H_4Br-4	H	MES ED_{50} 55 (ip) Met, 66% protn. at 67	Boswell et al. (1974)

H_2NCO	H	MES ED_{50} 46 (ip); Met, 45% protn. at 100	Boswell et al. (1974)
H_2NCO	H	MES ED_{50} 35 (ip); Met, ED_{50} 89 (ip)	Boswell et al. (1974)
MeNHCO	H	MES ED_{50} 80 (ip); Met, 80% protn. at 200	Boswell et al. (1974)
Me_2CO	$OC_6H_4CF_3$-3	MES ED_{50} 47 (ip); Met, 80% protn. at 200	Boswell et al. (1974)
EtNHCO	$OC_6H_4CF_3$-3	MES, 80% protn. at 100; Met, 40% protn. at 200	Boswell et al. (1974)
PhNCO	$OC_6H_4CF_3$-3	MES, 20% protn. at 100; Met, 20% protn. at 200	Boswell et al. (1974)
H_2NCO	OC_6H_4OMe-2	MES ED_{50} 109 (ip); Met, 40% protn. at 200	Boswell et al. (1974)
4-$MeOC_6H_4HNCO$	OC_6H_4OMe-2	MES, 20% protn. at 100; Met, 0% protn. at 100	Boswell et al. (1974)
MeNHCO	OC_6H_4OMe-2	MES, 100% protn. at 200; Met, 0% protn. at 200	Boswell et al. (1974)
Ph_2NCO	OC_6H_4OMe-2	MES, 100% protn. at 100; Met, 20% protn. at 100	Boswell et al. (1994)
Me_2NH	OC_6H_4F-4	MES ED_{50} 150 (ip); Met, 60% protn. at 150	Boswell et al. (1974)
$(CH_2)_2C(Ph)OH$ 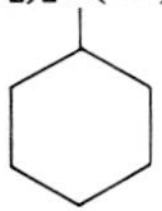	H	As active as luminol MES ED_{50} 16; Met ED_{50} 83	Dojtschinov (1970) Millichap et al. (1968)

| $CH_2CONHN=CHC_6H_4Cl$-4 | H | ES 30–50 (ip) | Tajana and Pozzi (1971) |
| 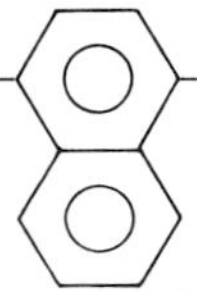 $CH_2CONHN=CH$ — (4-chloronaphthalen-1-yl) | H | ES 30–50 (ip) | Tajana and Pozzi (1971) |

(continued)

335

TABLE II—*Continued*

R	R'	R"	Activity	Reference
$CH_2CONHN=CHC_6H_4Me$-4	H	H	ES 30–50 (ip)	Tajana and Pozzi (1971)
$CH_2CONHN=CH$— (benzofuran, H_3C)	H	H	ES 30–50 (ip)	Tajana and Pozzi (1971)
$CONH_2$	PhCO	H	MES ED_{50} 88; Met ED_{50} 103	Helsey et al. (1969)
$CONH_2$	$4\text{-}FC_6H_4CO$	H	MES, 40% protn. at 100; Met, 40% protn. at 100	Helsley et al. (1969)
$CONH_2$	$3\text{-}CF_3C_6H_4CO$	H	MES, 30% protn. at 100; Met, 40% protn. at 200	Helsley et al. (1969)
$CONHMe$	$3\text{-}CF_3C_6H_4CO$	H	MES ED_{50} 60; Met, 40% protn. at 100	Helsley et al. (1969)
CO_2Et	Ph	H	MES, 40% protn. at 100; Met, 20% protn. at 100	Helsley et al. (1969)
$CH_2CH=C(Ph)C_6H_4Me$-4	H	H	MES ED_{50} 21; Met, partial protn. at 25	Saxena et al. (1969)

D. 2-Pyrrolidinones

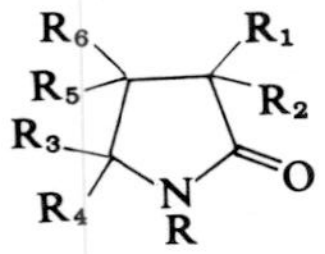

All R's are H except as noted	Activity	Reference
R_1 = Ar; R_2 = R	Active	Lutz and Schnider (1959, 1961)
R_1 = Ph; R_2 = 2-Pyr	Active	Hoffmann et al. (1956)
R_3 = Ph; R_4 = Et	Met, 70% protn. at 80	Perez de la Mora and Tapia (1973)
R_5 = Ar; R_6 = 2-Pyr	Active	Hoffmann et al. (1956)
R = 4-$SO_2NHC_6H_4$	Active	Pfirrmann and Hofstetter (1972)
R = 2-PhCO-4-ClC_6H_3	MES and Met ED_{50} 200–400	Wei and Bell (1972, 1973)
R_1 = Ph; R_2 = Et	MES and Met ED_{50} 60	Marshall (1958)
R_1 = Ph; R_2 = Me; R_5, R_6 = =O	Active	Miller (1958)
R_1 = Ph; R_2 = Et; R_5, R_6 = =O	Active	Miller (1958)
R_1 = Ph; R_2 = Pr; R_5, R_6 = =O	Active	Miller (1958)
R_1 = Ph; R_3 = Me; R_5, R_6 = =O	Active	Miller (1958)
R_1 = Ph; R_2 = R_3 = Me, R_5, R_6 = =O	Active	Miller (1958)
R_5, R_6 = —(CH$_2$)$_3$—; R_3, R_4 = =O	Active	Laboratoires Dausse (1969)
R_1, R_2 = =C(Me)NHAr; R_5, R_6 = =O	Active	Takiura et al. (1973)
R_1 = Ph; R_2 = Pyr; R_3, R_4 = =O	Active	Hoffmann et al. (1956)
R_1 = Ph; R_2 = Pyr; R_3, R_4 = =S	Active	Hoffmann et al. (1956)

(continued)

TABLE II—*Continued*

E. Isoindoles

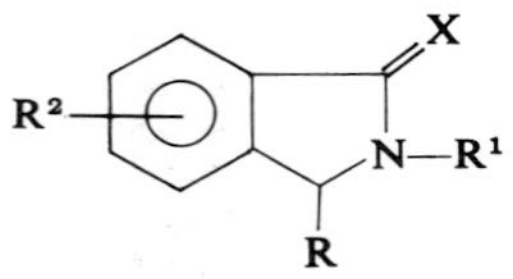

X	R	R¹	R²	Activity	Reference
H₂	R	Ar	R	Active	Sulkowski and Mascitti (1969)
O	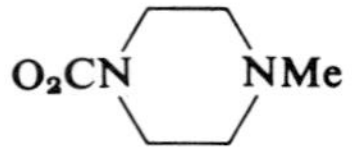 O₂CN—(piperazine)—NMe	Ar	H	Active	Challier et al. (1972)
O	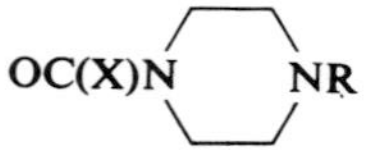 OC(X)N—(piperazine)—NR	3-Pyr	H	Active	Cotrel et al. (1972)
O	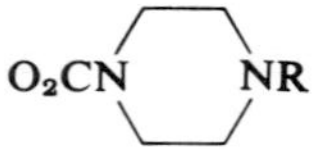 O₂CN—(piperazine)—NR	2-Quin	H	Active	Cotrel et al. (1973b)
O	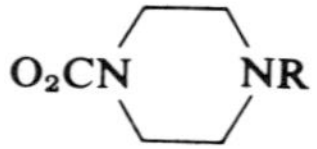 O₂CN—(piperazine)—NR	Heterocyclic	H	Active	Cotrel et al. (1974)
O	=O	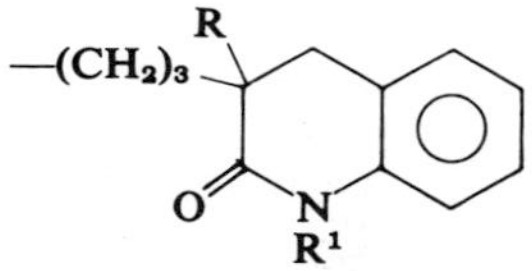 —(CH₂)₃—	H	Active	Mashimo et al. (1974a)

F. Miscellaneous

Structure	Activity	Reference
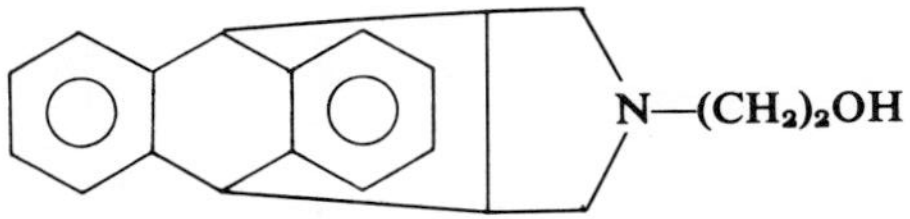 N—(CH$_2$)$_2$OH	Active	Schumann et al. (1964)
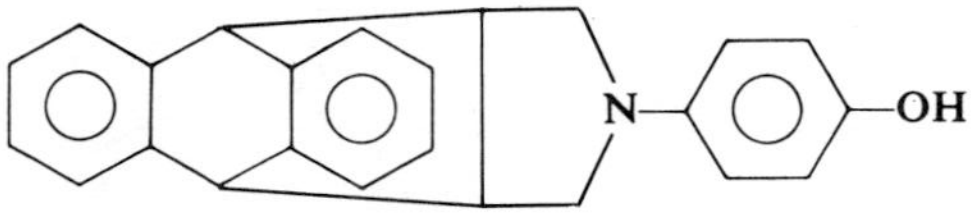 —OH	Active	Schumann et al. (1964)
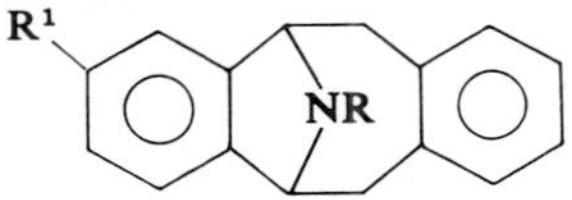 R^1 NR	Active	Roussel-Uclaf (1974); Nedelec and Frechet (1973)
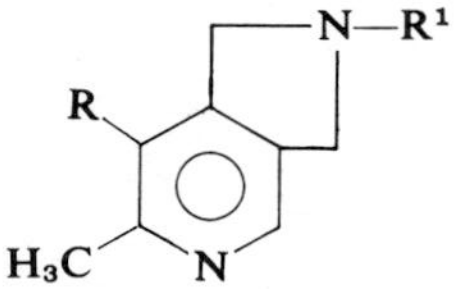 R N—R^1 H$_3$C	Active	Wright (1956)
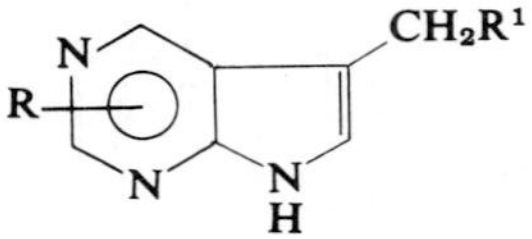 CH$_2$R^1 R N H	Active	Burroughs Wellcome & Co. (1965)
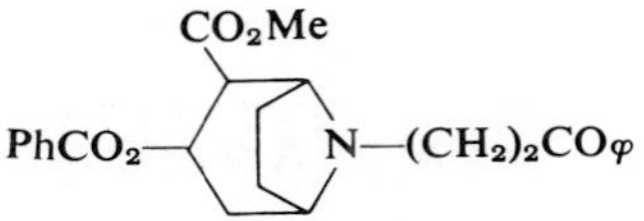 CO$_2$Me PhCO$_2$ N—(CH$_2$)$_2$COφ	MES and Met ED$_{50}$ 100–200	Sallay (1970)

(continued)

TABLE II—*Continued*

F. Miscellaneous

Structure	Activity	Reference
(pyridine bearing $N-CO_2Et$, R, R^1, Y)	Active	Song *et al.* (1962)
(pyrrolo-pyrimidine bearing NR^3R^4, R^1, R^2)	Active	Hitchings *et al.* (1962)
(SR-substituted pyrrolopyrimidine, N, H)	Active	Wellcome Foundation Ltd. (1964)
(O, $N-Ar$, $OCON$, $N-Me$ piperazine fused pyridinone)	Active	Challier *et al.* (1973)

	Activity	Reference
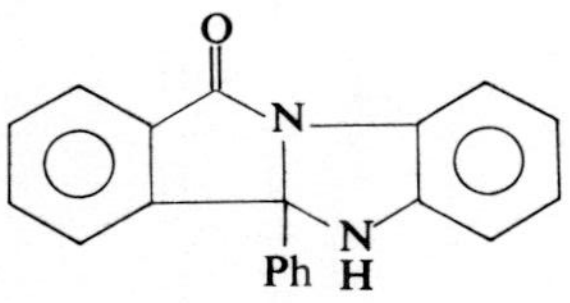	Active	Sulkowski (1969)
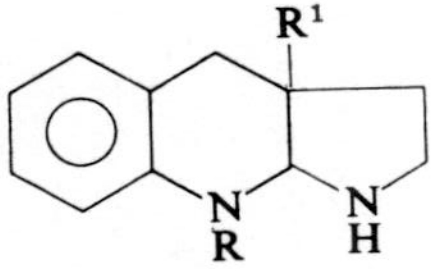	Active	Mashimo et al. (1974b)
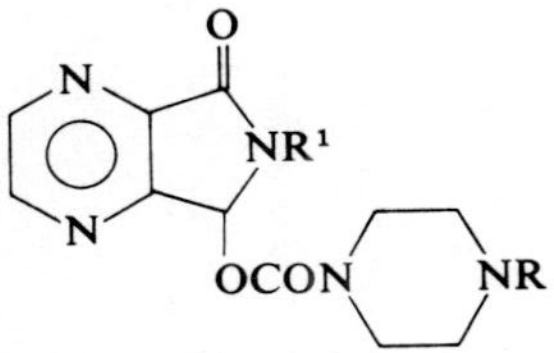	Active	Cotrel et al. (1973a)
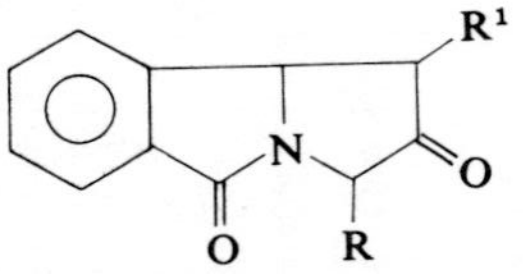	Active	Viscontini and Adank (1962)

(continued)

341

TABLE II—*Continued*

G. Indoles

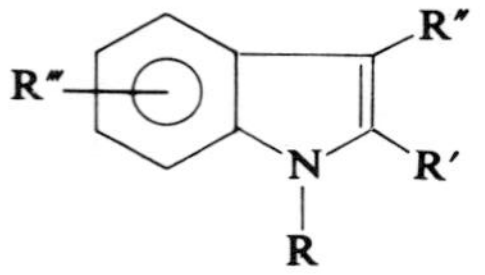

R	R'	R''	R''	Activity	Reference
H	H	$CH_2CH(Et)NH_2$	4-Cl	MES ED_{50} 150	Whittle and Young (1963)
H	H	$CH_2CH(Me)NH_2$	5-Cl	MES ED_{50} 100	Whittle and Young (1963)
H	H	$CH_2CH(Et)NH_2$	5-Cl	MES ED_{50} 150	Whittle and Young (1963)
H	H	$CH_2CH(Me)NH_2$	6-Cl	MES ED_{50} 100	Whittle and Young (1963)
H	H	$CH_2CH(Et)NH_2$	6-Cl	MES ED_{50} 70	Whittle and Young (1963)
H	H	$CH_2CH(Me)NH_2$	7-Cl	MES ED_{50} 66	Whittle and Young (1963)
H	H	$CH_2CH(Et)NH_2$	7-Cl	MES ED_{50} 100	Whittle and Young (1963)
H	H	$CH_2CH(Me)NH_2$	H	MES ED_{50} 60	Whittle and Young (1963)
H	H	$CH_2CH(Et)NH_2$	H	MES ED_{50} 32	Whittle and Young (1963)
H	H	2-MeCONH-5-ClC$_6$H$_3$	H	Met and MES, act. at 50–200	Freeman and Judd (1972)

		Structure / R		Activity	Reference
H	H	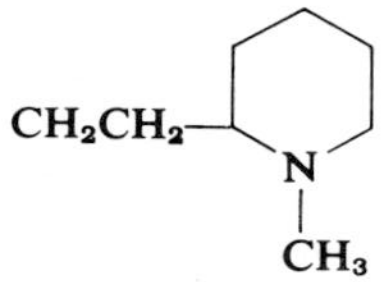 (CH₂CH₂ / N–CH₃ piperidine)	H	MES ED$_{50}$ 26 (ip); MES ED$_{50}$ 55 (po)	Julou et al. (1957); Julou et al. (1957)
R	H	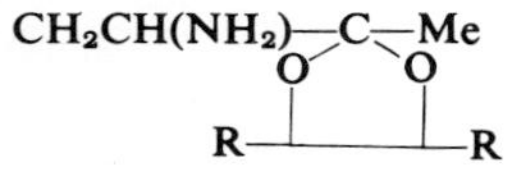 CH₂CH(NH₂)—C—Me (O, O, R)	R'	Active	Szmuszkovic and Anthony (1961a)
R	H	C(Ar)CH(R')CH(R'')NR''R''	R''	Active	Szmuszkovic and Anthony (1961b)
H	H	C(Me)=NO(CH₂)₂NH₂	H	Active	Philips' Gloeilampenfabricken (1970)
H	H	(CH₂)₂NHCOMe	5-OMe	Active	Anton-Jay (1971)
R	R	CH(OH)CH₂NHR	H	Active	Crowther and Smith (1966)
R	H	(CH₂)₂NR₂	5-OH	ES, active	Chou and Tu (1965)
H	CH₂N(Bu-n)₂	H	H	Active	Chou et al. (1966)
H	H	CH(OH)CH₂NMe₂	H	ES, 100% protn. at 100 (ip)	Singh and Bhandar (1973)
H	H	CH₂NH(CH₂)₂OH	H	ES, 100% protn. at 50 (ip)	Singh and Bhandar (1973)
H	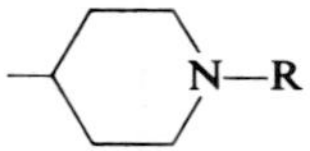 (N–R piperidine)	R	H	Active	Société des Usines Chimiques (1959b)
H	H	CONH-Nap-1	O(CH₂)₂Br	Met, 10% protn. at 100 (ip)	Gupta et al. (1975)
H	H	CONHC₆H₄Et-2	O(CH₂)₂Br	Met, 20% protn. at 100 (ip)	Gupta et al. (1975)
H	H	CONHC₆H₄Et-4	O(CH₂)₂Br	Met, 30% protn. at 100 (ip)	Gupta et al. (1975)

(continued)

343

TABLE II—*Continued*

R	R'	R"	(ring)	Activity	Reference
H	$CONHC_6H_3Me_2$-2,4	$O(CH_2)_2Br$	H	Met, 20% protn. at 100 (ip)	Gupta et al. (1975)
H	$CONHC_6H_3Me_2$-3,4	$O(CH_2)_2Br$	H	Met, 20% protn. at 100 (ip)	Gupta et al. (1975)
H	CONH-Nap-1	$O(CH_2)_2NHNH_2$	H	Met, 10% protn. at 100 (ip)	Gupta et al. (1975)
H	CONH-Nap-2	$O(CH_2)_2NHNH_2$	H	Met, 20% protn. at 100 (ip)	Gupta et al. (1975)
H	$CONHC_6H_4Et$-4	$O(CH_2)_2NHNH_2$	H	Met, 20% protn. at 100 (ip)	Gupta et al. (1975)
H	CO_2Et	$O(CH_2)_2(CH_2)_2NR_2$	H	Active	Nakanishi and Kobayashi (1974)
R	R	$(CH_2)_2N(Me)CH_2R$ [R defined by structure]	R	Active	Boch and Molle (1974)
H	Me	[decahydroquinolizidine–CH_2 structure]	5-OMe	ES, act. 200 (po)	Boido and Boidocanu (1973)
Ph	Me	$CONR_2$	5-OMe	Active	Fauran et al. (1974b)
H	Me	$(CH_2)_2NMe_2$	4-Me-5-Me	ES, act. 44 (ip)	Allen et al. (1973)
H	Me	$NHCH_2C(Me){=}CH_2$	4-Me-5-Me	ES, act. 37 (ip)	Allen et al. (1973)
H	Me	[N-methylpyrrolidine structure]	4-Me-5-Me	ES, act. 46 (ip)	Allen et al. (1973)
H	Me	$CH_2CONHNHCSNHC_6H_5$	H	Met, 20% protn. 0.2 LD_{50}	Rastogi et al. (1974)

H	Me	$CH_2CONHNHCSNHC_6H_4Me\text{-}2$	H	Met, 30% protn. 0.2 LD_{50}	Rastogi *et al.* (1974)
H	Me	$CH_2CONHNHCSNHC_6H_4Me\text{-}4$	H	Met, 30% protn. 0.2 LD_{50}	Rastogi *et al.* (1974)
H	Me	$CH_2CONHNHCSNHC_6H_4Cl\text{-}4$	H	Met, 30% protn. 0.2 LD_{50}	Rastogi *et al.* (1974)
H	Me	$CH_2CONHNHCSNHC_6H_4Br\text{-}4$	H	Met, 30% protn. 0.2 LD_{50}	Rastogi *et al.* (1974)
H	Me	$CH_2CONHNHCSNHC_6H_4I\text{-}4$	H	Met, 70% protn. 0.2 LD_{50}	Rastogi *et al.* (1974)
H	Me	$CH_2CONHNHCSNHC_6H_{11}$	H	Met, 50% protn. 0.2 LD_{50}	Rastogi *et al.* (1974)
H	Me	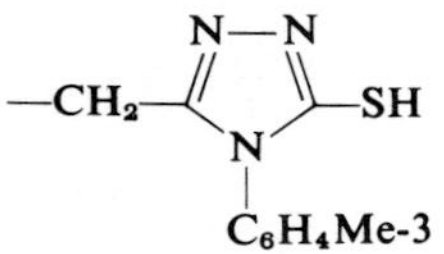 triazole ring ($-CH_2-$ / N–N / SH / N–$C_6H_4Me\text{-}3$)	H	Met, 30% protn. 0.2 LD_{50}	Rastogi *et al.* (1974)
H	Me	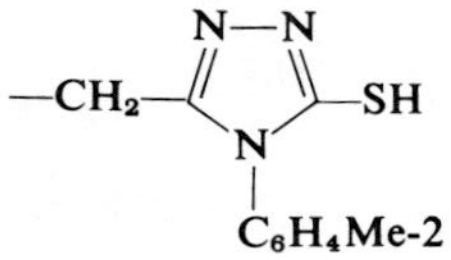 triazole ring ($-CH_2-$ / N–N / SH / N–$C_6H_4Me\text{-}2$)	H	Met, 20% protn. 0.2 LD_{50}	Rastogi *et al.* (1974)
H	Me	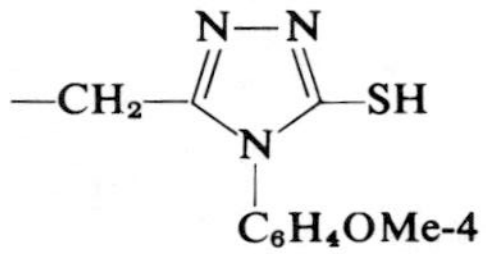 triazole ring ($-CH_2-$ / N–N / SH / N–$C_6H_4OMe\text{-}4$)	H	Met, 30% protn. 0.2 LD_{50}	Rastogi *et al.* (1974)
H	Me	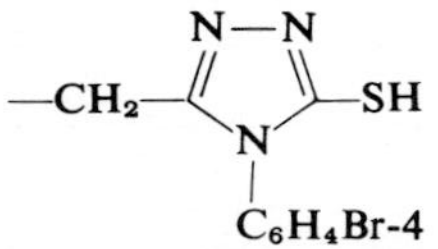 triazole ring ($-CH_2-$ / N–N / SH / N–$C_6H_4Br\text{-}4$)	H	Met, 30% protn. 0.2 LD_{50}	Rastogi *et al.* (1974)

(continued)

345

TABLE II—*Continued*

R	R'	R″	R‴	Activity	Reference
H	Me	triazole: —CH$_2$ / N—N / SH ; N—C$_6$H$_4$I-4	H	Met, 20% protn. 0.2 LD$_{50}$	Rastogi *et al.* (1974)
H	Me	triazole: —CH$_2$ / N—N / SH ; N—CH$_2$—CH=CH$_2$	H	Met, 20% protn. 0.2 LD$_{50}$	Rastogi *et al.* (1974)
H	Me	triazole: —CH$_2$ / N—N / SH ; N—C$_4$H$_9$-n	H	Met, 20% protn. 0.2 LD$_{50}$	Rastogi *et al.* (1974)
H	Ph	CH$_2$NH(CH$_2$)$_2$NMe$_2$	H	Met, 50% protn. at 100	Agarwal *et al.* (1974)
H	4-ClC$_6$H$_4$	CH$_2$NH(CH$_2$)$_3$NMe$_2$	H	Met, 45% protn. at 100	Agarwal *et al.* (1974)
H	4-MeC$_6$H$_4$	CH$_2$NH(CH$_2$)$_3$NMe$_2$	H	Met, 55% protn. at 100	Agarwal *et al.* (1974)
H	Ph	CH$_2$NH—(cyclopentyl)	H	Met, 45% protn. at 100	Agarwal *et al.* (1974)
H	4-ClC$_6$H$_4$	CH$_2$NH—(cyclopentyl)	H	Met, 52% protn. at 100	Agarwal *et al.* (1974)
H	4-MeC$_6$H$_4$	CH$_2$NH—(cyclopentyl)	H	Met, 55% protn. at 100	Agarwal *et al.* (1974)

H	Ph	CH_2NH–cyclohexyl	H	Met, 60% protn. at 100	Agarwal *et al.* (1974)
H	$4\text{-}ClC_6H_4$	CH_2NH–cyclohexyl	H	Met, 55% protn. at 100	Agarwal *et al.* (1974)
H	$4\text{-}MeC_6H_4$	CH_2NH–cyclohexyl	H	Met, 50% protn. at 100	Agarwal *et al.* (1974)
H	Me	$CH_2CONHNHCH_2C_6H_3(OMe)_2\text{-}3,4$	5-Me	Met, 60% protn. at 100	Agarwal *et al.* (1972)
H	Me	$CH_2CONHNHCH_2C_6H_3(OMe)_2\text{-}3,4$	H	Met, 70% protn. at 100	Agarwal *et al.* (1972)
H	Me	$CH_2CONHNHCH_2C_6H_3(OMe)_2\text{-}3,4$	5-MeO	Met, 75% protn. at 100	Agarwal *et al.* (1972)
H	Me	$CH_2CONHNHCH_2C_6H_2(OMe)_3\text{-}3,4,5$	5-Me	Met, 60% protn. at 100	Agarwal *et al.* (1972)
H	Me	$CH_2CONHNHCH_2C_6N_2(OMe)_3\text{-}3,4,5$	H	Met, 40% protn. at 100	Agarwal *et al.* (1972)
H	Me	$CH_2CONHNHCH_2C_6H_2(OMe)_3\text{-}3,4,5$	5-OMe	Met, 50% protn. at 100	Agarwal *et al.* (1972)
H	Me	$CH_2CONHN{=}CHC_6H_4OH\text{-}4$	H	Met, 40% protn. at 100	Nagar *et al.* (1972)
H	Me	$CH_2CONHN{=}CHC_6H_4OMe\text{-}4$	H	Met, 20% protn. at 100	Nagar *et al.* (1972)
H	Me	$CH_3CONHN{=}CHC_6H_4Cl\text{-}4$	H	Met, 20% protn. at 100	Nagar *et al.* (1972)
H	Me	$CH_2CONHN{=}CHC_6H_3OH\text{-}2\text{-}Cl\text{-}3$	H	Met, 20% protn. at 100	Nagar *et al.* (1972)
H	Me	$CH_2CONHN{=}CHC_6H_4NMe_2\text{-}4$	H	Met, 20% protn. at 100	Nagar *et al.* (1972)
R	R	$(CH_2)_2\text{-}Pyr\text{-}(2 \text{ and } 4)$	R	Active	American Home Products (1968); Freed and Archibald (1969)
H	OH	OH	H	MES ED_{50} 60; Met ED_{50} 60	Mueller and Schmiedel (1964)

(continued)

TABLE II—*Continued*

R	R'	R"	R‴	Activity	Reference
H	H	COMe	H	ES, 100 less act. 10 Pb	Keasling *et al.* (1964)
Me	H	COMe	H	ES, 100 less act. 10 Pb	Keasling *et al.* (1964)
H	Me	COMe	H	ES, 100 less act. 10 Pb	Keasling *et al.* (1964)
Me	Me	COMe	H	ES, 100 less act. 10 Pb	Keasling *et al.* (1964)
COMe	H	COMe	H	ES, 100 less act. 10 Pb	Keasling *et al.* (1964)
H	H	CH$_2$CH(Me)$_2$	H	ES, 100 less act. 10 Pb	Keasling *et al.* (1964)
H	H	CH$_2$COMe	H	ES, 100 less act. 10 Pb	Keasling *et al.* (1964)
H	H	COEt	H	ES, 100 more act. 10 Pb	Keasling *et al.* (1964)
Me	H	COEt	H	ES, 100 more act. 10 Pb	Keasling *et al.* (1964)
Me	H	COCHMe$_2$	H	ES, 100 more act. 10 Pb	Keasling *et al.* (1964)
Et	H	COCHMe$_2$	H	ES, 100 less act. 10 Pb	Keasling *et al.* (1964)
H	H	COCHMe$_2$	H	ES, 100 same act. 10 Pb	Keasling *et al.* (1964)
Me	H	COC(OH)Me$_2$	H	ES, 100 less act. 10 Pb	Keasling *et al.* (1964)
Et	H	CHOHC(OH)Me$_2$	H	ES, 100 less act. 10 Pb	Keasling *et al.* (1964)
H	H	COC(OH)Me$_2$	H	ES, 100 more act. 10 Pb	Keasling *et al.* (1964)
Me	H	CHOHC(OH)Me$_2$	H	ES, 100 more act. 10 Pb	Keasling *et al.* (1964)
Et	H	COC(OH)Me$_2$	H	ES, 100 less act. 10 Pb	Keasling *et al.* (1964)
Me	H	COC(OH)Et$_2$	H	ES, 100 less act. 10 Pb	Keasling *et al.* (1964)
H	H	COC(OH)Et$_2$	H	ES, 100 more act. 10 Pb	Keasling *et al.* (1964)
H	H	COC(OH)Et$_2$	H	ES, 100 less act. 10 Pb	Keasling *et al.* (1964)
H	H	COPr-*n*	H	ES, 100 less act. 10 Pb	Keasling *et al.* (1964)
H	H	CH$_2$COEt	H	ES, 100 less act. 10 Pb	Keasling *et al.* (1964)
H	Me	COCH$_2$CHMe$_2$	H	ES, 100 less act. 10 Pb	Keasling *et al.* (1964)
H	Me	COCH(Me)Et	H	ES, 100 less act. 10 Pb	Keasling *et al.* (1964)
H	H	(CH$_2$)$_2$COMe	H	ES, 100 less act. 10 Pb	Keasling *et al.* (1964)
Me	Me	COPh	H	ES, 100 less act. 10 Pb	Keasling *et al.* (1964)
Me	H	COCHPh$_2$	H	ES, 100 less act. 10 Pb	Keasling *et al.* (1964)
H	H	COC(OH)Ph$_2$	H	ES, 100 less act. 10 Pb	Keasling *et al.* (1964)

H. 2-Oxoindoles

Compound	Activity	Reference
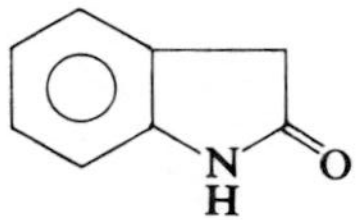	ES and Met, active MES ED$_{50}$ 50; Met ED$_{50}$ 56	Orcutt et al. (1964) Mueller and Schmiedel (1964)
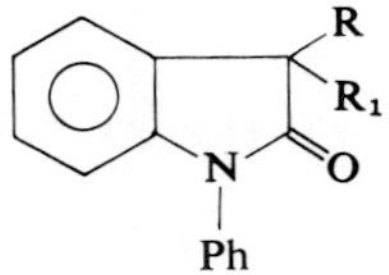	Active	Pelczarska (1969)
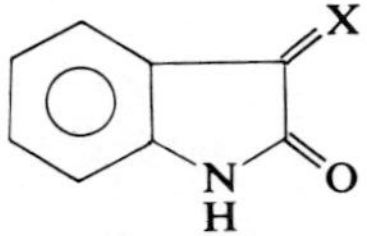	X = 0: MES 100% protn. at 400 X = NOH: MES 0% protn. at 400 X = (OH)$_2$: MES 33% protn. at 400	Sareen et al. (1962) Sareen et al. (1962) Sareen et al. (1962)

I. Miscellaneous indoles

Compound	Activity	Reference
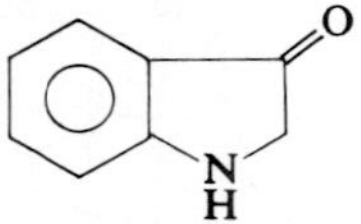	MES 33% protn. at 400	Sareen et al. (1962)
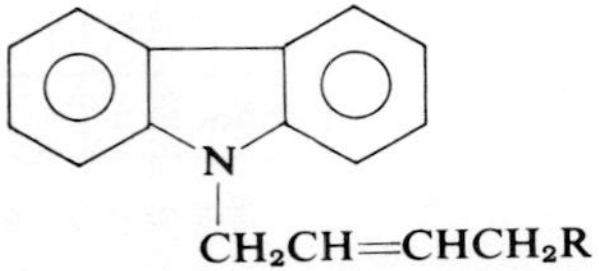 CH$_2$CH=CHCH$_2$R	Active	Schindler (1968)

(continued)

349

TABLE II—*Continued*

Compound	Activity	Reference
	R = Ph: MES ED_{50} 52 (ip) R = 4-MeOC$_6$H$_4$: MES ED_{50} 29 (ip) R = 4-ClC$_6$H$_4$: MES ED_{50} 34 (ip)	Demerson *et al.* (1974) Demerson *et al.* (1974) Demerson *et al.* (1974)
	MES ED_{50} 316; MET inactive at 400	Saxena *et al.* (1969)
	R = NEt$_2$: MES ED_{50} 18 (po)	Schindler (1970)
(cis): MES ED_{50} 15		Schindler (1970)
CH$_3$ (cis): MES ED_{50} 17		Schindler (1970)
CH$_3$ (trans): MES ED_{50} 16		Schindler (1970)

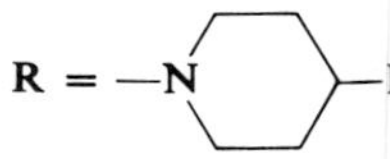	Et (trans): MES ED_{50} 17	Schindler (1970)
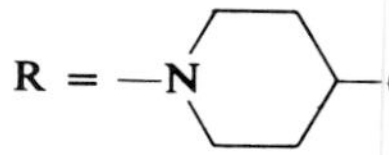	$(CH_2)_2OH$ (cis): MES ED_{50} 9	Schindler (1970)
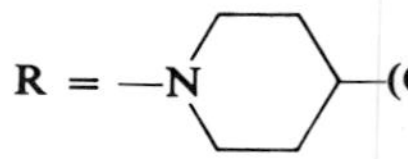	$(CH_2)_2OEt$ (cis): MES ED_{50} 13	Schindler (1970)
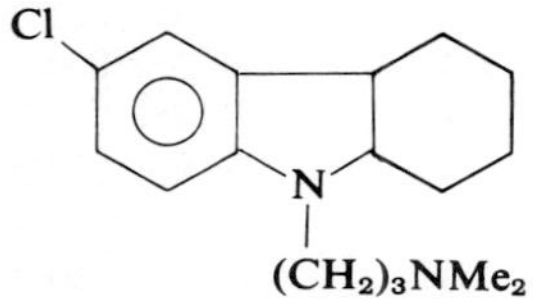	MES 100% protn. 0.2 LD_{50} (ip) MES, 20% protn. 0.1 LD_{50} (ip)	Shoeb *et al.* (1973)
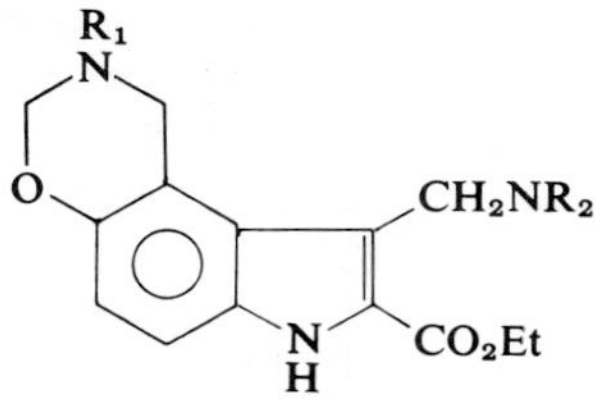	Active	Fauran *et al.* (1973b)
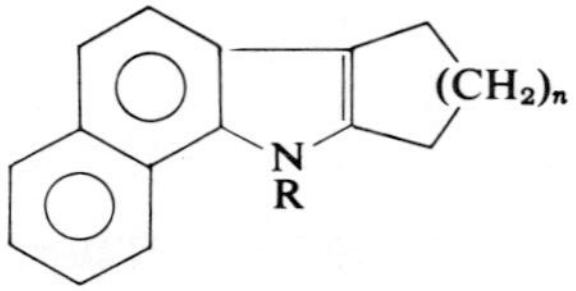	Active	Rice *et al.* (1965)

(*continued*)

TABLE II—*Continued*

R	R_1	R_2	R_3	R_4	R_5	% protn. 0.2 LD_{50} (ip)	% protn. 0.1 LD_{50} (ip)	Reference
$(CH_2)_2NC_4H_8$	H	H	F	H	H	80	20	Shoeb et al. (1973)
$(CH_2)_2NMe_2$	H	Cl	H	H	H	100	80	Shoeb et al. (1973)
$(CH_2)_2NC_4H_8$	H	Cl	H	H	H	60	0	Shoeb et al. (1973)
$(CH_2)_2NMe_2$	H	H	Cl	H	H	100	0	Shoeb et al. (1973)
$(CH_2)_2NMe_2$	H	H	Cl	H	H	60	20	Shoeb et al. (1973)
$(CH_2)_2NMe_2$	MeO	H	H	H	H	80	0	Shoeb et al. (1973)
$(CH_2)_2NC_4H_8$	MeO	H	H	H	H	100	0	Shoeb et al. (1973)
$(CH_2)_2NMe_2$	H	MeO	H	H	H	100	0	Shoeb et al. (1973)
$(CH_2)_2NC_4H_8$	H	MeO	H	H	H	100	0	Shoeb et al. (1973)
$(CH_2)_3NMe_2$	H	MeO	H	H	H	100	100 (ED_{50} 23.5)	Shoeb et al. (1973)
$(CH_2)_3NMe_2$	H	H	MeO	H	H	80	0	Shoeb et al. (1973)
$(CH_2)_2NMe_2$	H	Cl	H	MeO	H	80	0	Shoeb et al. (1973)
$(CH_2)_2NEt_2$	H	Cl	H	H	MeO	100	50	Shoeb et al. (1973)
$(CH_2)_2NC_4H_8$	H	Cl	H	H	MeO	80	20	Shoeb et al. (1973)
$(CH_2)_3NMe_2$	H	Cl	H	H	MeO	80	60 (ED_{50} 20.3)	Shoeb et al. (1973)

Compound	Activity	Reference
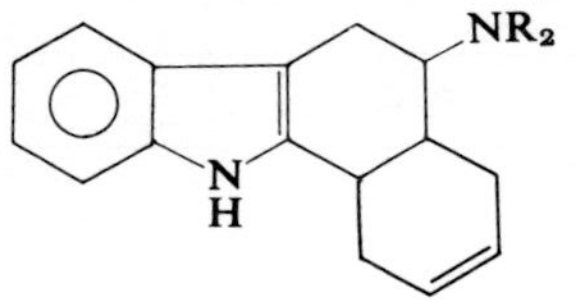 (structure: NR₂-substituted fused ring system with indole NH)	Active	Sallay (1966)
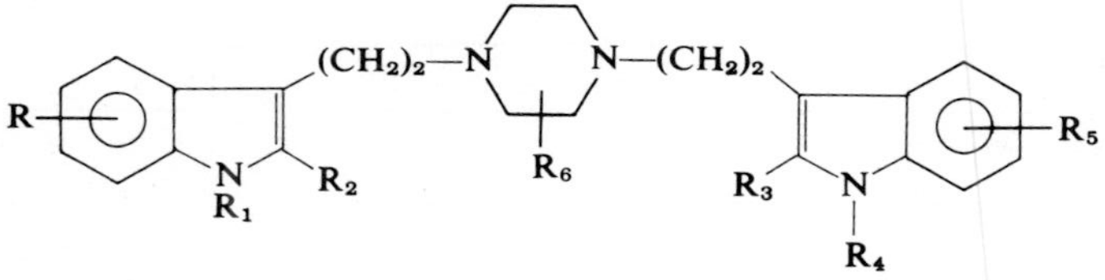 (structure: piperazine-linked bis-indole system with R, R₁, R₂, R₃, R₄, R₅, R₆)	Active	American Home Products (1968); Archibald and Freed (1969, 1971)

TABLE III FURAN DERIVATIVES

	A. Furans and benzofurans	
Compound	Activity	Reference
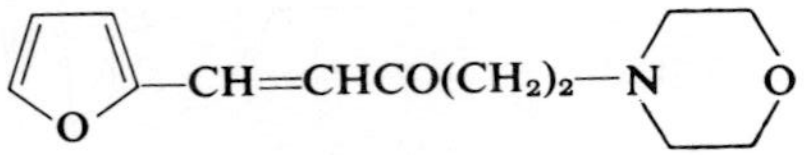 (furan)—CH=CHCO(CH₂)₂—N(morpholine)	Met, partial activity	Ottaviano and Pasqua (1959)
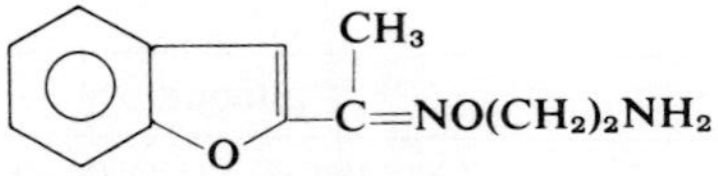 (benzofuran) CH₃—C=NO(CH₂)₂NH₂	Active	Philips' Gloeilampen Labrikien (1970)

(*continued*)

353

TABLE III—*Continued*

B. Tetrahydrofurans and benzotetrahydrofurans

Compound	Activity	Reference
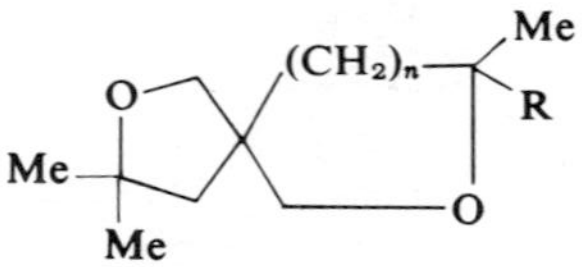	Active	Wasson and Parker (1963)
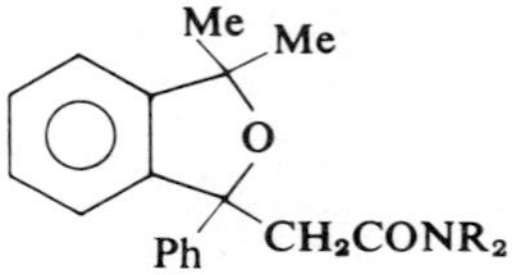	ES, 100% protn. at 200 (po); Met act. at 140 (sc)	Ratouis and Boissier (1971); Ratouis (1972)

C. γ-Butyrolactones

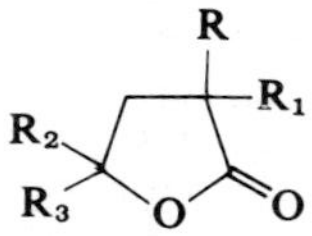

R	R_1	R_2	R_3	Activity	Reference
H	H	$CONH_2$	4-ClC_6H_4	Met, active at 287.5	Witkowska (1972)
$NHCO_2(CH_2)_3CH_3$	H	H	H	ES, 100% protn. at 250; Met inact.	Sandrini and Ferrari (1973); Sandrini (1974); Ferrari and Sandrini (1973)

Compound	Activity	Reference
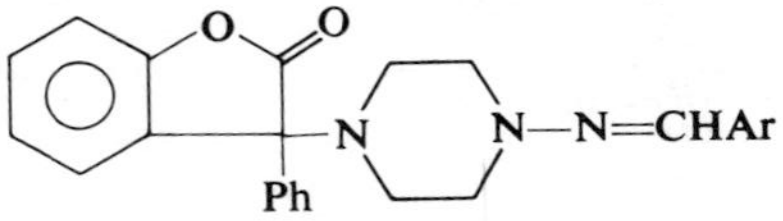	Active	Cusic *et al.* (1973, 1974)

TABLE IV THIOPHENE DERIVATIVES

Compound	Activity	Reference
H_3C—thiophene—$C(CH_3)$=$NOCH_2CH_2NH_2$	Active	Philips' Gloeilampenfabrieken (1970)
benzothiophene—$CONH$—$(CH_2)_n$—N(morpholine)	Active	Wright and Brabander (1970)
thiophene (R^2, R^3, $COAr$) substituted triazole (R^1, CH_2R, Z—N)	Z = N or CH: active	Shiroki et al. (1974)

C. WITH TWO NITROGENS

A number of pyrazoles, pyrazolines, and related five-membered rings with the nitrogen 1,2 are included in Table V. The anticonvulsant activity of several of the pyrazolines is unrelated to monoamine oxidase inhibition (Parmar *et al.*, 1974c) and to the inhibition of NAD-dependent oxidation (Singh *et al.*, 1974b). Despite the large interest in hydantoins, as indicated in Chapter 5, relatively little has appeared on imidazoles and related compounds, as can be seen in Table VI. The anticonvulsant activity of a group of imidazolones (Verma *et al.*, 1974) and benzimidazoles (Parmar *et al.*, 1972c) was unrelated to the MAO inhibitory ability of the compounds.

D. WITH TWO HETEROATOMS

Tables VII–X include a variety of five-membered heterocyclic compounds containing two heteroatoms. In view of the large amount of work, indicated in Chapter 5, on 2,4-oxazolidinediones, the lack of a large number of active 2-oxazolidinones and other oxazoles is noteworthy.

Since the report in 1956 by Charonnat and co-workers on the anticonvulsant activity of clomethiazole (the ethane disulfonate of the thiazole V), there have been a number of attempts to study the structure–activity relationships. While the oxazole isostere **VI** has the same anticonvulsant activity as **V**

(V)   (VI)

(Lindberg, 1966), other analogues are devoid of equivalent anticonvulsant effects, as indicated in Tables VIIIA, and IX,A (Lindberg, 1966, 1971a; Lindberg *et al.*, 1967, 1970, 1971). The work on these structure–activity effects has been reviewed (Lindberg, 1971b) as has the general pharmacology of clomethiazole (Lechat, 1966). Clomethiazole does not appear to be used clinically as an anticonvulsant, but it is used in the treatment of delirium tremens and other acute alcoholic states.

No correlation was found between anticonvulsant activity and the ability to inhibit NAD-dependent oxidations for several of the compounds in Table IX (Misra, 1974; Parmar *et al.*, 1972a).

E. WITH THREE AND FOUR HETEROATOMS

Tables XI–XVII include a variety of five-membered heterocyclic compounds containing three or four heteroatoms. The anticonvulsant activity of

TABLE V PYRAZOLE DERIVATIVES

A. Pyrazoles

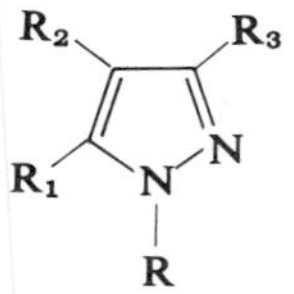

R	R₁	R₂	R₃	Activity	Reference
H	Ph	H	Me	Active	Laboratoire Millot (1964)
$CH_2CHR'OCONHR$	Me	H	Me	Active	Wolf (1968b)
MeCO	H	H	Undecyl	ES ED$_{50}$ 270	Karmas and Oroshnik (1960)
$ClCH_2CO$	H	H	Undecyl	ES ED$_{50}$ < 250	Karmas and Oroshnik (1960)
PhCO	H	H	Decyl	ES ED$_{50}$ 75–125	Karmas and Oroshnik (1960)
PhCO	H	H	Undecyl	ES ED$_{50}$ 130	Karmas and Oroshnik (1960)
PhCO	H	H	Dodecyl	ES ED$_{50}$ 400	Karmas and Oroshnik (1960)
CH_2OH	H	H	n-Decyl	ES ED$_{50}$ 125–250	Karmas and Mallory (1959)
CH_2OH	H	H	n-Nonyl	ES ED$_{50}$ 250–500	Karmas and Mallory (1959)
CH_2OH	H	H	n-Undecyl	ES ED$_{50}$ 100–125	Karmas and Mallory (1959)
CH_2OH	H	H	4-Methyldecyl	ES ED$_{50}$ 325	Karmas and Mallory (1959)
CH_2OH	H	H	4,8-Me₂nonen-7-yl	ES ED$_{50}$ 170	Karmas and Mallory (1959)
CH_2NEt_2	H	H	Nonyl	ES ED$_{50}$ 125–200	Karmas (1960a)
CH_2NEt_2	H	H	Decyl	ES ED$_{50}$ 75	Karmas (1960a)
CH_2NEt_2	H	H	Undecyl	ES ED$_{50}$ 104	Karmas (1960a)
CH_2NEt_2	H	H	Dodecyl	ES ED$_{50}$ 600–750	Karmas (1960a)
Me	Me	NO₂	Me	ES, active	Batulin (1968)
H	H	H	Ph	ES, active	Batulin (1968)
H	Ph	H	Me	ES, active	Batulin (1968)
H	H	Et	H	ES, active	Batulin (1968)
H	H	Me	H	Met, act. 200; MES, act. 100	Batulin et al. (1968)

(continued)

357

TABLE V—*Continued*

R	R_1	R_2	R_3	Activity	Reference
H	H	Et	H	Met, act. < 100; MES, act. 60	Batulin et al. (1968)
H	H	i-Pr	H	Met, act. < 100; MES, act. 100	Batulin et al. (1968)
H	H	C_5H_7	H	Met, act. 100; MES, act. 60	Batulin et al. (1968)
H	H	C_4H_9	H	Met, act. 100; MES, act. 50	Batulin et al. (1968)
H	NH_2	H	Ph	ES, active	Gladenko and Fortushnyi; and Osdene (1964)
H	NH_2	H	RSO_2	ES and Met, active	Santilli and Osdene (1970)
H	Ph	H	RSO_2	ES and Met, active	Santilli and Osdene (1970)
R	H	X	C(OH)R'R"	Active	Easton (1961)
H	H	Me	H	MES ED_{50} 125 (po)	Karmas (1960b)
H	H	Et	H	MES ED_{50} 96 (po)	Karmas (1960b)
H	H	Pr	H	MES ED_{50} 70 (po)	Karmas (1960b)
H	H	Bu	H	MES ED_{50} 75–100 (po)	Karmas (1960b)
H	H	Amyl	H	MES ED_{50} 50 (po)	Karmas (1960b)
H	H	Amyl	Me	MES ED_{50} 75–125 (po)	Karmas (1960b)
H	H	Hexyl	H	MES ED_{50} 75 (po)	Karmas (1960b)
H	H	Heptyl	H	MES ED_{50} 50 (po)	Karmas (1960b)
H	H	Octyl	H	MES ED_{50} 50–75 (po)	Karmas (1960b)
H	H	Octyl	Me	MES ED_{50} 50–75 (po)	Karmas (1960b)
H	H	Nonyl	H	MES ED_{50} 50–75 (po)	Karmas (1960b)
H	H	Decyl	H	MES ED_{50} 75 (po)	Karmas (1960b)
H	H	Decyl	Me	MES ED_{50} 75–125 (po)	Karmas (1960b)
H	H	Ph	H	MES ED_{50} 500 (po)	Karmas (1960b)
H	H	Ph	Me	MES ED_{50} 150 (po)	Karmas (1960b)
H	H	$PhCH_2$	H	MES ED_{50} 75–100 (po)	Karmas (1960b)
H	H	H	H	MES ED_{50} 89; Met ED_{50} 98	Owen et al. (1958)
H	H	H	Me	MES ED_{50} 67; Met ED_{50} 132	Owen et al. (1958)
H	H	H	Pr	MES ED_{50} 33; Met ED_{50} 77	Owen et al. (1958)
H	H	H	Bu	MES ED_{50} 15; Met ED_{50} 38	Owen et al. (1958)
H	H	H	Amyl	MES ED_{50} 37; Met ED_{50} 72	Owen et al. (1958)
H	H	H	Nonyl	MES ED_{50} 48; Met ED_{50} 142	Owen et al. (1958)
H	R	H	R'	MES and Met, active	Vikhlyaev et al. (1962)
H	H	H	H	Met ED_{50} 200	Polevoi et al. (1968)

				Met ED$_{50}$	Reference
C$_7$H$_{11}$	Me	Me	Me	Met ED$_{50}$ 100	Polevoi et al. (1968)
C$_7$H$_{15}$	Me	NHCOMe	Me	Met ED$_{50}$ 159	Polevoi et al. (1968)
PhCH$_2$	Me	NH$_2$	Me	Met ED$_{50}$ 251	Polevoi et al. (1968)
Ph	NH$_2$	H	NH$_2$	Met ED$_{50}$ 400	Polevoi et al. (1968)
PhCH$_2$CH$_2$	NH$_2$	H	NH$_2$	Met ED$_{50}$ 310	Polevoi et al. (1968)
Ph	NH$_2$	H	4-NH$_2$C$_6$H$_4$	Met ED$_{50}$ 100	Polevoi et al. (1968)
H	H	Me	Ph	Met ED$_{50}$ 100	Polevoi et al. (1968)
H	Me	H	Ph	Met ED$_{50}$ 126	Polevoi et al. (1968)
Ph	H	CO$_2$H	H	Met ED$_{50}$ 251	Polevoi et al. (1968)
H	NH$_2$	H	Ph	Met ED$_{50}$ 126	Polevoi et al. (1968)
C$_7$H$_{15}$	NH$_2$	H	4-NH$_2$C$_6$H$_4$	Met ED$_{50}$ 80	Polevoi et al. (1968)
C$_9$H$_{19}$	NH$_2$	H	4-NH$_2$C$_6$H$_4$	Met ED$_{50}$ 80	Polevoi et al. (1968)
PhCH$_2$	NH$_2$	H	4-NH$_2$C$_6$H$_4$	Met ED$_{50}$ 100	Polevoi et al. (1968)
3,4-(MeO)$_2$C$_6$H$_3$CH$_2$	NH$_2$	H	4-NH$_2$C$_6$H$_4$	Met ED$_{50}$ 159	Polevoi et al. (1968)
PhCH$_2$CH$_2$	NH$_2$	H	4-NH$_2$C$_6$H$_4$	Met ED$_{50}$ 200	Polevoi et al. (1968)
2-MeC$_6$H$_4$	NH$_2$	H	4-NH$_2$C$_6$H$_4$	Met ED$_{50}$ 126	Polevoi et al. (1968)
4-NH$_2$C$_6$H$_4$	NH$_2$	H	4-NH$_2$C$_6$H$_4$	Met ED$_{50}$ 400	Polevoi et al. (1968)
4-NO$_2$C$_6$H$_4$	NH$_2$	H	4-NH$_2$C$_6$H$_4$	Met ED$_{50}$ 1000	Polevoi et al. (1968)
2,4-(NO$_2$)$_2$C$_6$H$_3$	NH$_2$	H	4-NH$_2$C$_6$H$_4$	Met ED$_{50}$ 1000	Polevoi et al. (1968)
2-Nap	NH$_2$	H	4-NH$_2$C$_6$H$_4$	Met ED$_{50}$ 251	Polevoi et al. (1968)

B. Pyrazolines

Type I

Type II

Type I:

R	R$_1$	R$_2$	Activity	Reference
Ph	Me	H	ES ED$_{50}$ 89; Met ED$_{50}$ 116	Fiordalisi (1963, 1965); Oroshnik (1959)
Ph	Et	Me	ES, active at 25	Gittos et al. (1967)
Bu	Bu	Me	ES ED$_{50}$ 1000; Met ED$_{50}$ 750	Fiordalisi (1963, 1965)
Me	Me	H	ES ED$_{50}$ > 800; Met ED$_{50}$ > 800	Fiordalisi (1965)

(continued)

TABLE V—*Continued*

Type II:

Ar	Ar$_1$	Ar$_2$	Activity	Reference
Ph	3-MeCONHC$_6$H$_4$	Ph	Met, 30% protn. at 100	Singh et al. (1974b)
2-NO$_2$C$_6$H$_4$	3-MeCONHC$_6$H$_4$	Ph	Met, 40% protn. at 100	Singh et al. (1974b)
4-NO$_2$C$_6$H$_4$	3-MeCONHC$_6$H$_4$	Ph	Met, 30% protn. at 100	Singh et al. (1974b)
2,4-(NO$_2$)$_2$C$_6$H$_3$	3-MeCONHC$_6$H$_4$	Ph	Met, 40% protn. at 100	Singh et al. (1974b)
Ph	3-MeCONHC$_6$H$_4$	4-ClC$_6$H$_4$	Met, 60% protn. at 100	Singh et al. (1974b)
2-NO$_2$C$_6$H$_4$	3-MeCONHC$_6$H$_4$	4-ClC$_6$H$_4$	Met, 60% protn. at 100	Singh et al. (1974b)
4-NO$_2$C$_6$H$_4$	3-MeCONHC$_6$H$_4$	4-ClC$_6$H$_4$	Met, 40% protn. at 100	Singh et al. (1974b)
2,4-(NO$_2$)$_2$C$_6$H$_3$	3-MeCONHC$_6$H$_4$	4-ClC$_6$H$_4$	Met, 70% protn. at 100	Singh et al. (1974b)
Ph	3-MeCONHC$_6$H$_4$	4-MeOC$_6$H$_4$	Met, 40% protn. at 100	Singh et al. (1974b)
2-NO$_2$C$_6$H$_4$	3-MeCONHC$_6$H$_4$	4-MeOC$_6$H$_4$	Met, 50% protn. at 100	Singh et al. (1974b)
4-NO$_2$C$_6$H$_4$	3-MeCONHC$_6$H$_4$	4-MeOC$_6$H$_4$	Met, 60% protn. at 100	Singh et al. (1974b)
2,4-(NO$_2$)$_2$C$_6$H$_3$	3-MeCONHC$_6$H$_4$	4-MeOC$_6$H$_4$	Met, 80% protn. at 100	Singh et al. (1974b)
Ph	2,3,4-(OH)$_3$C$_6$H$_2$	Ph	Met, 50% protn. at 100	Parmar et al. (1974c)
Ph	2,3,4-(OH)$_3$C$_6$H$_2$	4-ClC$_6$H$_4$	Met, 90% protn. at 100	Parmar et al. (1974c)
Ph	2,3,4-(OH)$_3$C$_6$H$_2$	4-MeOC$_6$H$_4$	Met, 80% protn. at 100	Parmar et al. (1974c)
Ph	2,3,4-(OH)$_3$C$_6$H$_2$	3,4-(MeO)$_2$C$_6$H$_3$	Met, 60% protn. at 100	Parmar et al. (1974b)
Ph	2,3,4-(OH)$_3$C$_6$H$_2$	4-PhCH$_2$OC$_6$H$_4$	Met, 80% protn. at 100	Parmar et al. (1974c)
Ph	2,3,4-(OH)$_3$C$_6$H$_2$	PhCH=CH	Met, 80% protn. at 100	Parmar et al. (1974c)
Ph	4-ClC$_6$H$_4$CH$_2$	Ph	Met, 70% protn. at 100	Parmar et al. (1974c)
Ph	4-ClC$_6$H$_4$CH$_2$	4-ClC$_6$H$_4$	Met, 60% protn. at 100	Parmar et al. (1974c)
Ph	4-ClC$_6$H$_4$CH$_2$	3,4-Cl$_2$C$_6$H$_3$	Met, 50% protn. at 100	Parmar et al. (1974c)
Ph	4-ClC$_6$H$_4$CH$_2$	4-MeOC$_6$H$_4$	Met, 60% protn. at 100	Parmar et al. (1974c)
Ph	4-ClC$_6$H$_4$CH$_2$	4-HO-3-MeOC$_6$H$_3$	Met, 40% protn. at 100	Parmar et al. (1974c)
Ph	4-ClC$_6$H$_4$CH$_2$	4-HOC$_6$H$_4$	Met, 30% protn. at 100	Parmar et al. (1974c)
Ph	4-ClC$_6$H$_4$CH$_2$	3-MeC$_6$H$_4$	Met, 40% protn. at 100	Parmar et al. (1974c)
Ph	4-ClC$_6$H$_4$CH$_2$	PhCH=CH	Met, 40% protn. at 100	Parmar et al. (1974c)
Ph	4-ClC$_6$H$_4$CH$_2$	(furan-2-yl structure, —CH=CH attached to furan ring)	Met, 50% protn. at 100	Parmar et al. (1974c)

C. Miscellaneous Derivatives

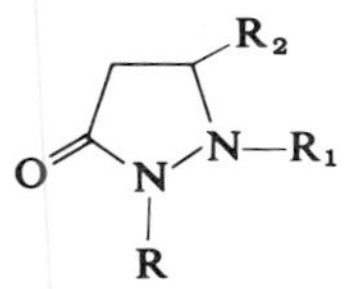

R	R_1	R_2	Activity	Reference
H	Me	Ph	MES ED$_{50}$ 30 (ip and po); Met ED$_{50}$ 125 (ip and po)	Bass et al. (1959)
Ph	H	Me	Met, active 150–200	Motovilov and Kozhevnikov (1968)
H	H	Ph	Met, active 150–200	Motovilov and Kozhevnikov (1968)
H	Me	Ph	Met active 150–200	Motovilov and Kozhevnikov (1968)

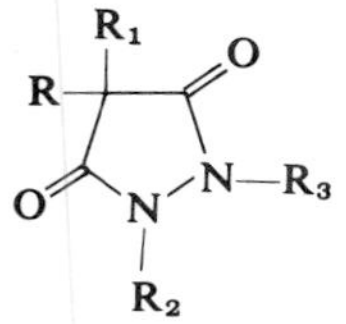

R	R_1	R_2	R_3	Activity	Reference
—(CH$_2$)$_3$—		H	Me	Met, 20% protn. at 500; MES, 0% protn. at 500	Kornet et al. (1974)
—(CH$_2$)$_3$—		H	Me	Met, 20% protn. at 500; MES, 0% protn. at 500	Kornet et al. (1974)
Et	Et	H	Me	Met, 40% protn. at 500; MES, 0% protn. at 500	Kornet et al. (1974)
Ph	H	H	Me	Met, 40% protn. at 500; MES, 0% protn. at 500	Kornet et al. (1974)
Ph	Me	H	Me	Met, 60% protn. at 500; MES, 0% protn. at 500	Kornet et al. (1974)
Ph	Et	H	Me	Met, 20% protn. at 500; MES, 0% protn. at 500	Kornet et al. (1974)
n-Bu	n-Bu	H	Me	Met, 20% protn. at 500; MES, 0% protn. at 500	Kornet et al. (1974)
Ph	Et	H	Et	Met, 40% protn. at 500; MES, 0% protn. at 500	Kornet et al. (1974)
Ph	Me	MeCO	Me	Met, 0% protn. at 500; MES, 20% protn. at 500	Kornet et al. (1974)

(continued)

361

TABLE V—Continued

Compound	Activity	Reference
	ES, active 300 (po)	Schenone et al. (1975)
	ES, active 300 (po)	Bondavalli et al. (1975)
	ES and Met, active	DeRidder (1970)
	ES and Met, active	DeRidder (1970)
	$R = C_6H_5$, $R_1 = C_6H_5$: MES $ED_{50} > 100$ $R = H$; $R_1 = NMe_2$: MES $ED_{50} > 100$	Boltze et al. (1963) Boltze et al. (1963)

TABLE VI IMIDAZOLE DERIVATIVES

A. Imidazoles

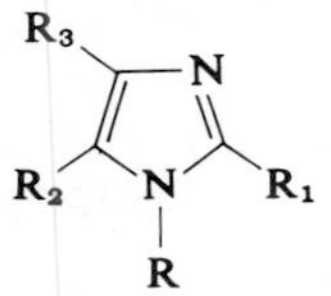

R	R_1	R_2	R_3	Activity	Reference
H	H	Me	Me	Met ED_{50} > 50 (iv)	Lindberg et al. (1970)
H	H	Et	Me	Met ED_{50} > 55 (iv)	Lindberg et al. (1970)
H	H	n-Pr	Me	Met ED_{50} > 28 (iv)	Lindberg et al. (1970)
H	H	i-Pr	Me	Met ED_{50} > 28 (iv)	Lindberg et al. (1970)
CH(Ph)Me	Me	CO_2Me	H	MES ED_{50} 100; Met ED_{50} 68	Godefroi and Platje (1972)
CH(Ph)Me	Me	CO_2Et	H	MES ED_{50} 147; Met ED_{50} 68	Godefroi and Platje (1972)
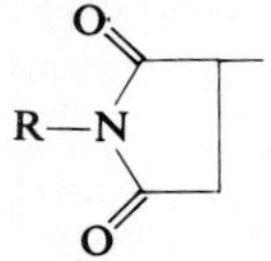 (succinimide)	R_1	R_2	H	Active	Hasegawa and Kotani (1974)
2-ArCO-4-$NO_2C_6H_3$	R_1	H	H	Active	Nakanishi et al. (1975)
2-ArCO-x-$R_4C_6H_3$	CH_2NMe_2	R_2	R_3	Active	Nakanishi et al. (1974h)

(continued)

364

TABLE VI—*Continued*

B. Benzimidazoles

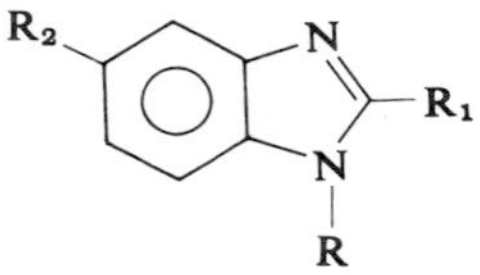

R	R₁	R₂	Activity	Reference
(CH₂)₂COAr	R₁		Active	Fauran et al. (1974a)
CH₂NHC₆H₄CONHNH₂-4	H	H	Met, 20% protn. at 100	Parmar et al. (1972c)
CH₂NHC₆H₄CONHNH₂-4	Me	H	Met, 10% protn. at 100	Parmar et al. (1972c)
CH₂NHC₆H₄CONHNH₂-4	Et	H	Met, 50% protn. at 100	Parmar et al. (1972c)
CH₂NHC₆H₄CONHNH₂-4	n-Pr	H	Met, 30% protn. at 100	Parmar et al. (1972c)
CH₂NHC₆H₄CONHNH₂-4	i-Pr	H	Met, 20% protn. at 100	Parmar et al. (1972c)
H	Et	NHCSNH₃	MES ED₅₀ 54; Met ED₅₀ 74	Arora et al. (1972); Gupta et al. (1972, 1973)
H	Et	NHCSNHC₆H₄Me-2	MES ED₅₀ 22; Met ED₅₀ 21	Arora et al. (1972); Gupta et al. (1972, 1973)
H	Et	NHCSNHC₆H₄Me-4	MES ED₅₀ 20; Met ED₅₀ 17	Arora et al. (1972); Gupta et al. (1972, 1973)
H	OH	NHCSNH₂	MES ED₅₀ 32; Met ED₅₀ 39	Arora et al. (1972); Gupta et al. (1972, 1973)
H	SH	NHCSNH₂	MES ED₅₀ 46; Met ED₅₀ 40	Arora et al. (1972); Gupta et al. (1972, 1973)

C. Miscellaneous derivatives

Compound	Activity	Reference
Ph₂C pyrazoline (Ph, Ph substituted 4,5-dihydroimidazole)	Active	Goodman (1956)
R-substituted imidazolone	R = OCH(Me)CH₂CH=CH₂: Met ED₅₀ 47 R = OC(=CH₂)Et: Active	Sumitomo Chemical Co., Ltd. (1963a) Sumitomo Chemical Co., Ltd. (1963b)
Ph, Ph substituted imidazolidinone (NH, C=O)	Active	Goodman (1956)

R = OCH(Me)CH₂CH=CH₂ — rendered as $R = OCH(Me)CH_2CH{=}CH_2$: Met ED$_{50}$ 47
$R = OC({=}CH_2)Et$: Active

R	R₁	Activity	Reference
H	2-CO₂Et	Met, 50% protn. at 100	Verma et al. (1974)
H	3-CO₂Et	Met, 40% protn. at 100	Verma et al. (1974)
H	4-CO₂Et	Met, 40% protn. at 100	Verma et al. (1974)
MeO	2-CO₂Et	Met, 20% protn. at 100	Verma et al. (1974)

(continued)

TABLE VI—*Continued*

R	R₁	Activity	Reference
MeO	3-CO_2Et	Met, 40% protn. at 100	Verma *et al.* (1974)
MeO	4-CO_2Et	Met, 70% protn. at 100	Verma *et al.* (1974)
Cl	2-CO_2Et	Met, 20% protn. at 100	Verma *et al.* (1974)
Cl	3-CO_2Et	Met, 40% protn. at 100	Verma *et al.* (1974)
Cl	4-CO_2Et	Met, 60% protn. at 100	Verma *et al.* (1974)
H	2-CONHNH₂	Met, 40% protn. at 100	Verma *et al.* (1974)
H	3-CONHNH₂	Met, 30% protn. at 100	Verma *et al.* (1974)
H	4-CONHNH₂	Met, 20% protn. at 100	Verma *et al.* (1974)
MeO	2-CONHNH₂	Met, 40% protn. at 100	Verma *et al.* (1974)
MeO	3-CONHNH₂	Met, 50% protn. at 100	Verma *et al.* (1974)
MeO	4-CONHNH₂	Met, 40% protn. at 100	Verma *et al.* (1974)
Cl	2-CONHNH₂	Met, 10% protn. at 100	Verma *et al.* (1974)
Cl	3-CONHNH₂	Met, 20% protn. at 100	Verma *et al.* (1974)
Cl	4-CONHNH₂	Met, 30% protn. at 100	Verma *et al.* (1974)

Compound	Activity	Reference
	Active	Vander Burg (1975)
	$^-$O—C(OH)(CF₃)₂: MES, v. act.; Met, active $^-$O—C(CF₂Cl)₂: MES, mod. act.; Met, inact.	Gilbert and Rumanowski (1971)
	$^-$O—C(OH)(CF₃)₂: MES, mod. act.; Met, mod. act. $^-$O—C(OH)(CF₂Cl)₂: MES, active; Met, active	Gilbert and Rumanowski (1971)

RCONH structure with N–Ar, (CH$_2$)$_n$	ES, active at 400	Bell and Gochman (1971)
spiro piperidine structure	Active	Maruyama et al. (1975)
benzimidazolone structure	Active	Clark and Pessolano (1960)
piperazine purine structure	ES and Met, active	Regnier et al. (1972)
thiazole–SO$_2$Me structure	MES, 60% protn. 0.3 LD$_{50}$; Met 8% protn. 0.3 LD$_{50}$	Almirante et al. (1966)
benzothiazole–SO$_2$Me structure	MES, 60% protn. 0.3 LD$_{50}$; Met, 70% protn. 0.3 LD$_{50}$	Almirante et al. (1966)

367

TABLE VI—*Continued*

R	R_1	R_2	Active	Reference
H	7-Me	CN	MES, 100% protn. 0.3 LD_{50}; Met, 50% protn. 0.3 LD_{50}	Almirante and Murmann (1967)
Me	H	CN	MES, 20% protn. 0.3 LD_{50}; Met, 11% protn. 0.3 LD_{50}	Almirante et al. (1969)
4-ClC$_6$H$_4$	H	CH$_2$CN	MES, 25% protn. 0.3 LD_{50}; Met, 50% protn. 0.3 LD_{50}	Almirante et al. (1969)
Me	H	CH$_2$CONH$_2$	MES, 25% protn. 0.3 LD_{50}; Met, 0% protn. 0.3 LD_{50}	Almirante et al. (1969)
4-ClC$_6$H$_4$	H	CH$_2$CONH$_2$	MES, 56% protn. 0.3 LD_{50}; Met, 90% protn. 0.3 LD_{50}	Almirante et al. (1969)
H	H	CO$_2$H	MES, 10% protn. 0.3 LD_{50}; Met, 10% protn. 0.3 LD_{50}	Almirante et al. (1969)
H	H	CH$_2$CO$_2$H	MES, 22% protn. 0.3 LD_{50}; Met, 0% protn. 0.3 LD_{50}	Almirante et al. (1969)
4-ClC$_6$H$_4$	H	CH$_2$CO$_2$H	MES, 0% protn. 0.3 LD_{50}; Met, 60% protn. 0.3 LD_{50}	Almirante et al. (1969)
Ph	H	H	MES, 10% protn. 0.3 LD_{50}; Met, 0% protn. 0.3 LD_{50}	Almirante et al. (1969)
4-MeC$_6$H$_4$	H	H	MES, 40% protn. 0.3 LD_{50}; Met, 20% protn. 0.3 LD_{50}	Almirante et al. (1969)
4-NO$_2$C$_6$H$_4$	H	H	MES, 30% protn. 0.3 LD_{50}; Met, 10% protn. 0.3 LD_{50}	Almirante et al. (1969)

$4\text{-MeOC}_6\text{H}_4$	H		MES, 100% protn. 0.3 LD_{50}; Met, 100% protn. 0.3 LD_{50}	Almirante et al. (1969)
$4\text{-MeSC}_6\text{H}_4$	H		MES, 10% protn. 0.3 LD_{50}; Met, 30% protn. 0.3 LD_{50}	Almirante et al. (1969)
$4\text{-MeSOC}_6\text{H}_4$	H		Met, 60% protn. 0.3 LD_{50}	Almirante et al. (1969)
$4\text{-MeSO}_2\text{C}_6\text{H}_4$	H		MES, 48% protn. 0.3 LD_{50}; Met, 36% protn. 0.3 LD_{50}	Almirante et al. (1969)
$4\text{-MeSO}_2\text{C}_6\text{H}_4$	5-Me		MES, 100% protn. 0.3 LD_{50}; Met, 60% protn. 0.3 LD_{50}	Almirante et al. (1969)
$4\text{-MeSO}_2\text{C}_6\text{H}_4$	7-Me		MES, 96% protn. 0.3 LD_{50}; Met, 83% protn. 0.3 LD_{50}	Almirante et al. (1969)
$4\text{-MeSO}_2\text{C}_6\text{H}_4$	H	Br	MES, 10% protn. 0.3 LD_{50}; Met, 20% protn. 0.3 LD_{50}	Almirante et al. (1969)
$4\text{-MeSO}_2\text{C}_6\text{H}_4$	H	NH_2	MES, 0% protn. 0.3 LD_{50}; Met, 30% protn. 0.3 LD_{50}	Almirante et al. (1969)
$4\text{-MeSO}_2\text{C}_6\text{H}_4$	H	NMe_2	MES, 40% protn. 0.3 LD_{50}; Met, 0% protn. 0.3 LD_{50}	Almirante et al. (1969)
$4\text{-MeSO}_2\text{C}_6\text{H}_4$	H	CH_3NMe_2	MES, 8% protn. 0.3 LD_{50}; Met, 16% protn. 0.3 LD_{50}	Almirante et al. (1969)
$4\text{-MeSO}_2\text{C}_6\text{H}_4$	H	CH_2N–(morpholino)	MES, 16% protn. 0.3 LD_{50}; Met, 32% protn. 0.3 LD_{50}	Almirante et al. (1969)
$4\text{-MeSO}_2\text{C}_6\text{H}_4$	H	CH_2N–(piperazinyl)$N(CH_2)_2OH$	MES, 0% protn. 0.3 LD_{50}; Met, 40% protn. 0.3 LD_{50}	Almirante et al. (1969)
$2\text{-MeSO}_2\text{C}_6\text{H}_4$	H	NO	MES, 0% protn. 0.3 LD_{50}; Met, 10% protn. 0.3 LD_{50}	Almirante et al. (1969)
$2\text{-MeSO}_2\text{C}_6\text{H}_4$	H	NH_2	MES, 0% protn. 0.3 LD_{50}; Met, 20% protn. 0.3 LD_{50}	Almirante et al. (1969)
$2\text{-MeSO}_2\text{C}_6\text{H}_4$	H	CH_2N–(morpholino)	MES, 100% protn. 0.3 LD_{50}; Met, 90% protn. 0.3 LD_{50}	Almirante et al. (1965)

(continued)

369

TABLE VI—*Continued*

R	R_1	R_2	Activity	Reference
2-MeSO$_2$C$_6$H$_4$	H	CH$_2$N(piperazine)N(CH$_2$)$_2$OH	MES, 0% protn. 0.3 LD$_{50}$; Met, 70% protn. 0.3 LD$_{50}$	Almirante *et al.* (1965)
4-MeSC$_6$H$_4$	H	CH$_2$N(morpholine)	MES, 64% protn. 0.3 LD$_{50}$; Met, 10% protn. 0.3 LD$_{50}$	Almirante *et al.* (1965)
4-MeSC$_6$H$_4$	H	CH$_2$N(piperazine)N(CH$_2$)$_2$OH	MES, 0% protn. 0.3 LD$_{50}$; Met, 20% protn. 0.3 LD$_{50}$	Almirante *et al.* (1965)
Ph	H	NH$_2$	MES, 0% protn. 0.3 LD$_{50}$; Met, 20% protn. 0.3 LD$_{50}$	Almirante *et al.* (1965)
4-MeC$_6$H$_4$	H	CH$_2$N(morpholine)	MES, 40% protn. 0.3 LD$_{50}$; Met, 70% protn. 0.3 LD$_{50}$	Almirante *et al.* (1965)
4-MeOC$_6$H$_4$	H	CH$_2$N(morpholine)	Met, 20% protn. 0.3 LD$_{50}$	Almirante *et al.* (1965)
4-NO$_2$C$_6$H$_4$	H	CH$_2$N(morpholine)	MES, 40% protn. 0.3 LD$_{50}$; Met, 90% protn. 0.3 LD$_{50}$	Almirante *et al.* (1965)

R	R₁	R₂	Activity	Reference
2-MeSO$_2$C$_6$H$_4$	H	H	MES, 24% protn. 0.3 LD$_{50}$; Met, 20% protn. 0.3 LD$_{50}$	Almirante *et al.* (1966)
4-MeSC$_6$H$_4$	H	H	MES, 0% protn. 0.3 LD$_{50}$; Met, 50% protn. 0.3 LD$_{50}$	Almirante *et al.* (1966)
4-MeSOC$_6$H$_4$	H	H	MES, 90% protn. 0.3 LD$_{50}$; Met, 80% protn. 0.3 LD$_{50}$	Almirante *et al.* (1966)
4-MeSO$_2$C$_6$H$_4$	H	H	MES, 0% protn. 0.3 LD$_{50}$; Met, 40% protn. 0.3 LD$_{50}$	Almirante *et al.* (1966)
2-MeSO$_2$C$_6$H$_4$	H	CH$_2$N[piperazine]N(CH$_2$)$_2$OH	MES, 10% protn. 0.3 LD$_{50}$; Met, 20% protn. 0.3 LD$_{50}$	Almirante *et al.* (1966)
4-MeSC$_6$H$_4$	H	CH$_2$N[morpholine, O]	MES, 72% protn. 0.3 LD$_{50}$; Met, 79% protn. 0.3 LD$_{50}$	Almirante *et al.* (1966)
4-MeSC$_6$H$_4$	H	CH$_2$N[piperazine]N(CH$_2$)$_2$OH	MES, 14% protn. 0.3 LD$_{50}$; Met, 19% protn. 0.3 LD$_{50}$	Almirante *et al.* (1966)
4-MeSOC$_6$H$_4$	H	CH$_2$N[morpholine, O]	MES, 80% protn. 0.3 LD$_{50}$; Met, 100% protn. 0.3 LD$_{50}$	Almirante *et al.* (1966)
4-MeSOC$_6$H$_4$	H	CH$_2$N[piperazine]N(CH$_2$)$_2$OH	MES, 0% protn. 0.3 LD$_{50}$; Met, 30% protn. 0.3 LD$_{50}$	Almirante *et al.* (1966)

(continued)

TABLE VI—*Continued*

R	R_1	R_2	Activity	Reference
4-MeSO$_2$C$_6$H$_4$	H	CH$_2$NMe$_2$	MES, 10% protn. 0.3 LD$_{50}$; Met, 10% protn. 0.3 LD$_{50}$	Almirante *et al.* (1966)
4-MeSO$_2$C$_6$H$_4$	H	CH$_2$N⟨morpholino⟩	MES, 60% protn. 0.3 LD$_{50}$; Met, 40% protn. 0.3 LD$_{50}$	Almirante *et al.* (1966)
4-MeSO$_2$C$_6$H$_4$	H	CH$_2$N⟨N(CH$_2$)$_2$OH⟩	MES, 0% protn. 0.3 LD$_{50}$; Met, 40% protn. 0.3 LD$_{50}$	Almirante *et al.* (1966)
4-MeSO$_2$C$_6$H$_4$	6-MeO	H	MES, 10% protn. 0.3 LD$_{50}$; Met, 0% protn. 0.3 LD$_{50}$	Almirante *et al.* (1966)

Compound	Activity	Reference
	R = H: MES, 11% protn. 0.3 LD$_{50}$; Met, 10% protn. 0.3 LD$_{50}$	Almirante *et al.* (1966)
	R = Cl: MES, 0% protn. 0.3 LD$_{50}$; Met, 20% protn. 0.3 LD$_{50}$	Almirante *et al.* (1966)
	R = MeO: MES, 0% protn. 0.3 LD$_{50}$; Met, 10% protn. 0.3 LD$_{50}$	Almirante *et al.* (1966)

TABLE VII ISOXAZOLE DERIVATIVES

R	R_1	Activity	Reference
CH(OH)CH$_2$NR$_2$	ArOH	Active	Kano and Takahashi (1974)
CH(OH)CH$_2$NR$_2$	R$_1$	Active	Hayashi (1973)
CH(OH)CH$_2$NR$_2$	Ph	Active	Hirai and Kawata (1974)
COCHRSMe	Ph	Active	Hirai and Kawata (1974)
COCHRSOMe	Ph	Active	Hirai and Kawata (1974)
4-Pyr	2-ClC$_6$H$_4$	MES ED$_{50}$ 190	Arena et al. (1975)
CH(OH)CH$_2$NR$_2$	R$_1$	Active	Takahashi (1974)

CH(OH)CH$_2$N	C$_6$H$_5$	Active	Takahashi (1975a, b)

Compound	Activity	Reference
(mixture)	ES, inactive at 500; Met, active at 200	Germane et al. (1975)

373

TABLE VIII   OXAZOLE DERIVATIVES

A. Oxazoles

R	R_1	R_2	Activity	Reference
H	Me	$(CH_2)_2Cl$	Met ED_{50} 30	Saeter and Lindberg (1968)
			Same activity as clomethiazole	Lindberg (1966)
H	Me	$(CH_2)_2Br$	Met ED_{50} 12 (iv)	Lindberg et al. (1970)
H	Me	CH_2Cl	Met ED_{50} 220 (po), 80 (ip), 52 (iv)	Lindberg et al. (1967)
Me	Me	$(CH_2)_2Cl$	Met ED_{50} 70 (iv)	Lindberg et al. (1967)
Ph	Me	$(CH_2)_2Cl$	Met ED_{50} 200 (iv)	Lindberg et al. (1967)
H	Me	$(CH_2)_2Cl$	Met ED_{50} 125 (iv)	Lindberg et al. (1967)
H	Me	$(CH_2)_2Cl$	Met ED_{50} 100 (iv)	Lindberg et al. (1967)
H	Me	Me	Met ED_{50} 90 (iv)	Lindberg et al. (1970)
H	Me	Et	Met ED_{50} 100 (iv)	Lindberg et al. (1970)
H	Me	n-Pr	Met ED_{50} 50 (iv)	Lindberg et al. (1970)
H	Me	i-Pr	Met ED_{50} 50 (iv)	Lindberg et al. (1970)
H	Me	i-Bu	Met ED_{50} 100 (iv)	Lindberg et al. (1970)
H	Me	CH_2OPr-i	Met ED_{50} 200 (iv)	Lindberg (1971a)
H	Ph	H	Met ED_{50} 180 (iv)	Lindberg et al. (1971)
H	Ph	Me	Met ED_{50} 110 (iv)	Lindberg et al. (1971)
H	Ph	Et	Met ED_{50} 114 (ip)	Lindberg et al. (1971)
NEt_2	Ph	Me	Met ED_{50} 53 (iv)	Lindberg et al. (1971)
NEt_2	Ph	Me	Met ED_{50} 36 (iv)	Lindberg et al. (1971)

B. 2-Oxazolidinones

R	R₁	R₂	R₃	R₄	Activity	Reference
=CH	R	R₂	R₃	R₄	Active	Cameron (1958)
H	H	R₂	Ar	CONHR	Active	Fauran *et al.* (1971a)
H	H	H	Ph	CONR₃	Active	Fauran *et al.* (1974d)
H	R₁	R₂	R₃	H	Active	Applegath and France (1958)
H	H	H	CH₂OC₆H₃(OMe)₂-2,6	H	ES, active	Lunsford (1965)
H	H	H	CH₂OCOR	Ph	Active	Huguet *et al.* (1972)

C. Miscellaneous derivatives

Compound	Activity	Reference
	Active	Chemische Werke Albert (1965)
	Active	Englisch *et al.* (1971)

(continued)

TABLE VIII—*Continued*

Compound	Activity	Reference
Ph, cyclohexyl N-oxazolidine structure	Met, 80% protn. at 30	Irwin *et al.* (1972)
Ph N—CH₂CH₂Ph oxazolidine structure	Met, 20% protn. at 10	Irwin *et al.* (1972)
NR, CCl₃ oxazolidinone structure	Active	Parke Davis and Co. (1959)
H₂NCONH benzoxazolone (N—H) structure	ES and Met, active	Orcutt *et al.* (1964)
Benzoxazolone (N—H) structure	Active	Clark and Pessolano (1967)
CH₂CH₂NR₂ benzoxazolone structure	Weak activity	Kaku *et al.* (1964)

Compound	R	Activity	Reference
$CH_2NHC_6H_4R$ (benzoxazole-2-thione)	2-CO_2Me	Met, 40% protn. at 100	Misra (1974)
	3-CO_2Et	Met, 20% protn. at 100	Misra (1974)
	4-CO_2Et	Met, 30% protn. at 100	Misra (1974)
	2-$CONHNH_2$	Met, 20% protn. at 100	Misra (1974)
	4-$CONHNH_2$	Met, 30% protn. at 100	Misra (1974)
(Cl-benzoxazol-2-amine)		Met, 90% protn. at 200	Sam (1961)
(benzoxazole NHR structure)		Active	Philippe (1973)
		Active	Sandoz, Ltd. (1965); Griot (1966)
(dimethoxy NR_2 structure)		Active	Fauran et al. (1974e, 1975)
		Active	Sulkowski (1967)

TABLE IX THIAZOLE DERIVATIVES

A. Thiazoles

R	R_1	R_2	Activity	Reference
H	Me	$(CH_2)_2Cl$	Met ED_{50} 700 (po), 118 (ip), 52 (iv)	Lindberg et al. (1967)
			Met, 100% protn. at 44; MES, 100% protn. at 88	Lechat et al. (1965)
			MES ED_{50} 79 (ip); Met, ED_{50} 68 (ip)	Guczoghy et al. (1972)
			MES and Met, active in rabbit	Charonnat et al. (1957)
			Met ED_{50} 13 (iv)	Lindberg et al. (1970)
H	$(CH_2)_2X$	Me	Active	Charonnat et al. (1958)
HO	Me	$(CH_2)_2Cl$	Active	Herbertz (1974)
NH_2	Me	$(CH_2)_2OH$	Active	Herbertz (1974)
NH_2	Me	$(CH_2)_2Cl$	Active	Herbertz (1974)
H	Me	$CH_2CHClCH_3$	Met ED_{50} 50 (iv)	Lindberg et al. (1967)
H	Me	CH_2Cl	Met ED_{50} 80 (iv)	Lindberg et al. (1967)
H	H	CH_2Cl	Met ED_{50} 170 (iv)	Lindberg et al. (1967)
H	H	$(CH_2)_2Cl$	Met, inact. 35; MES, inact. 71	Lechat et al. (1965)
H	Me	$(CH_2)_2Br$	Met ED_{50} > 200 (iv)	Lindberg et al. (1967)
H	Me	$(CH_2)_2NH_2$	Met ED_{50} > 150 (iv)	Lindberg et al. (1967)
H	Me	$(CH_2)_2NEt_2$	Met ED_{50} 70 (iv)	Lindberg et al. (1967)
H	Me	$(CH_2)_2NH(CH_2)_3NEt_2$	Met ED_{50} > 200 (iv)	Lindberg et al. (1967)
H	Me	$(CH_2)_2N$	Met ED_{50} 30 (iv)	Lindberg et al. (1967)
H	Me	$(CH_2)_2Cl$	Met ED_{50} > 100 (iv)	Lindberg et al. (1967)
			Met ED_{50} 100 (iv)	Lindberg et al. (1967)
			MES, 70% protn. at 76; Met, 100% protn. at 38	Lechat et al. (1965)

H	Me	(CH$_2$)$_4$Cl	MES, 90% protn. at 60; Met, 40% protn. at 30	Lechat et al. (1965)
H	Me	Me	Met ED_{50} 80 (iv)	Lindberg et al. (1970)
H	Me	Et	Met ED_{50} 20 (iv)	Lindberg et al. (1970)
H	Me	n-Pr	Met ED_{50} 45 (iv)	Lindberg et al. (1970)
H	Me	i-Pr	Met ED_{50} 50 (iv)	Lindberg et al. (1970)
H	Me	i-Bu	Met ED_{50} > 60 (iv)	Lindberg et al. (1970)
H	Et	H	Met ED_{50} 76 (iv)	Lindberg et al. (1970)
H	i-Bu	H	Met ED_{50} 60 (iv)	Lindberg et al. (1970)
H	Me	(CH$_2$)$_2$OH	Met ED_{50} > 200 (iv)	Lindberg (1971a)
H	Me	CHOHCH$_3$	Met ED_{50} 95 (iv)	Lindberg (1971a)
H	Me	CH$_2$CHOHCH$_3$	Met ED_{50} > 125 (iv)	Lindberg (1971a)
H	Me	CH$_2$OMe	Met ED_{50} > 120 (iv)	Lindberg (1971a)
H	Me	CH$_2$OEt	Met ED_{50} > 125 (iv)	Lindberg (1971a)
H	Me	CH$_2$OPr-i	Met ED_{50} > 130 (iv)	Lindberg (1971a)
H	Me	COMe	Met ED_{50} 100 (iv)	Lindberg (1971a)
H	Me	CH=CH$_2$	Met ED_{50} > 85 (iv)	Lindberg (1971a)
Me	Me	(CH$_2$)$_2$Cl	Met ED_{50} > 65 (iv)	Lindberg et al. (1971)
Cl	Me	(CH$_2$)$_2$Cl	Met ED_{50} 50 (iv)	Lindberg et al. (1971)
Ph	Me	(CH$_2$)$_2$Cl	Met ED_{50} > 140 (iv)	Lindberg et al. (1971)
PhCH$_2$NH	Me	(CH$_2$)$_2$Cl	Met ED_{50} > 50 (iv)	Lindberg et al. (1971)
H	Ph	(CH$_2$)$_2$Cl	Met ED_{50} > 140 (iv)	Lindberg et al. (1971)
4-ClC$_6$H$_4$	H	(CH$_2$)$_2$Cl	Met ED_{50} > 175 (iv)	Lindberg et al. (1971)
NH$_2$	Me	Pr	Met ED_{50} > 62 (iv)	Lindberg et al. (1971)
H	Ph	H	Met ED_{50} 150 (ip)	Lindberg et al. (1971)
H	Ph	Me	Met ED_{50} > 130 (iv)	Lindberg et al. (1971)
H	Ph	Et	Met ED_{50} > 33 (iv)	Lindberg et al. (1971)
NH$_2$	Ph	H	Met ED_{50} 75 (ip)	Lindberg et al. (1971)
NH$_2$	Ph	Me	Met ED_{50} > 75 (iv)	Lindberg et al. (1971)
Cl	Ph	Me	Met ED_{50} > 300 (iv)	Lindberg et al. (1971)
NH$_2$	Ph	Et	Met ED_{50} > 136 (ip)	Lindberg et al. (1971)

(continued)

TABLE IX—*Continued*

B. 4-Thiazolidinones

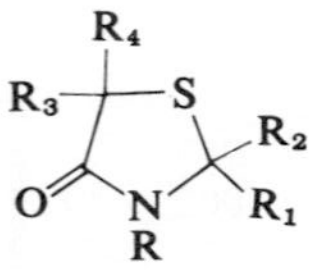

$R_3 = R_4 = H; R = $![furan-CH2] $-CH_2-; R_1, R_2 = N-N=CHAr$

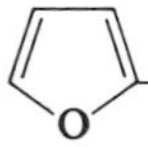

Ar	Activity	Reference
Ph	Met, 10% protn. at 100	Kumar et al. (1970)
2-ClC$_6$H$_4$	Met, 60% protn. at 100	Kumar et al. (1970)
4-ClC$_6$H$_4$	Met, 60% protn. at 100	Kumar et al. (1970)
3-NO$_2$C$_6$H$_4$	Met, 70% protn. at 100	Kumar et al. (1970)
3-HOC$_6$H$_4$	Met, 10% protn. at 100	Kumar et al. (1970)
2-HOC$_6$H$_4$	Met, 20% protn. at 100	Kumar et al. (1970)
2-MeOC$_6$H$_4$	Met, 20% protn. at 100	Kumar et al. (1970)
4-MeOC$_6$H$_4$	Met, 50% protn. at 100	Kumar et al. (1970)
4-HO-3-MeOC$_6$H$_3$	Met, 10% protn. at 100	Kumar et al. (1970)
3,4,5-(MeO)$_3$C$_6$H$_2$	Met, 0% protn. at 100	Kumar et al. (1970)
PhCH=CH	Met, 20% protn. at 100	Kumar et al. (1970)
4-Me$_2$NC$_6$H$_4$	Met, 20% protn. at 100	Kumar et al. (1970)
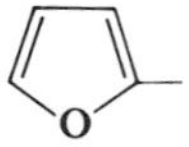 ![furan-Me]	Met, 40% protn. at 100	Kumar et al. (1970)

2-HO-3,5-Cl$_2$C$_6$H$_2$
$R_1 = R_2 = R_3 = H; R_4 = (CH_2)_2OR; R = R$

	Met, 50% protn. at 100	Kumar et al. (1970)
	Active	Surrey and Webb (1967)

$R_3 = R_4 = H; R_1, R_2 = $=NAr; $R = (CH_2)_3N$![morpholine]

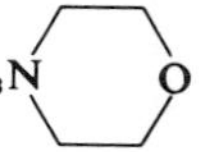

	Met, 30–80% protn. at 100	Chaudhari et al. (1975)

(continued)

TABLE IX—*Continued*

$R_3 = R_4 = H$; $R = 3,4\text{-}(MeO)_2H_6H_3$; $R_1, R_2 = =N-N=CHAr$

Ar	Activity	Reference
Ph	Met, 60% protn. at 100	Singh *et al.* (1974a)
2-ClC$_6$H$_4$	Met, 40% protn. at 100	Singh *et al.* (1974a)
4-ClC$_6$H$_4$	Met, 60% protn. at 100	Singh *et al.* (1974a)
3,4-Cl$_2$C$_6$H$_3$	Met, 30% protn. at 100	Singh *et al.* (1974a)
2-MeC$_6$H$_4$	Met, 60% protn. at 100	Singh *et al.* (1974a)
4-MeOC$_6$H$_4$	Met, 50% protn. at 100	Singh *et al.* (1974a)
3, 4-(Meo)$_2$C$_6$H$_3$	Met, 60% protn. at 100	Singh *et al.* (1974a)
3-MeO-4-EtOC$_6$H$_3$	Met, 20% protn. at 100	Singh *et al.* (1974a)
4-Me$_2$NC$_6$H$_4$	Met, 10% protn. at 100	Singh *et al.* (1974a)
PhCH=CH$_2$	Met, 70% protn. at 100	Singh *et al.* (1974a)

$R_3 = R_4 = H$; $R = 4\text{-}ClC_6H_4(CH_2)_2$; $R_2 = =NAr$

Ar	Activity	Reference
Ph	Met, 20% protn. at 100	Parmar *et al.* (1972a)
3-MeC$_6$H$_4$	Met, 30% protn. at 100	Parmar *et al.* (1972a)
4-MeC$_6$H$_4$	Met, 40% protn. at 100	Parmar *et al.* (1972a)
3,4-Me$_2$C$_6$H$_3$	Met, 20% protn. at 100	Parmar *et al.* (1972a)
2-MeOC$_6$H$_4$	Met, 20% protn. at 100	Parmar *et al.* (1972a)

$R_3 = H$; $R_4 = CH_2CO_2H$; $R_1, R_2 = =N-\triangleleft$

R	Activity	Reference
2-MeC$_6$H$_4$	Met, 80% protn. 0.2 LD$_{50}$	Nagar *et al.* (1973)
3-MeC$_6$H$_4$	Met, 30% protn. 0.2 LD$_{50}$	Nagar *et al.* (1973)
4-MeC$_6$H$_4$	Met, 20% protn. 0.2 LD$_{50}$	Nagar *et al.* (1973)
2-MeOC$_6$H$_4$	Met, 60% protn. 0.2 LD$_{50}$	Nagar *et al.* (1973)
4-MeOC$_6$H$_4$	Met, 30% protn. 0.2 LD$_{50}$	Nagar *et al.* (1973)
Cyclohexyl	Met, 80% protn. 0.2 LD$_{50}$	Nagar *et al.* (1973)

$R_3 = H$; $R_4 = CH_2CO_2H$; $R_1, R_2, = =N-\langle\rangle$

R	Activity	Reference
Ph	Met, 20% protn. 0.2 LD$_{50}$	Nagar *et al.* (1973)
4-ClC$_6$H$_4$	Met, 20% protn. 0.2 LD$_{50}$	Nagar *et al.* (1973)
4-IC$_6$H$_4$	Met, 40% protn. 0.2 LD$_{50}$	Nagar *et al.* (1973)
2-MeC$_6$H$_4$	Met, 40% protn. 0.2 LD$_{50}$	Nagar *et al.* (1973)
4-MeC$_6$H$_4$	Met, 20% protn. 0.2 LD$_{50}$	Nagar *et al.* (1973)
3-MeOC$_6$H$_4$	Met, 40% protn. 0.2 LD$_{50}$	Nagar *et al.* (1973)

(continued)

TABLE IX—*Continued*

$$R_3 = R_4 = H;\ R = 3,4\text{-}(MeO)_2C_6H_4(CH_2)_2;\ R_2 = NAr$$

Ar	Activity	Reference
Ph	Met, 30% protn. at 100	Dwivedi *et al.* (1972)
2-MeC$_6$H$_4$	Met, 70% protn. at 100	Dwivedi *et al.* (1972)
3-MeC$_6$H$_4$	Met, 30% protn. at 100	Dwivedi *et al.* (1972)
4-MeC$_6$H$_4$	Met, 40% protn. at 100	Dwivedi *et al.* (1972)
3,4-Me$_2$C$_6$H$_3$	Met, 10% protn. at 100	Dwivedi *et al.* (1972)
2-MeOC$_6$H$_4$	Met, 50% protn. at 100	Dwivedi *et al.* (1972)
4-MeOC$_6$H$_4$	Met, 10% protn. at 100	Dwivedi *et al.* (1972)
4-ClC$_6$H$_4$	Met, 60% protn. at 100	Dwivedi *et al.* (1972)
4-BrC$_6$H$_4$	Met, 30% protn. at 100	Dwivedi *et al.* (1972)
1-Nap	Met, 50% protn. at 100	Dwivedi *et al.* (1972)

C. Benzothiazoles

R	R$_1$	Activity	Reference
N=C(NHPr-*n*)NHC$_6$H$_4$Br-4	Br	ES ED 160 (po)	Bhargava and Shyam (1974)
NHC(=NH)NHCH$_2$Ph	Cl	ES ED$_{50}$ 80	Bhargava and Singh (1971)
NHC(=NMe)NHCH$_2$Ph	Br	ES ED$_{50}$ 30	Bhargava and Singh (1971)
SCONHNHCSNHAr	H	Active	Singh *et al.* (1975)

D. Miscellaneous derivatives

Compound	Activity	Reference
	Active	Surrey and Webb (1967)
	Active	Bellus (1973)

TABLE IX—*Continued*

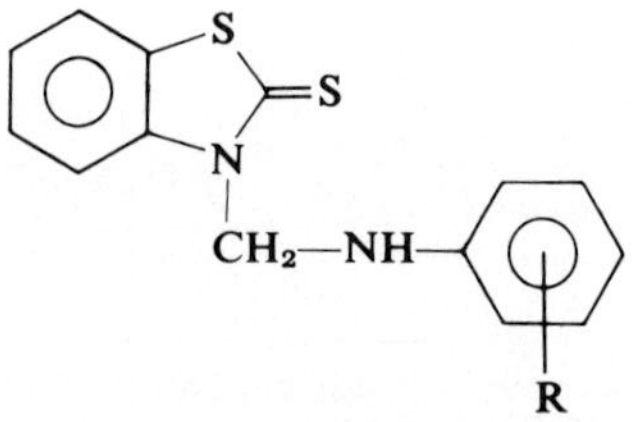

R	Activity	Reference
2-CO_2Me	Met, 40% protn. at 100	Misra (1974)
3-CO_3Et	Met, 10% protn. at 100	Misra (1974)
4-CO_2Et	Met, 20% protn. at 100	Misra (1974)
2-$CONHNH_2$	Met, 10% protn. at 100	Misra (1974)
3-$CONHNH_2$	Met, 20% protn. at 100	Misra (1974)
4-$CONHNH_2$	Met, 10% protn. at 100	Misra (1974)

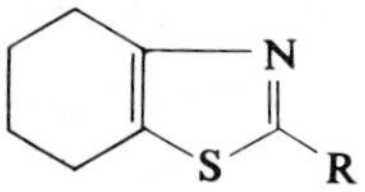

R	Activity	Reference
H	Met ED_{50} 60 (iv)	Lindberg *et al.* (1971)
NH_2	Met ED_{50} 50 (iv)	Lindberg *et al.* (1971)

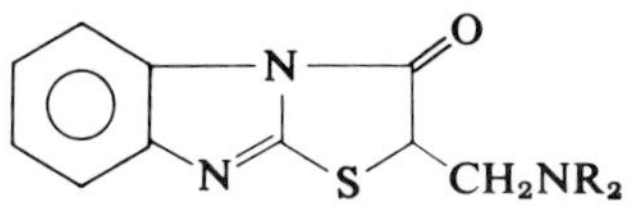

NR_2	Activity	Reference
NEt_2	ES convul. thresh. raised 15–20 mA	Singh (1969)
NMe_2	ES convul. thresh. raised 10–15 mA	Singh (1969)
NPh_2	ES convul. thresh. raised 40 mA	Singh (1969)
N(Ph)Et	ES convul. thresh. raised 15–20 mA	Singh (1969)
N(n-Pr)$_2$	ES convul. thresh. raised 15–20 mA	Singh (1969)
N(n-Bu)$_2$	ES convul. thresh. raised 40 mA	Singh (1969)
N(sec-Bu)$_2$	ES convul. thresh. raised 40 mA	Singh (1969)
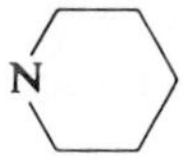	ES convul. thresh. raised 60 mA	Singh (1969)
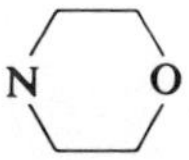	ES convul. thresh. raised 60 mA	Singh (1969)

(*continued*)

TABLE IX—*Continued*

R	Activity	Reference
Ph	ES convul. thresh. raised 15–20 mA	Singh (1970)
2-MeC$_6$H$_4$	ES convul. thresh. raised 15–20 mA	Singh (1970)
4-MeC$_6$H$_4$	ES convul. thresh. raised 15–20 mA	Singh (1970)
3-MeC$_6$H$_4$	ES convul. thresh. raised 15–20 mA	Singh (1970)
2-BrC$_6$H$_4$	ES convul. thresh. raised 40 mA	Singh (1970)
4-BrC$_6$H$_4$	ES convul. thresh. raised 40 mA	Singh (1970)
3-BrC$_6$H$_4$	ES convul. thresh. raised 40 mA	Singh (1970)
2-ClC$_6$H$_4$	ES convul. thresh. raised 60 mA	Singh (1970)
4-ClC$_6$H$_4$	ES convul. thresh. raised 60 mA	Singh (1970)
3-ClC$_6$H$_4$	ES convul. thresh. raised > 60 mA	Singh (1970)

TABLE X DIOXOLANE DERIVATIVES

A. Dioxolanes

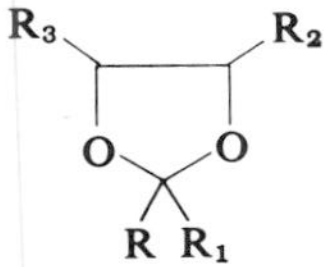

R	R_1	R_2	R_3	Activity	Reference
Et, Me	Ar	CH_2OH	H	Met, active	Chladt and Braunlich (1965)
CH_2NR_2	H	$CH_2OC_6H_4Me\text{-}2$	H	Active	Hallman et al. (1962)
$PhCH_2$	H	H	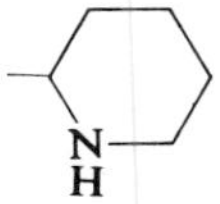 (2-methylpiperidinyl)	$MES\ ED_{50} < 80$	Hardie et al. (1966)
$PhCH_2$	$PhCH_2$	H	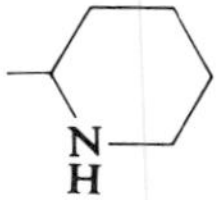 (2-methylpiperidinyl)	$MES\ ED_{50} > 50$	Hardie et al. (1966)
Ph	H	H	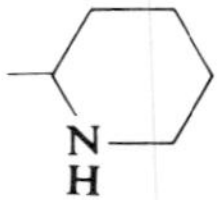 (2-methylpiperidinyl)	$MES\ ED_{50} > 20$	Hardie et al. (1966)
Ph	Me	H	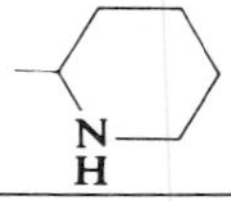 (2-methylpiperidinyl)	$MES\ ED_{50} > 100$	Hardie et al. (1966)

(continued)

TABLE X—*Continued*

R	R_1	R_2	R_3	Activity	Reference
Ph	Et (α)	H		MES ED_{50} 12.5	Hardie *et al.* (1966)
Ph	Et (β)	H		MES ED_{50} < 75	Hardie *et al.* (1966)
Ph	Ph (α)	H		MES ED_{50} 60	Hardie *et al.* (1966)
Ph	Ph (β)	H		MES ED_{50} > 100	Hardie *et al.* (1966)
Ph	Ph (α-d)	H		MES ED_{50} 50	Hardie *et al.* (1966)
Ph	Ph (α-l)	H		MES ED_{50} 75	Hardie *et al.* (1966)
Ph	4-ClC$_6$H$_4$	H		MES ED_{50} > 100	Hardie *et al.* (1966)

4-ClC$_6$H$_4$	4-ClC$_6$H$_4$	H		MES ED$_{50}$ > 150	Hardie *et al.* (1966)
Ph	2-Thienyl (α)	H		MES ED$_{50}$ > 50	Hardie *et al.* (1966)
Ph	2-Thienyl (β)	H		MES ED$_{50}$ > 100	Hardie *et al.* (1966)
C$_6$H$_{11}$	C$_6$H$_{11}$	H		MES ED$_{50}$ > 150	Hardie *et al.* (1966)
Me	Ph$_2$CH	H		MES ED$_{50}$ 50	Hardie *et al.* (1966)
Ph	PhCH$_2$	H		MES ED$_{50}$ 75	Hardie *et al.* (1966)
4-MeOC$_6$H$_4$	4-MeOC$_6$H$_4$	H		MES ED$_{50}$ > 200	Hardie *et al.* (1966)

(continued)

TABLE X—*Continued*

R	R_1	R_2	R_3	Activity	Reference
Ph	Ph	H	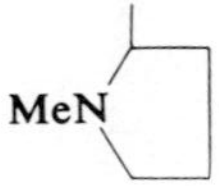 MeN (structure) (α)	MES ED_{50} 100	Hardie *et al.* (1966)
Ph	Ph	H	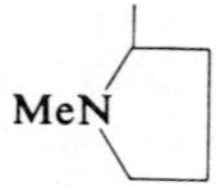 MeN (structure) (α-d)	MES ED_{50} 125	Hardie *et al.* (1966)
Ph	Ph	H	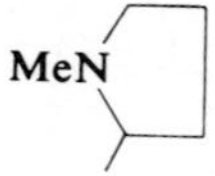 MeN (structure) (α-l)	MES ED_{50} > 75	Hardie *et al.* (1966)
Ph	Ph	H	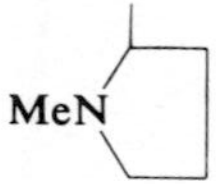 MeN (structure) (β)	MES ED_{50} > 75	Hardie *et al.* (1966)
Ph	Ph	H	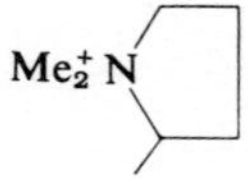 Me_2^+N (structure) I^-	MES ED_{50} > 150	Hardie *et al.* (1966)
Ph	Ph	H	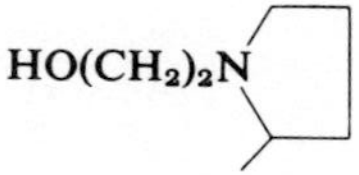 $HO(CH_2)_2N$ (structure)	MES ED_{50} > 75	Hardie *et al.* (1966)
Ph	Ph	H	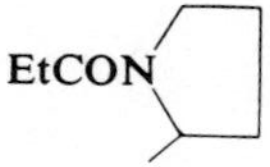 EtCON (structure) (α)	MES ED_{50} < 150	Hardie *et al.* (1966)
Ph	Ph	H	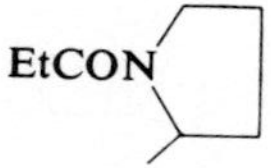 EtCON (structure) (β)	MES ED_{50} > 200	Hardie *et al.* (1966)

			Structure	Activity	Reference
Ph	Ph	H	n-PrN (α)	MES ED_{50} 100	Hardie et al. (1966)
Ph	Ph	H	n-PrN (β)	MES ED_{50} > 75	Hardie et al. (1966)
Ph	Ph	H	$ClCH_2CON$	MES ED_{50} >200	Hardie et al. (1966)
Ph	Ph	H	$PhCH_2N$	MES ED_{50} > 75	Hardie et al. (1966)
Ph	Ph	H	$PhCH_2N$	MES ED_{50} 120	Hardie et al. (1966)
Ph	Ph	H	$PhCH_2N$	MES ED_{50} 200	Hardie et al. (1966)
Ph	Ph	H	$PhCH_2N$	MES ED_{50} > 200	Hardie et al. (1966)
Ph	Ph	H	Et_2NCH_2CON	MES ED_{50} > 75	Hardie et al. (1966)

(continued)

TABLE X—*Continued*

R	R_1	R_2	R_3	Activity	Reference
Ph	Ph	H	Et_2NCH_2CON (2-methylcyclohexyl)	MES ED_{50} > 50	Hardie *et al.* (1966)
Ph	Ph	H	$Et_2N(CH_2)_2N$ (2-methylcyclohexyl)	MES ED_{50} > 37.5	Hardie *et al.* (1966)
Ph	Ph	H	Me–N^+–O^- (2-methylpiperidinium oxide)	MES ED_{50} 200	Hardie *et al.* (1966)
Ph	Ph	H	Me–N^+–O^- (2-methylpiperidinium oxide)	MES ED_{50} 150	
Ph	Ph	H	Et–N^+–O^- (2-methylpiperidinium oxide)	MES ED_{50} > 150	Hardie *et al.* (1966)
Ph	Ph	H	*i*-PrN (2-methylpiperidine)	MES ED_{50} 75	Hardie *et al.* (1966)
Alkyl	Alkyl	H	$ROCH_2$	Met and MES, active	Weiss and Ewing (1959)
Et	4-ClC_6H_4	H	$HOCH_2$	ES, 100% protn. at 0.5 LD_{50}	Melson (1962)

TABLE X—*Continued*

B. Miscellaneous derivatives

Compound	Activity	Reference
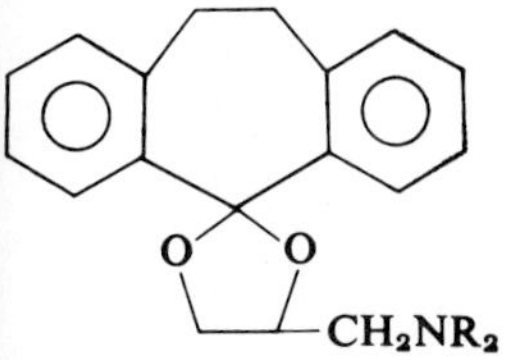	Active	Fauran *et al.* (1971b)
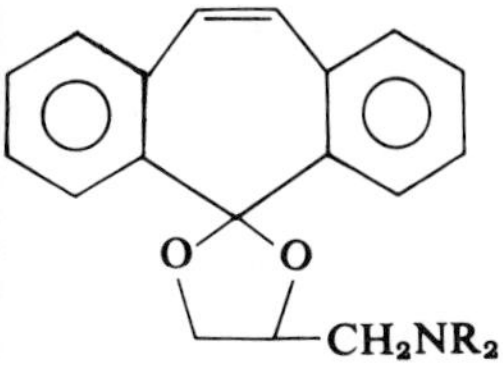	Active	Fauran *et al.* (1971b)
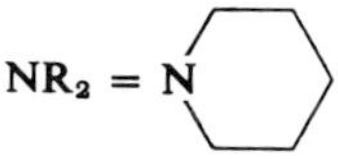 $NR_2 = $	ES, 90% protn. at 75 (po)	Fauran (1973a)
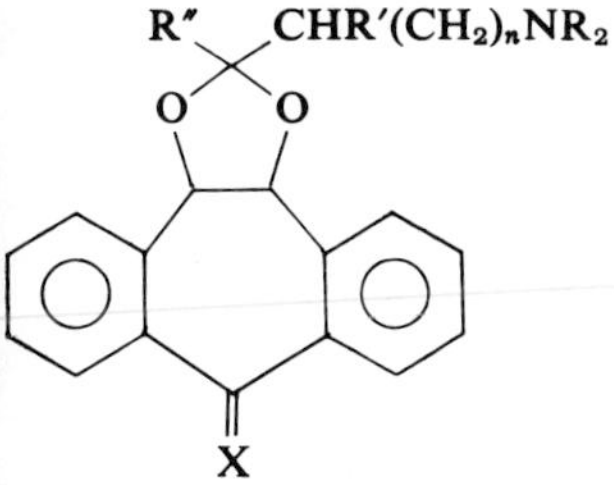	Active	Viterbo *et al.* (1972)
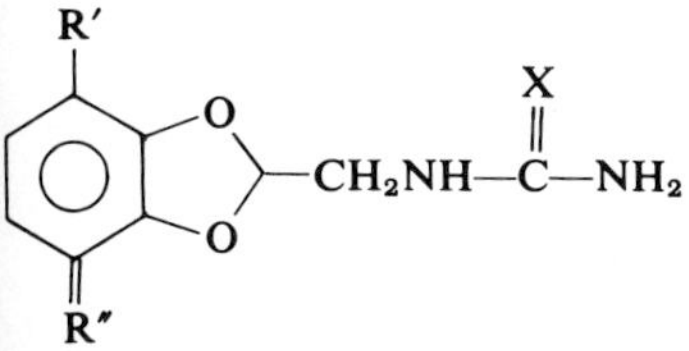	Active	Gardner and Willey (1964)

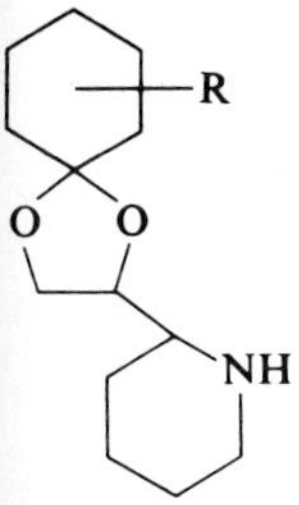 R = H: MES ED$_{50}$ > 75	Hardie *et al.* (1966)
R = 6-Me: MES ED$_{50}$ 150	Hardie *et al.* (1966)
R = 7-Me: MES ED$_{50}$ > 150	Hardie *et al.* (1966)
R = 8-Me: MES ED$_{50}$ > 150	Hardie *et al.* (1966)
R = 7,9-Me$_2$: MES ED$_{50}$ > 125	Hardie *et al.* (1966)
R = 6-Et: MES ED$_{50}$ > 200	Hardie *et al.* (1966)
R = 6-Cl: MES ED$_{50}$ 200	Hardie *et al.* (1966)
R = 8-Cl (α): MES ED$_{50}$ > 150	Hardie *et al.* (1966)
R = 8-Cl (β): MES ED$_{50}$ 200	Hardie *et al.* (1966)
R = 8-*t*-Bu: MES ED$_{50}$ 150	Hardie *et al.* (1966)
R = 8-Me-8-Ph: MES ED$_{50}$ < 100	Hardie *et al.* (1966)

TABLE XI 1,2,3-TRIAZOLES

Compound	Activity	Reference
	MES and Met, mod. act.	Gilbert and Rumanowsk (1971)
	Active	Wolf (1968a)

TABLE XII

A. Triazole derivatives

R	R_1	R_2	Activity	Reference
$CH_2CH(OH)R$	H, Me	H, Me	Active	Wolf (1968a)
4-R-2-ArCOC$_6$H$_3$	H, Me	CH_2R	Active	Takeda Chemical Industries, Ltd. (1974)

3-MeC$_6$H$_4$	H		MES ED$_{50}$ 62; Met ED$_{50}$ > 100	Ainsworth *et al.* (1962)
4-MeC$_6$H$_4$	H		MES ED$_{50}$ > 100; Met ED$_{50}$ > 100	Ainsworth *et al.* (1962)
2-MeOC$_6$H$_4$	H		MES ED$_{50}$ > 100; Met ED$_{50}$ > 100	Ainsworth *et al.* (1962)
3-MeOC$_6$H$_4$	H		MES ED$_{50}$ 80; Met ED$_{50}$ > 100	Ainsworth *et al.* (1962)
4-MeOC$_6$H$_4$	H		MES ED$_{50}$ > 100; Met ED$_{50}$ > 100	Ainsworth *et al.* (1962)
4-ClC$_6$H$_4$	H		MES ED$_{50}$ 42; Met ED$_{50}$ > 100	Ainsworth *et al.* (1962)
3-ClC$_6$H$_4$	H		MES ED$_{50}$ 72; Met ED$_{50}$ > 100	Ainsworth *et al.* (1962)
4-BrC$_6$H$_4$	H		MES ED$_{50}$ 36; Met ED$_{50}$ > 100	Ainsworth *et al.* (1962)
4-NO$_2$C$_6$H$_4$	H		MES ED$_{50}$ > 100; Met ED$_{50}$ > 100	Ainsworth *et al.* (1962)
2,4-Cl$_2$C$_6$H$_3$	H		MES ED$_{50}$ 37; Met ED$_{50}$ > 100	Ainsworth *et al.* (1962)
PhCH$_2$	H		MES ED$_{50}$ > 100; Met ED$_{50}$ > 100	Ainsworth *et al.* (1962)
Ph	SH	(CH$_2$)$_2$—benzimidazole	Met, 30% protn. at 100 (ip)	Parmar *et al.* (1972b)
3-MeC$_6$H$_4$	SH	(CH$_2$)$_2$—benzimidazole	Met, 70% protn. at 100 (ip)	Parmar *et al.* (1972b)
2-MeOC$_6$H$_4$	SH	(CH$_2$)$_2$—benzimidazole	Met, 70% protn. at 100 (ip)	Parmar *et al.* (1972b)
4-MeOC$_6$H$_4$	SH	(CH$_2$)$_2$—benzimidazole	Met, 70% protn. at 100 (ip)	Parmar *et al.* (1972b)
C$_6$H$_{11}$	SH	(CH$_2$)$_2$—benzimidazole	Met, 60% protn. at 100 (ip)	Parmar *et al.* (1972b)

(*continued*)

TABLE XII—*Continued*

R	R_1	R_2	Activity	Reference
$CH_2CH{=}CH_2$	SH	$(CH_2)_2$ benzimidazole	Met, 50% protn. at 100 (ip)	Parmar *et al.* (1972b)
Ph	SCH_2CO_2Et	$(CH_2)_2$ benzimidazole	Met, 40% protn. at 100 (ip)	Parmar *et al.* (1972b)
3-MeC_6H_4	SCH_2CO_2Et	$(CH_2)_2$ benzimidazole	Met, 40% protn. at 100 (ip)	Parmar *et al.* (1972b)
2-MeOC_6H_4	SCH_2CO_2Et	$(CH_2)_2$ benzimidazole	Met, 40% protn. at 100 (ip)	Parmar *et al.* (1972b)
4-MeOC_6H_4	SCH_2CO_2Et	$(CH_2)_2$ benzimidazole	Met, 80% protn. at 100 (ip)	Parmar *et al.* (1972b)
C_6H_{11}	SCH_2SO_2Et	$(CH_2)_2$ benzimidazole	Met, 60% protn. at 100 (ip)	Parmar *et al.* (1972b)

$CH_2CH{=}CH_2$	SCH_2CO_2Et	$(CH_2)_2$	Met, 50% protn. at 100 (ip)	Parmar et al. (1972b)
Ph	$SCH_2CONHNH_2$	$(CH_2)_2$	Met, 30% protn. at 100 (ip)	Parmar et al. (1972b)
$3\text{-}MeC_6H_4$	$SCH_2CONHNH_2$	$(CH_2)_2$	Met, 50% protn. at 100 (ip)	Parmar et al. (1972b)
$2\text{-}MeOC_6H_4$	$SCH_2CONHNH_2$	$(CH_2)_2$	Met, 40% protn. at 100 (ip)	Parmar et al. (1972b)
$4\text{-}MeOC_6H_4$	$SCH_2CONHNH_2$	$(CH_2)_2$	Met, 70% protn. at 100 (ip)	Parmar et al. (1972b)
C_6H_{11}	$SCH_2CONHNH_2$	$(CH_2)_2$	Met, 50% protn. at 100 (ip)	Parmar et al. (1972b)
$CH_2CH{=}CH_2$	$SCH_2CONHNH_2$	$(CH_2)_2$	Met, 60% protn. at 100 (ip)	Parmar et al. (1972b)
$2\text{-}C_6H_5COC_6H_4$	CH_2R_3	R_2	Active	Meguro et al. (1974)

(continued)

TABLE XII—*Continued*

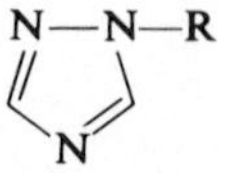

$$N\text{---}N\text{---}R$$

R	Activity	Reference
n-Pr	MES $ED_{50} > 200$; Met $ED_{50} > 200$	Ainsworth *et al.* (1962)
i-Pr	MES $ED_{50} > 200$; Met $ED_{50} > 200$	Ainsworth *et al.* (1962)
CH(Me)Et	MES $ED_{50} > 200$; Met $ED_{50} > 200$	Ainsworth *et al.* (1962)
Ph	MES ED_{50} 24; Met ED_{50} 52	Ainsworth *et al.* (1962)
n-Bu	MES ED_{50} 200; Met $ED_{50} > 200$	Ainsworth *et al.* (1962)
$4\text{-}NO_2C_6H_4$	MES ED_{50} 50; Met $ED_{50} > 100$	Ainsworth *et al.* (1962)
$4\text{-}NH_2C_6H_4$	MES ED_{50} 34; Met $ED_{50} > 100$	Ainsworth *et al.* (1962)
$4\text{-}MeCONHC_6H_4$	MES $ED_{50} > 100$; Met $ED_{50} > 100$	Ainsworth *et al.* (1962)
$4\text{-}ClC_6H_4$	MES ED_{50} 16; Met $ED_{50} > 100$	Ainsworth *et al.* (1962)
$PhCH_2$	MES ED_{50} 21; Met ED_{50} 41	Ainsworth *et al.* (1962)
$4\text{-}ClC_6H_4CH_2$	MES ED_{50} 22; Met ED_{50} 44	Ainsworth *et al.* (1962)
$1\text{-}NapCH_2$	MES ED_{50} 16; Met ED_{50} 85	Ainsworth *et al.* (1962)
$PhCH_2CH_2$	MES ED_{50} 53; Met ED_{50} 80	Ainsworth *et al.* (1962)
Ph (3-Me)	MES ED_{50} 34; Met ED_{50} 54	Ainsworth *et al.* (1962)
Ph (5-Me)	MES ED_{50} 70; Met ED_{50} 132	Ainsworth *et al.* (1962)

B. Miscellaneous derivatives

Compound	Activity	Reference
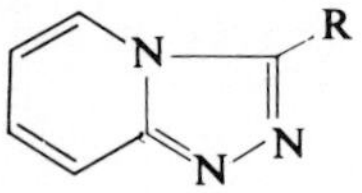	Active	Bicking (1959)
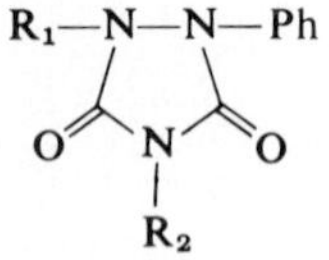	Met and MES $ED_{50} \leq 500$	Jacobson *et al.* (1972)

TABLE XIII   1,2,4-OXADIAZOLES

A. Oxadiazole derivatives

R	R_1	Activity	Reference
Cyclopropyl	Hetero-Ar	Active	Fanshawe and Safir (1974)
Hetero-Ar	Cyclopropyl	Active	Fanshawe and Safir (1974)
$2\text{-}ClC_6H_4$	4-Pyr	ES ED_{50} 13 (po)	Leszkovszky and Tardos (1970)
$4\text{-}ClC_6H_4$	4-Pyr	ES ED_{50} > 200 (po)	Leszkovszky and Tardos (1970)
Ph_2CHCH_2	4-Pyr	ES ED_{50} > 100 (po)	Leszkovszky and Tardos (1970)
4-Pyr	4-Pyr	ES ED_{50} > 100 (po)	Leszkovszky and Tardos (1970)
3-Pyr	4-Pyr	ES ED_{50} > 100 (po)	Leszkovszky and Tardos (1970)
Me	4-Pyr	ES ED_{50} > 100 (po)	Leszkovszky and Tardos (1970)
4-Pyr	$2\text{-}ClC_6H_4$	ES ED_{50} 56 (po)	Leszkovszky and Tardos (1970)
4-Pyr	$PhCH{=}CH$	ES ED_{50} > 200 (po)	Leszkovszky and Tardos (1970)
$4\text{-}NH_2C_6H_4$	3-Pyr	ES ED_{50} > 100 (po)	Leszkovszky and Tardos (1970)
3-Pyr	3-Pyr	ES ED_{50} 200 (po)	Leszkovszky and Tardos (1970)
$(CH_2)_2CON_2H_3$	3-Pyr	ES ED_{50} > 300 (ip)	Leszkovszky and Tardos (1970)
3-Pyr	2-Et-4-Pyr	ES ED_{50} > 50 (ip)	Leszkovszky and Tardos (1970)
$2\text{-}ClC_6H_4$	2-Pyr	ES ED_{50} 25 (po)	Leszkovszky and Tardos (1970)
$2\text{-}ClC_6H_4$	1-Me-4-Pyr$^+$	ES ED_{50} > 100 (po)	Leszkovszky and Tardos (1970)
1-Me-4-Pyr$^+$	$2\text{-}ClC_6H_4$	ES ED_{50} > 100 (po)	Leszkovszky and Tardos (1970)
$2\text{-}ClC_6H_4$	$CH(NH_2)Ph$	ES ED_{50} > 100 (sc)	Leszkovszky and Tardos (1970)
Ph_2CHCH_2	$CH(NH_2)Ph$	ES ED_{50} > 50 (sc)	Leszkovszky and Tardos (1970)
$(CH_2)_2CON_2H_3$	$2\text{-}ClC_6H_4$	ES ED_{50} > 200 (po)	Leszkovszky and Tardos (1970)
$O(CH_2)_2NEt_2$	$2\text{-}ClC_6H_4$	ES ED_{50} > 100 (ip)	Leszkovszky and Tardos (1970)

B. Miscellaneous derivatives

Compound	Activity	Reference
$R = H, Me$	ES, active	Lopresti and Safir (1958)

TABLE XIV 1,3,4-OXADIAZOLES

A. Oxadiazole derivatives

R	R_1	Activity	Reference
Ar	$ROCH_2$	Active	Thomas (1974)
Ar	CH_2CO_2R	Active	Buguet *et al.* (1974)
NHPh	$4\text{-}t\text{-Bu-2-Br}C_6H_3OCH_2$	Met, 30% protn. at 100	Parmar *et al.* (1974b)
$NHC_6H_4Me\text{-}2$	$4\text{-}t\text{-Bu-2-Br}C_6H_3OCH_2$	Met, 50% protn. at 100	Parmar *et al.* (1974b)
$NHC_6H_4Me\text{-}3$	$4\text{-}t\text{-Bu-2-Br}C_6H_3OCH_2$	Met, 50% protn. at 100	Parmar *et al.* (1974b)
$NHC_6H_4Me\text{-}4$	$4\text{-}t\text{-Bu-2-Br}C_6H_3OCH_2$	Met, 60% protn. at 100	Parmar *et al.* (1974b)
$NHC_6H_4OMe\text{-}2$	$4\text{-}t\text{-Bu-2-Br}C_6H_3OCH_2$	Met, 30% protn. at 100	Parmar *et al.* (1974b)
$NHC_6H_4OMe\text{-}4$	$4\text{-}t\text{-Bu-2-Br}C_6H_3OCH_2$	Met, 60% protn. at 100	Parmar *et al.* (1974b)
$NHC_6H_4Cl\text{-}4$	$4\text{-}t\text{-Bu-2-Br}C_6H_3OCH_2$	Met, 40% protn. at 100	Parmar *et al.* (1974b)
$NHC_6H_4Br\text{-}4$	$4\text{-}t\text{-Bu-2-Br}C_6H_3OCH_2$	Met, 70% protn. at 100	Parmar *et al.* (1974b)
$NHC_6H_4I\text{-}4$	$4\text{-}t\text{-Bu-2-Br}C_6H_3OCH_2$	Met, 60% protn. at 100	Parmar *et al.* (1974b)

B. Miscellaneous derivatives

R	Activity	Reference
4-*n*-Bu-carboxylate phenyl	Met, 10% protn. at 100 (ip)	Ram and Pandey (1974)
4-*i*-Bu-carboxylate phenyl	Met, 20% protn. at 100 (ip)	Ram and Pandey (1974)
$3\text{-}NO_2C_6H_4$	Met, 20% protn. at 100 (ip)	Ram and Pandey (1974)
$4\text{-}NO_2C_6H_4$	Met, 20% protn. at 100 (ip)	Ram and Pandey (1974)
4-Carboxyphenyl	Met, 20% protn. at 100 (ip)	Ram and Pandey (1974)

TABLE XV 1,2,3-THIADIAZOLES

Compound	Activity	Reference
	ES ED_{50} 185 (ip); Met ED_{50} 200	Ramsby *et al.* (1973)

TABLE XVI 1,3,4-THIADIAZOLES

A. Thiadiazole derivatives

R	R_1	Activity	Reference
SO_2NH_1	CH_3CONH	MES ED_{50} 40 (po), 60 (iv)	Pala and Sguanci (1960)
		MES ED_{50} 100 (ip)	Torchiana et al. (1973)
		MES ED_{50} 26	Rudzik and Mehnear (1966)
		MES ED_{50} 37 (ip)	Mennear and Rudzik (1968)
NH_2		Active	Lepetit (1959)
NH_2	OPr, OBu	Active	Clarkson (1964)
NH_2	2-MeOC_6H_4	Met act. > 200	Maffii et al. (1958)
NH_2		Met act. > 200; MES ED_{50} 70	Maffii et al. (1958)
NH_2		MES ED_{50} 150	Maffii et al. (1958)
NH_2	Ph	Met act. > 200; MES ED_{50} 20	Maffii et al. (1958)
NH_2	Et	MES ED_{50} > 200	Maffii et al. (1958)
NH_2	$3\text{-NO}_2C_6H_4$	MES ED_{50} > 200	Maffii et al. (1958)
NH_2	4-MeCONHC_6H_4	MES ED_{50} > 200	Maffii et al. (1958)
NH_2	3-MeO-4-HOC_6H_3	MES ED_{50} > 400	Maffii et al. (1958)
NH_2	2-ClC_6H_4	Met act. > 100; MES ED_{50} 75	Maffii et al. (1958)
NH_2	$PhCH{=}CH$	Met act. > 200; MES ED_{50} 75	Maffii et al. (1958)
MeCONH	Ph	MES ED_{50} > 200	Maffii et al. (1958)
$NHCO_2Et$	Ph	MES ED_{50} > 200	Maffii et al. (1958)
NH_2	2-MeC_6H_4	Met act. > 100; MES ED_{50} 75	Maffii et al. (1958)
H	Ph	Met act. > 200; MES ED_{50} 70	Maffii et al. (1958)
Me	Ph	Met act. > 200; MES ED_{50} 100	Maffii et al. (1958)
Ph	Ph	MES ED_{50} > 200	Maffii et al. (1958)
OH	Ph	MES ED_{50} 150	Maffii et al. (1958)
SH	Ph	MES ED_{50} > 200	Maffii et al. (1958)
SCH_2CO_2H	Ph	MES ED_{50} > 200	Maffii et al. (1958)
SCH_2CO_2Et	Ph	MES ED_{50} 200	Maffii et al. (1958)
NH_2	Cyclohexyl	MES ED_{50} 200	Maffii et al. (1958)

(continued)

TABLE XVI—*Continued*

B. Thiadiazolines

$$R_1-N-N$$
$$RN=\underset{S}{\overset{}{\diagup\!\!\diagdown}}-SO_2NH_2$$

R	R_1	Activity	Reference
3,4,5-(MeO)$_3$C$_6$H$_2$CO	Me	Met ED$_{50}$ 62 (ip)	Lukes and Nieforth (1975)
2,4,6-(MeO)$_3$C$_6$H$_2$CO	Me	Met ED$_{50}$ 54 (ip)	Lukes and Nieforth (1975)
2,4,5-(MeO)$_3$C$_6$H$_2$CO	Me	Met ED$_{50}$ 50 (ip)	Lukes and Nieforth (1975)
4-ClC$_6$H$_4$CO	Me	Met ED$_{50}$ 56 (ip)	Lukes and Nieforth (1975)
4-BrC$_6$H$_4$CO	Me	Met ED$_{50}$ 62 (ip)	Lukes and Nieforth (1975)
4-IC$_6$H$_4$CO	Me	Met ED$_{50}$ 52 (ip)	Lukes and Nieforth (1975)
PhCO	Me	Met ED$_{50}$ 62 (ip)	Lukes and Nieforth (1975)
CH$_3$CO	Me	Met ED$_{50}$ 54 (ip)	Lukes and Nieforth (1975)
		MES ED$_{50}$ 28 (ip)	Torchiana *et al.* (1973)
CH$_3$CO	Et	MES ED$_{50}$ 9 (po), 13 (iv)	Pala and Sguanci (1960)

C. Miscellaneous derivatives

Compound	Activity	Reference
Me—N—N / Ph—⟨ ⟩—S$^\ominus$ (S) ⊕	Active	Amann *et al.* (1974)
R—N—N / Ar—⟨ ⟩—S$^\ominus$ (S) ⊕	Active	Amann *et al.* (1975)

a number of oxadiazoles has been shown to be unrelated to their ability to inhibit oxidation of pyruvate, α-ketoglutarate, and succinate (Parmar *et al.*, 1974b).

The most noteworthy compound in this group is acetazolamide (**VII**). This compound has been known for some time (Bergstrom *et al.*, 1962) and has been used clinically. The usefulness of acetazolamide is limited because of the

$$CH_3CONH-\underset{S}{\overset{N-N}{\diagup\!\!\diagdown}}-SO_2NH_2$$

(**VII**)

rapid development of tolerance to its anticonvulsant effects. A large number of papers have appeared concerning the mechanism of action of acetazolamide (Gilbert *et al.*, 1971; Mazzanti, 1960; Mennear and Rudzik, 1966; Rauh and Gray, 1968; Rudzik and Mennear, 1966; Sakamoto, 1968;

TABLE XVII TETRAZOLE DERIVATIVES[a]

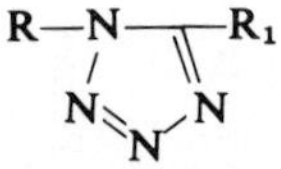

$$R-N-R_1$$

(structure: tetrazole ring with N—N, N, N)

R	R_1	Activity
Me	Ph	MES ED_{50} 242; 70% protn. at 300 (po)
		Met ED_{50} 516; 20% protn. at 300 (po)
Et	3-$NH_2C_6H_4$	MES ED_{50} 320; 30% protn. at 300 (po)
		Met ED_{50} 445; 20% protn. at 300 (po)
Ph	CH_2CHMe_3	MES ED_{50} 162; 80% protn. at 300 (po)
		Met ED_{50} 112; 100% protn. at 300 (po)
Ph	CH_2NMe	MES, 30% protn. at 1000 (po)
		Met, 10% protn. at 1000 (po)
Ph	CH(Me)NHMe	MES, 77% protn. at 1000 (po)
		Met, 40% protn. at 1000 (po)
3-$NH_2C_6H_4$	Et	MES ED_{50} 327; 40% protn. at 1000 (po)
		Met ED_{50} 217; 80% protn. at 1000 (po)
3-$NH_2C_6H_4$	n-Bu	MES, 10% protn. at 1000 (po)
		Met, 10% protn. at 1000 (po)
2-Nap	CH_2NEt_2	MES, 10% protn. at 1000 (po)
		Met, 10% protn. at 1000 (po)

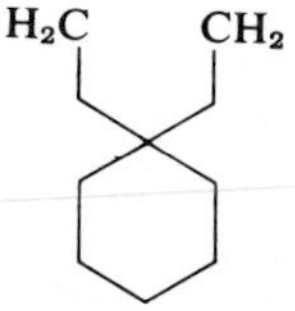

H_2C CH_2

(cyclohexane/spiro structure)

MES, 30% protn. at 1000 (po)
Met, 10% protn. at 1000 (po)

[a] Data from Mitchell (1964).

Torchiana *et al.*, 1973; Woodbury and Kemp, 1970). Acetazolamide selectively blocks, as does carbon dioxide, the monosynaptic action potential in the spinal cord. It acts primarily by causing carbon dioxide accumulation in the brain. The anticonvulsant effect is related directly to the inhibition of brain carbonic anhydrase. It involves largely adrenergic mechanisms within the central nervous system.

III. SIX-MEMBERED RINGS

A. WITH ONE HETEROATOM

Tables XVIII–XXI include various six-membered heterocyclic compounds with one heteroatom. The major emphasis has been on the screening of

TABLE XVIII   PIPERIDINE DERIVATIVES

A. Piperidines

R	R_1	Activity	Reference
(cyclohexyl)	H	MES ED_{50} 37	Millichap et al. (1968)
$CH_2CH_2C(Ph)OH$			
$CH_2CONHN{=}CHAr$	H	ES, act. 30–50 (ip)	Tajana and Pozzi (1971)
Ph—(cyclohexyl)	H	ES, act. 5; Met, inact. 40	Chen and Bohner (1961)
	$3\text{-}CF_3C_6H_4$	Active	Helsley (1971)
CONHR			
$(CH_2)_3COC_6H_4F\text{-}4$	R_1	Active	Hernestam et al. (1971)
$(CH_2)_3COC_6H_4F\text{-}4$	Me	Met and ES, active	Hernestam et al. (1974)
$(CH_2)_3COPh$	Me	Active	Ferrosan (1965)
(cyclohexyl)	Ph	Active	Pelz and Protiva (1967)
$(CH_2)_3OCOC(Ph)OH$			

	Ph	Met, active	Pelz and Protiva (1967)
N=CHPyr-4	CH(Ph)$_2$	MES ED$_{50}$ 8 (po); Met, inact.	Craig (1967)
N=CHPyr-3	CH(Ph)$_2$	MES ED$_{50}$ 27 (po); Met, inact.	Craig (1967)
N=CHPyr-4	CH(Ph)C$_6$H$_4$Cl-4	MES ED$_{50}$ 11 (po); Met, inact.	Craig (1967)
N=CHPyr-3	CH(Ph)C$_6$H$_4$Cl-4	MES ED$_{50}$ 28 (po); Met, inact.	Craig (1967)
CONH$_2$	Ph	MES ED$_{50}$ 32; Met, 0% protn. at 100	Helsley et al. (1969)
CONMe$_2$	Ph	MES, 40% protn. at 100; Met, 60% protn. at 200	Helsley et al. (1969)
CONH$_2$	C$_6$H$_4$F-4	MES ED$_{50}$ 73; Met, ED$_{50}$ 108	Helsley et al. (1969)
CONHMe	C$_6$H$_4$F-4	MES ED$_{50}$ 92; Met, 60% protn. at 200	Helsley et al. (1969)
CONMe$_2$	C$_6$H$_4$F-4	MES ED$_{50}$ 111; Met, 0% protn. at 100	Helsley et al. (1969)
CONH$_2$	4-MeOC$_6$H$_4$	MES, 30% protn. at 100; Met, 0% protn. at 200	Helsley et al. (1969)
CONHMe	3-CF$_3$C$_6$H$_4$	MES, 0% protn. at 50; Met, 40% protn. at 100	Helsley et al. (1969)
CH$_2$CONHCONHC$_6$H$_4$Me-2	Me	Met, 20% protn. at 100 (ip)	Gupta et al. (1974)
CH$_2$CONHCONHC$_6$H$_4$Me-3	Me	Met, 20% protn. at 100 (ip)	Gupta et al. (1974)
CH$_2$CONHCONHC$_6$H$_4$Me-4	Me	Met. 20% protn. at 100 (ip)	Gupta et al. (1974)
CH$_2$CONHCONHC$_6$H$_4$Me$_2$-3,4	Me	Met, 40% protn. at 100 (ip)	Gupta et al. (1974)
CH$_2$CONHCONHC$_6$H$_4$OMe-2	Me	Met, 30% protn. at 100 (ip)	Gupta et al. (1974)
CH$_2$CONHCONHC$_6$H$_4$OMe-4	Me	Met, 50% protn. at 100 (ip)	Gupta et al. (1974)
CH$_2$CONHCONHC$_6$H$_4$Cl-4	Me	Met, 20% protn. at 00 (ip)	Gupta et al. (1974)
CONHMe	OPh	MES, 0% protn. at 100 (ip); Met, 100% protn. at 200 (ip)	Boswell et al. (1974)
CONH$_2$	2-MeOC$_6$H$_4$O	MES, 20% protn. at 50; Met, 0% protn. at 200	Boswell et al. (1974)
CONH$_2$	3-CF$_3$C$_6$H$_4$O	MES ED$_{50}$ 69 (ip); Met ED$_{50}$ 88 (ip)	Boswell et al. (1974)
CONHMe	3-CF$_3$C$_6$H$_4$O	MES ED$_{50}$ 29 (ip); Met ED$_{50}$ 97 (ip)	Boswell et al. (1974)
CONMe$_2$	3-CF$_3$C$_6$H$_4$O	MES ED$_{50}$ 47 (ip); Met ED$_{50}$ 89 (ip)	Boswell et al. (1974)

(continued)

TABLE XVIII—*Continued*

R	R_1	Activity	Reference
$CONHC_4H_9$	$3\text{-}CF_3C_6H_4O$	MES, 40% protn. at 100 Met, 60% protn. at 200	Boswell et al. (1974) Boswell et al. (1974)
CONHEt	$3\text{-}CF_3C_6H_4O$	MES, 40% protn. at 33 Met, 0% protn. at 22	Boswell et al. (1974) Boswell et al. (1974)
CONHPh	$3\text{-}CF_3C_6H_4O$	MES, 40% protn. at 100 Met, 40% protn. at 200	Boswell et al. (1974) Boswell et al. (1974)
$CONHC_6H_4Cl\text{-}3$	$3\text{-}CF_3C_6H_4O$	MES, 20% protn. at 100 Met, 20% protn. at 100	Boswell et al. (1974) Boswell et al. (1974)
$CONH_2$	$4\text{-}CF_3C_6H_4O$	MES ED_{50} 32; Met ED_{50} 37	Boswell et al. (1974)
CONHMe	$4\text{-}CF_3C_6H_4O$	MES ED_{50} 36; Met ED_{50} 20	Boswell et al. (1974)
$CONMe_2$	$4\text{-}CF_3C_6H_4O$	MES ED_{50} 28; Met ED_{50} 64	Boswell et al. (1974)

R	Other substituents[a]	Activity	Reference
$CH_2CONHC_6H_3Me_2\text{-}2,6$	R_3 = OCOMe	MES, 100% protn. at 400	Zenitz (1964)
$CH_2CONHCONHC_6H_4Me\text{-}2$	R_1 = Me	Met, 50% protn. at 100 (ip)	Gupta et al. (1974)
$CH_2CONHCONHC_6H_4Me\text{-}3$	R_1 = Me	Met, 30 protn. at 100 (ip)	Gupta et al. (1974)
$CH_2CONHCONHC_6H_4Me\text{-}4$	R_1 = Me	Met, 50 protn. at 100 (ip)	Gupta et al. (1974)
$CH_2CONHCONHC_6H_3Me_2\text{-}3,4$	R_1 = Me	Met, 60% protn. at 100 (ip)	Gupta et al. (1974)
$CH_2CONHCONHC_6H_4OMe\text{-}2$	R_1 = Me	Met, 30% protn. at 100 (ip)	Gupta et al. (1974)
$CH_2CONHCONHC_6H_4OMe\text{-}4$	R_1 = Me	Met, 20% protn. at 100 (ip)	Gupta et al. (1974)
$CH_2CONHCONHC_6H_4Cl\text{-}2$	R_1 = Me	Met, 30% protn. at 100 (ip)	Gupta et al. (1974)

CH$_2$CONHCONHC$_6$H$_4$Me-2	R$_2$ = Me	Met, 60% protn. at 100 (ip)	Gupta *et al.* (1974)
CH$_2$CONHCONHC$_6$H$_4$Me-4	R$_2$ = Me	Met, 60% protn. at 100 (ip)	Gupta *et al.* (1974)
CH$_2$CONHCONHC$_6$H$_3$Me$_2$-3,4	R$_2$ = Me	Met, 40% protn. at 100 (ip)	Gupta *et al.* (1974)
CH$_2$CONHCONHC$_6$H$_4$OMe-2	R$_2$ = Me	Met, 60% protn. at 100 (ip)	Gupta *et al.* (1974)
CH$_2$CONHCONHC$_6$H$_4$Cl-2	R$_2$ = Me	Met, 10% protn. at 100 (ip)	Gupta *et al.* (1974)
H	R$_1$ = C(OH)Ph$_2$ (S)	MES ED$_{50}$ 38	Portoghese *et al.* (1968)
H	R$_1$ = C(OH)Ph$_2$ (R)	MES ED$_{50}$ 55	Portoghese *et al.* (1968)
R	R$_2$ = O$_2$CCHPh$_2$	Active	Mochizuki *et al.* (1974)
(CH$_2$)$_n$OCH$_2$C(=CH$_2$)Ar	R$_1$ = Me	ES, active	Elpern and Bandurco (1972)
NH$_2$	R$_4$ = OH; R$_5$ = Ph	MES ED$_{50}$ 38	Harper *et al.* (1967)
Me	R$_2$ = OCOPh; R$_3$ = Ph	Active	Hirata *et al.* (1974)
Me	R$_4$, R$_5$ = [structure]	ES, 90% protn. at 30; Met, none	Sharma *et al.* (1968)
Me	R$_4$, R$_5$ = [structure with S]	ES, 60% protn. at 20; Met, none	Sharma *et al.* (1968)
Me	R$_4$, R$_5$ = [structure]	Active	Houlihan and Nadelson (1972)
Et	R$_2$ = OCOCH(C$_6$H$_5$)$_2$	Active	Fujimoto (1975)

(*continued*)

TABLE XVIII—*Continued*

B. Miscellaneous derivatives

Compound	Activity	Reference
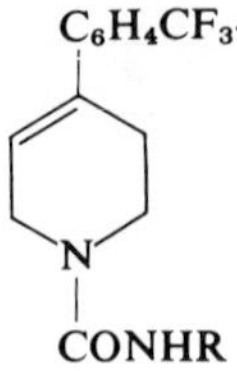C6H4CF3-3 N CONHR	Active	Helsley (1971)
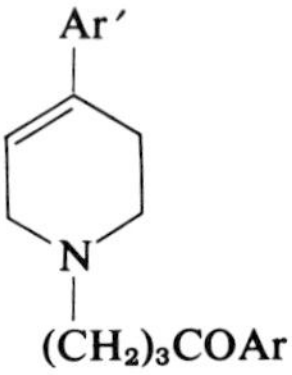Ar′ N (CH2)3COAr	Active	Janssen (1961)
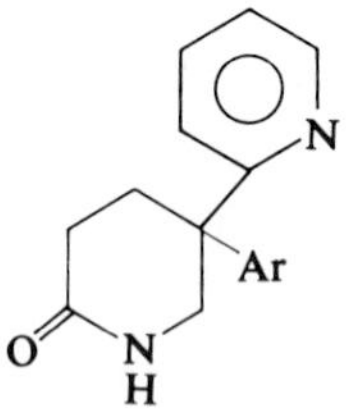N Ar O N H	Active	Hoffmann *et al.* (1956)
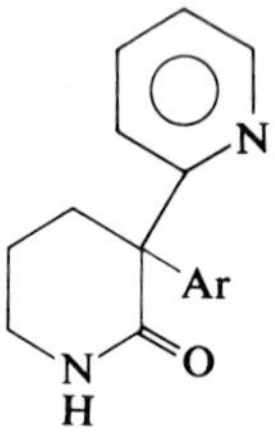N Ar N H O	Active	Hoffmann *et al.* (1956)

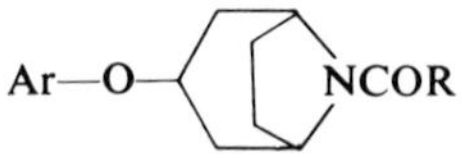
Ar—O
NCOR

Ar	R	Activity	Reference
3-$CF_3C_6H_4$	NH_2 (α)	MES ED_{50} 23 (ip); Met ED_{50} 47 (ip)	Boswell *et al.* (1974)
3-$CF_3C_6H_4$	NH_2 (β)	MES ED_{50} 29 (ip); Met ED_{50} 47 (ip)	Boswell *et al.* (1974)
3-$CF_3C_6H_4$	NHMe (α)	MES ED_{50} 43 (ip); Met ED_{50} 53 (ip)	Boswell *et al.* (1974)
3-$CF_3C_6H_4$	NHME (β)	MES ED_{50} 28 (ip); Met ED_{50} 72 (ip)	Boswell *et al.* (1974)
4-$CF_3C_6H_4$	NH_2 (α)	MES ED_{50} 15 (ip); Met ED_{50} 33 (ip)	Boswell *et al.* (1974)
4-$CF_3C_6H_4$	NHEt (α)	MES ED_{50} 36 (ip); Met ED_{50} 34 (ip)	Boswell *et al.* (1974)
3-$CF_3C_6H_4$	NMe_2 (β)	MES ED_{50} 15 (ip); Met, 80% protn. at 200	Boswell *et al.* (1974)

TABLE XVIII—*Continued*

Compound	Activity	Reference
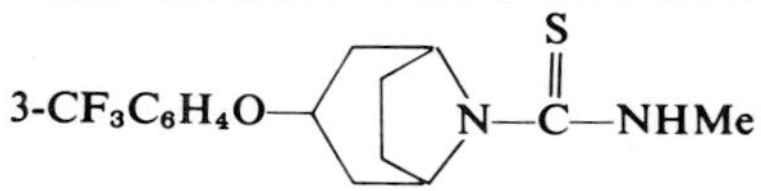	MES ED_{50} 74 (ip); Met, 0% protn. at 179	Boswell *et al.* (1974)
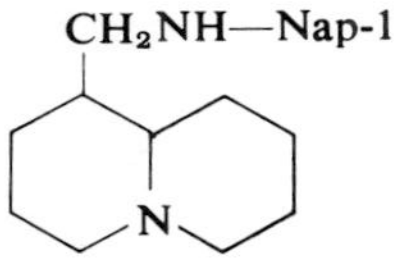	ES, active at 100	Boido and Sparatore (1974)
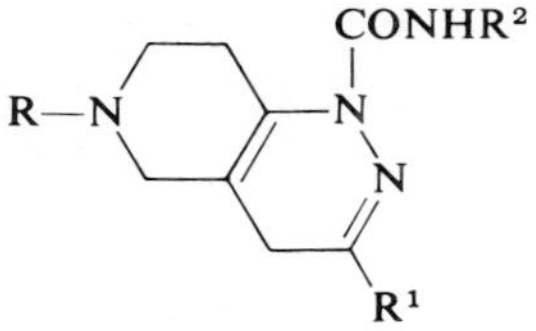	Active	Nakanishi *et al.* (1973a, 1974c,d,e,f)
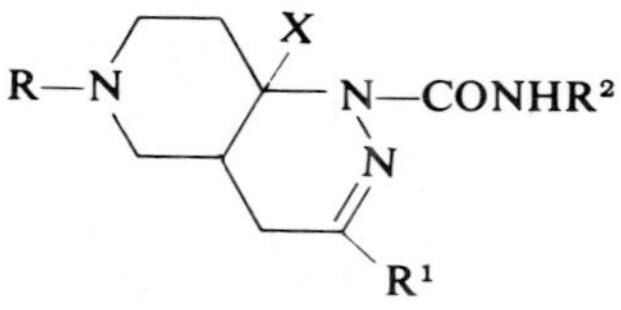	Active	Nakanishi *et al.* (1974e,f)
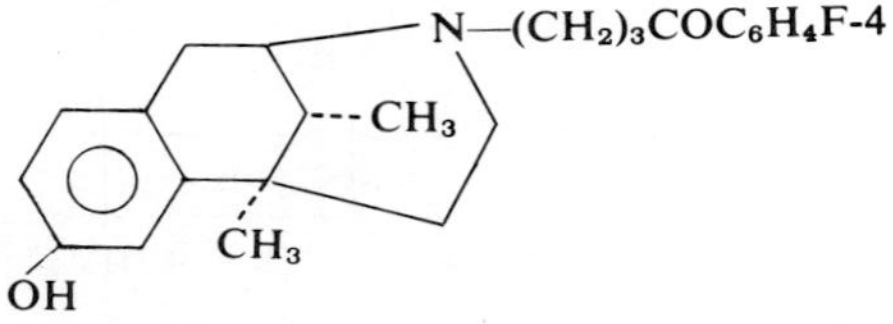	sl. act.	Yamamoto *et al.* (1975)

(*continued*)

TABLE XVIII—*Continued*

Compound	Activity	Reference
	Met, active	Nedelec *et al.* (1973a)
	R = H: MES ED$_{50}$ 20 (po) R = Me: MES ED$_{50}$ 63 (po) R = various: Active	Gootjes *et al.* (1972) Gootjes *et al.* (1972) Dobson and Davis (1971)

R	R$_1$	R$_2$	X	Activity	Reference
H	H	OH	O	Active	Dobson and Davis (1970a,b)
H	OH	H	H$_2$	ES, active; Met. act. 1/300 LD$_{50}$	Davis and Dobson (1972)
H	OH	=O	O	ES, active	Davis and Dobson (1969)
R	R$_1$	H	H$_2$	Active	Russel (1971)

a All R's are H except as noted.

TABLE XIX PYRIDINE DERIVATIVES

A. Pyridines[a]

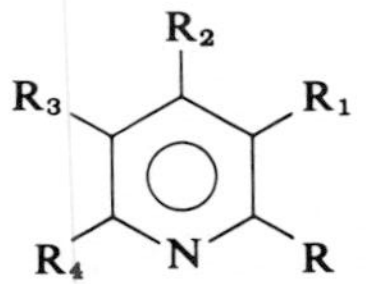

R	R_1	R_2	Activity	Reference
Me	Et	H	Met ED_{50} > 50 (iv)	Lindberg (1971a)
Me	CH_2CH_2Cl	H	Met ED_{50} > 350 (ip), 85 (iv)	Lindberg et al. (1967)
$(CH_2)_3Cl$	H	H	Met ED_{50} 65 (iv)	Lindberg et al. (1967)
H	$(CH_2)_3Cl$	H	Met ED_{50} 65 (iv)	Lindberg et al. (1967)
H	H	$(CH_2)_3Cl$	Met ED_{50} 50 (iv)	Lindberg et al. (1967)
$(CH_2)_2Cl$	H	H	Met ED_{50} 100 (iv)	Lindberg et al. (1967)
H	$(CH_2)_2Cl$	H	Met ED_{50} 115 (iv)	Lindberg et al. (1967)
$(CH_2)_2Cl$	H	H; R_4 = Me	Met ED_{50} 60 (iv)	Lindberg et al. (1967)
CH_2Cl	H	H; R_4 = Me	Met ED_{50} 110 (iv)	Lindberg et al. (1967)
H	H	$NH(CH_2)_2Ph$	MES, 60% protn. at 5 (ip)	Jain et al. (1968)
H	NH_2	$NH(CH_2)_2C_6H_4OMe-4$	MES, 20% protn. at 38 (ip)	Jain et al. (1968)

(continued)

TABLE XIX—*Continued*

R	R_1	R_2	Activity	Reference
$NH(CH_2)_2C_6H_3(OMe)_2$-3,4	NH_2	H	MES, 40% protn. at 100 (ip)	Jain *et al.* (1968)
H	NH_2	$NH(CH_2)_2Ph$	MES, 40% protn. at 38 (ip)	Jain *et al.* (1968)
H; R_3 = NO_2	NO_2	$NH(CH_2)_2N$⬡	Met, active	Vohra *et al.* (1965)
H; R_3 = Br	NO_2	$NH(CH_2)_2N$⬡	Met, active	Vohra *et al.* (1965)
H	NO_2	$NH(CH_2)_2Ph$	Met, active	Vohra *et al.* (1965)
H; R_3 = Br	NH_2	$NH(CH_2)_2N$⬡	ES, active	Vohra *et al.* (1965)
H	NH_2	$-N\!\!\underset{}{\bigcirc}\!\!NC_6H_4CF_3$-3	MES ED_{50} 12.6 (po), 7.6 (ip); Met, 90% protn. at 20	Ahmad (1967)
$PhCH_2N(CH_2)_2NMe_2$	H	H	MES ED_{50} 43; Met, inact. 50	Saxena *et al.* (1969)
$4\text{-}ClC_6H_4N(CH_2)_2NMe_2$	H	H	MES, inact.; Met partially act. 80	Saxena *et al.* (1969)
NH_2	CONHR	H	Active	Chesnokov *et al.* (1973)
Cl	H	CONH▷; R_4 = RO	Active	Dufour (1973)

H	$Ph(CH_2)_2NH$	NH_2	MES, 70% protn. at 50 (ip); Met, 70% protn. at 50	Ahmad et al. (1966)
H	NH_2	$Ph(CH_2)_2NH$	MES, 70% protn. at 50; Met, 70% protn. at 50	Ahmad et al. (1966)
H	NH_2	$PhCH_2CH(Me)NH$	MES, 25% protn. at 40; Met, 40% protn. at 40	Ahmad et al. (1966)
H	NH_2	[piperazine N–NPh]	MES, 100% protn. at 40; Met, 100% protn. at 40	Ahmad et al. (1966)
H	H	COC_6H_4F-4	MES ED_{50} 3.51 moles/kg	Breen et al. (1973)
H	H	$COC_6H_4CF_3$-3	MES ED_{50} 3.43 moles/kg	Breen et al. (1973)
H	H	COC_6H_4OMe-2	MES ED_{50} 3.41 moles/kg	Breen et al. (1973)
H	H	COC_6H_4Me-2	MES ED_{50} 3.41 moles/kg	Breen et al. (1973)
H	H	$COPh$	MES ED_{50} 3.39 moles/kg	Breen et al. (1973)
H	H	COC_6H_4OMe-4	MES ED_{50} 3.27 moles/kg	Breen et al. (1973)
H	H	$COC_6H_3Me_2$-2,5	MES ED_{50} 3.25 moles/kg	Breen et al. (1973)
H	H	COC_6H_4Cl-4	MES ED_{50} 3.24 moles/kg	Breen et al. (1973)
H	H	COC_6H_4Me-4	MES ED_{50} 3.19 moles/kg	Breen et al. (1973)
H	H	COC_6H_4Bu-t-4	MES ED_{50} 3.17 moles/kg	Breen et al. (1973)

(continued)

TABLE XIX—*Continued*

R	R_1	R_2	Activity	Reference
H	H	$COC_6H_4NO_2$-4	MES ED_{50} 3.07 moles/kg	Breen *et al.* (1973)
H	H	$COC_6H_4SO_2NH_2$-4	MES ED_{50} 2.56 moles/kg	Breen *et al.* (1973)
H	H	COC_6H_4OH-2	MES ED_{50} 2.70 moles/kg	Breen *et al.* (1973)
H	H	CH_2COR	Active	Brust *et al.* (1966)
H	H	$CH_2CH(OH)R$	Active	Brust *et al.* (1966)
H	H	$CH_2C(NR_2)RCH_2$Pyr-4	Active	Brust *et al.* (1970)
Me	HO	CHO, R_3 = 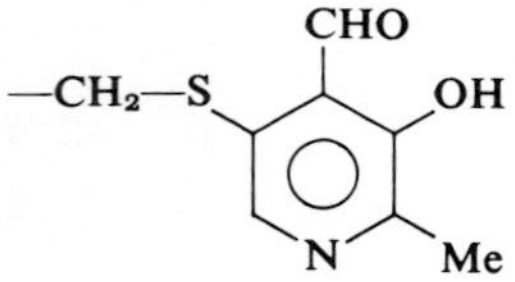	Active	Merck (1965)
$CH_2NHCOC_6H_4Me_2$-3,5	H	H	Active	Martinez-Roldan *et al.* (1974)
H	$CH_2NHCOC_6H_4Me_2$-3,5	H	Active	Martinez-Roldan *et al.* (1974)
H	H	$CH_2NHCOC_6H_4Me_2$-3,5	Active	Martinez-Roldan *et al.* (1974)
H	H	COPh	MES ED_{50} 35	Frank *et al.* (1971)
H	H	COMe	MES ED_{50} 150	Frank *et al.* (1971)
H	H	COEt	MES ED_{50} 200	Frank *et al.* (1971)
H	H	COPr-*n*	MES ED_{50} 99	Frank *et al.* (1971)
H	H	CONu-*n*	MES ED_{50} 75	Frank *et al.* (1971)
H	H	COC_5H_{11}-*n*	MES ED_{50} 149	Frank *et al.* (1971)
H	H	COC_6H_{13}-*n*	MES ED_{50} 87	Frank *et al.* (1971)
H	H	COC_7H_{15}-*n*	MES ED_{50} 225	Frank *et al.* (1971)
H	H	COC_6H_{11}	MES ED_{50} 98	Frank *et al.* (1971)

			Activity	Reference
NHPh	CONHPh	H	Active	Mikhalev et al. (1975)
NHC$_4$H$_9$-n	CONHPh	H	Active	Mikhalev et al. (1975)
NHC$_6$H$_4$OMe-4	CONHPh	H	Active	Mikhalev et al. (1975)
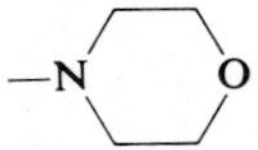 (morpholino ring)	CONHPh	H	Active	Mikhalev et al. (1975)
H	C(=NH)NHC$_6$H$_4$CF$_3$-3	H	MES ED$_{50}$ 42; Met ED$_{50}$ 60	Raynaud and Gouret (1972)
H	C(=NH)NHC$_6$H$_3$Cl-3-Me-4	H	MES ED$_{50}$ 130	Raynaud and Gouret (1972)
H	C(=NH)NHC$_6$H$_3$Cl$_2$-3,4	H	MES ED$_{50}$ 21; Met ED$_{50}$ 95	Raynaud and Gouret (1972)
H	C(=NH)NHC$_6$H$_4$OMe-2	H	MES, 10% protn. at 100	Raynaud and Gouret (1972)
H	C(=NH)NHC$_6$H$_4$OMe-4	H	Met, 10% protn. at 100	Raynaud and Gouret (1972)
H	C(=NH)NHC$_6$H$_3$(OMe)$_2$-2,5	H	MES, 50% protn. at 100	Raynaud and Gouret (1972)
H	C(=NH)NHC$_6$H$_4$Me-4	H	MES, 40% protn. at 100	Raynaud and Gouret (1972)
H	C(=NH)NHNap-1	H	MES ED$_{50}$ 20	Raynaud and Gouret (1972)
H	C(=NH)NHNap-2	H	MES ED$_{50}$ 50	Raynaud and Gouret (1972)
H	H	C(=NH)NHC$_6$H$_4$CF$_3$-3	MES ED$_{50}$ 20	Raynaud and Gouret (1972)
H	H	C(=NH)NHC$_6$H$_3$Cl-3-Me-4	MES, 10% protn. at 100	Raynaud and Gouret (1972)
H	H	C(=NH)NHC$_6$H$_4$Cl-4	MES, 30% protn. at 100	Raynaud and Gouret (1972)

(continued)

413

TABLE XIX—*Continued*

R	R_1	R_2	Activity	Reference
H	H	$C(=NH)NHC_6H_3Cl_2$-3,4	MES ED_{50} 70; Met ED_{50} 145	Raynaud and Gouret (1972)
H	H	$C(=NH)NHC_6H_3(OMe)_2$-2,5	MES, 10% protn. at 100	Raynaud and Gouret (1972)
H	H	$C(=NH)NHC_6H_4OH$-2	MES, 20% protn. at 100	Raynaud and Gouret (1972)
H	H	$C(=NH)NHNap$-1	MES, 30% protn. at 100	Raynaud and Gouret (1972)
H	H	$C(=NH)NHNap$-2	MES, 50% protn. at 100	Raynaud and Gouret (1972)
n-BuO	CONHNHMe	n-BuO	Met and ES, active at 35 (ip)	Parravicini et al. (1975)
n-BuO	CONMeNHMe	n-BuO	Met and ES, active at 75 (ip)	Parravicini et al. (1975)
n-BuO	CON(morpholine) 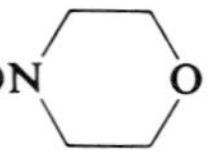	n-BuO	Met and ES, active at 150 (ip)	Parravicini et al. (1975)

B. Miscellaneous derivatives

Compound	Activity	Reference
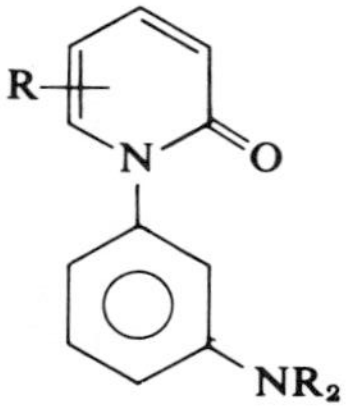	Active	Scudi et al. (1960a)

Structure	Activity	Reference
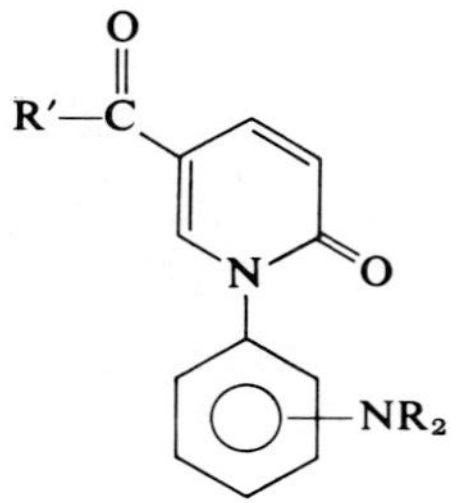 (pyridone structure with $R'\text{-}C(=O)$ and NR_2)	Active	Scudi *et al.* (1960b)
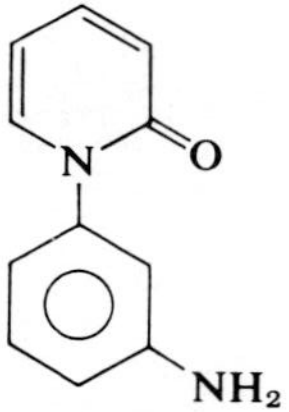 (pyridone structure with NH_2)	Met, active	Steiner and Himwich (1963)
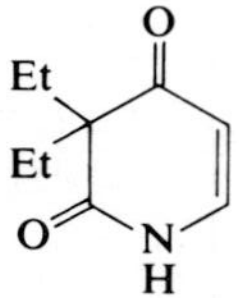 (Et, Et substituted piperidinedione structure)	ES, 70% protn. at 50; Met, active at 50	Osumi *et al.* (1967)
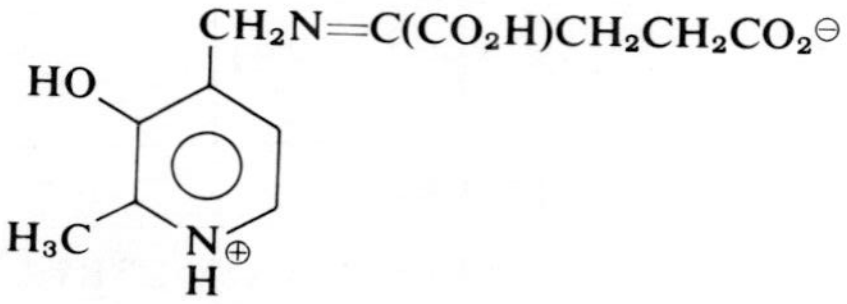 (pyridinium structure: $CH_2N\!=\!C(CO_2H)CH_2CH_2CH_2CO_2^{\ominus}$, HO, H_3C, $\overset{\oplus}{N}H$)	Active	Martinez-Roldan and Fernandez (1973, 1974a,b)

(continued)

415

TABLE XIX—*Continued*

Compound	Activity	Reference
	Active	Martinez-Roldan and Fernandez (1973, 1974a,b)
	Active	Mathes and DaVanzo (1963)
	Active	Schumann (1965)
	Met, active	Carboni *et al.* (1975)

Compound	X	R	R_1	Activity	Reference
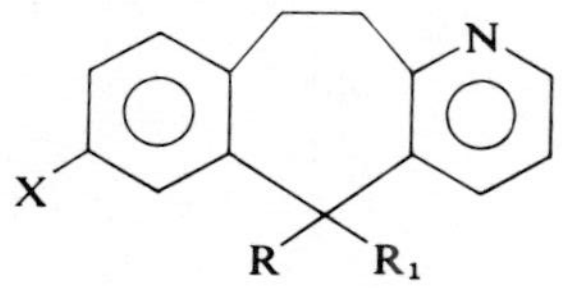	H	=NOCOEt		Active	vander Stelt et al. (1971)
	H	=NOCONHMe		Active	vander Stelt et al. (1971)
	H	OH	C≡CH	Active	vander Stelt et al. (1971)
	H	H	$CONH_2$	Active	vander Stelt et al. (1971)
	Cl	=O		MES ED_{50} 150; Met ED_{50} 220	vander Stelt et al. (1972)
	Cl	H	OH	MES ED_{50} 63; Met ED_{50} 200	vander Stelt et al. (1972)
	HO	H	OH	MES ED_{50} 200; Met ED_{50} 200	vander Stelt et al. (1972)
	H	H	OH	MES ED_{50} 38; Met ED_{50} 170	vander Stelt et al. (1972)
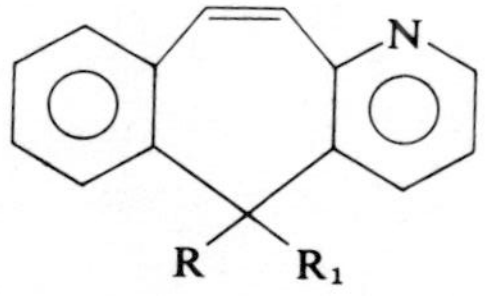		=NOCOEt		Active	vander Stelt et al. (1971)
		=NOCONHMe		Active	vander Stelt et al. (1971)
		H	NH_2	Active	vander Stelt et al. (1971)
		H	$CONH_2$	Active	vander Stelt et al. (1971)
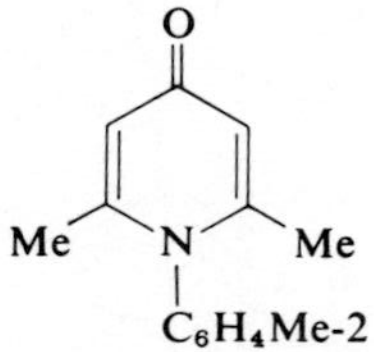				MES ED_{50} > 100	Boltze et al. (1963)

C. Quinoline derivatives

Compound	Activity	Reference
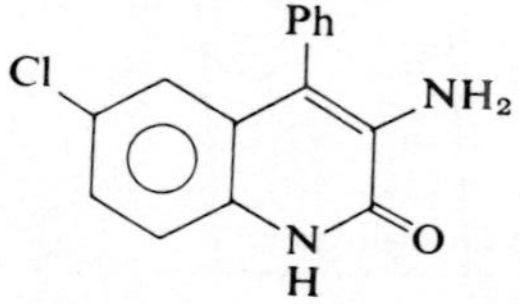	Active	Sulkowski (1962)

(continued)

417

TABLE XIX—*Continued*

Compound	Activity	Reference
	ES, active	Wei and Bell (1970)
	ES, active	Otto (1970)
	Active	Thyagarajan *et al.* (1963)
	MES ED_{50} 199 (ip)	Daruwala *et al.* (1974)
	R = H: MES ED_{50} 324 (ip) R = Me: MES ED_{50} 118 (ip) R = Et: MES ED_{50} 100 (ip)	Daruwala *et al.* (1974) Daruwala *et al.* (1974) Daruwala *et al.* (1974)

Compound	X	R	Activity	Reference
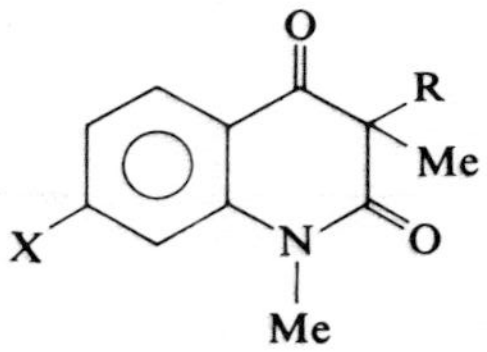	H	Me	MES ED$_{50}$ 76 (ip)	Daruwala et al. (1974)
	Cl	Me	MES ED$_{50}$ 168 (ip)	Daruwala et al. (1974)
	OMe	Me	MES ED$_{50}$ 236 (ip)	Daruwala et al. (1974)
	H	Et	MES ED$_{50}$ 107 (ip)	Daruwala et al. (1974)
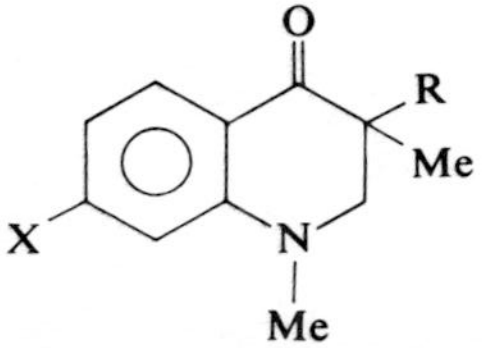	H	Cl	MES ED$_{50}$ 134 (ip)	Daruwala et al. (1974)
	Me	Cl	MES ED$_{50}$ 138 (ip)	Daruwala et al. (1974)
	Me	OMe	MES ED$_{50}$ 160 (ip)	Daruwala et al. (1974)

D. Isoquinoline derivatives

Compound	Activity	Reference
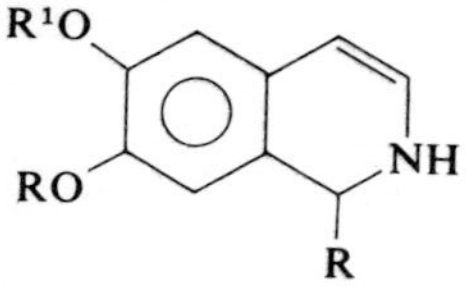	Active	Jansen et al. (1974)
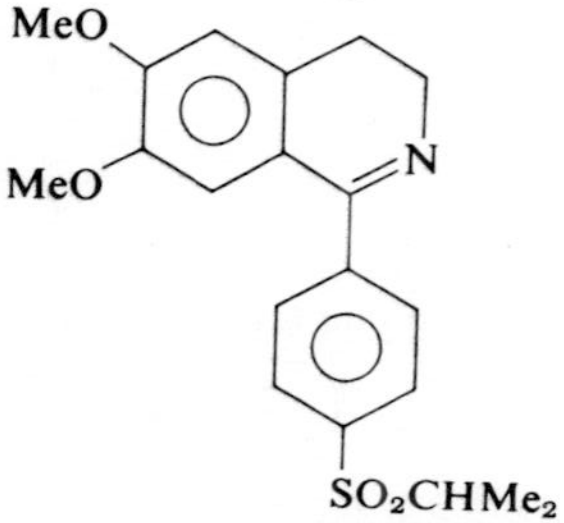	Met ED$_{50}$ 250; MES ED$_{50}$ 200	Chodnekar and Blum (1968)

(continued)

419

TABLE XIX—*Continued*

Compound	Activity	Reference
	R = H: MES, sl. act.; Met, inact. R = COMe: MES, mod. act.; Met, sl. act.	Neumeyer *et al.* (1973) Neumeyer *et al.* (1973)
	Active	Kutter *et al.* (1974)
	Active	Deak *et al.* (1972); Gy and Gyan (1974a,b)
	R = H: MES ED_{50} 150 (ip) R = $PhCH_2$: MES ED_{50} > 300 (ip)	Aeberli *et al.* (1967) Aeberli *et al.* (1967)

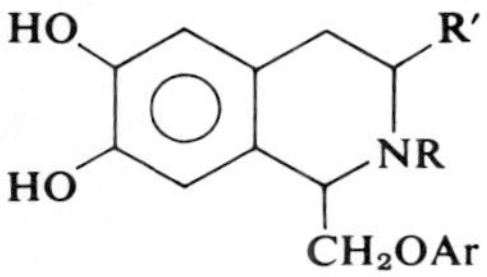	Active	Kishimoto *et al.* (1974a,b)
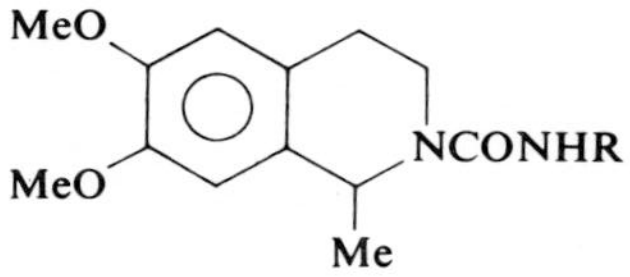	Active	Takayama *et al.* (1973a,b)
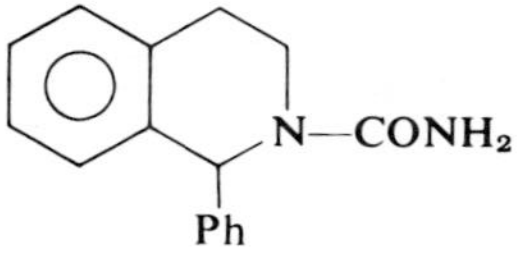	Active	Takayama *et al.* (1973a,b)
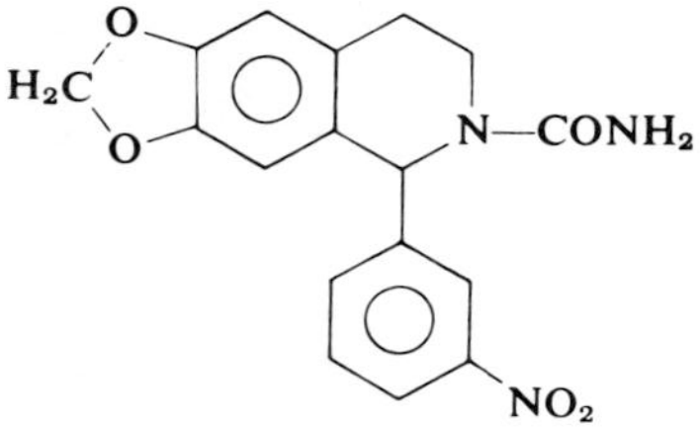	Active	Takayama *et al.* (1973a,b)
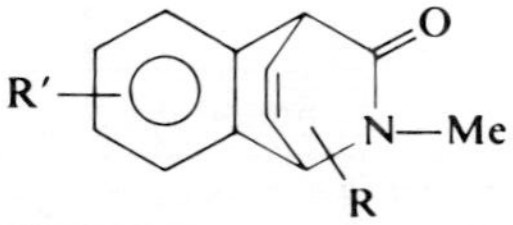	Active	Giurgea (1972)

(*continued*)

TABLE XIX—*Continued*

Compound	Activity	Reference
	Active	Parke Davis & Co. (1961); Godefroi (1962)
	$R = Ph(CH_2)_2$: Met ED_{50} 50 (ip) $R = Ph$: Met ED_{50} 57 (ip)	Archer and Schulenberg (1972a,b,c) Archer and Schulenberg (1972a,b,c)
	$X = H$: MES ED_{50} 15; Met, inact. $X = Cl$: MES ED_{50} 34; Met, inact.	Coyne and Cusic (1968) Coyne and Cusic (1968)
	Active	Kunstmann and Kaiser (1975)

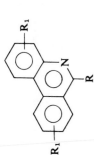

R^b	Activity	Reference
4-Et$_2$N(CH$_2$)$_2$OC$_6$H$_4$	Met ED$_{50}$ 18 (po); MES ED$_{50}$ 18 (po)	Ashford *et al.* (1971)
3-Et$_2$N(CH$_2$)$_2$OC$_6$H$_4$	Met ED$_{50}$ 8 (po); MES ED$_{50}$ 23 (po)	Ashford *et al.* (1971)
2-Et$_2$N(CH$_2$)$_2$OC$_6$H$_4$	Met ED$_{50}$ > 40 (po); MES ED$_{50}$ 62 (po)	Ashford *et al.* (1971)
4-Et$_2$N(CH$_2$)$_2$SC$_6$H$_4$	Met ED$_{50}$ 16 (po); MES ED$_{50}$ 15 (po)	Ashford *et al.* (1971)
4-Et$_2$N(CH$_2$)$_2$NHC$_6$H$_4$	Met ED$_{50}$ 25 (po); MES ED$_{50}$ 50 (po)	Ashford *et al.* (1971)
4-Et$_2$N(CH$_2$)$_3$OC$_6$H$_4$	Met ED$_{50}$ 20 (po); MES ED$_{50}$ 29 (po)	Ashford *et al.* (1971)
4-Me$_2$N(CH$_2$)$_2$OC$_6$H$_4$	Met ED$_{50}$ 11 (po); MES ED$_{50}$ 43 (po)	Ashford *et al.* (1971)
4-Me$_2$N(CH$_2$)$_3$OC$_6$H$_4$	Met ED$_{50}$ 12 (po); MES ED$_{50}$ 25 (po)	Ashford *et al.* (1971)
4-(PhCH$_2$)$_2$N(CH$_2$)$_2$OC$_6$H$_4$	Met ED$_{50}$ 100–200 (po); MES ED$_{50}$ > 200 (po)	Ashford *et al.* (1971)
![4-N(CH$_2$)$_2$OC$_6$H$_4$ piperidine]	Met ED$_{50}$ 11 (po); MES ED$_{50}$ < 25 (po)	Ashford *et al.* (1971)
![4-N(CH$_2$)$_2$OC$_6$H$_4$ morpholine]	Met ED$_{50}$ 23 (po); MES ED$_{50}$ 55 (po)	Ashford *et al.* (1971)
4-EtNH(CH$_2$)$_2$OC$_6$H$_4$	Met ED$_{50}$ 12 (po); MES ED$_{50}$ 24 (po)	Ashford *et al.* (1971)
4-H$_2$N(CH$_2$)$_2$OC$_6$H$_4$	Met ED$_{50}$ 13 (po); MES ED$_{50}$ 16 (po)	Ashford *et al.* (1971)
4-Et$_2$N—⟨phenyl⟩—OC$_6$H$_4$	Met ED$_{50}$ > 200 (po); MES ED$_{50}$ > 200 (po)	Ashford *et al.* (1971)
4-Et$_2$N(CH$_2$)$_2$OC$_6$H$_4$, R$_1$ = 3,8-(NO$_2$)$_2$	Met ED$_{50}$ > 200 (po); MES ED$_{50}$ > 200 (po)	Ashford *et al.* (1971)
4-Et$_2$N(CH$_2$)$_2$OC$_6$H$_4$, R$_1$ = 8-(CH$_2$)$_2$NEt$_2$	Met ED$_{50}$ > 200 (po); MES ED$_{50}$ > 200 (po)	Ashford *et al.* (1971)

(*continued*)

423

TABLE XIX—*Continued*

R^b	Activity	Reference
$4\text{-Et}_2\text{N}(CH_2)_2OC_6H_4$, $R_1 = 3,8\text{-}(NH_2)_2$	Met $ED_{50} > 200$ (po); MES $ED_{50} > 200$ (po)	Ashford *et al.* (1971)
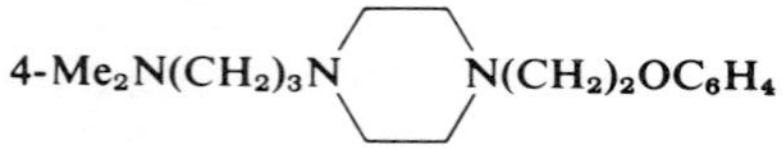 $4\text{-Me}_2\text{N}(CH_2)_3\text{N}\!\!\diagdown\!\!\text{N}(CH_2)_2OC_6H_4$	Met $ED_{50} > 200$ (po); MES $ED_{50} > 200$ (po)	Ashford *et al.* (1971)
$NH\text{-}4\text{-Et}_2\text{N}(CH_2)_2OC_6H_4$	Met ED_{50} 18–25 (po); MES $ED_{50} > 100$ (po)	Ashford *et al.* (1971)
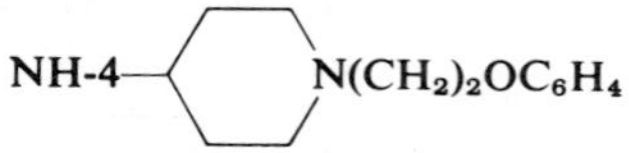 $NH\text{-}4\!\!\diagdown\!\!\text{N}(CH_2)_2OC_6H_4$	Met ED_{50} 14 (po); MES ED_{50} 70 (po)	Ashford *et al.* (1971)
$(CH_2)_2\text{-}4\text{-Et}_2\text{N}(CH_2)_2OC_6H_4$	Met ED_{50} 54 (po); MES ED_{50} 100 (po)	Ashford *et al.* (1971)
$CH_2\text{-}4\text{-Et}_2\text{N}(CH_2)_2OC_6H_4$	Met ED_{50} 19 (po); MES ED_{50} 28 (po)	Ashford *et al.* (1971)

[a] R_3, $R_4 = H$ unless otherwise noted.
[b] $R_1 = H$ except as noted.

TABLE XX   PYRAN DERIVATIVES

A. Monocyclic compounds

Compound	R	Activity	Reference
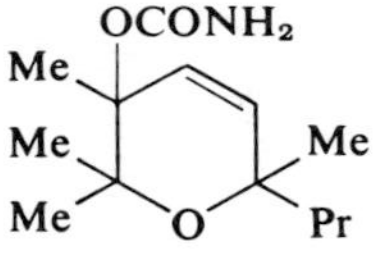 (pyran structure: OCONH₂, Me, Me, Me, Me, Pr)		Met and ES, active	Khaldarov and Lebedeva (1973)

Compound		Reference
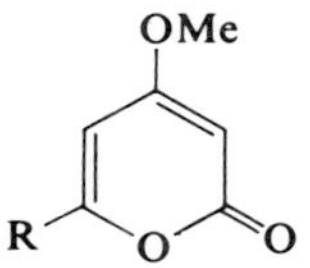 PhCH=CH	MES ED$_{50}$ 4.3 (iv), 180 (ip)	Meyer and Kretzchmar (1969)
Ph(CH$_2$)$_2$	MES ED$_{50}$ 4.4 (iv), 90 (ip)	Meyer and Kretzchmar (1969)
3,4-CH$_2$O$_2$C$_6$H$_3$CH=CH	MES ED$_{50}$ 5.7 (iv), 3700 (ip)	Meyer and Kretzchmar (1969)
3,4-CH$_2$O$_2$C$_6$H$_3$(CH$_2$)$_2$	MES ED$_{50}$ 8.2 (iv), 45 (ip)	Meyer and Kretzchmar (1969)
4-MeOC$_6$H$_4$CH=CH	MES ED$_{50}$ 10.6 (iv), 1000 (ip)	Meyer and Kretzchmar (1969)
4-MeOC$_6$H$_4$(CH$_2$)$_2$	MES ED$_{50}$ 7.6 (iv), 190 (ip)	Meyer and Kretzchmar (1969)
Me	MES ED$_{50}$ 64 (iv), 108 (ip)	Meyer and Kretzchmar (1969)
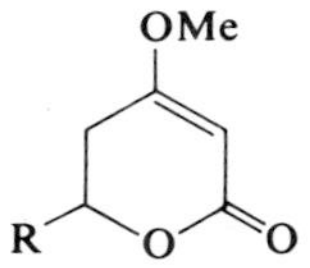 Me	MES ED$_{50}$ 104 (iv), 135 (ip)	Meyer and Kretzchmar (1969)
Ph(CH$_2$)$_2$	MES ED$_{50}$ 3.4 (iv), 28.7 (ip)	Meyer and Kretzchmar (1969)
PhCH=CH	MES ED$_{50}$ 4.2 (iv), 21.3 (ip)	Meyer and Kretzchmar (1969)
3,4-CH$_2$O$_2$C$_6$H$_3$(CH$_2$)$_2$	MES ED$_{50}$ 6.2 (iv), 23.5 (ip)	Meyer and Kretzchmar (1969)
3,4-CH$_2$O$_2$C$_6$H$_3$CH=CH	MES ED$_{50}$ 4.7 (iv), 19 (ip)	Meyer and Kretzchmar (1969)
4-MeOC$_6$H$_4$(CH$_2$)$_2$	MES ED$_{50}$ 8.5 (iv), 125 (ip)	Meyer and Kretzchmar (1969)
4-MeOC$_6$H$_4$CH=CH	MES ED$_{50}$ 13.5 (iv), 58 (ip)	Meyer and Kretzchmar (1969)

B. Other pyrans

Compound	Activity	Reference
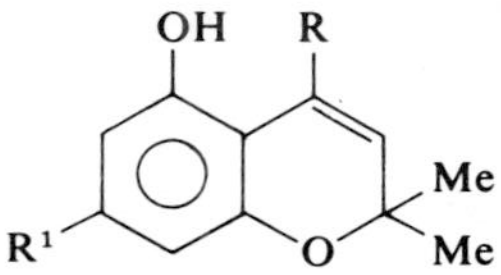	Active	Gardner and Tickle (1972)
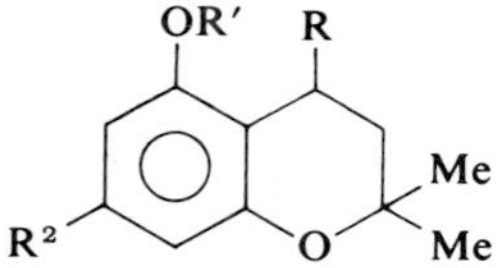	Active	Hadley (1973)
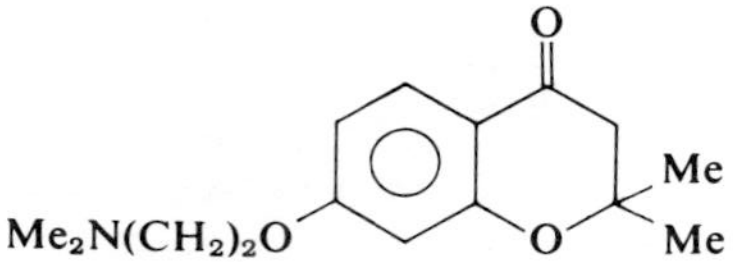	Active	Razdan and Mehta (1973)

(continued)

425

TABLE XX—*Continued*

Compound	Activity	Reference
CONH₂	MES ED₅₀ 54 (ip); 53 (po); Met ED₅₀ 45 (po)	Davis *et al.* (1964)
	Active	Winn *et al.* (1975)
	Active	Chaturvedi *et al.* (1974)

TABLE XX—*Continued*

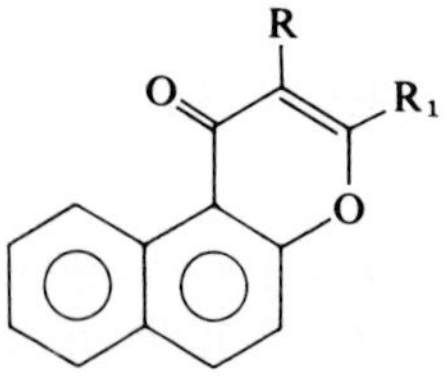

R	R_1	Activity	Reference
H	NEt_2	Met ED_{50} 45.6 (os)	Ermili *et al.* (1974a)
H	NMEt	Met ED_{50} 41.7 (os)	Ermili *et al.* (1974a)
H	NPr_2	Met ED_{50} 76.3 (os)	Ermili *et al.* (1974a)
H	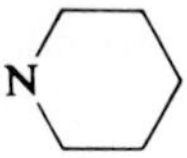 N(piperidine)	Met ED_{50} 50.8 (os)	Ermili *et al.* (1974a)
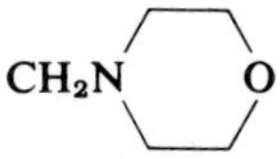 CH_2N(morpholine)	NMe_2	Met ED_{50} 45.5 (os)	Ermili *et al.* (1974b)
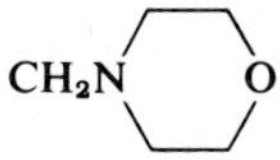 CH_2N(morpholine)	NEt_2	Met ED_{50} 37.3 (os)	Ermili *et al.* (1974b)
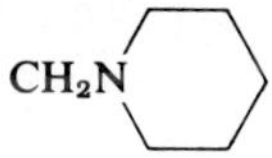 CH_2N(piperidine)	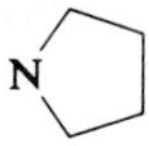 N(pyrrolidine)	Met ED_{50} 22.8 (os)	Ermili *et al.* (1974b)
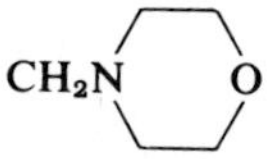 CH_2N(morpholine)	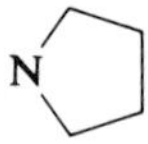 N(pyrrolidine)	Met ED_{50} 48.8 (os)	Ermili *et al.* (1974b)
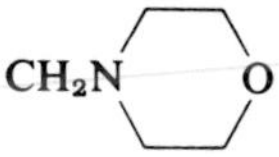 CH_2N(morpholine)	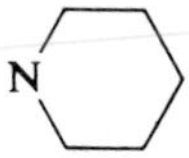 N(piperidine)	Met ED_{50} 50.2 (os)	Ermili *et al.* (1974b)

piperidines and pyridines. None of these compounds has been studied in any detail, although **VIII** has been reported (Ahmad, 1967) to be a better anti-convulsant in animals than diphenylhydantoin sodium. The benzopyran derivatives are discussed in Chapter 6.

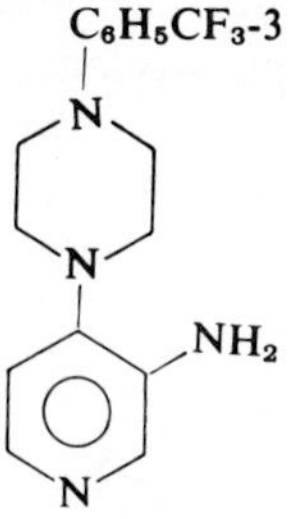

(VIII)

B. WITH MORE THAN ONE HETEROATOM

Tables XXII–XXXVI include various six-membered heterocyclic compounds with more than one heteroatom. Compounds such as the barbiturates and those related to primidone are included in Chapter 5.

A large number of benzhydrylpiperazines appear in Table XXIV. Some of these exhibit a profile of activity equal to or better than that of diphenylhydantoin (Craig, 1967). Studies indicate that assessment of 1-benzylhydryl-4-(6-methyl-2-pyridylmethylenimino)piperazine in primates is warranted (Edmonds and Stark, 1974; Edmonds *et al.*, 1974). The anticonvulsant activity of a series of piperazines was found to be independent of their ability to selectively inhibit NAD-dependent oxidations (Singh *et al.*, 1974c), while the anticonvulsant activity of another group of piperazines was independent of their ability to inhibit the oxidation of pyruvic acid (Chaturvedi *et al.*, 1975).

Sulthiame (**IX**), which was introduced in Europe in the sixties (Engelmeier, 1960; Flugel *et al.*, 1960; Raffauf, 1960), has been used for several years for the treatment of psychomotor seizures. Good results have also been reported in other forms of epilepsy. Like acetazolamide, sulthiame is a powerful inhibitor of carbonic anhydrase. The therapeutic index for sulthiame was

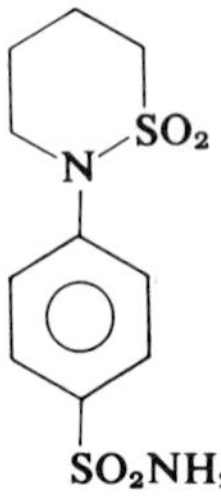

(IX)

found in the electroshock test to be 140 times greater than that of diphenylhydantoin (Wirth *et al.*, 1960). Clinical studies reveal that this drug, in addition to its effectiveness in patients with major motor and/or psychomotor epilepsy, does not possess a high incidence of serious untoward reactions (Livingston *et al.*, 1967b).

As can be seen from Table XXIII,B a tremendous number of 4-quinazolones have been prepared in studies of analogues of methaqualone (**X**).

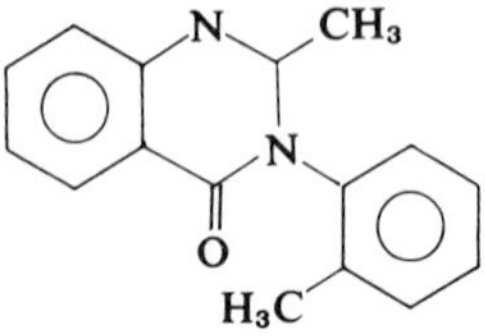

(X)

TABLE XXI THIOPYRAN DERIVATIVES

X	R	R_1	Activity	Reference
H	H	$CONH_2$	Met ED_{50} 29 (po); MES ED_{50} 34 (ip), 66 (po)	Davis *et al.* (1964)
Cl	$=CH(CH_2)_2NMe_2$		Met and ES, active 5–15 (po)	Dobrescu *et al.* (1974)
H	$=CH(CH_2)_2N$⟩N(CH_2)_2OH		MES ED_{50} 144; Met, partial protn. at 50	Saxena *et al.* (1969)

TABLE XXII PYRIDAZINE DERIVATIVES

A. 3-Pyridazones

R	R_1	R_2	R_3	Activity	Reference
H	H	Me	R	Met, active	Hammann (1960)
Ph	X	H	OMe	Active	Druey and Eichenberger (1957)
CH_2COX	R	R	R	Active	Engelbrecht and Lenke (1960)
$(CH_2)_2NO$	Me	H	Ph	ES, active	Laborit et al. (1965)
$(CH_2)_2Ar$	X	NRNHR'	H	Active	Linder (1973)
$2\text{-}F\text{-}5\text{-}CF_3C_6H_3$	Cl	$N(Me)NH_2$	H	Active	Linder (1974)

B. Phthalazines

R	R_1	Activity	Reference
Me	Ar	Active	Sullivan (1965)
CH_2CONMe_2	R	Active	Engelbrecht and Lenke (1960)
C_6H_5	$CH{=}CHC_6H_5$	MES $ED_{50} > 200$	Boltze et al. (1963)
$2\text{-}MeC_6H_4$	Me	MES ED_{50} 118	Boltze et al. (1963)

TABLE XXIII PYRIMIDINE DERIVATIVES

A. Pyrimidines

Compound	Activity	Reference
(NR$_2$, CONHR^1, R^2)	Active	Kim and Santilli (1970)
Ph-CHCH$_2$NH— pyrimidine, OH	MES ED$_{50}$ 125 (ip); Met ED$_{50}$ 70 (ip)	O'Dell et al. (1963)
(R^1, R)	ES, active	Hardtmann and Ott (1972, 1974)
(HN, CHR^1, Ar)	Active	Schwan et al. (1972)

(continued)

TABLE XXIII—*Continued*

Compound	Activity	Reference
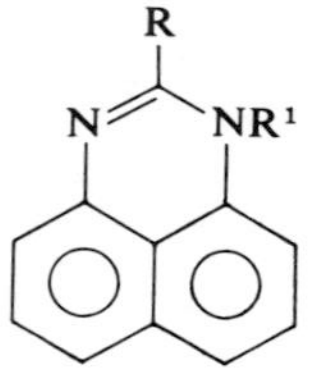	Met, active	Paragamian (1970)
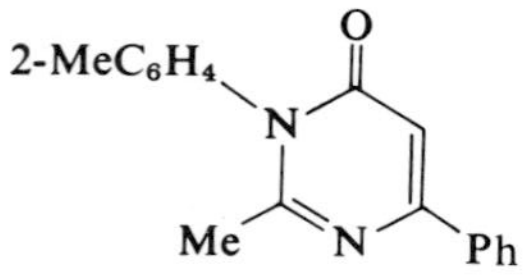	MES ED_{50} 98	Boltze *et al.* (1973)

B. 4-Quinazolones

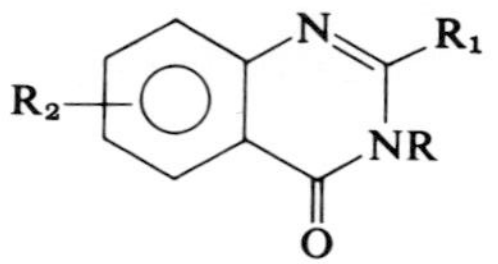

R	R_1	R_2	Activity	Reference
Ar	R_1	6-R_2	Active	Breuer *et al.* (1967)
2,4-$Cl_2C_6H_3$	H	H	Active	Hurmer and Vernin (1969)
2-MeC_6H_4	CH=CH-3-Pyr	H	Active	Karamchand Premchand Private Ltd. (1972, 1973)
Pyr	Pyr	H	Active	Noda *et al.* (1974)
Ar	R_1	R_2	Active	Olin Mathieson Chemical Corp. (1964)

	8-R2		
Et	H	Met ED$_{50}$ 54	Classe and Mos (1967)
R	H	Active	Philips' Gloeilampen-fabrieken (1965)
Ar	Me	Active	Stefanova et al. (1972)
2-MeC$_6$H$_4$	Me	Met and MES, active	Takagi et al. (1960)
		MES ED$_{50}$ 50 (ip); Met ED$_{50}$ 45 (ip)	Soncin (1961)
		Met ED$_{50}$ 28 (po)	Weaver et al. (1963)
		MES ED$_{50}$ 37 (ip); Met ED$_{50}$ 35 (ip)	Ochiai et al. (1972)
		MES ED$_{50}$ 50; Met ED$_{50}$ 70	Hurmer and Vernin (1967)
		MES ED$_{50}$ 19 (po); Met ED$_{50}$ 20 (po)	Gujral et al. (1957)
		MES ED$_{50}$ 30.5; Met ED$_{50}$ 16	Zilbermints (1964)
		MES ED$_{50}$ 115; Met ED$_{50}$ 37	Bonati and Rosati (1965)
		MES ED$_{50}$ 50	Boissier et al. (1967)
		MES ED$_{50}$ 50; Met ED$_{50}$ 70	Boltze et al. (1963)
		MES ED$_{50}$ 45; Met ED$_{50}$ 30	Leszkovszky et al. (1965)
		MES ED$_{50}$ 68	Swift et al. (1960)
		Met, 100% protn. at 50 (po)	Hisano et al. (1972)
		Met ED$_{50}$ 25–100	Breuer et al. (1971)
		Met, 3.3 × troxidone	Bianchi and David (1960)
CH=CH-hetero-Ar	H	Active	Troponwerke Dinklage & Co. (1964)
3-MeOC$_6$H$_4$	n-Pr	MES ED$_{50}$ 75	Somasekhara et al. (1972)
2-MeC$_6$H$_4$	n-Pr	MES and Met, 25% protn. at 200	Somasekhara et al. (1972)
2-MeC$_6$H$_4$	CH$_2$F	MES ED$_{50}$ 25 (ip); Met ED$_{50}$ 27 (ip)	Ochiai et al. (1972)
2-MeC$_6$H$_4$	CH=CH-2-Pyr	MES ED$_{50}$ 14.5; Met ED$_{50}$ 145 (ip)	Boltze et al. (1965)
2-ClC$_6$H$_4$	CH$_2$OMe	MES ED$_{50}$ 26.5	Kozhevnikov et al. (1970)
Ar	CH$_2$OMe	Active	Kozhevnikov et al. (1970)

8-Cl

R or 2-MeC$_6$H$_4$

(continued)

433

TABLE XXIII—*Continued*

R	R_1	R_2	Activity	Reference
4-ClC$_6$H$_4$	CH$_2$OMe	6-Br	Active	Kozhevnikov et al. (1970)
C$_6$H$_5$	Me	H	Met ED$_{50}$ 24 (po); MES ED$_{50}$ 46 (po)	Gujral et al. (1957)
C$_6$H$_5$	Et	H	Met ED$_{50}$ 102 (po); MES ED$_{50}$ 58 (po)	Gujral et al. (1957)
2-pyr	Me	H	Met ED$_{50}$ 60 (po); MES ED$_{50}$ 295 (po)	Bonati and Rosati (1965)
2-(3-MePyr)	Me	H	Met ED$_{50}$ 26 (po); MES ED$_{50}$ 128 (po)	Bonati and Rosati (1965)
2-(4-MePyr)	Me	H	Met ED$_{50}$ 340 (po); MES ED$_{50}$ 370 (po)	Bonati and Rosati (1965)
2-(6-MePyr)	Me	H	Met ED$_{50}$ 127 (po); MES ED$_{50}$ 158 (po)	Bonati and Rosati (1965)
2-(4,6-Me$_2$Pyr)	Me	H	Met ED$_{50}$ 339 (po); MES ED$_{50}$ 285 (po)	Bonati and Rosati (1965)
2-(5-ClPyr)	Me	H	Met ED$_{50}$ 29; MES ED$_{50}$ 128	Bonati and Rosati (1965)
2-(5-ClPyr)	Et	H	Met ED$_{50}$ 63; MES ED$_{50}$ 133	Bonati and Rosati (1965)
2-(5-BrPyr)	Me	H	Met ED$_{50}$ 30; MES ED$_{50}$ 100	Bonati and Rosati (1965)
2-(3,5-Cl$_2$Pyr)	Me	H	Met ED$_{50}$ 1500; MES ED$_{50}$ > 2000	Bonati and Rosati (1965)
4-NH$_2$C$_6$H$_4$	i-Pr	H	Active	Heusner et al. (1969)
i-Pr	Me	H	Met ED$_{50}$ 110 (ip); MES ED$_{50}$ 78 (ip)	Dua et al. (1967)
n-Bu	Me	H	Met ED$_{50}$ 70 (ip); MES ED$_{50}$ 50 (ip)	Dua et al. (1967)
2-MeC$_6$H$_4$	H	H	Met ED$_{50}$ 90 (ip)	Hurmer and Vernin (1967)
2-Me-3-ClC$_6$H$_3$	H	H	Met ED$_{50}$ 75 (ip)	Hurmer and Vernin (1967)
2-Me-3-ClC$_6$H$_3$	Me	H	Met ED$_{50}$ 84 (ip); MES ED$_{50}$ 29 (ip)	Hurmer and Vernin (1967)

2-EtC$_6$H$_4$	H		Met ED$_{50}$ > 200 (ip); MES ED$_{50}$ 80 (ip)	Hurmer and Vernin (1967)
2,4-Cl$_2$C$_6$H$_3$	H		Met ED$_{50}$ 30 (ip); MES ED$_{50}$ 135 (ip)	Hurmer and Vernin (1967)
2,3-Cl$_2$C$_6$H$_3$	H		Met ED$_{50}$ 180 (ip); MES ED$_{50}$ > 200 (ip)	Hurmer and Vernin (1967)
2-BrC$_6$H$_4$	H		Met ED$_{50}$ 50 (ip)	Hurmer and Vernin (1967)
2-Me-4-ClC$_6$H$_3$	H		Met ED$_{50}$ 100 (ip); MES ED$_{50}$ 250 (ip)	Hurmer and Vernin (1967)
2-Me-4-ClC$_6$H$_3$	Me		Met ED$_{50}$ 65 (ip); MES ED$_{50}$ 30 (ip)	Hurmer and Vernin (1967)
2-ClC$_6$H$_4$	Me		MES ED$_{50}$ 52	Boissier et al. (1967)
3-ClC$_6$H$_4$	Me		MES ED$_{50}$ 160	Boissier et al. (1967)
4-ClC$_6$H$_4$	Me		MES ED$_{50}$ 100	Boissier et al. (1967)
2,3-Cl$_2$C$_6$H$_3$	Me		MES ED$_{50}$ > 372	Boissier et al. (1967)
2,4-Cl$_2$C$_6$H$_3$	Me		MES ED$_{50}$ 50	Boissier et al. (1967)
2,5-Cl$_2$C$_6$H$_3$	Me		MES ED$_{50}$ 175	Boissier et al. (1967)
2,6-Cl$_2$C$_6$H$_3$	Me		MES ED$_{50}$ > 372	Boissier et al. (1967)
2-Cl-3-MeC$_6$H$_3$	Me		MES ED$_{50}$ > 372	Boissier et al. (1967)
2-Cl-4-MeC$_6$H$_3$	Me		MES ED$_{50}$ 130	Boissier et al. (1967)
2-Cl-5-MeC$_6$H$_3$	Me		MES ED$_{50}$ > 372	Boissier et al. (1967)
2-Cl-6-MeC$_6$H$_3$	Me		MES ED$_{50}$ 200	Boissier et al. (1967)
3-MeC$_6$H$_4$	Me		MES ED$_{50}$ 310	Boissier et al. (1967)
2-Me-4-ClC$_6$H$_3$	Me		MES ED$_{50}$ 52	Boissier et al. (1967)
2-Me-6-ClC$_6$H$_3$	Me		MES ED$_{50}$ 200	Boissier et al. (1967)
C$_6$H$_5$	H		MES ED$_{50}$ 25–100	Breuer and Roesch (1971)
2-MeC$_6$H$_5$	H		MES ED$_{50}$ 25–100	Breuer and Roesch (1971)
4-NH$_2$C$_6$H$_4$	H		MES ED$_{50}$ 10–25	Breuer and Roesch (1971)
2-Me-4-NH$_2$C$_6$H$_3$	H		MES ED$_{50}$ 10–25	Breuer and Roesch (1971)
2-Me-4-NH$_2$C$_6$H$_3$	Me		MES ED$_{50}$ < 10	Breuer and Roesch (1971)
2-Me-4-NH$_2$C$_6$H$_3$	H	6-Cl	MES ED$_{50}$ 10–25	Breuer and Roesch (1971)
2-Me-4-NH$_2$C$_6$H$_3$	Me	6-Me	MES ED$_{50}$ 25–100	Breuer and Roesch (1971)
2-Me-4-MeNHC$_6$H$_3$	Me		MES ED$_{50}$ 10–25	Breuer and Roesch (1971)

(continued)

TABLE XXIII—*Continued*

R	R_1	R_2	Activity	Reference
2-Me-4-Me$_2$NC$_6$H$_3$	Me	H	MES ED$_{50}$ 25–100	Breuer and Roesch (1971)
2-MeC$_6$H$_4$	Me	5-NH$_2$	MES ED$_{50}$ 25–100	Breuer and Roesch (1971)
2-MeC$_6$H$_4$	Me	6-NH$_2$	MES ED$_{50}$ 10–25	Breuer and Roesch (1971)
2-MeC$_6$H$_4$	Me	7-NH$_2$	MES ED$_{50}$ 25–100	Breuer and Roesch (1971)
2-MeC$_6$H$_4$	H	6-NH$_2$	MES ED$_{50}$ 10–25	Breuer and Roesch (1971)
2-MeC$_6$H$_4$	Et	6-NH$_2$	MES ED$_{50}$ < 10	Breuer and Roesch (1971)
2-MeC$_6$H$_4$	n-Pr	6-NH$_2$	MES ED$_{50}$ 10–25	Breuer and Roesch (1971)
2-MeC$_6$H$_4$	i-Pr	6-NH$_2$	MES ED$_{50}$ 25–100	Breuer and Roesch (1971)
2-MeC$_6$H$_4$	n-Bu	6-NH$_2$	MES ED$_{50}$ 10–25	Breuer and Roesch (1971)
2-MeC$_6$H$_4$	i-Bu	6-NH$_2$	MES ED$_{50}$ 25–100	Breuer and Roesch (1971)
C$_6$H$_5$	Me	6-NH$_2$	MES ED$_{50}$ 25–100	Breuer and Roesch (1971)
3-MeC$_6$H$_4$	Me	6-NH$_2$	MES ED$_{50}$ 25–100	Breuer and Roesch (1971)
4-MeC$_6$H$_4$	Me	6-NH$_2$	MES ED$_{50}$ 10–25	Breuer and Roesch (1971)
2-EtC$_6$H$_4$	Me	6-NH$_2$	MES ED$_{50}$ 10–25	Breuer and Roesch (1971)
2-FC$_6$H$_4$	Me	6-NH$_2$	MES ED$_{50}$ 10–25	Breuer and Roesch (1971)
2-ClC$_6$H$_4$	Me	6-NH$_2$	MES ED$_{50}$ < 10	Breuer and Roesch (1971)
2-CF$_3$C$_6$H$_4$	Me	6-NH$_2$	MES ED$_{50}$ 10–25	Breuer and Roesch (1971)
2-MeOC$_6$H$_4$	Me	6-NH$_2$	MES ED$_{50}$ 25–100	Breuer and Roesch (1971)
2-MeO$_2$CC$_6$H$_4$	Me	6-NH$_2$	MES ED$_{50}$ 25–100	Breuer and Roesch (1971)
2-NO$_2$C$_6$H$_4$	Me	6-NH$_2$	MES ED$_{50}$ 10–25	Breuer and Roesch (1971)
2,4-Me$_2$C$_6$H$_3$	Me	6-NH$_2$	MES ED$_{50}$ 10–25	Breuer and Roesch (1971)
2-Me-4-FC$_6$H$_3$	Me	6-NH$_2$	MES ED$_{50}$ $\approx$ 10	Breuer and Roesch (1971)
2-Me-4-ClC$_6$H$_3$	Me	6-NH$_2$	MES ED$_{50}$ < 10	Breuer and Roesch (1971)
2-Me-4-BrC$_6$H$_3$	Me	6-NH$_2$	MES ED$_{50}$ 10–25	Breuer and Roesch (1971)
2-Me-4-NO$_2$C$_6$H$_3$	Me	6-NH$_2$	MES ED$_{50}$ 10–25	Breuer and Roesch (1971)
2-Me-4-Me$_2$NC$_6$H$_3$	Me	6-NH$_2$	MES ED$_{50}$ 25–100	Breuer and Roesch (1971)
2-MeC$_6$H$_4$	Me	6-CHONH	MES ED$_{50}$ 25–100	Breuer and Roesch (1971)
2-MeC$_6$H$_4$	Me	6-MeCONH	MES ED$_{50}$ 25–100	Breuer and Roesch (1971)
2-MeC$_6$H$_4$	Me	6-Et$_2$NCH$_2$CONH	MES ED$_{50}$ 25–100	Breuer and Roesch (1971)

2-MeC$_6$H$_4$	Me	6-MeNH	MES ED$_{50}$ 25–100	Breuer and Roesch (1971)
2-MeC$_6$H$_4$	Me	6-C$_6$H$_5$CH=N	MES ED$_{50}$ 25–100	Breuer and Roesch (1971)
2-MeC$_6$H$_4$	Me	HOCH$_2$CONH	MES ED$_{50}$ 25–100	Breuer and Roesch (1971)
2-HOCH$_2$C$_6$H$_4$	Me	MeCONH	MES ED$_{50}$ 25–100	Breuer and Roesch (1971)
2-Me-4-NH$_2$C$_6$H$_3$	Me	H	MES ED$_{50}$ < 10	Breuer and Roesch (1971)
2-Me-Cl-C$_6$H$_3$	Me	6-NH$_2$	MES ED$_{50}$ < 10	Breuer and Roesch (1971)
Ar	Me	H	Met, active	Lietz and Matthies (1964)
Ar	CH$_2$OCOR$_3$	6- or 8-R$_2$	Active	Kozhevnikov et al. (1975)
(CHR$_3$)$_n$CO$_2$Et	Me	6- or 8-R$_2$	ES, active	Misra and Prakash (1974)
2-MeC$_6$H$_4$	Me	6-Cl	Met ED$_{50}$ 70; MES ED$_{50}$ 96	Leszkovszky et al. (1965)
2-Me-4-ClC$_6$H$_3$	Me	H	Met ED$_{50}$ 71; MES ED$_{50}$ 80	Leszkovszky et al. (1965)
2-Me-4-BrC$_6$H$_3$	Me	H	Met ED$_{50}$ 75; MES ED$_{50}$ 125	Leszkovszky et al. (1965)
2-Me-4-ClC$_6$H$_3$	n-Pr	H	Met ED$_{50}$ 50; MES ED$_{50}$ 75	Leszkovszky et al. (1965)
2-MeC$_6$H$_5$	CH=CHC$_6$H$_5$	H	Met ED$_{50}$ 150; MES ED$_{50}$ > 200	Leszkovszky et al. (1965)
2-MeC$_6$H$_5$	CH=CH-2-Pyr	H	Met ED$_{50}$ 71; MES ED$_{50}$ 86	Leszkovszky et al. (1965)
2-MeC$_6$H$_5$	CH=CH-2-Pyr	6-Cl	Met ED$_{50}$ 50	Leszkovszky et al. (1965)
2-MeC$_6$H$_5$	CH=CH-2-Fur	H	Met ED$_{50}$ > 150; MES ED$_{50}$ > 150	Leszkovszky et al. (1965)
C$_6$H$_5$	Me	H	Met ED$_{50}$ 70; MES ED$_{50}$ 95	Leszkovszky et al. (1965)
2-MeC$_6$H$_4$ (=O is =S)	Me	H	Met ED$_{50}$ 150; MES ED$_{50}$ 54	Leszkovszky et al. (1965)
2-Me-3-ClC$_6$H$_3$	Me	H	Met ED$_{50}$ 84; MES ED$_{50}$ 29	Boltze et al. (1963)
2-Me-4-ClC$_6$H$_3$	Me	H	Met ED$_{50}$ 63; MES ED$_{50}$ 30	Boltze et al. (1963)
2-Me-5-ClC$_6$H$_3$	Me	H	Met ED$_{50}$ > 200; MES ED$_{50}$ 82	Boltze et al. (1963)
2-Me-6-ClC$_6$H$_3$	Me	H	Met ED$_{50}$ 150; MES ED$_{50}$ 170	Boltze et al. (1963)
2,3-Me$_2$C$_6$H$_3$	Me	H	MES ED$_{50}$ > 100	Boltze et al. (1963)
2,4-Me$_2$C$_6$H$_3$	Me	H	MES ED$_{50}$ > 100	Boltze et al. (1963)
2,6-Me$_2$C$_6$H$_3$	Me	H	MES ED$_{50}$ > 100	Boltze et al. (1963)
4-ClC$_6$H$_4$	Me	H	Met ED$_{50}$ 80; MES ED$_{50}$ 72	Boltze et al. (1963)
4-BrC$_6$H$_4$	Me	H	Met ED$_{50}$ 76; MES ED$_{50}$ 33	Boltze et al. (1963)
2-Me-3-NH$_2$C$_6$H$_3$	Me	H	MES ED$_{50}$ > 100	Boltze et al. (1963)
2-Me-5-NH$_2$C$_6$H$_3$	Me	H	MES ED$_{50}$ > 100	Boltze et al. (1963)

(continued)

TABLE XXIII—*Continued*

R	R_1	R_2	Activity	Reference
2-Me-3-NO$_2$C$_6$H$_3$	Me	H	Met ED$_{50}$ > 100	Boltze *et al.* (1963)
2-Me-5-NO$_2$C$_6$H$_3$	Me	H	Met ED$_{50}$ > 200; MES ED$_{50}$ > 100	Boltze *et al.* (1963)
2-Me-6-NO$_2$C$_6$H$_3$	Me	H	Met ED$_{50}$ > 400; MES ED$_{50}$ 150	Boltze *et al.* (1963)
2-NO$_2$C$_6$H$_4$	Me	H	Met ED$_{50}$ 66; MES ED$_{50}$ 29	Boltze *et al.* (1963)
4-NO$_3$C$_6$H$_4$	Me	H	Met ED$_{50}$ 90; MES ED$_{50}$ 113	Boltze *et al.* (1963)
2-HOC$_6$H$_4$	Me	H	Met ED$_{50}$ 130; MES ED$_{50}$ 44	Boltze *et al.* (1963)
4-HOC$_6$H$_4$	Me	H	Met ED$_{50}$ > 200; MES ED$_{50}$ > 100	Boltze *et al.* (1963)
4-EtOC$_6$H$_4$	Me	H	Met ED$_{50}$ > 100	Boltze *et al.* (1963)
2-EtO-4-MeC$_6$H$_3$	Me	H	Met ED$_{50}$ > 200; MES ED$_{50}$ > 100	Boltze *et al.* (1963)
2-EtO-6-ClC$_6$H$_3$	Me	H	Met ED$_{50}$ > 200; MES ED$_{50}$ > 100	Boltze *et al.* (1963)
2,5-(EtO)$_2$-4-ClC$_6$H$_2$	Me	H	Met ED$_{50}$ > 200; MES ED$_{50}$ > 100	Boltze *et al.* (1963)
2-C$_6$H$_5$O-5-ClC$_6$H$_3$	Me	H	Met ED$_{50}$ > 100	Boltze *et al.* (1963)
CH(OH)CCl$_3$	Me	H	Met ED$_{50}$ > 200; MES ED$_{50}$ > 200	Boltze *et al.* (1963)
CH$_2$-2-Pyr	Me	H	Met ED$_{50}$ > 100	Boltze *et al.* (1963)
	Me	H	Met ED$_{50}$ > 200; MES ED$_{50}$ > 100	Boltze *et al.* (1963)
NH$_2$	Me	H	Met ED$_{50}$ > 200; MES ED$_{50}$ > 100	Boltze *et al.* (1963)
NMe$_2$	Me	H	Met ED$_{50}$ > 200; MES ED$_{50}$ > 100	Boltze *et al.* (1963)

4-ClC$_6$H$_4$CH$_2$NH	Me	Met ED$_{50}$ > 200; MES ED$_{50}$ > 100	Boltze et al. (1963)
4-ClC$_6$H$_4$CH=N	Me	Met ED$_{50}$ > 200; MES ED$_{50}$ > 100	Boltze et al. (1963)
C$_6$H$_5$NH	Me	MES ED$_{50}$ > 100	Boltze et al. (1963)
C$_6$H$_5$NCOMe	Me	MES ED$_{50}$ > 100	Boltze et al. (1963)
Phthalimido	Me	Met ED$_{50}$ > 200; MES ED$_{50}$ > 100	Boltze et al. (1963)
2-CF$_3$C$_6$H$_4$	Me	Met ED$_{50}$ 76; MES ED$_{50}$ 76	Boltze et al. (1963)
3-CF$_3$C$_6$H$_4$	Me	MES ED$_{50}$ > 200	Boltze et al. (1963)
2-ClC$_6$H$_5$	Me	Met ED$_{50}$ 50; MES ED$_{50}$ 75	Boltze et al. (1963)
1-(4-BrNap)	Me	MES ED$_{50}$ > 200	Boltze et al. (1963)
2-Me-3-MeCONH	Me	MES ED$_{50}$ > 100	Boltze et al. (1963)
2-Pyr	Me	Met ED$_{50}$ > 200; MES ED$_{50}$ 110	Boltze et al. (1963)
2-NH$_2$C$_6$H$_4$	Me	Met ED$_{50}$ 88; MES ED$_{50}$ 46	Boltze et al. (1963)
C$_6$H$_5$NCOC$_6$H$_5$	Me	MES ED$_{50}$ > 100	Boltze et al. (1963)
3-FC$_6$H$_4$	Me	Met ED$_{50}$ 78; MES ED$_{50}$ 88	Boltze et al. (1963)
2-Me-3-n-PrOC$_6$H$_3$	Me	MES ED$_{50}$ > 100	Boltze et al. (1963)
2-CF$_3$-4-BrC$_6$H$_3$	Me	Met ED$_{50}$ > 100; MES ED$_{50}$ 59	Boltze et al. (1963)
4-FC$_6$H$_4$	Me	Met ED$_{50}$ 52; MES ED$_{50}$ 75	Boltze et al. (1963)
2-EtO$_2$CNHC$_6$H$_4$	Me	Met ED$_{50}$ > 200; MES ED$_{50}$ 82	Boltze et al. (1963)
2,3-Cl$_2$C$_6$H$_3$	Me	MES ED$_{50}$ > 200	Boltze et al. (1963)
1-(4-ClNap)	Me	MES ED$_{50}$ > 200	Boltze et al. (1963)
Et$_2$NCH$_2$CH$_2$OC$_6$H$_4$	Me	MES ED$_{50}$ > 200	Boltze et al. (1963)
2-Me-4-FC$_6$H$_3$	Me	Met ED$_{50}$ 62; MES ED$_{50}$ 62	Boltze et al. (1963)
2-Me-3-FC$_6$H$_3$	Me	Met ED$_{50}$ 40; MES ED$_{50}$ 76	Boltze et al. (1963)
2-Me-3-BrC$_6$H$_3$	Me	Met ED$_{50}$ 31; MES ED$_{50}$ 63	Boltze et al. (1963)
2-Me-3-IC$_6$H$_3$	Me	Met ED$_{50}$ 77; MES ED$_{50}$ 48	Boltze et al. (1963)
2-Me-3-NCC$_6$H$_3$	Me	Met ED$_{50}$ 90; MES ED$_{50}$ 46	Boltze et al. (1963)
2-FC$_6$H$_4$	Me	Met ED$_{50}$ 35; MES ED$_{50}$ 39	Boltze et al. (1963)

(continued)

439

TABLE XXIII—*Continued*

R	R_1	R_2	Activity	Reference
2-$Et_2NCOC_6H_4$	Me	H	MES ED_{50} > 200	Boltze et al. (1963)
2-$MeO_2CC_6H_4$	Me	H	MES ED_{50} 84	Boltze et al. (1963)
$C_6H_5CH_2CH(Me)$	Me	H	Met ED_{50} > 200; MES ED_{50} > 100	Boltze et al. (1963)
$C_6H_5CH_2CH_2CH(Me)$	Me	H	Met ED_{50} > 200; MES ED_{50} > 100	Boltze et al. (1963)
(structure: CH_2CH_2—N, Me, O, N)	Me	H	Met ED_{50} > 200; MES ED_{50} > 100	Boltze et al. (1963)
H	Me	H	MES ED_{50} > 200	Boltze et al. (1963)
Me	Me	H	MES ED_{50} > 200	Boltze et al. (1963)
2-MeC_6H_4	Et	H	Met ED_{50} 128; MES ED_{50} 53	Boltze et al. (1963)
2-Me-3-ClC_6H_3	Et	H	Met ED_{50} 150; MES ED_{50} 70	Boltze et al. (1963)
2-Me-4-ClC_6H_3	Et	H	Met ED_{50} > 100; MES ED_{50} 56	Boltze et al. (1963)
2-Me-6-ClC_6H_3	Et	H	Met ED_{50} 100; MES ED_{50} 91	Boltze et al. (1963)
2-Me-4-ClC_6H_3	$C_6H_5CH=CH$	H	MES ED_{50} > 100	Boltze et al. (1963)
2-MeC_6H_4	3-$NO_2C_6H_4CH=CH$	H	MES ED_{50} > 100	Boltze et al. (1963)
2-MeC_6H_4	3,4-$CH_2O_2C_6H_3CH=CH$	H	MES ED_{50} > 100	Boltze et al. (1963)
2-MeC_6H_4	4-$MeOC_6H_4CH=CH$	H	MES ED_{50} > 100	Boltze et al. (1963)
2-MeC_6H_4	4-$ClC_6H_4CH=CH$	H	MES ED_{50} > 100	Boltze et al. (1963)
2-MeC_6H_4	$C_6H_5CH=CH$	H	Met ED_{50} > 2500; MES ED_{50} 19	Boltze et al. (1963)
2-MeC_6H_4	2-PyrCH=CH	H	Met ED_{50} 145; MES ED_{50} 14.5	Boltze et al. (1963)
2-Me-4-ClC_6H_3	2-PyrCH=CH	H	MES ED_{50} > 100	Boltze et al. (1963)
2-Me-3-ClC_6H_3	$C_6H_5CH=CH$	H	MES ED_{50} > 100	Boltze et al. (1963)
2-MeC_6H_4	3-PyrCH=CH	H	Met ED_{50} 27; MES ED_{50} 15	Boltze et al. (1963)

Me	2-PyrCH=CH	H	MES ED_{50} > 100	Boltze et al. (1963)
2-Me-3-ClC$_6$H$_3$	2-PyrCH=CH	H	MES ED_{50} > 100	Boltze et al. (1963)
2-MeC$_6$H$_4$	3-(1-Me$^+$Pyr)CH=CH$^-$I	H	MES ED_{50} > 100	Boltze et al. (1963)
2-MeC$_6$H$_4$	4-PyrCH=CH	H	Met ED_{50} 68; MES ED_{50} 39	Boltze et al. (1963)
2-MeC$_6$H$_4$	2-FurCH=CH	H	Met ED_{50} > 200; MES ED_{50} 175	Boltze et al. (1963)
2-MeC$_6$H$_4$	2-ThiopCH=CH	H	MES ED_{50} > 100	Boltze et al. (1963)
2-ClC$_6$H$_4$	3-PyrCH=CH	H	Met ED_{50} > 200; MES ED_{50} 19	Boltze et al. (1963)
2-MeC$_6$H$_4$	2-(6-MePyr)CH=CH	H	Met ED_{50} > 200; MES ED_{50} 50	Boltze et al. (1963)
2-MeC$_6$H$_4$	2-QuinCH=CH	H	MES ED_{50} > 100	Boltze et al. (1963)
2-ClCH$_2$C$_6$H$_4$	CH$_2$Cl	H	Met ED_{50} > 200; MES ED_{50} 100	Boltze et al. (1963)
CH$_2$CH$_2$NEt$_2$	C$_6$H$_5$CH$_2$	H	Met ED_{50} > 200; MES ED_{50} 37	Boltze et al. (1963)
2-MeC$_6$H$_4$	CH$_2$CH(OH)CCl$_3$	H	Met ED_{50} > 100; MES ED_{50} 55	Boltze et al. (1963)
2-MeC$_6$H$_4$	CH$_2$CH$_2$N⬡	H	Met ED_{50} > 100; MES ED_{50} 34	Boltze et al. (1963)
2-Me-3-ClC$_6$H$_3$	CH$_2$CH$_2$N⬡	H	Met ED_{50} > 100; MES ED_{50} 38	Boltze et al. (1963)
2-MeC$_6$H$_4$	2-PyrCHBrCHBr	H	MES ED_{50} > 100	Boltze et al. (1963)
2-MeC$_6$H$_4$	2-PyrC≡C	H	MES ED_{50} > 100	Boltze et al. (1963)
Me	CHCl$_2$	H	MES ED_{50} > 100	Boltze et al. (1963)
2-MeC$_6$H$_4$	Me	6-Cl	MES ED_{50} > 100	Boltze et al. (1963)
2-MeC$_6$H$_4$	Me	7-Cl	MES ED_{50} > 100	Boltze et al. (1963)
2-Me-3-ClC$_6$H$_3$	Me	6-NO$_2$	MES ED_{50} > 100	Boltze et al. (1963)
2-Me-4-ClC$_6$H$_3$	Me	6-NO$_2$	MES ED_{50} > 100	Boltze et al. (1963)
2-MeC$_6$H$_4$	Me	6-NO$_2$	MES ED_{50} > 100	Boltze et al. (1963)

(continued)

TABLE XXIII—*Continued*

R	R$_1$	R$_2$	Activity	Reference
2-MeC$_6$H$_4$	Me	6,7-(MeO)$_2$	MES ED$_{50}$ > 100	Boltze *et al.* (1963)
2-MeC$_6$H$_4$	Me	6,7-CH$_2$O$_2$	MES ED$_{50}$ 140	Boltze *et al.* (1963)
2-MeC$_6$H$_4$ (=O is =S)	Me	H	MES ED$_{50}$ > 200	Boltze *et al.* (1963)
2-Me-3-ClC$_6$H$_3$	Me	H	MES ED$_{50}$ > 100	Boltze *et al.* (1963)
2-ClC$_6$H$_4$ (=O is =S)	Me	H	MES ED$_{50}$ > 100	Boltze *et al.* (1963)
4-BrC$_6$H$_4$ (=O is =S)	Me	H	MES ED$_{50}$ > 100	Boltze *et al.* (1963)
4-BrC$_6$H$_4$	Me	H	Met ED$_{50}$ 30; MES ED$_{50}$ 140	Bianchi and David (1960)
2-MeOC$_6$H$_4$	Me	H	2.2 × troxidone	Bianchi and David (1960)
4-MeOC$_6$H$_4$	Me	H	2.1 × troxidone	Bianchi and David (1960)
2-EtOC$_6$H$_4$	Me	H	2.0 × troxidone	Bianchi and David (1960)
3-EtOC$_6$H$_4$	Me	H	<0.5 × troxidone	Bianchi and David (1960)
4-EtOC$_6$H$_4$	Me	H	<0.3 × troxidone	Bianchi and David (1960)
2-ClC$_6$H$_4$	Me	H	10.0 × troxidone	Bianchi and David (1960)
3-ClC$_6$H$_4$	Me	H	7.0 × troxidone	Bianchi and David (1960)
4-ClC$_6$H$_4$	Me	H	13.0 × troxidone	Bianchi and David (1960)
2-BrC$_6$H$_4$	Me	H	14.0 × troxidone	Bianchi and David (1960)
3-BrC$_6$H$_4$	Me	H	1.5 × troxidone	Bianchi and David (1960)
4-BrC$_6$H$_4$	Me	H	14.0 × troxidone	Bianchi and David (1960)
4-IC$_6$H$_4$	Me	H	6.7 × troxidone	Bianchi and David (1960)
4-FC$_6$H$_4$	Me	H	2.6 × troxidone	Bianchi and David (1960)
2,4-Cl$_2$C$_6$H$_3$	Me	H	2.1 × troxidone	Bianchi and David (1960)
2,5-Cl$_2$C$_6$H$_3$	Me	H	14.0 × troxidone	Bianchi and David (1960)
2,6-Me$_2$C$_6$H$_3$	Me	H	4.5 × troxidone	Bianchi and David (1960)
3,5-Me$_2$C$_6$H$_3$	Me	H	1.3 × troxidone	Bianchi and David (1960)
2,3-Me$_2$-4-BrC$_6$H$_2$	Me	H	2.5 × troxidone	Bianchi and David (1960)
C$_6$H$_5$	Et	H	2.0 × troxidone	Bianchi and David (1960)
2-ClC$_6$H$_4$	Et	H	2.0 × troxidone	Bianchi and David (1960)
4-BrC$_6$H$_4$	Et	H	<2.5 × troxidone	Bianchi and David (1960)
4-BrC$_6$H$_4$	Pr	H	2.4 × troxidone	Bianchi and David (1960)

Me	C_6H_5	H	3.0 × troxidone	Bianchi and David (1960)
Me	2-MeC_6H_4	H	7.4 × troxidone	Bianchi and David (1960)
Me	4-ClC_6H_4	H	<0.7 × troxidone	Bianchi and David (1960)
Me	2-BrC_6H_4	H	6.3 × troxidone	Bianchi and David (1960)
Me	4-BrC_6H_4	H	<1.0 × troxidone	Bianchi and David (1960)
Et	C_6H_5	H	1.3 × troxidone	Bianchi and David (1960)
$CH_2CHOHCH_2OH$	C_6H_5	H	2.3 × troxidone	Bianchi and David (1960)
Et	4-BrC_6H_4	H	<0.7 × troxidone	Bianchi and David (1960)
2-MeC_6H_4 (=O is =S)	Me	H	2.3 × troxidone	Bianchi and David (1960)
4-ClC_6H_4 (=O is =S)	Me	H	<0.7 × troxidone	Bianchi and David (1960)
2-BrC_6H_4 (=O is =S)	Me	H	<0.7 × troxidone	Bianchi and David (1960)
4-BrC_6H_4 (=O is =S)	Me	H	<0.7 × troxidone	Bianchi and David (1960)
4-BrC_6H_4	Me	5,6,7,8-F_4	Met, 20% protn. at 100 (ip)	Joshi et al. (1975)
2-MeC_6H_4	Me	5,6,7,8-F_4	Met, 20% protn. at 100 (ip)	Joshi et al. (1975)
C_6H_5	Et	5,6,7,8-F_4	Met, 20% protn. at 100 (ip)	Joshi et al. (1975)
C_6H_5	C_6H_5	7-F	Met, 40% protn. at 100 (ip)	Joshi et al. (1975)
2-MeC_6H_4	C_6H_5	7-F	Met, 20% protn. at 100 (ip)	Joshi et al. (1975)
2-MeC_6H_4	Me	6-F	Met, 20% protn. at 100 (ip)	Joshi et al. (1975)
2-MeC_6H_5	Me	7-F	Met, 60% protn. at 100 (ip)	Joshi et al. (1975)
4-FC_6H_4	$CH_2{=}CHCH_2S$	5,6,7,8-F_4	Met, 20% protn. at 100 (ip)	Joshi et al. (1975)
4-FC_6H_4 (O is =S)	SH	5,6,7,8-F_4	Met, 20% protn. at 100 (ip)	Joshi et al. (1975)
4-FC_6H_4	n-PrS	5,6,7,8-F_4	Met, 100% protn. at 100 (ip)	Joshi et al. (1975)
2-Pyrimidyl	Me	H	Met, 70% protn. at 100 (ip)	Chaturvedi and Parmar (1972b)
2-Pyrimidyl	Me	6-Cl	Met, 50% protn. at 100 (ip)	Chaturvedi and Parmar (1972b)
2-Pyrimidyl	Me	6-Br	Met, 60% protn. at 100 (ip)	Chaturvedi and Parmar (1972b)
2-Pyrimidyl	Me	6-I	Met, 50% protn. at 100 (ip)	Chaturvedi and Parmar (1972b)
2-Pyrimidyl	Me	6,8-Cl_2	Met, 40% protn. at 100 (ip)	Chaturvedi and Parmar (1972b)

(continued)

TABLE XXIII—*Continued*

R	R_1	R_2	Activity	Reference
2-Pyrimidyl	Me	$6,8\text{-}I_2$	Met, 20% protn. at 100 (ip)	Chaturvedi and Parmar (1972b)
3-*N*-Piperidino-Pr	Me	H	Met, 60% protn. at 100 (ip)	Chaturvedi and Parmar (1972b)
3-*N*-Piperidino-Pr	Me	6-I	Met, 30% protn. at 100 (ip)	Chaturvedi and Parmar (1972b)
3-*N*-Piperidino-Pr	Me	$6,8\text{-}Cl_2$	Met, 20% protn. at 100 (ip)	Chaturvedi and Parmar (1972b)
3-*N*-Piperidino-Pr	Me	$6,8\text{-}I_2$	Met, 10% protn. at 100 (ip)	Chaturvedi and Parmar (1972b)
$2,5\text{-}(MeO)_2\text{-}4\text{-}ClC_6H_2$	Me	H	Met, 30% protn. at 100 (ip)	Chaturvedi and Parmar (1972b)
$2,5\text{-}(MeO)_2\text{-}4\text{-}ClC_6H_2$	Me	6-Cl	Met, 40% protn. at 100 (ip)	Chaturvedi and Parmar (1972b)
$2,5\text{-}(MeO)_2\text{-}4\text{-}ClC_6H_2$	Me	6-I	Met, 50% protn. at 100 (ip)	Chaturvedi and Parmar (1972b)
$2,5\text{-}(MeO)_2\text{-}4\text{-}ClC_6H_2$	Me	$6,8\text{-}Cl_2$	Met, 50% protn. at 100 (ip)	Chaturvedi and Parmar (1972b)
$2,5\text{-}(MeO)_2\text{-}4\text{-}ClC_6H_2$	Me	$6,8\text{-}I_2$	Met, 30% protn. at 100 (ip)	Chaturvedi and Parmar (1972b)
C_6H_5	SCH_2CO_2Et	H	Met, 40% protn. at 100 (ip)	Dwivedi and Parmar (1972)
C_6H_5	$SCH_2CONHNH_2$	H	Met, 60% protn. at 100 (ip)	Dwivedi and Parmar (1972)
$2\text{-}MeC_6H_4$	SCH_2CO_2Et	H	Met, 40% protn. at 100 (ip)	Dwivedi and Parmar (1972)
$2\text{-}MeC_6H_4$	$SCH_2CONHNH_2$	H	Met, 50% protn. at 100 (ip)	Dwivedi and Parmar (1972)
$3\text{-}MeC_6H_4$	SCH_2CO_2Et	H	Met, 50% protn. at 100 (ip)	Dwivedi and Parmar (1972)
$3\text{-}MeC_6H_4$	$SCH_2CONHNH_2$	H	Met, 10% protn. at 100 (ip)	Dwivedi and Parmar (1972)
$4\text{-}MeC_6H_4$	SCH_2CO_2Et	H	Met, 50% protn. at 100 (ip)	Dwivedi and Parmar (1972)
$4\text{-}MeC_6H_4$	$SCH_2CONHNH_2$	H	Met, 30% protn. at 100 (ip)	Dwivedi and Parmar (1972)
$3,4\text{-}Me_2C_6H_3$	SCH_2CO_2Et	H	Met, 70% protn. at 100 (ip)	Dwivedi and Parmar (1972)

3,4-Me$_2$C$_6$H$_3$	SCH$_2$CONHNH$_2$	H	Met, 20% protn. at 100 (ip)	Dwivedi and Parmar (1972)
2,4-Me$_2$C$_6$H$_3$	Me	6,8-Cl$_2$	Met, 20% protn. at 100 (ip)	Nagar and Parmar (1971)
2,4-Me$_2$C$_6$H$_3$	Me	6,8-I$_2$	Met, 40% protn. at 100 (ip)	Nagar and Parmar (1971)
CH$_2$CH$_2$N⟨ring⟩NH	Me	6-Cl	Met, 70% protn. at 100 (ip)	Parmar et al. (1974a)
CH$_2$CH$_2$N⟨ring⟩NH	Me	6-Br	Met, 50% protn. at 100 (ip)	Parmar et al. (1974a)
CH$_2$CH$_2$N⟨ring⟩NH	Me	6-I	Met, 30% protn. at 100 (ip)	Parmar et al. (1974a)
CH$_2$CH$_2$N⟨ring⟩NH	Me	6,8-Cl$_2$	Met, 30% protn. at 100 (ip)	Parmar et al. (1974a)
CH$_2$CH$_2$N⟨ring⟩NCOMe	Me	6-Br	Met, 10% protn. at 100 (ip)	Parmar et al. (1974a)
CH$_2$CH$_2$N⟨ring⟩NCOMe	Me	6,8-Cl$_2$	Met, 50% protn. at 100 (ip)	Parmar et al. (1974a)
CH$_2$CH$_2$N⟨ring⟩NCOPh	Me	6,8-Cl$_2$	Met, 40% protn. at 100 (ip)	Parmar et al. (1974a)
CH$_2$CH$_2$N⟨ring⟩N—CO—(2-furanyl)	Me	6,8-Cl$_2$	Met, 20% protn. at 100 (ip)	Parmar et al. (1974a)
CH$_2$CH$_2$N⟨ring⟩NCOC$_6$H$_2$(OMe)$_3$	Me	6-Br	Met, 30% protn. at 100 (ip)	Parmar et al. (1974a)

(continued)

TABLE XXIII—*Continued*

R	R_1	R_2	Activity	Reference
CH_2CH_2N⟨⟩$NCOC_6H_2(OMe)_3$	Me	6,8-Cl$_2$	Met, 20% protn. at 100	Parmar *et al.* (1974a)
4-CH$_2$=CHCH$_2$OC$_6$H$_4$	Me	H	Met, 20% protn. at 100	Parmar *et al.* (1970)
4-CH$_2$=CHCH$_2$OC$_6$H$_4$	Me	6-Cl	Met, 10% protn. at 100	Parmar *et al.* (1970)
4-CH$_2$=CHCH$_2$OC$_6$H$_4$	Me	6-Br	Met, 10% protn. at 100	Parmar *et al.* (1970)
4-CH$_2$=CHCH$_2$OC$_6$H$_4$	Me	6-I	Met, 10% protn. at 100	Parmar *et al.* (1970)
4-CH$_2$=CHCH$_2$OC$_6$H$_4$	Me	6,8-Cl$_2$	Met, 10% protn. at 100	Parmar *et al.* (1970)
4-OH-3-CH$_2$CH=CHC$_6$H$_3$	Me	H	Met, 30% protn. at 100	Parmar *et al.* (1970)
4-OH-3-CH$_2$CH=CHC$_6$H$_3$	Me	6-Cl	Met, 10% protn. at 100	Parmar *et al.* (1970)
4-OH-3-CH$_2$CH=CHC$_6$H$_3$	Me	6-Br	Met, 10% protn. at 100	Parmar *et al.* (1970)
4-OH-3-CH$_2$CH=CHC$_6$H$_3$	Me	6-I	Met, 20% protn. at 100	Parmar *et al.* (1970)
4-OH-3-CH$_2$CH=CHC$_6$H$_3$	Me	6,8-Cl$_2$	Met, 10% protn. at 100	Parmar *et al.* (1970)
4-OH-3-CH$_2$CH=CHC$_6$H$_3$		6,8-Br$_2$	Met, 10% protn. at 100	Parmar *et al.* (1970)
4-MeSO$_2$NHC$_6$H$_4$	Me	6-Br	Met, 60% protn. at 100	Singh *et al.* (1972)
4-MeSO$_2$NHC$_6$H$_4$	Me	6-I	Met, 60% protn. at 100	Singh *et al.* (1972)
4-MeSO$_2$NHC$_6$H$_4$	Me	6-Cl	Met, 60% protn. at 100	Singh *et al.* (1972)
4-MeC$_6$H$_4$SO$_2$NHC$_6$H$_4$-4	Me	6-Br	Met, 40% protn. at 100	Singh *et al.* (1972)
4-MeC$_6$H$_4$SO$_2$NHC$_6$H$_4$-4	Me	6-I	Met, 20% protn. at 100	Singh *et al.* (1972)
4-MeOC$_6$H$_4$SO$_2$NHC$_6$H$_4$-4	Me	6-Cl	Met, 20% protn. at 100	Singh *et al.* (1972)
4-MeOC$_6$H$_4$SO$_2$NHC$_6$H$_4$-4	Me	6-Br	Met, 60% protn. at 100	Singh *et al.* (1972)
4-MeOC$_6$H$_4$SO$_2$NHC$_6$H$_4$-4	Me	6-I	Met, 40% protn. at 100	Singh *et al.* (1972)
4-FC$_6$H$_4$SO$_2$NHC$_6$H$_4$-4	Me	6-Br	Met, 40% protn. at 100	Singh *et al.* (1972)
4-FC$_6$H$_4$SO$_2$NHC$_6$H$_4$-4	Me	6-I	Met, 40% protn. at 100	Singh *et al.* (1972)
4-FC$_6$H$_4$SO$_2$NHC$_6$H$_4$-4	Me	6-Cl	Met, 80% protn. at 100	Singh *et al.* (1972)
4-BrC$_6$H$_4$SO$_2$NHC$_6$H$_4$-4	Me	6-I	Met, 20% protn. at 100	Singh *et al.* (1972)
2-MeC$_6$H$_4$	2-Pyr	H	Met, 30% protn. at 200 (po)	Hisano *et al.* (1972)
2-MeC$_6$H$_4$	4-Pyr	H	Met, 100% protn. at 150 (po)	Hisano *et al.* (1972)
C$_6$H$_5$	4-Pyr	H	Met, 90% protn. at 100 (po)	Hisano *et al.* (1972)

3-MeC$_6$H$_4$	4-Pyr	H	Met, 90% protn. at 100 (po)	Hisano *et al.* (1972)
4-MeC$_6$H$_4$	4-Pyr	H	Met, 60% protn. at 100 (po)	Hisano *et al.* (1972)
4-MeOC$_6$H$_4$	4-Pyr	H	Met, 40% protn. at 100 (po)	Hisano *et al.* (1972)
2-MeC$_6$H$_4$	3-Pyr	H	Met, 100% protn. at 100 (po)	Hisano *et al.* (1972)
C$_6$H$_5$	EtS	H	MES, 67% protn. at 600 (po)	Glasser *et al.* (1971)
C$_6$H$_5$CH$_2$CH$_2$	EtS	H	MES, 100% protn. at 100 (po)	Glasser *et al.* (1971)
C$_6$H$_5$CH$_2$CH$_2$	SCH$_2$CO$_2$H	H	MES, 33% protn. at 600 (po)	Glasser *et al.* (1971)
C$_6$H$_5$	SCH$_2$CO$_2$H	H	MES, 100% protn. at 600 (po)	Glasser *et al.* (1971)
CH$_2$CO$_2$Et	Me	H	Met, 10% protn. at 160 (po)	Barthwal *et al.* (1973)
CH$_2$CONHNH$_2$	Me	H	Met, 10% protn. at 160 (po)	Barthwal *et al.* (1973)
CH$_2$CO$_2$Et	Me	6-Cl	Met, 20% protn. at 160 (po)	Barthwal *et al.* (1973)
CH$_2$CONHNH$_2$	Me	6-Cl	Met, 20% protn. at 160 (po)	Barthwal *et al.* (1973)
CH$_2$CO$_2$Et	Me	6-Br	Met, 10% protn. at 320 (po)	Barthwal *et al.* (1973)
CH$_2$CONHNH$_2$	Me	6-Br	Met, 20% protn. at 160 (po)	Barthwal *et al.* (1973)
CH$_2$CO$_2$Et	Me	6-I	Met, 20% protn. at 80 (po)	Barthwal *et al.* (1973)
CH$_2$CONHNH$_2$	Me	6-I	Met, 30% protn. at 80 (po)	Barthwal *et al.* (1973)
CH$_2$CO$_2$Et	Me	6,8-Cl$_2$	Met, 30% protn. at 320 (po)	Barthwal *et al.* (1973)
CH$_2$CONHNH$_2$	Me	6,8-Cl$_2$	Met, 50% protn. at 320 (po)	Barthwal *et al.* (1973)
CH$_2$CO$_2$Et	Me	6,8-Br$_2$	Met, 30% protn. at 320 (po)	Barthwal *et al.* (1973)
CH$_2$CONHNH$_2$	Me	6,8-Br$_2$	Met, 40% protn. at 80 (po)	Barthwal *et al.* (1973)
CH$_2$CONHNH$_2$	Me	H	Met, 50% protn. at 80 (po)	Barthwal *et al.* (1973)
CH$_2$CONHNHCSNHC$_6$H$_4$Me-3	Me	H	Met, 50% protn. at 320 (po)	Barthwal *et al.* (1973)
CH$_2$CONHNHCSNHC$_6$H$_4$Me-4	Me	H	Met, 60% protn. at 160 (po)	Barthwal *et al.* (1973)
CH$_2$CONHNHCSNHC$_6$H$_4$OMe-4	Me	6-Br	Met, 50% protn. at 320 (po)	Barthwal *et al.* (1973)
CH$_2$CONHNHCSNHC$_6$H$_4$Me-3	Me	6-Br	Met, 50% protn. at 80 (po)	Barthwal *et al.* (1973)
CH$_2$CONHNHCSNHC$_6$H$_4$OMe-4	Me	6,8-Cl$_2$	Met, 70% protn. at 320 (po)	Barthwal *et al.* (1973)
CH$_2$CONHNHCSNHC$_6$H$_4$Me-3	Me	6,8-Cl$_2$	Met, 50% protn. at 80 (po)	Barthwal *et al.* (1973)
CH$_2$CONHNHCSNHC$_6$H$_4$Me-4	Me	6,8-Cl$_2$	Met, 50% protn. at 320 (po)	Barthwal *et al.* (1973)
H_2C–⟨N=N, O ring⟩–NHC$_6$H$_4$Me-3	Me	H	Met, 30% protn. at 160 (po)	Barthwal *et al.* (1973)
H_2C–⟨N=N, O ring⟩–NHC$_6$H$_4$Me-4	Me	H	Met, 60% protn. at 320 (po)	Barthwal *et al.* (1973)

(continued)

TABLE XXIII—Continued

Compound	R	R_2	Activity	Reference
H_2C— (oxadiazole) —NHC_6H_4OMe-4	Me	H	Met, 20% protn. at 320 (po)	Barthwal et al. (1973)
H_2C— (oxadiazole) —NHC_6H_4Me-3	Me	6-Br	Met, 40% protn. at 80 (po)	Barthwal et al. (1973)
H_2C— (oxadiazole) —NHC_6H_4OMe-4	Me	6-Br	Met, 50% protn. at 160 (po)	Barthwal et al. (1973)
H_2C— (oxadiazole) —NHC_6H_4Me-3	Me	$6,8-Cl_2$	Met, 50% protn. at 80 (po)	Barthwal et al. (1973)
H_2C— (oxadiazole) —NHC_6H_4Me-4	Me	$6,8-Cl_2$	Met, 30% protn. at 320 (po)	Barthwal et al. (1973)
H_2C— (oxadiazole) —NHC_6H_4OMe-4	Me	$6,8-Cl_2$	Met, 70% protn. at 320 (po)	Barthwal et al. (1973)
$4-BrC_6H_4$	Me	6-Br	Met, 25% protn. at 300 (po) MES, 10% protn. at 200 (po)	Mehta and Malhotra (1966) Mehta and Malhotra (1966)
$4-BrC_6H_4$	Me	6-Cl	MES, 40% protn. at 300 (po) Met, 40% protn. at 300 (po)	Mehta and Malhotra (1966) Mehta and Malhotra (1966)
$2-MeC_6H_4$	Me	6-Cl-8-Br	Met, 70% protn. at 200 (po) MES, 75% protn. at 300 (po)	Mehta and Malhotra (1966) Mehta and Malhotra (1966)
$2-MeC_6H_4$	Me	6-Cl	MES, 100% protn. at 200 (po) MES, 90% protn. at 300 (po)	Mehta and Malhotra (1966) Mehta and Malhotra (1966)

3-OH-4-$CONHNH_2C_6H_3$	Me	6-Cl	Met, 30% protn. at 100 (po)	T. K. Gupta *et al.* (1973)
			MES, 30% protn. at 100 (po)	T. K. Gupta *et al.* (1973)
3-OH-4-$CONHNH_2C_6H_3$	Me	6-Br	Met, 10% protn. at 100 (po)	T. K. Gupta *et al.* (1973)
			MES, 10% protn. at 100 (po)	T. K. Gupta *et al.* (1973)
3-OH-4-$CONHNH_2C_6H_3$	Me	6-I	Met, 40% protn. at 100 (po)	T. K. Gupta *et al.* (1973)
			MES, 30% protn. at 100 (po)	T. K. Gupta *et al.* (1973)
3-OH-4-$CONHNH_2C_6H_3$	Me	6,8-Cl_2	Met, 20% protn. at 100 (po)	T. K. Gupta *et al.* (1973)
3-OH-4-$CONHNH_2C_6H_3$	Me	6,8-Br_2	Met, 40% protn. at 100 (po)	T. K. Gupta *et al.* (1973)
			MES, 60% protn. at 100 (po)	T. K. Gupta *et al.* (1973)
3-OH-4-$CONHNH_2C_6H_3$	Me	6,8-I_2	MES, 30% protn. at 100 (po)	T. K. Gupta *et al.* (1973)
			Met, 40% protn. at 100 (po)	T. K. Gupta *et al.* (1973)
3-OH-4-$CONHNH_2C_6H_3$	Me	H	Met, 10% protn. at 100 (po)	T. K. Gupta *et al.* (1973)
			MES, 30% protn. at 100 (po)	T. K. Gupta *et al.* (1973)

C. Miscellaneous quinazolines

Compound	Activity	Reference
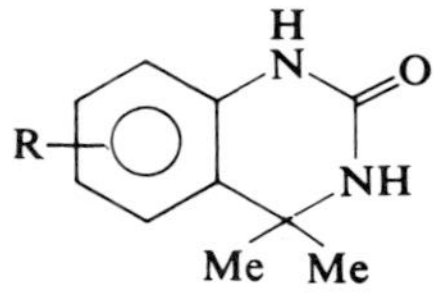	Met and ES, active	Bernardi *et al.* (1970)
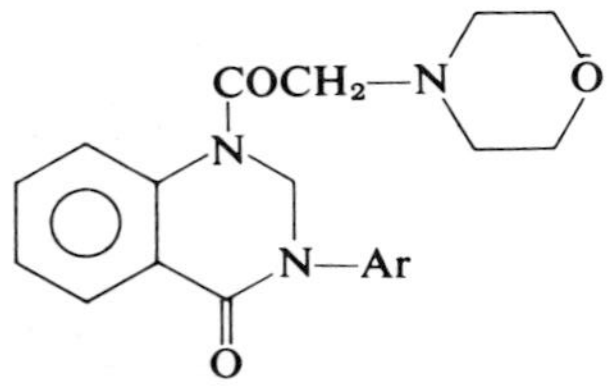	Active	Bonola *et al.* (1968)
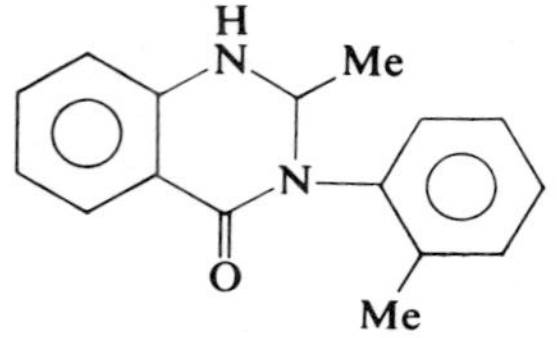	MES ED_{50} > 100	Boltze *et al.* (1963)

(*continued*)

TABLE XXIII—*Continued*

Compound	Activity	Reference
	MES ED$_{50}$ > 100	Boltze *et al.* (1963)
	Active	Danielsson *et al.* (1968)
	Active Met and ES	Glasser *et al.* (1971)
	Active	Berlin *et al.* (1974); Pfeifer and Pohlmann (1974)

TABLE XXIV   PIPERAZINE DERIVATIVES

A. Piperazines[a]

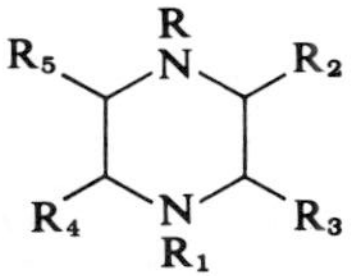

R	R_1	Activity	Reference
SO_2NH_2	Ar	Active	Hofmann (1956)
$CO(CH_2)_6CH_3$	$4\text{-}FC_6H_4CO(CH_2)_3$	Met, active	Rajsner et al. (1975)
$R(CH_2)_n$	$(CH_2)_2CH$ 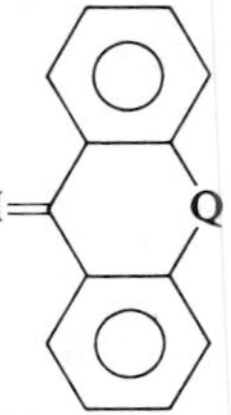	Active	Nakanishi et al. (1972d)
H	$(CH_2)_nO_2CAr$	Active	Kato et al. (1974)
$4\text{-}t\text{-}BuC_6H_4CH_2$	$CH(Ph)C_6H_4Cl\text{-}4$	MES ED_{50} 46	Saxena et al. (1969)
Me	$CH(Ph)C_6H_4Cl\text{-}4$	MES ED_{50} 121	Saxena et al. (1969)
$(CH_2)_2O(CH_2)_2OH$	$CH(Ph)C_6H_4Cl\text{-}4$	MES ED_{50} 31	Saxena et al. (1969)
$3\text{-}MeC_6H_4CH_2$	$CH(Ph)C_6H_4Cl\text{-}4$	MES ED_{50} 52	Saxena et al. (1969)
Me	$CH(Et)CO_2C_6H_3Me_2\text{-}2,6$	ES and Met, active	Coscia et al. (1968)
$N=CRR'$	$(CH_2)_nCH(Ar)Ar'$	ES and Met, active	Cusic and Levon (1965)
NHR	$CH(Ph)Ar$	ES and Met, active	Cusic and Levon (1964)
CH_2COR	$COCH=CHR'$	Active	Fauran et al. (1972)
$CH_2CONHCHMe_2$	$COCH=CH$ 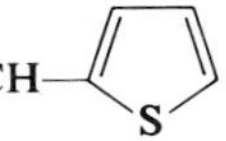	Met ED_{50} 75 (po)	Fauran et al. (1974f)

(continued)

451

TABLE XXIV—*Continued*

R	R_1	Activity	Reference
MeCHCH₂Ph	MeCHCH₂Ph	Met ED₅₀ 16.5 (sc)	Fauran *et al.* (1974f)
		MES ED₅₀ 11 (sc), 84 (po)	Stille *et al.* (1957)
COR	CH₂Ar	Active	Weber *et al.* (1974)
CONH₂	COR	Active	Goldman and Williams (1956)
CH₂Ph	COC₆H₃Cl-2-NH₂-4	Active	Jacob and Joseph (1959)
R	CH₂C₆H₄XPh-2	Active	Protiva *et al.* (1974a)
N=X	CH₂Ar	Active	Protiva *et al.* (1974b)
N=C(R)R'	CH(Ar)C₆H₄X-4	Active	LeVon and Cusie (1963)
CO₂Et	CH(Ph) 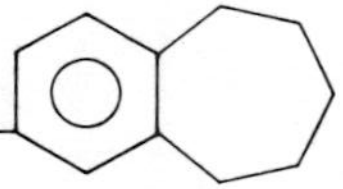	Met, sl. act.	Vejdelek *et al.* (1973a)
CH₂Ph	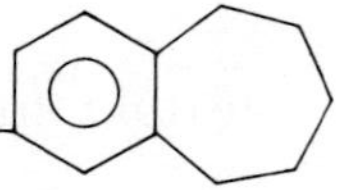 H₂C	Met, act. at 300	Vejdelek *et al.* (1974)
4-ClC₆H₄CH₂	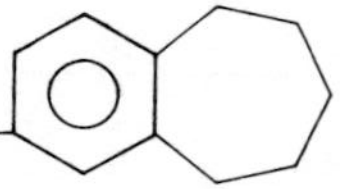 H₂C	Met, sl. act.; ES, act. at 300	Vejdelek *et al.* (1974)
2-MeOC₆H₄CH₂	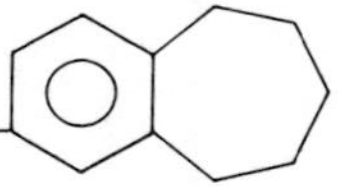 H₂C	Met, act. at 200	Vejdelek *et al.* (1974)
2-PhCH₂C₆H₄CH₂	CHMe₂	Met, active	Kopicova *et al.* (1972)
2-PhCH₂C₆H₄CH₂	NO	Met, active	Kopicova *et al.* (1972)
2-PhCH₂C₆H₄CH₂	N=CHC₆H₃(OMe)₂	ES, active	Kopicova *et al.* (1972)

452

Substituent	Substituent(s)	Activity	Reference
$CH_2C{\equiv}CH$		Met and ES, active	Vejdelek et al. (1973b)
$(CH_2)_3Ph$		Met and ES, active	Vejdelek et al. (1973b)
$(CH_2)_2CN$		Met and ES, active	Vejdelek et al. (1973b)
$COCH_3$		Met and ES, active	Vejdelek et al. (1973b)
CH_2Ph		Met and ES, active	Vejdelek et al. (1973b)
$N{=}CHPh$	$CHPh_2$	MES ED_{50} > 50 (po)	Craig (1967)
$N{=}CHPh$	$CH(Ph)C_6H_4Cl\text{-}4$	MES ED_{50} 44 (po)	Craig (1967)
$N{=}CHPyr\text{-}4$	$CHPh_2$	MES ED_{50} 4.9 (po)	Craig (1967)
$N{=}CHC_6H_3O_2CH_2\text{-}3,4$	$CH(Ph)C_6H_4Cl\text{-}4$	MES ED_{50} 16 (po)	Craig (1967)
$N{=}CHPyr\text{-}2\text{-}Me\text{-}6$	$CHPh_2$	MES ED_{50} 6.2 (po)	Craig (1967)
$N{=}CHPyr\text{-}3$	$CH(Ph)C_6H_4Cl\text{-}4$	MES ED_{50} 3.7 (po)	Craig (1967)
$N{=}CHPyr\text{-}2$	$CHPh_2$	MES ED_{50} 10 (po)	Craig (1967)
$N{=}CHC_6H_4OH\text{-}4$	$CH(Ph)C_6H_4Cl\text{-}4$	MES ED_{50} 3.7 (po)	Craig (1967)
$N{=}CHPyr\text{-}4$	$CH(Ph)C_6H_4Cl\text{-}4$	MES ED_{50} 8.2 (po)	Craig (1967)
$N{=}CHC_6H_4OH\text{-}4$	$CH(Ph)C_6H_4Cl\text{-}4$	MES ED_{50} 6.2 (po)	Craig (1967)
$N{=}CHC_6H_4CN\text{-}4$	$CHPh_2$	MES ED_{50} 2.9 (po)	Craig (1967)
$N{=}CHPyr\text{-}4\text{-}NO$	$CH(Ph)C_6H_4Cl\text{-}4$	MES ED_{50} 3.3 (po)	Craig (1967)
$N{=}CHPyr\text{-}4\text{-}NO$			

(continued)

TABLE XXIV—*Continued*

R	R_1	Activity	Reference
$N=CHPyr-4$	$CH(Ph)C_6H_4Me-4$	MES ED_{50} 5.5 (po)	Craig (1967)
$N=CHPh$	$CH(Ph)C_6H_4Br-4$	MES ED_{50} 39 (po)	Craig (1967)
$N=CHPyr-4$	$CH(Ph)C_6H_4Br-4$	MES ED_{50} 4.2 (po)	Craig (1967)
$N=CHPyr-4$	$CHPh_2$	MES ED_{50} 8.4 (po)	Craig (1967)
$N=CHPyr-3$	$CHPh_2$	MES ED_{50} 27 (po)	Craig (1967)
$N=CHPyr-4$	$CH(Ph)C_6H_4Cl-4$	MES ED_{50} 10.8 (po)	Craig (1967)
$N=CHPyr-3$	$CH(Ph)C_6H_4Cl-4$	MES ED_{50} 28 (po)	Craig (1967)
$3-CF_3C_6H_4$	H	MES, 80% protn. 0.25 LD_{50}	Jain et al. (1967)
$3-MeOC_6H_4$	H	MES, 40% protn. 0.25 LD_{50}	Jain et al. (1967)
$4-FC_6H_4$	H	MES, 60% protn. 0.25 LD_{50}	Jain et al. (1967)
$2,4-(MeO)_2C_6H_4$	H	MES, 40% protn. 0.25 LD_{50}	Jain et al. (1967)
$4-Pyr-3-NO_2$	Ph	MES, 60% protn. 0.25 LD_{50}	Jain et al. (1967)
$4-Pyr-3-NH_2$	Ph	MES, 20% protn. 0.25 LD_{50}	Jain et al. (1967)
$4-Pyr-3-NO_2$	$4-ClC_6H_4$	MES, 60% protn. 0.25 LD_{50}	Jain et al. (1967)
$4-Pyr-3-NH_2$	$4-ClC_6H_4$	MES, 20% protn. 0.25 LD_{50}	Jain et al. (1967)
$4-Pyr-3-NH_2$	$4-MeC_6H_4$	MES, 60% protn. 0.25 LD_{50}	Jain et al. (1967)
$4-Pyr-3-NH_2$	$3,4-(MeO)_2C_6H_3$	MES, 60% protn. 0.25 LD_{50}	Jain et al. (1967)
$4-Pyr-3-NO_2$	$2,4-(MeO)_2C_6H_3$	MES, 20% protn. 0.25 LD_{50}	Jain et al. (1967)
$4-Pyr-3-NH_2$	$2,4-(MeO)_2C_6H_3$	MES, 20% protn. 0.25 LD_{50}	Jain et al. (1967)
$4-Pyr-NO$	Ph	MES, 100% protn. 0.25 LD_{50} Met, 20% protn. at 20 (ip)	Jain et al. (1967)
$4-Pyr$	Ph	MES, 60% protn. 0.25 LD_{50}	Jain et al. (1967)
$4-Pyr-3-NO_2$	$4-MeOC_6H_4$	MES, 100% protn. 0.25 LD_{50} Met, 20% protn. at 20 (ip)	Jain et al. (1967)
$4-Pyr-3-NH_2$	$4-MeOC_6H_4$	MES, 100% protn. 0.25 LD_{50} Met, 100% protn. at 20 (ip)	Jain et al. (1967)
$4-Pyr-3-NO_2$	$4-NO_2C_6H_4$	MES, 60% protn. 0.25 LD_{50}	Jain et al. (1967)
$4-Pyr-3-NH_2$	$4-NH_2C_6H_4$	MES, 20% protn. 0.25 LD_{50}	Jain et al. (1967)

(*continued*)

4-Pyr-3-NO2	CH3	MES, 20% protn. 0.25 LD50	Jain *et al.* (1967)
(CH2)2NHC(=S)NHPh	4-NO2C6H4CO	Met, 20% protn. at 100 (ip)	Singh *et al.* (1974c)
(CH2)2NHC(=S)NHC6H4Me-2	4-NO2C6H4CO	Met, 60% protn. at 100 (ip)	Singh *et al.* (1974c)
(CH2)2NHC(=S)NHC6H4Me-3	4-NO2C6H4CO	Met, 40% protn. at 100 (ip)	Singh *et al.* (1974c)
(CH2)2NHC(=S)NHC6H4Me-4	4-NO2C6H4CO	Met, 30% protn. at 100 (ip)	Singh *et al.* (1974c)
(CH2)2NHC(=S)NHC6H4OMe-2	4-NO2C6H4CO	Met, 30% protn. at 100 (ip)	Singh *et al.* (1974c)
(CH2)2NHC(=S)NHC6H4OMe-4	4-NO2C6H4CO	Met, 40% protn. at 100 (ip)	Singh *et al.* (1974c)
(CH2)2NHC(=S)NHC6H4Cl-4	4-NO2C6H4CO	Met, 10% protn. at 100 (ip)	Singh *et al.* (1974c)
(CH2)2NHC(=S)NHC6H4Br-4	4-NO2C6H4CO	Met, 40% protn. at 100 (ip)	Singh *et al.* (1974c)
(CH2)2NHC(=S)NHC6H4I-4	4-NO2C6H4CO	Met, 30% protn. at 100 (ip)	Singh *et al.* (1974c)
(CH2)2NHC(=S)NHNap-1	4-NO2C6H4CO	Met, 60% protn. at 100 (ip)	Singh *et al.* (1974c)
(CH2)2NHC(=S)NHPh	3-NO2C6H4CO	Met, 20% protn. at 100 (ip)	Singh *et al.* (1974c)
(CH2)2NHC(=S)NHC6H4Me-3	3-NO2C6H4CO	Met, 30% protn. at 100 (ip)	Singh *et al.* (1974c)
(CH2)2NHC(=S)NHC6H4Me-4	3-NO2C6H4CO	Met, 10% protn. at 100 (ip)	Singh *et al.* (1974c)
(CH2)2NHC(=S)NHC6H4OMe-4	3-NO2C6H4CO	Met, 20% protn. at 100 (ip)	Singh *et al.* (1974c)
(CH2)2NHC(=S)NHC6H4Cl-4	3-NO2C6H4CO	Met, 20% protn. at 100 (ip)	Singh *et al.* (1974c)
(CH2)2NHC(=S)NHC6H4Br-4	3-NO2C6H4CO	Met, 30% protn. at 100 (ip)	Singh *et al.* (1974c)
(CH2)2NHC(=S)NHC6H4I-4	3-NO2C6H4CO	Met, 40% protn. at 100 (ip)	Singh *et al.* (1974c)
(CH2)2NHC(=S)NHNap-1	3-NO2C6H4CO	Met, 50% protn. at 100 (ip)	Singh *et al.* (1974c)
EtNHCONH(CH2)3	(CH2)3NHCONHEt	Met, 50% protn. at 100 (ip)	Chaturvedi *et al.* (1975)
PhNHCONH(CH2)3	(CH2)3NHCONHPh	Met, 50% protn. at 100 (ip)	Chaturvedi *et al.* (1975)
2-MeC6H4NHCONH(CH2)3	(CH2)3NHCONHC6H4Me-2	Met, 50% protn. at 100 (ip)	Chaturvedi *et al.* (1975)
3-MeC6H4NHCONH(CH2)3	(CH2)3NHCONHC6H4Me-3	Met, 60% protn. at 100 (ip)	Chaturvedi *et al.* (1975)
4-MeC6H4NHCONH(CH2)3	(CH2)3NHCONHC6H4Me-4	Met, 40% protn. at 100 (ip)	Chaturvedi *et al.* (1975)
2-ClC6H4NHCONH(CH2)3	(CH2)3NHCONHC6H4Cl-2	Met, 40% protn. at 100 (ip)	Chaturvedi *et al.* (1975)
3-ClC6H4NHCONH(CH2)3	(CH2)3NHCONHC6H4Cl-3	Met, 30% protn. at 100 (ip)	Chaturvedi *et al.* (1975)
4-ClC6H4NHCONH(CH2)3	(CH2)3NHCONHC6H4Cl-4	Met, 20% protn. at 100 (ip)	Chaturvedi *et al.* (1945)
4-BrC6H4NHCONH(CH2)3	(CH2)3NHCONHC6H4Br-4	Met, 40% protn. at 100 (ip)	Chaturvedi *et al.* (1975)
2-MeOC6H4NHCONH(CH2)3	(CH2)3NHCONHC6H4OMe-2	Met, 70% protn. at 100 (ip)	Chaturvedi *et al.* (1975)
4-MeOC6H4NHCONH(CH2)3	(CH2)3NHCONHC6H4OMe-4	Met, 40% protn. at 100 (ip)	Chaturvedi *et al.* (1975)
2-EtOC6H4NHCONH(CH2)3	(CH2)3NHCONHC6H4OEt-2	Met, 50% protn. at 100 (ip)	Chaturvedi *et al.* (1975)
4-EtOC6H4NHCONH(CH2)3	(CH2)3NHCONHC6H4OEt-4	Met, 70% protn. at 100 (ip)	Chaturvedi *et al.* (1975)

TABLE XXIV—*Continued*

R	R$_1$	Activity	Reference
PhNHC(=S)NH(CH$_2$)$_3$	(CH$_2$)$_3$NHC(=S)NHPh	Met, 20% protn. at 100 (ip)	Chaturvedi and Parmar (1972a)
CH$_2$=CHCH$_2$NHC(=S)NH(CH$_2$)$_3$	(CH$_2$)$_3$NHC(=S)NHCH$_2$CH=CH$_2$	Met, 60% protn. at 100 (ip)	Chaturvedi and Parmar (1972a)
EtNHC(=S)NH(CH$_2$)$_3$	(CH$_2$)$_3$NHC(=S)NHET	Met, 50% protn. at 100 (ip)	Chaturvedi and Parmar (1972a)
2-MeC$_6$H$_4$NHC(=S)NH(CH$_2$)$_3$	(CH$_2$)$_3$NHC(=S)NHC$_6$H$_4$Me-2	Met, 50% protn. at 100 (ip)	Chaturvedi and Parmar (1972a)
3-MeC$_6$H$_4$NHC(=S)NH(CH$_2$)$_3$	(CH$_2$)$_3$NHC(=S)NHC$_6$H$_4$Me-3	Met, 50% protn. at 100 (ip)	Chaturvedi and Parmar (1972a)
4-MeC$_6$H$_4$NHC(=S)NH(CH$_2$)$_3$	(CH$_2$)$_3$NHC(=S)NHC$_6$H$_4$Me-4	Met, 20% protn. at 100 (ip)	Chaturvedi and Parmar (1972a)
3,4-Me$_2$C$_6$H$_3$NHC(=S)NH(CH$_2$)$_3$	(CH$_2$)$_3$NHC(=S)NHC$_6$H$_3$Me$_2$-3,4	Met, 30% protn. 100 (ip)	Chaturvedi and Parmar (1972a)
4-ClC$_6$H$_4$NHC(=S)NH(CH$_2$)$_3$	(CH$_2$)$_3$NHC(=S)NHC$_6$H$_4$Cl-4	Met, 50% protn. 100 (ip)	Chaturvedi and Parmar (1972a)
2-MeOC$_6$H$_4$NHC(=S)NH(CH$_2$)$_3$	(CH$_2$)$_3$NHC(=S)NHC$_6$H$_4$OMe-2	Met, 40% protn. 100 (ip)	Chaturvedi and Parmar (1972a)
4-MeOC$_6$H$_4$NHC(=S)NH(CH$_2$)$_3$	(CH$_2$)$_3$NHC(=S)NHC$_6$H$_4$OMe-4	Met, 40% protn. 100 (ip)	Chaturvedi and Parmar (1972a)
N=CH— (with R)	[structure with (CH$_2$)$_n$] R$_3$, R$_5$ = R	Active	Cusic and Yonan (1968)
RCO	(CH$_2$)$_m$OCOR$_6$, R$_3$ = (CH$_2$)$_n$ (n = 1 or 2)	Active	Kato *et al.* (1975a,b,c)

TABLE XXIV—*Continued*

B. Miscellaneous derivatives

Compound	Activity	Reference
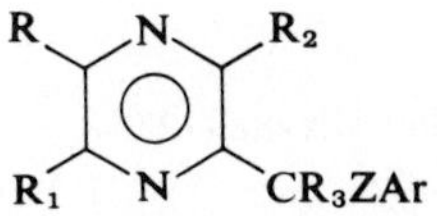	Active	Akkermann *et al.* (1963)
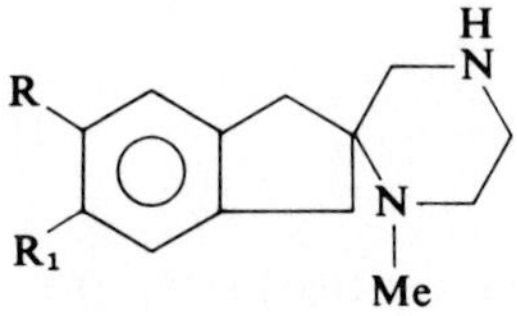	Active	Kato and Koshinaka (1974a)
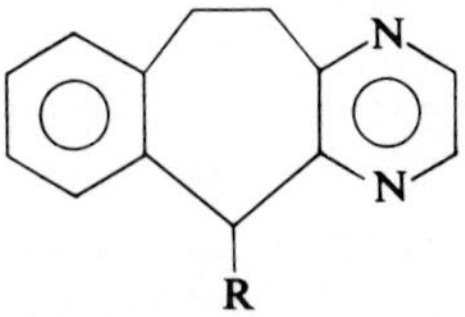	Active	Eberle (1975)
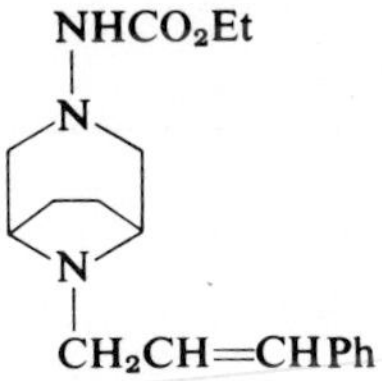	Active	Fontanella *et al.* (1972)
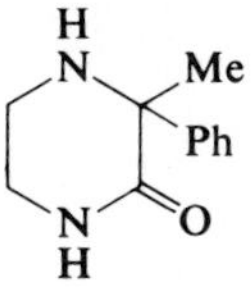	Active	Melone *et al.* (1961)
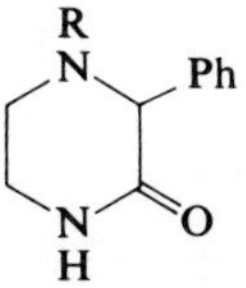	Active	Roderick *et al.* (1966)
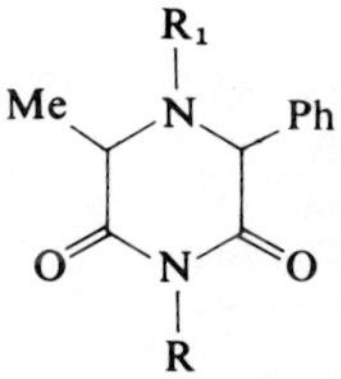	Active	Safir and Hlavka (1956b)

(*continued*)

TABLE XXIV—*Continued*

Compound	Activity	Reference
	Active	Safir and Hlavka (1956a)
	Active	Safir and Hlavka (1956c)
	Active	Field and Sternback (1971a)

[a] R_2, R_3, R_4, R_5 = H unless otherwise noted.

TABLE XXV 2,3-OXAZINE DERIVATIVES[a]

X	R	Activity
NO_2	H	MES ED_{50} 75
NO_2	Me	MES ED_{50} 75
NO_2	$(CH_2)_2OCONH_2$	MES ED_{50} 50
NO_2	$(CH_2)_2$Pyr-4	MES ED_{50} 50
NH_2	Me	MES ED_{50} 75
Cl	Me	MES ED_{50} 100

[a] Data from Pifferi *et al.* (1969).

TABLE XXVI 1,3-OXAZINE DERIVATIVES

Compound	Activity	Reference
	Active	Fauran *et al.* (1974c)
	Active	Testa (1960)
	Met, active	Boissier *et al.* (1972a); Farbwerke Hoechst (1969)
	R = Et: Met ED_{50} 165 (po) R = *i*-Pr: Met ED_{50} 300 R = H: Met ED_{50} < 300 R = Me: Met ED_{50} 200	Kuch (1973) Kuch (1973) Kuch (1973) Kuch (1973)
	Active	Bernardi *et al.* (1969)

R	R_1	R_2	Activity	Reference
MeCONH₂	H	H	Met ED_{50} > 200 (ip); MES, inactive	DeMarchi (1971)
	Ph	H	Met ED_{50} 105 (ip); MES ED_{50} 135 (ip)	DeMarchi (1971)
Me	Ph	H	Met ED_{50} > 200 (ip); MES ED_{50} 143 (ip)	DeMarchi (1971)
	Ph	Cl	Met ED_{50} 78 (ip); MES ED_{50} 52 (ip)	DeMarchi (1971)
Me	Ph	Cl	Met ED_{50} > 200 (ip); MES ED_{50} 200 (ip)	DeMarchi (1971)
MeCONH₂	Ph	Cl	Met ED_{50} > 200 (ip); MES ED_{50} 200 (ip)	DeMarchi (1971)
	Ph	NO₂	Met ED_{50} > 200 (ip); MES ED_{50} 200 (ip)	DeMarchi (1971)
Me	Ph	NO₂	Met ED_{50} > 200 (ip); MES ED_{50} 200 (ip)	DeMarchi (1971)

TABLE XXVII MORPHOLINE DERIVATIVES

A. Morpholines

R	R_1	R_2	R_3	Activity	Reference
i-Pr	CH_2ONap-1	H	H	MES ED_{50} 100 (po)	Greenwood et al. (1975)
i-Pr	2-CH_2=$CHCH_2OC_6H_4OCH_2$	H	H	MES ED_{50} 100 (po)	Greenwood et al. (1975)
i-Pr	3-$CF_3C_6H_4OCH_2$	H	H	MES ED_{50} 75 (po)	Greenwood et al. (1975)
i-Pr	3-$MeC_6H_4OCH_2$	H	H	MES ED_{50} 100 (po)	Greenwood et al. (1975)
H	2-$MeOC_6H_4OCH_2$	H	H	MES ED_{50} 100 (po)	Greenwood et al. (1975)
H	2-$EtOC_6H_4OCH_2$	H	H	MES ED_{50} 30 (po)	Greenwood et al. (1975)
H	2-n-$PrOC_6H_4OCH_2$	H	H	MES ED_{50} 30–100 (po)	Greenwood et al. (1975)
H	2-CH_2=$CHCH_2OC_6H_4OCH_2$	H	H	MES ED_{50} 30 (po)	Greenwood et al. (1975)
H	2-$PhOC_6H_4OCH_2$	H	H	MES ED_{50} 100 (po)	Greenwood et al. (1975)
H	4-$MeOC_6H_4OCH_2$	H	H	MES ED_{50} 100 (po)	Greenwood et al. (1975)
$(CH_2)_3COPh$	H	H	H	MES ED_{50} 20 (sc), 200 (po)	Squires and Lassen (1968)
$CH_2CH(Me)C(Ph)_2OH$	H	Me	Me	Active	Moffett (1968a)

B. Miscellaneous derivatives

Compound	Activity	Reference
	Met, 10% protn. at 100	Irwin *et al.* (1972)
	Active	Pesson (1972)
	R = H: Met, 10% protn. at 200 (ip) R = Me: Met, 10% protn. at 140 (ip)	Pesson (1972) Pesson (1972)

461

TABLE XXVIII 1,2-THIAZINE DERIVATIVES

A. Monocyclic systems		
Compound	Activity	Reference

MES, 65% protn. at 50 (po); MES ED_{50} 35 — Wirth *et al.* (1960)

Ar	Activity	Reference
4-NH$_2$C$_6$H$_4$	MES ED_{50} 105	Friebel (1960)
3-NH$_2$C$_6$H$_4$	MES ED_{50} 155	Friebel (1960)
4-MeO-3-NH$_2$C$_6$H$_3$	MES ED_{50} 500	Friebel (1960)
4-EtO-3-NH$_2$C$_6$H$_3$	MES ED_{50} 248; Met ED_{50} 300	Friebel (1960)
4-BuOC$_6$H$_4$	MES ED_{50} 500; Met ED_{50} 306	Friebel (1960)
2-Pyr	MES ED_{50} 470; Met ED_{50} 340	Friebel (1960)
PhCH$_2$	MES ED_{50} 220; Met ED_{50} 400	Friebel (1960)

Compound	Activity	Reference

MES ED_{50} 150; Met ED_{50} 22 — Friebel and Sommer (1960)

Active — Helferich (1959)

B. Bicyclic systems

R	Activity	Reference
H	MES, 70% protn. at > 150 (ip), > 150 (po)	Sianesi *et al.* (1973b)
Me	MES, 70% protn. at 230 (ip), > 230 (po)	Sianesi *et al.* (1973b)
Et	MES, 70% protn. at 300 (ip), > 300 (po)	Sianesi *et al.* (1973b)
n-Pr	MES, 70% protn. at > 520 (ip), > 520 (po)	Sianesi *et al.* (1973b)
i-Pr	MES, 70% protn. at 75 (ip), 150 (po)	Sianesi *et al.* (1973b)
n-Bu	MES, 70% protn. at > 174 (ip), > 174 (po)	Sianesi *et al.* (1973b)
$CH_2CH=CH_2$	MES, 70% protn. at 100 (ip), > 100 (po)	Sianesi *et al.* (1973b)
$CH_2C\equiv CH$	MES, 70% protn. at 300 (ip), 300 (po)	Sianesi *et al.* (1973b)
CH_2Ph	MES, 70% protn. at > 300 (ip), > 300 (po)	Sianesi *et al.* (1973b)

R	Activity	Reference
CH_2CONH_2	MES ED_{50} 50	Sianesi *et al.* (1973a)
$CH_2CONHMe$	MES ED_{50} 230	Sianesi *et al.* (1973a)
$CH_2CONHPr$-*n*	MES ED_{50} 28	Sianesi *et al.* (1973a)
$CH_2CONHCH_2CH=CH_2$	MES ED_{50} 50	Sianesi *et al.* (1973a)
$CH_2CON(Pr$-*i*$)_2$	MES ED_{50} 87	Sianesi *et al.* (1973a)
$C(Me)_2CONH_2$	MES ED_{50} 300	Sianesi *et al.* (1973a)
$C(Me)_2CONHPr$-*i*	MES ED_{50} 65	Sianesi *et al.* (1973a)
$CH_2CONHNH_2$	MES ED_{50} 150	Sianesi *et al.* (1973a)
$CH_2CONHNHEt$	MES ED_{50} 133	Sianesi *et al.* (1973a)
$CH_2CONHN=CHMe$	MES ED_{50} 130	Sianesi *et al.* (1973a)

R	Activity	Reference
H	MES, 70% protn. at > 150 (ip), > 150 (po)	Sianesi *et al.* (1973b)
Me	MES, 70% protn. at 100 (ip), 200 (po)	Sianesi *et al.* (1973b)
Et	MES, 70% protn. at 130 (ip), > 130 (po)	Sianesi *et al.* (1973b)
n-Pr	MES, 70% protn. at 200 (ip), 200 (po)	Sianesi *et al.* (1973b)
i-Pr	MES, 70% protn. at > 300 (ip), > 300 (po)	Sianesi *et al.* (1973b)
n-Bu	MES, 70% protn. at 300 (ip), 300 (po)	Sianesi *et al.* (1973b)
$CH_2CH=CH_2$	MES, 70% protn. at 160 (ip), > 160 (po)	Sianesi *et al.* (1973b)
$CH_2C\equiv CH$	MES, 70% protn. at > 300 (ip), > 300 (po)	Sianesi *et al.* (1973b)
CH_2Ph	MES, 70% protn. at > 300 (ip), > 300 (po)	Sianesi *et al.* (1973b)

TABLE XXIX 1,3-THIAZINE DERIVATIVES

Compound	Activity	Reference
	Active	Surrey (1964)
	Active	Sterling Drug Inc. (1959)
	Active	Gesler and Surrey (1958)
	Active	Gesler and Surrey (1958)

TABLE XXX 1,4-THIAZINE DERIVATIVES

A. Thiamorpholines

Compound	Activity	Reference
	Active	Skinner and Bicking (1957)
	Active	Skinner and Elmslie (1959)

TABLE XXX—*Continued*

B. Phenothiazines[a]

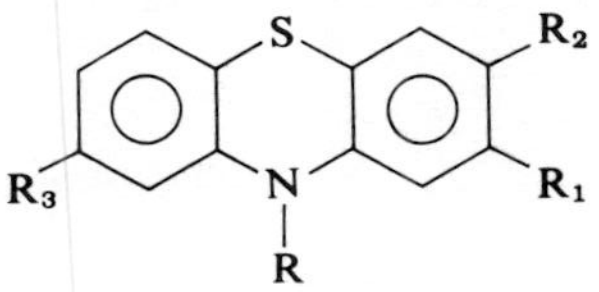

R	R₁	Activity	Reference
H (R₂ = SO₂NH₂) CONH₂	H (R₂ = SO₂NH₂)	Active Active MES, 100% protn. at 400 Active Active	T. Watanabe et al. (1973a,b) Naka et al. (1972) Naka et al. (1974) Kitano et al. (1973) Mercier et al. (1957)
H (R₃ = SO₂NH₂) (CH₂)₃NMe₂	SO₂NH₂ COMe		
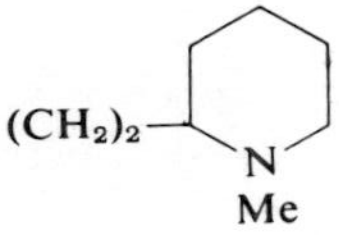 (CH₂)₂–(1-methylpiperidin-2-yl)	SO₂Me	Met, active	Maruyama et al. (1967a)
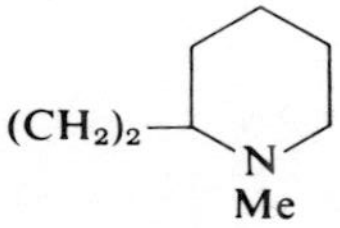 (CH₂)₂–(1-methylpiperidin-2-yl)	SMe	Met, active	Maruyama et al. (1967a,b)
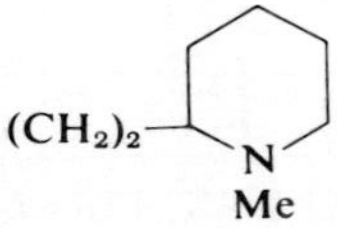 (CH₂)₂–(1-methylpiperidin-2-yl)	SOMe	Active	Maruyama et al. (1967b)

(continued)

TABLE XXX—*Continued*

R	R_1	Activity	Reference
$(CH_2)_2$— (2-methyl-1-methylpiperidine ring)	OMe	Active	Maruyama *et al.* (1968)
$(CH_2)_3N$— (4-methylpiperidine ring)	SEt	Met, active at 100	Maruyama *et al.* (1965)
$(CH_2)_3NMe_2$	OMe	Met, active	Georges *et al.* (1958)
$(CH_2)_3NMe_2$	Cl	Active	Georges *et al.* (1958)
CON— (morpholine ring)	H	Active	Georges *et al.* (1958)
H_2C— (1-methyl-4-piperidyl ring, NMe)	H	MES, active	Sharma *et al.* (1967)
$(CH_2)_2N$— (4-hydroxypiperidine ring, OH)	CN	MES, active	Sharma *et al.* (1967)
CH_3N (pyrrolidine ring)	H	MES, active	Sharma *et al.* (1967)
$CH_2CH(Me)\overset{+}{N}Me_2R\overset{-}{X}$	H	Active	Wunderlich *et al.* (1964)
$CONH_2$	H	Met ED_{50} 20 (po); MES ED_{50} 31 (ip), 34.5 (po)	Davis *et al.* (1964)
R	H	ES, active	Singh *et al.* (1969)
$CH_2CH(Me)NMe_2$	H	MES ED_{50} 24; Met, partially act. at 200	Saxena *et al.* (1969)

C. Miscellaneous derivatives

Compound	Activity	Reference
(phenothiazine structure with –CONH$_2$)	Active	Scholler (1958)
(phenothiazine structure with CH$_2$CHNMe$_2$ / CH$_3$)	MES ED$_{50}$ 58; Met, inactive	Saxena et al. (1969)

[a] R$_2$, R$_3$ = H unless otherwise noted.

467

TABLE XXXI   DIOXANES AND THIODIOXANES

Compound	Activity	Reference
HOCH$_2$ and HOCH$_2$ with dioxane ring bearing CCl$_3$	Active	Société d'Exploitation des Laboratoires Bottu (1961)
benzodioxane with C—CH$_3$ and NOH	Active	Judd and Biel (1963)
dithiine fused pyrrolone with O$_2$C—N piperazine NR′ and N—R, O	Active	Jeanmart et al. (1974)

TABLE XXXII   1,2,3-TRIAZINES

Ar	Activity	Reference
2-Me-4-ClC$_6$H$_3$	Met, active	Satzinger (1967)
2-Me-4-MeOC$_6$H$_3$	Met, active	Satzinger (1967)
2-Me-4-Et$_2$NC$_6$H$_3$	Met, as active as trimethadione	Satzinger (1967)
2-FC$_6$H$_4$	Active	Satzinger (1968)

TABLE XXXIII 1,2,4-TRIAZINES

R	Activity	Reference
SPh	ES, inact; Met, sl. act.	Prince (1966)
SCH$_2$Ph	ES, sl. act.; Met, inact.	Prince (1966)
S(CH$_2$)$_5$Ph	ES, active; Met, sl. act.	Prince (1966)
S(CH$_2$)$_3$Ph	ES, sl. act.; Met. sl. act.	Prince (1966)

R	R$_1$	R$_2$	R$_3$	Activity	Reference
2-ClC$_6$H$_4$	Me	H	Ph	MES, 65% protn. at 50 (ip)	Trepanier et al. (1966b)
4-MeC$_6$H$_4$	Me	H	Ph	MES, 75% protn. at 50 (ip)	Trepanier et al. (1966b)
2-MeC$_6$H$_4$	Me	H	Ph	MES, 85% protn. at 50 (ip)	Trepanier et al. (1966b)
Ph	H	H	Ph	MES, 25% protn. at 200 (ip)	Trepanier et al. (1966b)
3-Pyr	Me	H	Ph	MES, 95% protn. at 200 (ip)	Trepanier et al. (1966b)
Ph	H	Me	Me	MES, 25% protn. at 100 (ip)	Trepanier et al. (1966b)

TABLE XXXIV 1,3,5-TRIAZINE DERIVATIVES

R	R₁	R₂	Activity	Reference
MeO	Me	NHNH$_2$	Met, 17% protn. at 100 (ip)	Tsujikawa et al. (1975b)
MeO	Et	NHMe	Met, 50% protn. at 100 (ip)	Tsujikawa et al. (1975b)
MeO	Pr	NHEt	Met, 41% protn. at 100 (ip)	Tsujikawa et al. (1975b)
Me$_2$CHO	Et	NHEt	Met, 17% protn. at 100 (ip)	Tsujikawa et al. (1975b)
C$_4$H$_9$O	Me	NHEt	Met, 83% protn. at 100 (ip)	Tsujikawa et al. (1975b)
HO	Me	NHEt	Met, 17% protn. at 100 (ip)	Tsujikawa et al. (1975b)
MeO	CH$_2$Ph	NH$_2$	Met, 67% protn. at 100 (ip)	Tsujikawa et al. (1975a)
MeO	CF$_3$	NH$_2$	Met, 50% protn. at 100 (ip)	Tsujikawa et al. (1975a)
NMe$_2$	CH(Me)CH$_2$N⟨piperazinyl⟩NPh	NH$_2$	Met, 50% protn. at 100 (ip)	Tsujikawa et al. (1975a)
NMe$_2$	(CH$_2$)$_3$N⟨piperazinyl⟩NPh	NH$_2$	Met, 17% protn. at 100 (ip)	Tsujikawa et al. (1975a)
CHOHR	NR$_2$	NH$_2$	Met, active	Aron-Samuel and Sterne (1969)
3-Pyr	NEtC$_6$H$_4$Me-2	NH$_2$	Met, active	Shapiro et al. (1960b)
CH$_2$NHCONH$_2$	NHR	NH$_2$	Met, active	Shapiro et al. (1960c)
MeOCH$_2$CH$_2$	NHAr	NH$_2$	Met, v. act.	Shapiro et al. (1960a)
EtO(CH$_2$)$_2$	NHC$_6$H$_4$Me-3	NH$_2$	Met, v. act.	Shapiro et al. (1960a)
MeO(CH$_2$)$_2$	NEtAr	NH$_2$	Met, v. act.	Shapiro et al. (1960a)
CH$_2$OH	NHAr	NH$_2$	Met, v. act.	Shapiro et al. (1959)
CH$_2$OH	NEtC$_6$H$_4$Me-2	NH$_2$	Met, v. act.	Shapiro et al. (1959)
CH$_2$OMe	NHAr	NH$_2$	Met, active	Shapiro et al. (1959)
CH(Me)OMe	NHAr	NH$_2$	Met, active	Shapiro et al. (1959)
(CH$_2$)$_2$OMe	NRAr	NH$_2$	Met, active	Shapiro et al. (1959)
(CH$_2$)$_2$OEt	NRAr	NH$_2$	Met, active	Shapiro et al. (1959)

TABLE XXXV 1,3,4-OXADIAZINE DERIVATIVES[a]

R	R$_1$	Activity	Reference
4-Pyr (R$_3$ = Me)	Ph	MES, 60% protn. at 100	Trepanier *et al.* (1965)
4-Pyr	H	MES, 30% protn. at 50	Trepanier *et al.* (1965)
4-Pyr	Me	MES, 55% protn. at 50	Trepanier *et al.* (1965)
4-pyr (R$_2$ = Me)	Me	MES, 50% protn. at 100	Trepanier *et al.* (1965)
4-Pyr	Ph	MES, 30% protn. at 50	Trepanier *et al.* (1965)
2-Pyr (R$_3$ = Me)	Ph	MES, 90% protn. at 200	Trepanier *et al.* (1965)
3-Pyr	Ph	MES, 20% protn. at 100	Trepanier *et al.* (1965)
4-Pyr (R$_3$ = Me)	Ph	MES, 50% protn. at 100	Trepanier *et al.* (1965)
Ar	H	ES, protn. at 200	Trepanier (1969)
Ph	H	MES, 90% protn. at 200 (ip)	Trepanier *et al.* (1966a)
4-ClC$_6$H$_4$	H	MES, 50% protn. at 100 (ip)	Trepanier *et al.* (1966a)
		MES, 100% protn. at 200 (ip)	Trepanier *et al.* (1966a)
4-MeOC$_6$H$_4$	H	MES, 30% protn. at 200 (ip)	Trepanier *et al.* (1966a)
2-ClC$_6$H$_4$	H	MES, 10% protn. at 100 (ip)	Trepanier *et al.* (1966a)
		MES, 100% protn. at 200 (ip)	Trepanier *et al.* (1966a)
3,4,5-(MeO)$_3$C$_6$H$_2$	H	MES, 40% protn. at 200 (ip)	Trepanier *et al.* (1966a)
3,4-Cl$_2$C$_6$H$_3$	H	MES, 10% protn. at 200 (ip)	Trepanier *et al.* (1966a)
4-MeC$_6$H$_4$	H	MES, 10% protn. at 200 (ip)	Trepanier *et al.* (1966a)

[a] R$_2$, R$_3$ = H unless otherwise noted.

Compounds of this type can be synthesized conveniently by acid-catalyzed condensation of *N*-acylanthranilic acids with primary amines or by cyclization of *o*-aminobenzamides. Several studies of structure–activity relationships have appeared with each author reaching a conclusion based on a limited number of compounds. In view of the fact that a variety of screening techniques were used it is difficult to reach any broad conclusions. Substituents on the benzo ring or reduction of the double bond are not desirable. The 2-methyl group can be displaced by other alkyl groups and a number of other aryl groups can be used on the 3 position. All things considered, methaqualone and its 3-(2-chorophenyl) analogue appear to be the best anticonvulsant compounds in the series. Methaqualone, despite its activity in animal screens, does not appear to be used clinically as an anticonvulsant but has some use as a hypnotic. An excellent review of this compound has appeared (Brown and Goenechea, 1973).

Quinazolones with 1,3,4-oxadiazole substituents have anticonvulsant activity which is related to some extent to their MAO and acetylcholinesterase inhibiting properties (Barthwal *et al.*, 1973).

TABLE XXXVI   1,2,4-OXADIAZINE AND 1,2,4-THIADIAZINE DERIVATIVES

Compound	Activity	Reference
	Active	Bernstein and Losee (1966)
	Active	Beiersdorf (1974); Cohnen (1974)
	MES ED_{50} 100	Boltze *et al.* (1963)
	Active	Cohnen (1975)

IV. SEVEN-MEMBERED AND LARGER RINGS (EXCEPT FOR DIAZEPINES)

With the exception of the diazepines and related compounds the large-membered rings are included in Tables XXXVII–XLII. Compound **XI** shows anticonvulsant activity in a number of laboratory tests and was taken to clinical trial (Waring and Whittle, 1969). In man, however, **XI** did not produce any anticonvulsant effects over and above that produced by existing treatment. Compound **XII** was subjected to a neuropharmacological profile (Babington and Horovitz, 1973) which compared it favorably with carbamazepine and diphenylhydantoin as a possible antiepileptic.

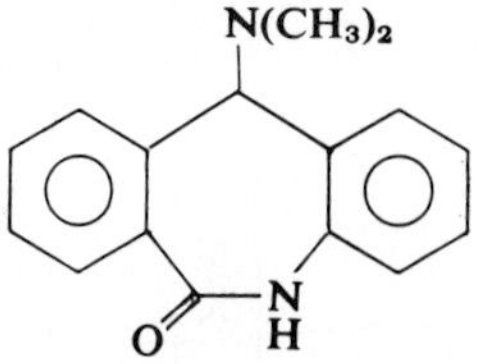

N(CH₃)₂ structure **(XI)** and structure **(XII)**

(XI) 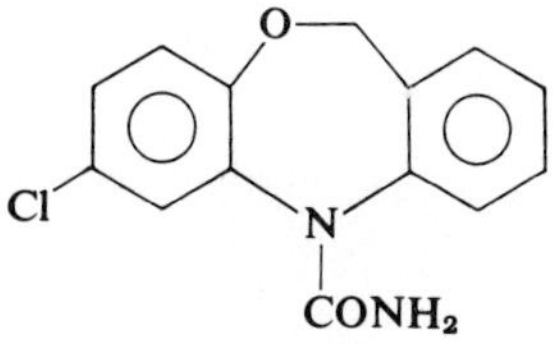   (XII)

The most promising compound in this large-ring group, however, is carbamazepine (**XIII**). This compound was originally introduced for the treatment of trigeminal neuralgia (Blom, 1962). The effect on cats (Julien,

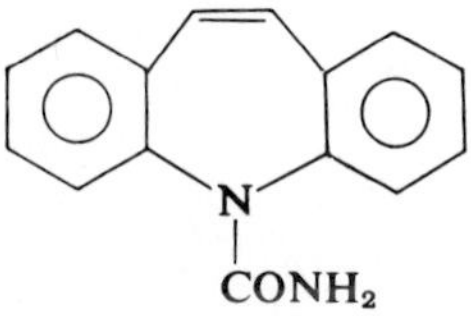

(XIII)

1973), the metabolism (Baker *et al.*, 1973), its mode of action (Hollister and Julien, 1974), and the plasma and tissue levels (Morselli *et al.*, 1971) of carbamazepine have been reported. It has been introduced into clinical trial in the treatment of epilepsy and these results have been reviewed (Livingston *et al.*, 1967a). The drug was approved as an anticonvulsant in 1974. The compound is an effective anticonvulsant in the control of psychomotor epilepsy. A variety of related structures have been prepared, and in addition to those listed in Table XXXVII it should be noted that some eight- (Pala *et al.*, 1971; Coyne and Cusic, 1968) and nine-membered (Pala *et al.*, 1971) analogues of carbamazepine are inactive.

V. DIAZEPINES AND RELATED COMPOUNDS

These compounds are listed in Table XLIII and the tables following XLIII.

The chemistry and pharmacology of the benzodiazepines have been extensively reviewed (Childress and Gluckman, 1964; Sternbach and Randall, 1966; Garattini *et al.*, 1973; Greenblatt and Shader, 1974; Randall *et al.*, 1976).

The synthesis of the marketed benzodiazepines has been reviewed (Randall *et al.*, 1976). The first of the useful 1,4-benzodiazepines, chlordiazepoxide (**XIV**), was prepared by ring enlargement of a quinazoline *N*-oxide (Sternbach *et al.*, 1961). Diazepam (**XV**) has been obtained from **XIV** and also be a wide

TABLE XXXVII AZEPINE DERIVATIVES

A. Benzazepines

Compound	Activity	Reference
(structure, R₁O-substituted benzazepine, N–R)	Active	Koo (1970)

B. Dibenz[b,f]azepines

Structure I and Structure II

R	R₁	Activity	Reference
Type I[a]			
$CONH_2$	H	MES ED_{50} 20	Coyne and Cusic (1968)
		MES ED_{50} 19 (ip), 20.5 (po); Met ED_{50} 21.5 (po)	Davis et al. (1964)
$CONHR$	H	MES ED_{50} 118 (po); Met ED_{50} 20 (po)	Theobald et al. (1967)
$CONHR$	$R_1, R_2 = $ —CH_2—	Active	Roehnert and Carstens (1973)
Me	NHR	Active	Morita and Kawashima (1973)
		Active	Linares (1972)

R		Activity	Reference
	H	Active	Geigy (1962); Schindler and Prins (1964)
Me	NH₂	Active	Fouche and Leger (1972)
Me (R₃ = Cl)	NH₂	Active	Fouche and Leger (1971)
CO(CH₂)₂N⟨piperidine⟩ (CONH₂)	H	Active	Nakanishi and Taira (1973)
H	(CH₂)₂NR₂	Active	Schindler and Blattner (1966)
H	(CH₂)₃N(Me)R	Active	Schindler and Blattner (1966)
(CH₂)₃NMe₂	H	MES ED_{50} 14 (ip); Met, synergism	Theobald et al. (1967)
(CH₂)₂NMe₂	H	MES ED_{50} 18 (ip); Met, synergism	Theobald et al. (1967)
(CH₂)₄NMe₂	H	MES ED_{50} 27 (ip); Met, synergism	Theobald et al. (1967)
(CH₂)₃NHMe	H	MES ED_{50} 18 (ip); Met, synergism	Theobald et al. (1967)
CH₂CH(Me)CH₂NMe₂	H	MES ED_{50} 38 (ip); Met, synergism	Theobald et al. (1967)
CH₂CH(Me)NMe₂	H	MES ED_{50} 19 (ip); Met, synergism	Theobald et al. (1967)
(CH₂)₃NMe₂ (R₃ = Cl)	H	MES ED_{50} 29 (ip); Met, synergism	Theobald et al. (1967)

Type II[a]

R		Activity	Reference
CONH₂	H	MES ED_{50} 11.7 (ip), 18.8 (po); Met ED_{50} 11.5 (po)	Davis et al. (1964)
		MES ED_{50} 16 (po); Met ED_{50} 20 (po)	Theobald et al. (1967)
		ES ED_{50} 19 (po); Met ED_{50} 88 (po)	Yale (1968)
CONH₂ (R₃ = Cl)	H	MES ED_{50} 260 (po); Met ED_{50} 88 (po)	Theobald et al. (1967)
CONHR	H	Active	Roehnert and Carstens (1973)
CONR₂	H	Active	Schindler (1960)
(CH₂)₃NMe₂	H	MES ED_{50} 21 (ip); Met, synergism	Theobald et al. (1967)
(CH₂)₃N⟨piperazine⟩N(CH₂)₂OH	H	MES ED_{50} 34 (ip)	Theobald et al. (1967)
R	H	Active	Schindler and Prins (1964); Société des Usines Chimiqués Rhone-Poulenc (1958); Geigy (1962)

(continued)

475

TABLE XXXVII—*Continued*

R	R₁	Activity	Reference
(CH₂)₃N⟨N-CH₃ piperazine⟩	H	Active	Société des Usines Chimiques Rhone-Poulenc (1959a)
Me	CH₂R	Active	Nedelec et al. (1973b)

C. Dibenz[b,e]azepines[b]

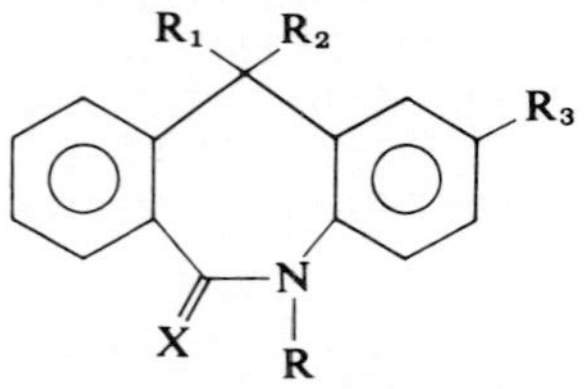

R	R_2	R_3	Activity	Reference
CONHNH₂	H (X = H₂)	H	MES ED_{50} 27	Coyne and Cusic (1968)
R	$R_2, R_1 = {=}N(CH_2)_2NR_2$	H	Active	Farbenfabriken Bayer (1969)
H	NR_2	R	Active	Imperial Chemical Industries Ltd, (1964)
H	NMe_2	H	MES ED_{50} 42; Met ED_{50} 38	Waring and Whittle (1969)
H	NEt_2	H	MES ED_{50} 60; Met ED_{50} 25	Waring and Whittle (1969)
H	$N(Pr\text{-}n)_2$	H	MES ED_{50} 118; Met ED_{50} 50–100	Waring and Whittle (1969)
H	$N(Me)CH_2CH_2OH$	H	MES ED_{50} 160	Waring and Whittle (1969)
H	NHEt	H	MES ED_{50} 44	Waring and Whittle (1969)
H	NHPr-*n*	H	MES ED_{50} > 250; Met ED_{50} 25	Waring and Whittle (1969)
H	NMe_2	Cl	MES ED_{50} 34; Met ED_{50} 100	Waring and Whittle (1969)
H	NMe_2	Br	MES ED_{50} 49; Met ED_{50} 50	Waring and Whittle (1969)
H	NEt_2	Cl	MES ED_{50} 63; Met ED_{50} 50–100	Waring and Whittle (1969)

				Reference
H	NCO₂Et (piperazine)	H	MES ED$_{50}$ > 250; Met ED$_{50}$ 200	Waring and Whittle (1969)
H	Ph (succinimide)	H	MES ED$_{50}$ > 250; Met ED$_{50}$ 50	Waring and Whittle (1969)
H	(piperidine)	H	MES ED$_{50}$ > 250; Met ED$_{50}$ 200	Waring and Whittle (1969)
H	(phthalimide)	H	MES ED$_{50}$ 50	Waring and Whittle (1969)
H		H	MES ED$_{50}$ > 250; Met ED$_{50}$ 200	Waring and Whittle (1969)
Me	NMe₂	H	MES, 100% protn. at 80	Waring and Whittle (1969)
Et	NMe₂	H	MES, 100% protn. at 100	Waring and Whittle (1969)
CH₂CH=CH₂	NMe₂	H	MES, 40% protn. at 100	Waring and Whittle (1969)
Bu-n	NMe₂	H	MES, 20% protn. at 100	Waring and Whittle (1969)
PhCH₂	NMe₂	H	MES, 40% protn. at 100	Waring and Whittle (1969)
CO₂Et	NMe₂	H	MES, 20% protn. at 100	Waring and Whittle (1969)
CH₂CONH₂	NMe₂	H	MES, 60% protn. at 100	Waring and Whittle (1969)
Me	(piperidine)	H	MES ED$_{50}$ 8	Waring and Whittle (1969)
Et	(piperidine)	H	MES ED$_{50}$ 8	Waring and Whittle (1969)

(continued)

TABLE XXXVII—*Continued*

R	R_2	R_3	Activity	Reference
$CH_2CH=CH_2$	(piperidine, N)	H	MES ED_{50} 22	Waring and Whittle (1969)
Pr-n	(piperidine, N)	H	MES ED_{50} 60	Waring and Whittle (1969)

[a] R_2, R_3 = H unless otherwise noted.
[b] R_1 = H, X = =O unless otherwise noted.

TABLE XXXVIII OXEPINE DERIVATIVES

R	R_1	Activity	Reference
$=CH(CH_2)_2NMe_2$		Met, active	Protiva *et al.* (1972)
H	$O(CH_2)_2NMe_2$ (trans)	Met ED_{50} 5	Protiva *et al.* (1972)
H	$O(CH_2)_2NMe_2$ (cis)	Met, active	Protiva *et al.* (1972)

Compound	Activity	Reference
CONH$_2$	Active	Niigata et al. (1974a)

R	X	Z	Activity	Reference
CONR$_2$ piperazine $-N\!\!\!\diagdown\!\!\!NR$	H$_2$	H	Active	Niigata et al. (1974a)
	O	R$_1$	Active	Geigy (1966)

Compound	Activity	Reference
CH(CH$_2$)$_2$NMe$_2$	Met ED$_{50}$ 7.6 (ip); MES ED$_{50}$ 20 (ip)	Wohlfarth-Ribbentrup and Schaumann (1969)

TABLE XXXIX THIEPINE DERIVATIVES

Compound	Activity	Reference
	Met, active	Sindelar *et al.* (1972)
	Active	Geigy (1966)
	R = OH, R_1 = Me: active R, R_1 = =CH$_2$: active	Umio and Ueda (1972a) Umio and Ueda (1972b)

TABLE XL OXAZEPINE DERIVATIVES

X	Activity	Reference
Cl	MES ED$_{50}$ 14 (po); Met ED$_{50}$ 105 (po)	Yale (1968)
H	MES ED$_{50}$ 29 (po); Met ED$_{50}$ 75 (po)	Yale (1968)

TABLE XL—*Continued*

R	R_1	R_2	Z	Activity	Reference
$(CH_2)_n NEt_2$	Cl	H	O	Active	Société d'Etudes Scientifiques et Industrielles de l'Ile-de-France (1966)
$CONH_2$	H	H	H_2	MES $ED_{50} > 50$	Coyne and Cusic (1968)
$CONHNR_2$	H	H	H_2	MES, $>20\%$ protn.	Coyne and Cusic (1970)
$CONHNH_2$	H	H	H_2	MES ED_{50} 24; Met, inact.	Coyne and Cusic (1968)
$CONHNH_2$	H	Cl	H_2	MES ED_{50} 14.8; Met, inact.	Coyne and Cusic (1968)
CONHN—NMe (piperidine)	H	H	H_2	MES $ED_{50} > 50$; Met, inact.	Coyne and Cusic (1968)
CONHNHCOMe	H	H	H_2	MES ED_{50} 27; Met, inact.	Coyne and Cusic (1968)
$CONHNMe_2$	H	Cl	H_2	MES ED_{50} 29; Met, inact.	Coyne and Cusic (1968)
CONHNHCOMe	H	Cl	H_2	MES ED_{50} 42; Met, inact.	Coyne and Cusic (1968)
CONMeNHMe	H	Cl	H_2	MES ED_{50} 50; Met, inact.	Coyne and Cusic (1968)

TABLE XLI   THIAZEPINE DERIVATIVES

Compound	Activity	Reference
	$R = COEt$: Met ED_{50} 45 (ip) $R = CO\triangleleft$: Met ED_{50} 11 $R = COCF_3$: Met ED_{50} 9	Dickinson (1972) Dickinson (1972) Dickinson (1972)
	Met ED_{50} 34.5 (ip)	Dickinson (1972)
	$X = S$, SO, SO_2: active	Hoffmann-La Roche & Co. (1965c)
	Active	Kathawala (1974)
	Met, active	Nacci *et al.* (1973)

TABLE XLII EIGHT- AND TEN-MEMBERED RINGS

Compound	Activity	Reference
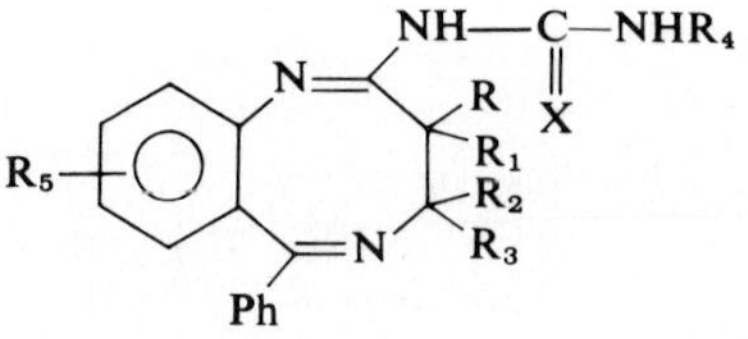	Active	Kuwada *et al.* (1973b)
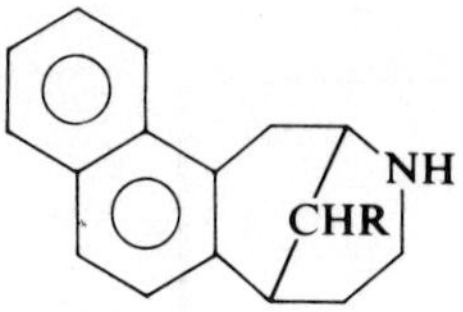	Active	Albertson (1968)

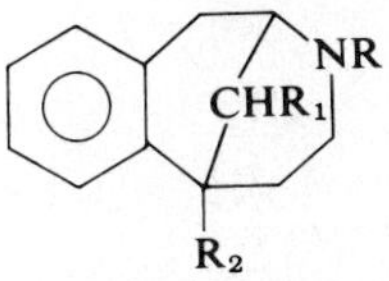

R	R_1	Activity	Reference
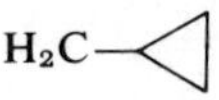 $H_2C-\triangleleft$	Me	MES ED_{50} 11 (ip), 26 (po); Met ED_{50} 2.3 (ip, 3.3 (po)	Albertson (1968)
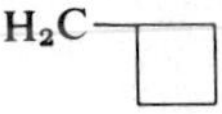 $H_2C-\square$	Me	MES ED_{50} 30 (ip); Met ED_{50} 13 (ip)	Albertson (1968)
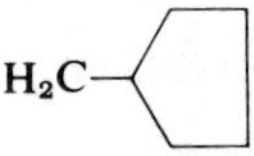 $H_2C-\pentagon$	Me	MES, inact.; Met ED_{50} 12 (ip)	Albertson (1968)

Compound	Activity	Reference
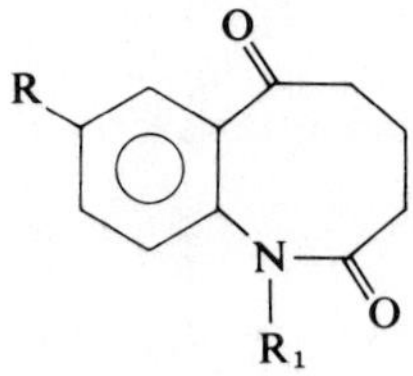	Active	Okamoto *et al.* (1974)
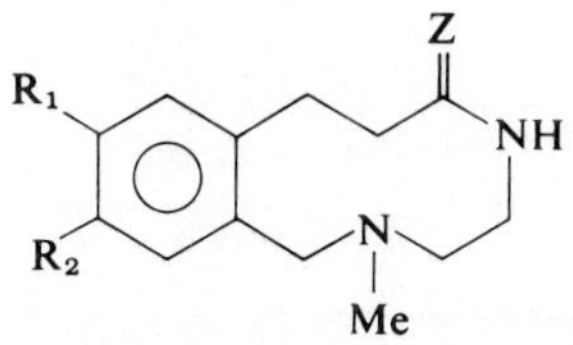	Active	Kato and Koshinaka (1974b)

(*continued*)

483

TABLE XLII—*Continued*

Compound	Activity	Reference
Active	Active	Kuwada *et al.* (1973a,b)
Active	Active	Kuwada *et al.* (1973a,b)
Active	Active	Kuwada *et al.* (1973a,b)
Active	Active	Kuwada *et al.* (1973a,b)
Active	Active	Field and Sternback (1971a)
Active	Active	Sulkowski (1964)

TABLE XLIII DIAZEPINE DERIVATIVES

A. 1,3-Diazepines

Compound	X	n	Activity	Reference
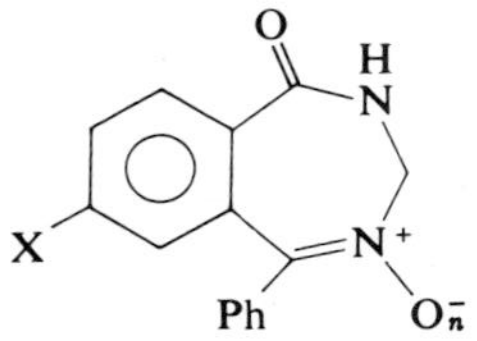	H	0	Met ED_{50} 24	Golik (1975)
	H	1	Met ED_{50} 28	Golik (1975)
	Cl	0	Met ED_{50} 1.5; MES ED_{50} 25	Golik (1975)

Compound	NRR_1	Activity	Reference
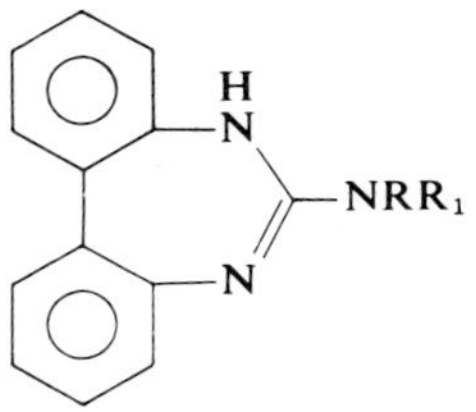	NHPr-i	MES ED_{50} 50–100 (po)	Kreighbaum and Scarborough (1964)
	NMe_2	MES ED_{50} 25 (po)	Kreighbaum and Scarborough (1964)
	NEt_2	MES ED_{50} 12 (po)	Kreighbaum and Scarborough (1964)
	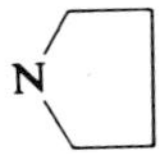	MES ED_{50} 50–100 (po)	Kreighbaum and Scarborough (1964)
	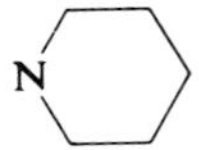	MES ED_{50} 50–100 (po)	Kreighbaum and Scarborough (1964)
	Miscellaneous	Active	Kreighbaum and Scarborough (1965)

(continued)

485

TABLE XLIII—Continued

B. 1H-1,4-Benzodiazepines

n	X	Ar	R	R_1	R_2	Activity	Reference
0	Cl	2-FC$_6$H$_4$	Me	SEt	H	Met ED$_{50}$ 0.18 (sc)	Earley and Fryer (1975)
0	Cl	2-FC$_6$H$_4$	Me	H	H	Met ED$_{50}$ 17.6	Earley and Fryer (1975)
0	Cl	C$_6$H$_5$	H	CONH$_2$	H	Met ED$_{50}$ 1.7	Coffen and Fryer (1974a)
0	Cl	C$_6$H$_5$	H	CN	H	Met ED$_{50}$ 2.5	Coffen and Fryer (1974a)
0	X	Ar	R	SR$_3$	R_2	Active	Earley et al. (1973)
1	Cl	C$_6$H$_5$	CH$_2$OH	N(Me)CH$_2$OH	H	Active	Shenoy (1974b)
0	Cl	C$_6$H$_5$	H	OK	CO$_2$K	Met ED$_{50}$ 1.7 (po), 1.0 (ip), 1.2 (sc); MES ED$_{50}$ 4.5 (po), 5.0 (ip), 2.0 (sc)	Schmitt et al. (1969)
0	NO$_2$	C$_6$H$_5$	H	OK	CO$_2$K	Met ED$_{50}$ 0.5 (po); MES ED$_{50}$ 3.2 (po)	Schmitt et al. (1969)

C. 3H-1,4-Benzodiazepines

X	Ar	R	R_1	Activity	Reference
With n = 0					
Cl	C$_6$H$_5$	CN	H	Active	Coffen and Fryer (1975)
Cl	C$_6$H$_5$	CONH$_2$	H	Active	Coffen and Fryer (1975)

Cl	$2\text{-}FC_6H_4$	CN	H	Active	Coffen and Fryer (1975)
Cl	$2\text{-}FC_6H_4$	$CONH_2$	H	Active	Coffen and Fryer (1975)
H	Ar	NHR_2 ($8\text{-}CF_3$)	H	Active	Sternbach and Saucy (1964)
Cl	C_6H_5	NR_2R_3	H	Active	Archer et al. (1964)
Cl	C_6H_5	SMe	H	Active	Archer et al. (1964)
R_2	Ar	NHR_3	R_1	Active	Keller et al. (1964b,c)
Cl	Ar	(ring, $-N$…NR, O)	H	Active	Moffett (1974)
Cl	C_6H_5	NHMe	H	Met ED_{50} 75 (po); MES ED_{50} 75 (po)	Sternbach and Randall (1966)
Cl	C_6H_5	$NH(CH_2)_3CH_3$	H	Met ED_{50} 50 (po); MES ED_{50} 300 (po)	Sternbach and Randall (1966)
Cl	C_6H_5	NH_2	H	Met ED_{50} 1.6 (po)	Childress and Gluckman (1964)
H	C_6H_5	NHMe	H	Met ED_{50} > 50	Childress and Gluckman (1964)
Cl	C_6H_5	NHMe	H	Met ED_{50} 5.5	Childress and Gluckman (1964)
Me	C_6H_5	NHMe	H	Met ED_{50} > 50	Childress and Gluckman (1964)
Cl	C_6H_5	NH_2	OH	Met ED_{50} 25 (po); MES ED_{50} 40 (po)	Childress and Gluckman (1964)
Cl	C_6H_5	NHMe	OH	Met ED_{50} 31 (po); MES ED_{50} 28 (po)	Childress and Gluckman (1964)
Cl	C_6H_5	NHCONHMe	H	MES ED_{50} > 50 (po)	Moffett and Rudzik (1973)
Cl	C_6H_5	NMeCONHMe	H	Met ED_{50} > 50 (po); MES ED_{50} > 50 (po)	Moffett and Rudzik (1973)
Cl	C_6H_5	NHCONHCOMe	H	MES ED_{50} > 50 (po)	Moffett and Rudzik (1973)
Cl	C_6H_5	$NHCONHCO_2Et$	H	Met ED_{50} > 50 (po); MES ED_{50} > 50 (po)	Moffett and Rudzik (1973)
Cl	$2\text{-}ClC_6H_4$	$NHCONHCO_2Et$	H	Met ED_{50} 12 (po); MES ED_{50} > 200 (po)	Moffett and Rudzik (1973)
Cl	C_6H_5	$NHCONHCH_2CH_2Cl$	H	MES ED_{50} > 50 (po)	Moffett and Rudzik (1973)

(continued)

TABLE XLIII—*Continued*

X	Ar	R	R_1	Activity	Reference
Cl	C_6H_5	$NMeCONHCH_2CH_2Cl$	H	Met ED_{50} > 50 (po); MES ED_{50} > 50 (po)	Moffett and Rudzik (1973)
Cl	$2\text{-}ClC_6H_4$	$NHCONHCH_2CH_2Cl$	H	Met ED_{50} 18 (po); MES ED_{50} > 200 (po)	Moffett and Rudzik (1973)
Cl	C_6H_5	$NHCONHCH_2CO_2Et$	H	Met ED_{50} > 50 (po); MES ED_{50} > 50 (po)	Moffett and Rudzik (1973)
Cl	C_6H_5	2-imidazolidinone (N-linked)	H	Met ED_{50} 20 (po); MES ED_{50} > 50 (po)	Moffett and Rudzik (1973)
Cl	$2\text{-}ClC_6H_5$	2-imidazolidinone (N-linked)	H	Met ED_{50} 16 (po); MES ED_{50} > 25 (po)	Moffett and Rudzik (1973)
Cl	$2\text{-}ClC_6H_4$	$N\text{-}(CH_2)NMe_2$ 2-imidazolidinone (N-linked)	H	Met ED_{50} 32 (po); MES ED_{50} 112 (po)	Moffett and Rudzik (1973)
Cl	C_6H_5	$NHOCON$ (imidazole)	H	MES ED_{50} 50 (ip); Met ED_{50} 12 (ip)	Hester and Rudzik (1974)
Cl	C_6H_5	$NHOH$	H	MES ED_{50} 100 (ip); Met ED_{50} 12.5 (ip)	Hester and Rudzik (1974)
Cl	C_6H_5	$NHOCH_2CH{=}CH_2$	H	MES ED_{50} > 100 (ip); Met ED_{50} 50 (ip)	Hester and Rudzik (1974)
Cl	C_6H_5	$NHOCMe_3$	H	MES ED_{50} > 100 (ip); Met ED_{50} > 100 (ip)	Hester and Rudzik (1974)
Cl	C_6H_5	$NHO(CH_2)_2NEt_2$	H	MES ED_{50} > 100 (ip); Met ED_{50} > 50 (ip)	Hester and Rudzik (1974)
Cl	C_6H_5	$NHOCH_2CO_2Et$	H	MES ED_{50} > 100 (ip); Met ED_{50} > 100 (ip)	Hester and Rudzik (1974)
Cl	C_6H_5	$NHO(CH_2)_2NC_4H_8$	H	MES ED_{50} > 200 (ip); Met ED_{50} 89 (ip)	Hester and Rudzik (1974)
Cl	$2\text{-}ClC_6H_4$	$NHOMe$	H	MES ED_{50} > 100 (ip); Met ED_{50} 2.1 (ip)	Hester and Rudzik (1974)
Cl	$2\text{-}ClC_6H_4$	$NHOCH_2CH{=}CH_2$	H	MES ED_{50} > 200 (ip); Met ED_{50} 0.8 (ip)	Hester and Rudzik (1974)
Cl	C_6H_5	$NHOMe$	H	MES ED_{50} > 100 (ip); Met ED_{50} 22 (ip)	Hester and Rudzik (1974)

With n = 1

Br	2-pyr	NHMe	H	Active	Fryer *et al.* (1963)
CF_3	C_6H_5	NHMe	H	Active	Gordon *et al.* (1963)
Cl	C_6H_5	NC_4H_8	H	Active	Hoffmann-LaRoche & Co. (1965a)
NO_2	C_6H_5	NHMe	H	Active	Keller *et al.* (1962, 1964a)
X	Ar	NHR_2	H	Active	Keller *et al.* (1964b,c)
X	Ar	NR_2R_3	H	Active	Reeder (1962)
Cl	C_6H_5	$NMeCH(OH)CH_2R_3$	H	Active	Shenoy (1974a)
H	Ar	NHR_2 (8-CF_3)	H	Active	Sternbach and Saucy (1964)
NO_2	C_6H_5	NH_2	H	Met ED_{50} 35 (po); MES ED_{50} 112 (po)	Sternbach *et al.* (1963)
NO_2	C_6H_5	NHMe	H	Met ED_{50} 5 (po); MES ED_{50} 183 (po)	Sternbach *et al.* (1963)
Cl	C_6H_5	NH_2	H	Met ED_{50} 3.6 (po)	Childress and Gluckman (1964)
H	C_6H_5	NHMe	H	Met ED_{50} > 50 (po)	Childress and Gluckman (1964)
Cl	C_6H_5	$NHCH_2C_6H_5$	H	Met ED_{50} 8 (po)	Childress and Gluckman (1964)
Cl	2-Thio	NHMe	H	Met ED_{50} 23 (po)	Childress and Gluckman (1964)
Cl	C_6H_5	NHEt	H	Met ED_{50} 31 (po); MES ED_{50} 67 (po)	Sternbach and Randall (1966)
Cl	C_6H_5	$NH(CH_2)_3CH_3$	H	Met ED_{50} 50 (po); MES ED_{50} 200 (po)	Sternbach and Randall (1966)
Cl	C_6H_5	NMeCOMe	H	Met ED_{50} 15 (po); MES ED_{50} 150 (po)	Sternbach and Randall (1966)
Cl	C_6H_5	NHMe (chlordiazepoxide[a])	H	Met ED_{50} 6.3; MES ED_{50} 104	Kido *et al.* (1970)
				Met ED_{50} 7 (po); MES ED_{50} 26.5 (po)	Sternbach *et al.* (1963)
				Met ED_{50} 7 (po); MES ED_{50} 26.5 (po)	Takagi *et al.* (1970)
				Met ED_{50} 18 (po); MES ED_{50} 92 (po)	Sternbach and Randall (1966)
				Met ED_{50} 3.7 (po); MES ED_{50} 14 (po)	Childress and Gluckman (1964)

(continued)

TABLE XLIII—*Continued*

X	Ar	R	R₁	Activity	Reference
				Met ED_{50} 2.9 (po); MES ED_{50} 22 (po)	Barzaghi *et al.* (1973)
				Met ED_{50} 10 (po); MES ED_{50} 17 (po)	Ferrini *et al.* (1974)
				Met ED_{50} 5 (ip); MES ED_{50} 28 (ip)	Lemke *et al.* (1972)
				Met ED_{50} 3.7 (po); MES ED_{50} 17 (po)	Gluckman (1971)
				MES ED_{50} 15 (ip)	McEvoy *et al.* (1968)
				Met ED_{50} 7.5 (po); MES ED_{50} 28.6 (po)	Nakajima *et al.* (1970)
				Met ED_{50} 4.6 (ip)	Nakanishi *et al.* (1973e)
				Met ED_{50} 8 (po)	Yamamoto *et al.* (1972); Walser and Fryer (1974)
				Met, 100% protn. at 50; MES, 80% protn. at 20	Marmo *et al.* (1971)

D. 1,3-Dihydro-2*H*-1,4-benzodiazepin-2-ones

X	R	Ar	Activity	Reference
With n = 0; R₁ = H				
X	$CH_2CH_2XCH_2R_2$	Ar	Met, active	Hoffmann-LaRoche & Co. (1974)
X	$(CH_2)_nX(CH_2)_mR_2$	Ar	Active	Jaunin and Hellerbach (1975a)
X	$CH_2CH_2R_2$	Ar	Active	Jaunin and Hellerbach (1975b)

X	CH$_2$CH$_2$XCH$_2$CONH$_2$	Ar	Active	Jaunin and Hellerbach (1975c)
X	CH$_2$CH$_2$XCH$_2$R$_2$	Ar	Active	Jaunin and Hellerbach (1975d)
Cl	(CH$_2$)$_n$R$_2$	Ar	Active	Sumitomo Chemical Co., Ltd. (1974c)
Cl	CH$_2$CH$_2$OMe	2,6-F$_2$C$_6$H$_3$	Active	Yamamoto et al. (1974b)
NR$_2$OR$_3$	R	Ar	Active	Fryer and Walser (1975a)
Cl	CH$_2$CF$_3$	Ar (=O is =S)	Active	Steinman (1972)
Cl	Me	C$_6$H$_5$ (=O is =NH)	Active	Takeda Chemical Industries Ltd. (1973)
Cl	Me	Ar (O= is =Z)	Active	Sternbach and Ning (1975)
Cl	CH$_2$C≡CH	C$_6$H$_5$	3.8 × Diazepam	Podesva and Vagi (1975)
Br	H	2-Pyr	Active	Hindley and McClymont (1975)
I	R	2-FC$_6$H$_4$	Active	Field and Sternbach (1975a–g)
X	R	2-Pyr	Active	Chase (1975)
Cl	Me	2-(4-ClPyr)	Active	Aries (1975)
X	R	2-NO$_2$C$_6$H$_4$	Active	Sternbach et al. (1962b)
X	R	Ar	Active	Sternbach et al. (1962a)
X	H (7,8-CH$_2$O$_2$)	C$_6$H$_5$	Active	Sumitomo Chemical Co., Ltd. (1974a)
X	R	Ar	Active	Sumitomo Chemical Co., Ltd. (1974b)
X	(CH$_2$)$_m$CH(OR$_2$)(CH$_2$)$_n$OR$_3$	Ar	Active	Sumitomo Chemical Co., Ltd. (1975)
X	CH$_2$C≡CH	Ar	Active	Tenconi et al. (1974)
Cl	CH$_2$CF$_3$	C$_6$H$_5$	Met, active	Topliss (1972)
R$_2$CO	R	Ar	Active	Wehrli et al. (1971)
MeCO	R	Ar	Active	Wehrli et al. (1974)
Cl	(CH$_2$)$_3$COC$_6$H$_4$F-2	Ar	Active	Welstead (1972a,b)
X	CH$_2$CH$_2$R$_2$	Ar	Active	Yamamoto et al. (1973b)

(continued)

491

TABLE XLIII—*Continued*

X	R	Ar	Activity	Reference
X	$CH_2CH_2SO_nR_2$	Ar	Active	Yamamoto et al. (1973a)
Cl	CH_2R_2	Ar	Active	Yamamoto et al. (1974a)
X	H	C_6H_5	Active	Andronati et al. (1970)
X	R	2-Pyrm	Active	Archer et al. (1970)
X	$CH_2CONR_2R_3$	Ar	Active	Archer and Sternbach (1966)
Cl	H (=O is =S)	C_6H_5	Active	Archer et al. (1964)
X	R	Ar	Active	Berger et al. (1962)
NO_2	R	Ar	Active	Boemches (1974)
X	R	R_3	Active	Boemches (1973)
X	H	C_6H_5	Active	Bogatskii et al. (1973)
X	R	Ar	Met, active	Hellerbach et al. (1974)
X	CHR_2OR_3	Ar	Active	Hellerbach and Walser, 1970; Hellerbach et al. (1972); Hellerbach and Walser (1972)
$N(R_2)_2$	$(CH_2)_nOR_3$	Ar	Active	Hellerbach and Walser (1973)
X	R	2-Pyr	Active	Hindley et al. (1973)
X	R	Ar	Active	Hoffmann-LaRoche & Co. (1964a)
Cl	R	Ar	Active	Hoffmann-LaRoche & Co. (1964b)
X	R	Ar	Active	Hoffmann et al. (1966a,b)
Cl	R	$2\text{-}FC_6H_4$	Active	Inaba et al. (1974)
X	$(CH_2)_nYZ$	Ar	Active	Jaunin and Hellerbach (1972)
X	R	Ar	Active	Kariss and Newmark (1963, 1964)

Cl	H	2-MeSC_6H_4	Active	Keller et al. (1963)
CF_3O	Me	C_6H_5	Active	McEvoy and Allen (1970)
Cl	$C(=X)NHR_2$	C_6H_5	Active	Metlesics and Sternbach (1974)
X	R	C_6H_5	Active	Ning and Sternbach (1972b)
CR_2R_3OH	R	Ar	Active	Ning and Sternbach (1972c)
MeCO	H	Ar	Active	Ning and Sternbach (1973b)
MeCO	R	Ar	Active	Ning and Sternbach (1974a)
Cl	R	Ar	Active	Okamoto et al. (1972)
H	H	C_6H_5	Met ED_{50} > 800 (po); MES ED_{50} 30 (po)	Sternbach and Randall (1966)
			Met ED_{50} 36 (po)	Childress and Gluckman (1964)
F	H	C_6H_5	Met ED_{50} > 60 (po)	DeAngelis et al. (1974a)
			Met ED_{50} > 800 (po); MES ED_{50} 23 (po)	Sternbach and Randall (1966)
Cl	H	C_6H_5	Met ED_{50} 6 (po); MES ED_{50} 25 (po)	Sternbach and Randall (1966)
(N-demethyldiazepam)			Met ED_{50} 0.9 (po)	Childress and Gluckman (1964)
			Met ED_{50} 0.9	Bell et al. (1968a)
			Met ED_{50} 2.5 (ip); MES ED_{50} 142 (ip)	Lemke et al. (1972)
			Met ED_{50} 1.2 (po)	DeAngelis et al. (1974a)
			Met ED_{50} 3.0 (so)	DeAngelis et al. (1974b)
			Met ED_{50} 2.9 (po); MES ED_{50} 5 (po), 2.5 (ip)	Schmitt et al. (1969)
Br	H	C_6H_5	Met ED_{50} 1.7 (po); MES ED_{50} 3.7 (po)	Sternbach and Randall (1966)

(continued)

TABLE XLIII—*Continued*

X	R	Ar	Activity	Reference
NO_2	H	C_6H_5	Met ED_{50} 0.5 (po); MES ED_{50} 8.4 (po)	Sternbach and Randall (1966)
	(nitrazepam)		Met ED_{50} 0.5 (po); MES ED_{50} 8 (po)	Sternbach et al. (1963)
			Met ED_{50} 0.2 (ip)	Nakanishi et al. (1973e)
			Met ED_{50} 0.75 (po); MES ED_{50} 8.4 (po)	Nakajima et al. (1970)
			Met ED_{50} 3.3; MES ED_{50} 35	Christmas and Maxwell (1970)
CF_3	H	C_6H_5	Met ED_{50} 1 (po); MES ED_{50} 5 (po)	Sternbach and Randall (1966)
H	H (8-Cl)	C_6H_5	Met ED_{50} 334 (po); MES ED_{50} 160 (po)	Sternbach and Randall (1966)
H	H (9-NO_2)	C_6H_5	Met ED_{50} > 800 (po); MES ED_{50} 400 (po)	Sternbach and Randall (1966)
Me	H	C_6H_5	Met ED_{50} 175 (po); MES ED_{50} 167 (po)	Sternbach and Randall (1966)
			Met ED_{50} > 50 (po)	Childress and Gluckman (1964)
NMe_2	H	C_6H_5	Met ED_{50} 42 (po); MES ED_{50} 367 (po)	Sternbach and Randall (1966)
CN	H	C_6H_5	Met ED_{50} 1.3 (po); MES ED_{50} 34 (po)	Sternbach and Randall (1966)
CF_3O	H (=O is =S)	C_6H_5	MES ED_{50} 20 (ip)	McEvoy et al. (1968)
SO_2NH_2	H	C_6H_5	MES ED_{50} > 200	Moffett and Rudzik (1971)
SO_2NMe_2	H	C_6H_5	MES ED_{50} > 200	Moffett and Rudzik (1971)
Cl	H	2-FC_6H_4	Met ED_{50} 0.08 (po); MES ED_{50} 1.5 (po)	Sternbach and Randall (1966)
			Met ED_{50} 0.32 (ip); MES ED_{50} 50 (ip)	Lemke et al. (1972)

Cl	H	$2\text{-}ClC_6H_4$	Met ED_{50} 0.4 (po); MES ED_{50} 13 (po)	Sternbach and Randall (1966)
			Met ED_{50} 0.6 (po)	DeAngelis et al. (1974a)
			Met ED_{50} 0.28; MES ED_{50} 29.7	Swinyard and Castellion (1966)
NO_2	H	C_6H_4	Met ED_{50} 0.14; MES ED_{50} 60	Swinyard and Castellion (1966)
Cl	H	$2\text{-}ClC_6H_4$	Met ED_{50} 0.17 (ip); MES ED_{50} 23 (ip)	Lemke et al. (1972)
Cl	H	$2\text{-}MeC_6H_4$	Met ED_{59} 7.7 (po); MES ED_{50} 21 (po)	Sternbach and Randall (1966)
Cl	H	$2\text{-}MeOC_6H_4$	Met ED_{50} 7.5 (po); MES ED_{50} 30 (po)	Sternbach and Randall (1966)
Cl	H	$3\text{-}FC_6H_4$	Met ED_{50} 4.2 (po); MES ED_{50} 20 (po)	Sternbach and Randall (1966)
Cl	H	$3\text{-}MeOC_6H_4$	Met ED_{50} 1.8 (po); MES ED_{50} 102 (po)	Sternbach and Randall (1966)
Cl	H	$4\text{-}FC_6H_4$	Met ED_{50} > 800 (po); MES ED_{50} 50 (po)	Sternbach and Randall (1966)
Cl	H	$4\text{-}ClC_6H_4$	Met ED_{50} > 800 (po); MES ED_{50} 300 (po)	Sternbach and Randall (1966)
NO_2	H	$2\text{-}FC_6H_4$	Met ED_{50} 0.96 (po); MES ED_{50} 20 (po)	Sternbach and Randall (1966)
NO_2	H	$2\text{-}ClC_6H_4$	Met, 100% protn. at 0.07 (ip); MES ED_{50} 84. (po)	Blum et al. (1973)
NO_2	H	$2\text{-}CF_3C_6H_4$	Met ED_{50} 0.036; MES ED_{50} > 2400	Swinyard and Castellion (1966)
I	H	$2\text{-}FC_6H_4$	Met ED_{50} 0.11, MES ED_{50} >2400	Swinyard and Castellion (1966)
			MES ED_{50} 1.6	Field and Sternbach (1971b, 1972, 1973)
Cl	H	$2,6\text{-}F_2C_6H_3$	Met ED_{50} 0.14 (ip); MES ED_{50} 63 (ip)	Lemke et al. (1972)

(continued)

495

TABLE XLIII—Continued

X	R	Ar	Activity	Reference
Cl	Me	C_6H_5	Met ED_{50} 1.4 (po); MES ED_{50} 6.4 (po)	Sternbach and Randall (1966); Sternbach et al. (1974)
		(diazepam[a])	Met ED_{50} 0.9 (po); MES ED_{50} 3.4 (po)	Childress and Gluckman (1964)
			Met ED_{50} 1.4 (po); MES ED_{50} 6.5 (po)	Takagi et al. (1970)
			Met ED_{50} 1.4 (po)	Walser and Fryer (1974)
			Met ED_{50} 1.2; MES ED_{50} 35	Kido et al. (1970)
			MES ED_{50} 11 (ip)	McEvoy et al. (1968)
			Met ED_{50} 0.9 (ip)	Nakanishi et al. (1973c)
			Met ED_{50} 3.0 (po); MES ED_{50} 14 (po)	Nakajima et al. (1970)
			Met ED_{50} 0.4 (po); MES ED_{50} 3.4 (po)	Gluckman (1971)
			Met ED_{50} 1.5 (po); MES ED_{50} 5.5 (po)	Ferrini et al. (1974)
			Met ED_{50} 4.2; MES ED_{50} 48	Christmas and Maxwell (1970)
			MES ED_{50} 2	Dobrescu and Coeugniet (1971)
			Met ED_{50} 4.75 (po)	DeAngelis et al. (1974b)
			Met ED_{50} 1.75 (po); MES ED_{50} 5 (po)	Schmitt et al. (1969)
			Met ED_{50} 0.8 (ip); MES ED_{50} 50 (ip)	Hester (1975)
NO_2	Me	C_6H_5	Met ED_{50} 0.6 (po); MES ED_{50} 1.5 (po)	Sternbach and Randall (1966)
		(nitrazepam)	Met ED_{50} 0.18 (po); MES ED_{50} 15 (po)	Sakai et al. (1972)

NMe$_2$	Me	C$_6$H$_5$	Met ED$_{50}$ 5.9 (po); MES ED$_{50}$ 92 (po)	Sternbach and Randall (1966)
CN	Me	C$_6$H$_5$	Met ED$_{50}$ 1.2 (po); MES ED$_{50}$ 14 (po)	Sternbach and Randall (1966)
NHSO$_2$Me	Me	C$_6$H$_5$	MES ED$_{50}$ > 200	Moffett and Rudzik (1971)
NMeSO$_2$Me	Me	C$_6$H$_5$	MES ED$_{50}$ > 100	Moffett et al. (1971)
H	Me	C$_6$H$_5$	Met ED$_{50}$ > 800 (po); MES ED$_{50}$ 50 (po)	Sternbach et al. (1974)
X	Me	Ferrocene	Met ED$_{50}$ > 800 (po)	Kalish et al. (1975)
NO$_2$	Me	2-FC$_6$H$_4$	Met ED$_{50}$ 0.12 (po); MES ED$_{50}$ 12 (po)	Sternbach and Randall (1966)
I	Me	2-FC$_6$H$_4$	MES ED$_{50}$ 1.3	Field and Sternbach (1971b, 1972, 1973)
Cl	Me	2-ClC$_6$H$_4$	Met ED$_{50}$ 0.42 (po); MES ED$_{50}$ 15 (po)	Sternbach and Randall (1966)
			Met ED$_{50}$ 0.10; MES ED$_{50}$ 80	Swinyard and Castellion (1966)
Cl	H	2-ClC$_6$H$_4$	Met ED$_{50}$ 0.10 (po); MES ED$_{50}$ 4 (po)	Childress and Gluckman (1964)
Cl	Me	2-FC$_6$H$_5$	Met ED$_{50}$ 0.10 (po); MES ED$_{50}$ 4.7 (po)	Childress and Gluckman (1964)
NO$_2$	Me	2-FC$_6$H$_4$	Met ED$_{50}$ 0.24 (po); MES ED$_{50}$ 1.9 (po)	Asami et al. (1974)
Cl	Me	4-FC$_6$H$_4$	Met ED$_{50}$ 0.02; MES ED$_{50}$ 2.7	Swinyard and Castellion (1966)
Cl	Me	C$_6$H$_5$	Met ED$_{50}$ 800 (po); MES ED$_{50}$ 83 (po)	Sternbach et al. (1974)
Cl	Et	C$_6$H$_5$	Met ED$_{50}$ 4 (po); MES ED$_{50}$ 8.3 (po)	Sternbach and Randall (1966)
			Met ED$_{50}$ 1.0 (po); MES ED$_{50}$ 9.4 (po)	Childress and Gluckman (1964)
Cl	CH$_2$C≡CH	C$_6$H$_5$	Met ED$_{50}$ 0.72 (po); MES ED$_{50}$ 14.6 (po)	Scrollini et al. (1975)

(continued)

497

TABLE XLIII—*Continued*

X	R	Ar	Activity	Reference
Cl	$CH_2C_3H_5$	C_6H_5	Met ED_{50} 3.2 (po); MES ED_{50} 24.6 (po)	Robichaud *et al.* (1970)
NO_2	CONHMe (prazepam)	C_6H_5	Met, 100% protn. at 8 (ip); MES ED_{50} 0.75 (po); MES ED_{50} 9.2 (po)	Boissier *et al.* (1972b) Nakajima *et al.* (1970)
Cl	CH_2CMe_3	C_6H_5	Met ED_{50} 22 (po); MES ED_{50} 600 (po)	Sternbach and Randall (1966)
Cl	$(CH_2)_2CHMe_2$	C_6H_5	Met ED_{50} 3.5 (po); MES ED_{50} 100 (po)	Sternbach and Randall (1966)
Cl	$CH_2CONHMe$	C_6H_5	Met ED_{50} 0.5 (po); MES ED_{50} 15 (po)	Sternbach and Randall (1966)
Cl	NH_2	$2\text{-}ClC_6H_4$	Met ED_{50} 0.42 (po); MES ED_{50} 20.8 (po)	Sternbach and Randall (1966)
Cl	$(CH_2)_2NEt_2$	$2\text{-}ClC_6H_4$	Met ED_{50} 22 (po); MES ED_{50} 150 (po)	Sternbach and Randall (1966)
Cl	$CH_2CH_2NEt_2$ (flurazepam)	$2\text{-}FC_6H_4$	Met ED_{50} 1.6 (po); Met ED_{50} 1.6 (po); MES ED_{50} 85 (po)	Walser and Fryer (1974) Sakai *et al.* (1971, 1972)
Cl	$CH_2CH_2NMe_2$	$2\text{-}ClC_6H_4$	Met ED_{50} 7 (po)	Walser and Fryer (1974)
Cl	$CH_2CH_2NOEt_2$	$2\text{-}FC_6H_4$	Met ED_{50} 1.1 (po)	Walser and Fryer (1974)
Cl	$CH_2CH_2NOEt_2$	$2\text{-}ClC_6H_4$	Met ED_{50} 10.6 (po)	Walser and Fryer (1974)
Cl	$CH{=}CH_2$	$2\text{-}FC_6H_4$	Met ED_{50} 0.36 (po)	Walser and Fryer (1974)
Cl	$CH{=}CH_2$	$2\text{-}ClC_6H_4$	Met ED_{50} 0.67 (po)	Walser and Fryer (1974)
H	$CH_2CH_2N(OH)Et$	$2\text{-}FC_6H_4$	Met ED_{50} 1.4 (po)	Walser and Fryer (1974)
Cl	CH_2CH_2OEt	$2\text{-}FC_6H_4$	Met ED_{50} 0.1 (po)	Inaba *et al.* (1971)
Cl	CH_2CHCH_2 (with epoxide O)	$2\text{-}FC_6H_4$	Met ED_{50} 0.13 (po)	Yamamoto *et al.* (1972)
Cl	H_2C (tetrahydrofuranyl, O)	$2\text{-}FC_6H_4$	Met ED_{50} 0.7 (po)	Yamamoto *et al.* (1972)

Cl	CH$_2$CH$_2$SO$_2$Me	2-FC$_6$H$_4$	Met ED$_{50}$ 0.25 (po); MES ED$_{50}$ 23 (po)	Asami *et al.* (1975)
Cl	H (=O is =S)	C$_6$H$_5$	Met ED$_{50}$ 40 (po); MES ED$_{50}$ 800 (po)	Sternbach and Randall (1966)
Cl	Me (=O is =S)	C$_6$H$_5$	Met ED$_{50}$ 9.2 (po); MES ED$_{50}$ 123 (po)	Sternbach and Randall (1966)
Br	H	Me	Met ED$_{50}$ > 800 (po); MES ED$_{50}$ 100 (po)	Sternbach and Randall (1966)
Cl	C$_6$H$_{13}$	C$_6$H$_{13}$	Met ED$_{50}$ 150 (po); MES ED$_{50}$ 334 (po)	Sternbach and Randall (1966)
Cl	H	2-Thioph.	Met ED$_{50}$ 100 (po); MES ED$_{50}$ 150 (po)	Sternbach and Randall (1966)
Cl	H	2-Pyr	Met ED$_{50}$ 0.5 (po); MES ED$_{50}$ 14 (po)	Sternbach and Randall (1966)
Br	H	2-Pyr	Met ED$_{50}$ 0.7 (po); MES ED$_{50}$ 34 (po)	Sternbach and Randall (1966)
Br	(CH$_2$)$_3$NMe$_2$	2-Pyr	Met ED$_{50}$ 84 (po); MES ED$_{50}$ 667 (po)	Sternbach and Randall (1966)
CF$_3$	H	2-Pyr	Met ED$_{50}$ 1 (po); MES ED$_{50}$ 12 (po)	Sternbach and Randall (1966)
N$_3$	H	C$_6$H$_5$	Met ED$_{50}$ 4.5 (po); MES ED$_{50}$ 8 (po)	Ning *et al.* (1973)
N$_3$	H	2-CF$_3$C$_6$H$_4$	Met ED$_{50}$ 2.6 (po); MES ED$_{50}$ 11 (po)	Ning *et al.* (1973)
N$_3$	H	2-ClC$_6$H$_4$	Met ED$_{50}$ 1.1 (po); MES ED$_{50}$ 20 (po)	Ning *et al.* (1973)
N$_3$	Me	C$_6$H$_5$	Met ED$_{50}$ 2.8 (po); MES ED$_{50}$ 12 (po)	Ning *et al.* (1973)
N$_3$	Me	2-FC$_6$H$_4$	Met ED$_{50}$ 0.9 (po); MES ED$_{50}$ 8 (po)	Ning *et al.* (1973)
N$_3$	CH$_2$CH$_2$OH	C$_6$H$_5$	Met ED$_{50}$ 3.2 (po); MES ED$_{50}$ 11 (po)	Ning *et al.* (1973)

(continued)

TABLE XLIII—*Continued*

X	R	Ar	Activity	Reference
Cl	$CONHCH_2CH=CH_2$	C_6H_5	Met ED_{50} 1.6 (ip); MES ED_{50} 23 (ip)	Moffett and Rudzik (1972)
CN	$CONHCH_2CH=CH_2$	C_6H_5	Met ED_{50} > 25 (ip)	Moffett and Rudzik (1972)
Cl	$CONHCH_2CH=CHMe$	C_6H_5	Met ED_{50} 3.2 (ip); MES ED_{50} > 100 (ip)	Moffett and Rudzik (1972)
Cl	$CONHC_3H_5$	C_6H_5	Met ED_{50} 18 (ip); MES ED_{50} 200 (ip)	Moffett and Rudzik (1972)
Cl	$CONHC_6H_{11}$	C_6H_5	Met ED_{50} > 25 (ip)	Moffett and Rudzik (1972)
Cl	$CONHCH_2CH_2Cl$	C_6H_5	Met ED_{50} 2.8 (ip); MES ED_{50} 50 (ip)	Moffett and Rudzik (1972)
Cl	$CONHCH_2CO_2Et$	C_6H_5	Met ED_{50} 10 (ip); MES ED_{50} > 50 (ip)	Moffett and Rudzik (1972)
Cl	$CONHMe$	C_6H_5	Met ED_{50} 2.2 (ip); MES ED_{50} > 50 (ip)	Moffett and Rudzik (1972)
Cl	CH_2CH_2OEt	C_6H_5	Met ED_{50} 4 (po); MES ED_{50} 10 (po)	Lamdan *et al.* (1970)
Cl	$CH_2CH_2OBu\text{-}n$	C_6H_5	Met ED_{50} 4 (po); MES ED_{50} 12 (po)	Lamdan *et al.* (1970)
Cl	$CH_2CH_2OC_6H_5$	C_6H_5	Met ED_{50} 40 (po); MES ED_{50} 400 (po)	Lamdan *et al.* (1970)
Cl	$(CH_2)_3OC_6H_5$	C_6H_5	Met ED_{50} 85 (po); MES ED_{50} > 500 (po)	Lamdan *et al.* (1970)
Cl	$CH_2CH_2OC_6H_4Me\text{-}p$	C_6H_5	Met ED_{50} 30 (po); MES ED_{50} 65 (po)	Lamdan *et al.* (1970)
Cl	$CH_2CH_2OC_6H_4NH_2\text{-}p$	C_6H_5	Met ED_{50} 15 (po); MES ED_{50} 75 (po)	Lamdan *et al.* (1970)
Cl	$CH_2CH_2OC_6H_4Cl\text{-}p$	C_6H_5	Met ED_{50} 57 (po); MES ED_{50} > 500 (po)	Lamdan *et al.* (1970)
Cl	$CH_2CH_2OC_6H_4NO_2\text{-}p$	C_6H_5	Met ED_{50} 92 (po); MES ED_{50} 160 (po)	Lamdan *et al.* (1970)

Cl	CH$_2$CH$_2$SC$_6$H$_5$	C$_6$H$_5$	Met ED$_{50}$ 15 (po); MES ED$_{50}$ 80 (po)	Lamdan *et al.* (1970)
Cl	CH$_2$CH$_2$SO$_2$C$_6$H$_5$	C$_6$H$_5$	Met ED$_{50}$ 18 (po); MES ED$_{50}$ 70 (po)	Lamdan *et al.* (1970)
Cl	CH$_2$CH$_2$OC$_{10}$H$_7$-2	C$_6$H$_5$	Met ED$_{50}$ 25 (po); MES ED$_{50}$ 500 (po)	Lamdan *et al.* (1970)
Cl	CH$_2$CF$_3$	C$_6$H$_5$	Met ED$_{50}$ 2.5 (po)	Steinman *et al.* (1973)
Cl	CH$_2$CF$_3$	C$_6$H$_5$ (=O is =S)	Met ED$_{50}$ 5 (po)	Steinman *et al.* (1973)
Cl	CH$_2$CF$_3$	2-ClC$_6$H$_4$	Met ED$_{50}$ 1 (po)	Steinman *et al.* (1973)
Cl	CH$_2$CF$_3$	2-FC$_6$H$_4$	Met ED$_{50}$ 0.1 (po)	Steinman *et al.* (1973)
Cl	CH$_2$CF$_3$	2-FC$_6$H$_4$ (=O is =S)	Met ED$_{50}$ 0.4 (po)	Steinman *et al.* (1973)
H	CH$_2$CF$_3$	C$_6$H$_5$	Met ED$_{50}$ 100 (po)	Steinman *et al.* (1973)
NO$_2$	CH$_2$CF$_3$	3-NO$_2$C$_6$H$_4$	Met ED$_{50}$ 60 (po)	Steinman *et al.* (1973)
Cl	CH$_2$CF$_3$	C$_6$H$_5$	Met ED$_{50}$ 30 (po)	Steinman *et al.* (1973)
Cl	CH$_2$CF$_2$CF$_3$	C$_6$H$_5$	Met ED$_{50}$ 30 (po)	Steinman *et al.* (1973)
NO$_2$	(CH$_2$)$_2$NMe$_2$	C$_6$H$_5$	Met ED$_{50}$ 6.3 (po); MES ED$_{50}$ 35 (po)	Sternbach *et al.* (1965)
CF$_3$	(CH$_2$)$_2$NMe$_2$	C$_6$H$_5$	Met ED$_{50}$ 7.1 (po); MES ED$_{50}$ 200 (po)	Sternbach *et al.* (1965)
Cl	CHMeCH$_2$NMe$_2$	C$_6$H$_5$	Met ED$_{50}$ 6.5 (po); MES ED$_{50}$ 22 (po)	Sternbach *et al.* (1965)
Cl	(CH$_2$)$_2$NEt$_2$	C$_6$H$_5$	Met ED$_{50}$ 5 (po); MES ED$_{50}$ 48 (po)	Sternbach *et al.* (1965)
Cl	(CH$_2$)$_2$NEt$_2$	C$_6$H$_5$	Met ED$_{50}$ 3.2 (po); MES ED$_{50}$ 50 (po)	Sternbach *et al.* (1965)
Cl	(CH$_2$)$_2$NEt$_2$	2-ClC$_6$H$_4$	Met ED$_{50}$ 22 (po); MES ED$_{50}$ 150 (po)	Sternbach *et al.* (1965)
Cl	(CH$_2$)$_2$NEt$_2$	2-FC$_6$H$_4$	Met ED$_{50}$ 1.6 (po); MES ED$_{50}$ 83 (po)	Sternbach *et al.* (1965)
Br	(CH$_2$)$_2$NEt$_2$	2-Pyr	Met ED$_{50}$ 3 (po); MES ED$_{50}$ 300 (po)	Sternbach *et al.* (1965)
Cl	(CH$_2$)$_2$NC$_4$H$_8$	C$_6$H$_5$	Met ED$_{50}$ > 400 (po); MES ED$_{50}$ 133 (po)	Sternbach *et al.* (1965)

(continued)

TABLE XLIII—*Continued*

X	R	Ar	Activity	Reference
Cl	$(CH_2)_2NC_5H_{10}$	C_6H_5	Met ED$_{50}$ 15 (po); MES ED$_{50}$ 150 (po)	Sternbach *et al.* (1965)
Cl	$(CH_2)_2N$—[ring]—NH	C_6H_5	Met ED$_{50}$ 21 (po); MES ED$_{50}$ 334 (po)	Sternbach *et al.* (1965)
Cl	$(CH_2)_2N$—[ring]—O	C_6H_5	Met ED$_{50}$ 8.9 (po); MES ED$_{50}$ 96 (po)	Sternbach *et al.* (1965)
Cl	$(CH_2)_2N$—[ring]—NMe	C_6H_5	Met ED$_{50}$ 8.4 (po); MES ED$_{50}$ 150 (po)	Sternbach *et al.* (1965)
Cl	$(CH_2)_2N$—[ring]—NMe	$2\text{-}FC_6H_4$	Met ED$_{50}$ 9.7 (po); MES ED$_{50}$ 200 (po)	Sternbach *et al.* (1965)
Cl	$(CH_2)_3NHMe$	$2\text{-}FC_6H_4$	Met ED$_{50}$ 7.5 (po); MES ED$_{50}$ 300 (po)	Sternbach *et al.* (1965)
Cl	$(CH_2)_3NMe_2$	C_6H_5	Met ED$_{50}$ 150 (po); MES ED$_{50}$ > 800 (po)	Sternbach *et al.* (1965)
NO$_2$	$(CH_2)_3NMe_2$	C_6H_5	Met ED$_{50}$ 18.8 (po); MES ED$_{50}$ 400 (po)	Sternbach *et al.* (1965)
Cl	$(CH_2)_3NMe_2$	$2\text{-}FC_6H_5$	Met ED$_{50}$ 6.5 (po); MES ED$_{50}$ 334 (po)	Sternbach *et al.* (1965)
Br	$(CH_2)_3NMe_2$	2 Pyr	Met ED$_{50}$ 73 (po); MES ED$_{50}$ 400 (po)	Sternbach *et al.* (1965)
Cl	$(CH_2)_3NEt_2$	C_6H_5	Met ED$_{50}$ 300 (po); MES ED$_{50}$ > 400 (po)	Sternbach *et al.* (1965)
Cl	$(CH_2)_3NEt_2$	$2\text{-}FC_6H_5$	Met ED$_{50}$ 35 (po); MES ED$_{50}$ 339 (po)	Sternbach *et al.* (1965)

X	R₂ (structure)	Ar	Activity	Reference
Cl	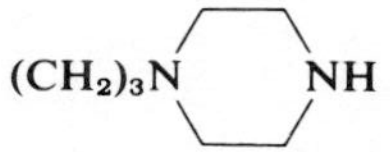 $(CH_2)_3N$—NH	$2\text{-}FC_6H_4$	Met ED_{50} 75 (po); MES ED_{50} > 100 (po)	Sternbach et al. (1965)
Cl	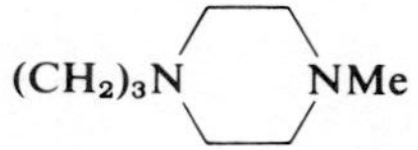 $(CH_2)_3N$—NMe	C_6H_5	Met ED_{50} 78 (po); MES ED_{50} 226 (po)	Sternbach et al. (1965)
Cl	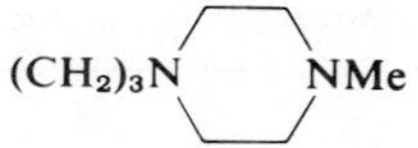 $(CH_2)_3N$—NMe	$2\text{-}FC_6H_4$	Met ED_{50} 16 (po); MES ED_{50} 175 (po)	Sternbach et al. (1965)
Cl	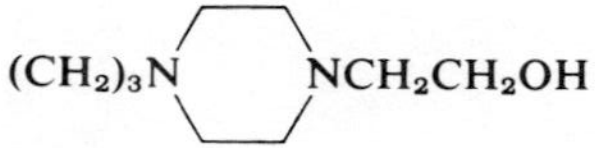 $(CH_2)_3N$—NCH_2CH_2OH	C_6H_5	Met ED_{50} 52 (po); MES ED_{50} 300 (po)	Sternbach et al. (1965)
Cl	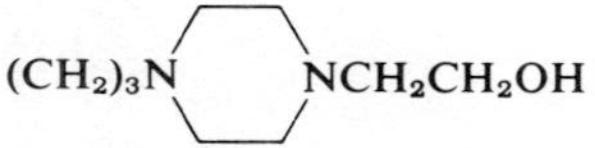 $(CH_2)_3N$—NCH_2CH_2OH	$2\text{-}FC_6H_5$	Met ED_{50} 14 (po); MES ED_{50} 200 (po)	Sternbach et al. (1965)
Cl	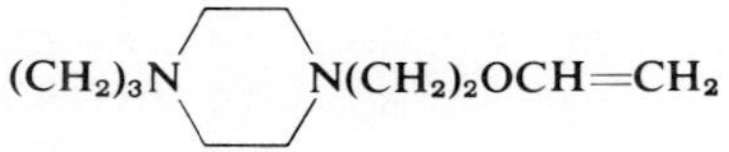 $(CH_2)_3N$—$N(CH_2)_2OCH{=}CH_2$	$2\text{-}FC_6H_4$	Met ED_{50} 16 (po); MES ED_{50} 400 (po)	Sternbach et al. (1965)

With n = 1; R₁ = H

X	R	Ar	Activity	Reference
X	R	C_6H_5	Active	Ning and Sternbach (1972b)
Cl	H	Ar	Active	Berger et al. (1962)
Cl	CH_2CONMe_2	C_6H_5	Active	Archer and Sternbach (1966)
H (8-CF₃)	R	Ar	Active	Sternbach and Saucy (1964)
Cl	H	C_6H_5	Met ED_{50} 6 (po): MES ED_{50} 25 (po)	Sternbach and Randall (1966)
			Met ED_{50} 2 (po)	Childress and Gluckman (1964)
H	H	C_6H_5	Met ED_{50} > 50 (po)	Childress and Gluckman (1964)

(continued)

503

TABLE XLIII—*Continued*

X	R	Ar	Activity	Reference
Me	H	C_6H_5	Met ED$_{50}$ 38 (po)	Childress and Gluckman (1964)
Cl	Me	C_6H_5	Met ED$_{50}$ 2.2 (po)	Childress and Gluckman (1964)
Cl	H	2-ClC$_6$H$_4$	Met ED$_{50}$ 2.0 (po); MES ED$_{50}$ >40 (po)	Childress and Gluckman (1964)
Cl	Me	2ClC$_6$H$_4$	Met ED$_{50}$ 0.65 (po); MES ED$_{50}$ 15 (po)	Childress and Gluckman (1964)
Cl	H	2-Thiop	Met ED$_{50}$ 20 (po)	Childress and Gluckman (1964)
Cl	CH$_2$CH$_2$NOEt$_2$	2-FC$_6$H$_4$	Met ED$_{50}$ 28 (po)	Walser and Fryer (1974)
Cl	CH=CH$_2$	2-FC$_6$H$_4$	Met ED$_{50}$ 7.7 (po)	Walser and Fryer (1974)
Cl	(CH$_2$)$_2$NMe$_2$	C_6H_5	Met ED$_{50}$ 17 (po); MES ED$_{50}$ 265 (po)	Sternbach et al. (1965)
Cl	CH$_2$CF$_3$	C_6H_5	Met ED$_{50}$ 1.7 (po)	Steinman et al. (1973)
Cl	CH$_2$CF$_3$	2-ClC$_6$H$_4$	Met ED$_{50}$ 17 (po)	Steinman et al. (1973)
Cl	CH$_2$CF$_3$	2-FC$_6$H$_4$	Met ED$_{50}$ 5 (po)	Steinman et al. (1973)
N$_3$	H	C_6H_4	Met ED$_{50}$ 8.9 (po); MES ED$_{50}$ 48 (po)	Ning et al. (1973)

With n = 0 and an R_1 substituent

X	R	R_1	Ar	Activity	Reference
Cl	H	R_1	C_6H_5	Active	Sunjic et al. (1975)
Cl	R	OR$_2$	Ar	Active	Kajfez et al. (1975)
X	R	=Z	Ar	Active	Pieper et al. (1974a,d,e)
X	R	CH$_2$OR$_2$	Ar	Active	Pieper et al. (1974c)
X	R	R_1	Ar	Active	Reeder and Sternbach (1964a); Reeder et al. (1962)

X			Ar	Activity	Reference
X	R	R₂, R₃	Ar	Active	Pieper et al. (1974b)
H	R (8-CF₃)	R₁	Ar	Active	Sternbach and Saucy (1964)
Cl	Me	OR₂	C₆H₅	Active	Sternbach and Stempel (1969)
X	H	OR₂	Ar	Active	Bell (1965a)
Cl	H	OH	C₆H₅	Active	Bell (1965b)
Cl	H	Me, N(R₂)₂	C₆H₅	Active	Bell (1968)
H	H	R₁	C₆H₅	Active	Ning and Sternbach (1972a)
CH(OH)Me	R	OR₂	Ar	Active	Ning and Sternbach (1973a)
X	(CH₂)ₙCO₂Y	R₁	Ar	Active	Earley et al. (1971)
X	H	OCOR₂	Ar	Active	Bell et al. (1965a)
Cl	H	SR₂	C₆H₅	Active	Bell et al. (1964b)
H	(CH₂)ₙN(R₂)₂	R₁	2-ClC₆H₄	Active	Beton (1974)
X	R	R₁	Pyr	Active	Fryer et al. (1963)
X	R	CO₂R₂	Ar	Active	Hellerbach et al. (1972)
Cl	H	R₁	C₆H₅	Active	Sunjic et al. (1975)
X	H	R₁	Ar	Active	Schmitt et al. (1966)
X	R	R₁	Ar	Active	Broger et al. (1972); Keller et al. (1964b,c,d)
Cl	H	OH (oxazepam[a])	C₆H₅	Met ED₅₀ 0.6 (po); MES ED₅₀ 3.1 (po)	Gluckman (1971)
				Met ED₅₀ 3; MES ED₅₀ 25	Christmas and Maxwell (1970)
				MES ED₅₀ 5.1 (po), 2.3 (ip)	Klupp and Kahling (1965)
				Met ED₅₀ 0.9 (po); MES ED₅₀ 1.3 (po)	Childress and Gluckman (1964)
				Met ED₅₀ 6.9 (ip)	Nakanishi et al. (1973e)
				Met ED₅₀ 7.8 (os)	DeAngelis et al. (1974b)
				Met, 100% protn. at 10 (os)	Mucci et al. (1965)

(continued)

505

TABLE XLIII—*Continued*

X	R	R_1	Ar	Activity	Reference
CF_3O	H	OH	C_6H_5	Met ED_{50} > 50	McEvoy (1968)
Cl	H	OH (lorazepam)	$2\text{-}ClC_6H_4$	Met ED_{50} 0.07 (po); MES ED_{50} 2.0 (po)	Gluckman (1971)
				Met ED_{50} 0.07 (po); MES ED_{50} 2.0 (po)	Childress and Gluckman (1964)
				Met, 100% protn. at 10; MES, 90% protn. at 5	Marmo et al. (1971)
X	R	R_1	Ar	Active	Bogatskii et al. (1970)
Cl	H	Me	C_6H_5	Met ED_{50} 6.5 (po)	Childress and Gluckman (1964)
Cl	Me	OH (temazepam)	C_6H_5	Met ED_{50} 0.7 (po); MES ED_{50} 2.6 (po)	Childress and Gluckman (1964)
				Met ED_{50} 6.4 (po); MES ED_{50} 4.0 (po)	Ferrini et al. (1974)
Cl	H	OEt	C_6H_5	Met ED_{50} 5.7 (po)	Childress and Gluckman (1964)
Cl	Me	OH	$2\text{-}ClC_6H_4$	Met ED_{50} 0.09 (po); MES ED_{50} 2.4 (po)	Childress and Gluckman (1964)
Cl	CH_2CH_2OH	OH	$2\text{-}FC_6H_4$	Met ED_{50} 0.096 (ip); MES ED_{50} 3.0 (ip)	Tamagnone et al. (1974)
Cl	H	OCOMe	C_6H_4	Met ED_{50} 2.6 (po)	Childress and Gluckman (1964)
Cl	H	OCOMe	$2\text{-}ClC_6H_4$	Met ED_{50} 0.26 (po); MES ED_{50} 3.7 (po)	Childress and Gluckman (1964)
Cl	H	CO_2K	C_6H_5	Met ED_{50} 1.7 (po); MES ED_{50} 4.6 (po)	Brunaud et al. (1970)
				Met ED_{50} 2.5 (po), 2.5 (ip); MES ED_{50} 5 (po), 2.5 (ip)	Schmitt et al. (1969)
NO_2	H	CO_2K	C_6H_5	Met ED_{50} 0.3 (po); MES ED_{50} 3 (po)	Schmitt et al. (1969)

Cl	Me	OCONMe$_2$	C$_6$H$_5$	Met ED$_{50}$ 5.8 (os); MES ED$_{50}$ 60 (os)	Ferrini et al. (1974)
Cl	H, + form	OCO(CH$_2$)$_2$CO$_2$Na	C$_6$H$_5$	Met ED$_{50}$ 0.77 (iv)	Mussini et al. (1972)
Cl	H, − form	OCO(CH$_2$)$_2$CO$_2$Na	C$_6$H$_5$	Met ED$_{50}$ 2.68 (iv)	Mussini et al. (1972)
Cl	H, ± form	OCO(CH$_2$)$_2$CO$_2$Na	C$_6$H$_5$	Met ED$_{50}$ 1.29 (iv)	Mussini et al. (1972)
Cl	H	OCO(CH$_2$)$_2$CO$_2$H	C$_6$H$_5$	Met ED$_{50}$ 0.95 (os)	Duchene-Marullaz et al. (1967)
Cl	H	OCO(CH$_2$)$_2$CO$_2^-$ Me$_2^+$NH(CH$_2$)$_2$OH	C$_6$H$_5$	Met ED$_{50}$ 2.76 (ip) Met ED$_{50}$ 3.69 (ip) Met ED$_{50}$ 5.0 (ip)	Babbini et al. (1969) Babbini et al. (1969) DeMarchi and Tamagnone (1971)
Cl	H	OCOCH(Pr-n)$_2$	C$_6$H$_5$	Met ED$_{50}$ 360	DeMarchi and Torrielli (1968)
Cl	CONHMe	OCOMe	C$_6$H$_5$	Met ED$_{50}$ 28 (ip); MES ED$_{50}$ > 50 (ip)	Moffett and Rudzik (1972)
Cl	CH$_2$CF$_3$	OCOMe	C$_6$H$_5$	Met ED$_{50}$ 10 (po)	Steinman et al. (1973)
Cl	CH$_2$CF$_3$	OH	C$_6$H$_5$	Met ED$_{50}$ 1.2 (po)	Steinman et al. (1973)
Cl	CH$_2$CF$_3$	OCOMe	2-FC$_6$H$_4$	Met ED$_{50}$ 0.8 (po)	Steinman et al. (1973)
Cl	H	NPyr Cl$^-$ (N$^+$)	2-ClC$_6$H$_4$	Met ED$_{50}$ 13.6; MES ED$_{50}$ 3.5	Kovac et al. (1974)
Cl	H	NPyr Cl$^-$ (N$^+$)	C$_6$H$_5$	Met ED$_{50}$ 17.0; MES ED$_{50}$ 4.0	Kovac et al. (1974)
Cl	Me	NPyr Cl$^-$ (N$^+$)	C$_6$H$_5$	Met ED$_{50}$ 15.6; MES ED$_{50}$ 3.7	Kovac et al. (1974)
Cl	H	—N$^+$ NMe Cl$^-$ (imidazole)	2-ClC$_6$H$_5$	Met ED$_{50}$ 5.3; MES ED$_{50}$ 5.7	Kovac et al. (1974)
Cl	H	—N$^+$ NMe Cl$^-$ (imidazole)	C$_6$H$_5$	Met ED$_{50}$ 5.6; MES ED$_{50}$ 6.0	Kovac et al. (1974)
Cl	Me	—N$^+$ NMe Cl$^-$ (imidazole)	C$_6$H$_5$	Met ED$_{50}$ 7.5; MES ED$_{50}$ 7.9	Kovac et al. (1974)

(continued)

507

TABLE XLIII—*Continued*

X	R	R$_1$	Ar	Activity	Reference
Cl	H	imidazolium, —NEt, Cl⁻	2-ClC$_6$H$_4$	Met ED$_{50}$ 4.3; MES ED$_{50}$ 4.7	Kovac *et al.* (1974)
Cl	H	imidazolium, —NEt, Cl⁻	C$_6$H$_5$	Met ED$_{50}$ 5.9; MES ED$_{50}$ 6.3	Kovac *et al.* (1974)
Cl	Me	imidazolium, —NEt, Cl⁻	C$_6$H$_5$	Met ED$_{50}$ 5.0; MES ED$_{50}$ 5.6	Kovac *et al.* (1974)
Cl	H	pyridinium, CONH$_2$	2-ClC$_6$H$_4$	Met ED$_{50}$ 6.0; MES ED$_{50}$ 0.70	Kovac *et al.* (1974)
Cl	H	pyridinium, Cl⁻, CONH$_2$	2-ClC$_6$H$_4$	Met ED$_{50}$ 5.8; MES ED$_{50}$ 0.60	Kovac *et al.* (1974)
Cl	Me	pyridinium, Cl⁻, CONH$_2$	C$_6$H$_5$	Met ED$_{50}$ 6.5; MES ED$_{50}$ 0.80	Kovac *et al.* (1974)
Cl	H	pyridinium, CONEt$_2$, Cl⁻	2-ClC$_6$H$_4$	Met ED$_{50}$ 7.3; MES ED$_{50}$ 1.6	Kovac *et al.* (1974)
Cl	H	pyridinium, CONEt$_2$, Cl⁻	C$_6$H$_5$	Met ED$_{50}$ 7.0; MES ED$_{50}$ 1.2	Kovac *et al.* (1974)

Cl	H	morpholine–CH₂CH₂OH, Cl⁻	$2\text{-ClC}_6\text{H}_4$	Met ED$_{50}$ 20.5; MES ED$_{50}$ 10.3	Kovac *et al.* (1974)
Cl	H	morpholine–CH₂CH₂OH, Cl⁻	C_6H_5	Met ED$_{50}$ 19.0; MES ED$_{50}$ 9.6	Kovac *et al.* (1974)
Cl	H	imidazole, Me, N–CH₂CH₂Br, NO₂, Cl⁻	$2\text{-ClC}_6\text{H}_4$	Met ED$_{50}$ 10.1; MES ED$_{50}$ 2.0	Kovac *et al.* (1974)
Cl	H	imidazole, Me, N–CH₂CH₂Br, NO₂, Cl⁻	C_6H_5	Met ED$_{50}$ 7.7; MES ED$_{50}$ 6.5	Kovac *et al.* (1974)
Cl	Me	imidazole, Me, N–CH₂CH₂Br, NO₂, Cl⁻	C_6H_5	Met ED$_{50}$ 6.0; MES ED$_{50}$ 5.0	Kovac *et al.* (1974)
Cl	H	OH	C_6H_5	Met ED$_{50}$ 0.6 (po); MES ED$_{50}$ 3.1 (po)	Bell *et al.* (1968b)
Cl	Me	OH	C_6H_5	Met ED$_{50}$ 0.7 (po); MES ED$_{50}$ 2.6 (po)	Bell *et al.* (1968b)
Cl	H	OH	$2\text{-ClC}_6\text{H}_5$	Met ED$_{50}$ 0.07 (po); MES ED$_{50}$ 2.0 (po)	Bell *et al.* (1968b)
Cl	Me	OH	$2\text{-ClC}_6\text{H}_5$	Met ED$_{50}$ 0.09 (po); MES ED$_{50}$ 2.4 (po)	Bell *et al.* (1968b)

(continued)

TABLE XLIII—*Continued*

X	R	R_1	Ar	Activity	Reference
Cl	$CH_2C_3H_5$	OH	C_6H_5	Met ED_{50} 6.2 (po); MES ED_{50} 13 (po)	Bell *et al.* (1968b)
H	H	OCOMe	C_6H_5	Met ED_{50} 31 (po); MES ED_{50} 71 (po)	Bell *et al.* (1968b)
Cl	H	OCOMe	C_6H_5	Met ED_{50} 2.6 (po); MES ED_{50} 3.8 (po)	Bell *et al.* (1968b)
Cl	Me	OCOMe	C_6H_5	Met ED_{50} 3.4 (po); MES ED_{50} 2.3 (po)	Bell *et al.* (1968b)
Cl	$CH_2C_3H_5$	OCOMe	C_6H_5	Met ED_{50} 4.5 (po); MES ED_{50} 25 (po)	Bell *et al.* (1968b)
Cl	H	OCOMe	$2\text{-}ClC_6H_4$	Met ED_{50} 0.3 (po); MES ED_{50} 3.7 (po)	Bell *et al.* (1968b)
Cl	H	OCOMe, Me	C_6H_5	Met ED_{50} 127 (po);	Bell *et al.* (1968b)
Cl	H	$OCOC_6H_5$	C_6H_5	Met ED_{50} 1.2 (po); MES ED_{50} > 40 (po)	Bell *et al.* (1968b)
Cl	H	$OCOCH_2Cl$	C_6H_5	Met ED_{50} 2.0 (po); MES ED_{50} 13 (po)	Bell *et al.* (1968b)
Cl	H	$OCOCH_2C_4H_8ON$	C_6H_5	Met ED_{50} 0.8 (po); MES ED_{50} 7.5 (po)	Bell *et al.* (1968b)
Cl	H	$OCOCH_2NC_5H_5Cl$	C_6H_5	Met ED_{50} 0.8 (po); MES ED_{50} 8.2 (po)	Bell *et al.* (1968b)
Cl	H	$OCOCH_2CH_2CO_2H$	C_6H_5	Met ED_{50} 1.1 (po); MES ED_{50} 17 (po)	Bell *et al.* (1968b)
Cl	H	$OCOCH_2CH_2CO_2H$	$2\text{-}ClC_6H_5$	Met ED_{50} 0.05 (po); MES ED_{50} 5.7 (po)	Bell *et al.* (1968b)
Cl	COMe	OCOMe	C_6H_5	Met ED_{50} 0.9 (po); MES ED_{50} 4.8 (po)	Bell *et al.* (1968b)
Cl	H	$OCOCH_2CH_2C_5H_9$	C_6H_5	Met ED_{50} 30 (po); MES ED_{50} 127 (po)	Bell *et al.* (1968b)

Cl	COMe	OCOMe	2-ClC$_6$H$_4$	Met ED$_{50}$ 0.4 (po); MES ED$_{50}$ 2.3 (po)	Bell et al. (1968b)
Cl	COCH$_2$Cl	OCOMe	C$_6$H$_5$	Met ED$_{50}$ 6.0 (po); MES ED$_{50}$ 40 (po)	Bell et al. (1968b)
Cl	H	OMe	C$_6$H$_5$	Met ED$_{50}$ 6.0 (po)	Bell et al. (1968b)
Cl	Me	OMe	C$_6$H$_5$	Met ED$_{50}$ 0.4 (po); MES ED$_{50}$ 0.9 (po)	Bell et al. (1968b)
Cl	H	OMe	2-ClC$_6$H$_4$	Met ED$_{50}$ 0.5 (po); MES ED$_{50}$ 2.2 (po)	Bell et al. (1968b)
Cl	Me	OMe	2-ClC$_6$H$_4$	Met ED$_{50}$ 0.4 (po); MES ED$_{50}$ 0.7 (po)	Bell et al. (1968b)
Cl	H	OEt	C$_6$H$_5$	Met ED$_{50}$ 5.7 (po)	Bell et al. (1968b)
Cl	H	OEt	2-ClC$_6$H$_4$	Met ED$_{50}$ 0.5 (po); MES ED$_{50}$ 2.6 (po)	Bell et al. (1968b)
Cl	H	OCH$_2$CO$_2$Et	C$_6$H$_5$	Met ED$_{50}$ > 127 (po)	Bell et al. (1968b)
Cl	H	OCH$_2$CO$_2$H	C$_6$H$_5$	Met ED$_{50}$ 75 (po); MES ED$_{50}$ > 40 (po)	Bell et al. (1968b)
Cl	H	Cl	C$_6$H$_5$	Met ED$_{50}$ 0.2 (po); MES ED$_{50}$ 3.0 (po)	Bell et al. (1968b)
Cl	H	Cl	2-ClC$_6$H$_4$	Met ED$_{50}$ 0.2 (po); MES ED$_{50}$ 1.4 (po)	Bell et al. (1968b)
Cl	Me	Cl	2-ClC$_6$H$_4$	Met ED$_{50}$ 0.2 (po)	Bell et al. (1968b)
Cl	H	SH	C$_6$H$_5$	Met ED$_{50}$ 45 (po); MES ED$_{50}$ 25 (po)	Bell et al. (1968b)
Cl	H	SCOMe	C$_6$H$_5$	Met ED$_{50}$ 13 (po); MES ED$_{50}$ 100 (po)	Bell et al. (1968b)
Cl	H	SCH$_2$CH$_2$NEt$_2$	C$_6$H$_5$	Met ED$_{50}$ 400 (po)	Bell et al. (1968b)
Cl	H	SC$_3$H$_4$NS	C$_6$H$_5$	Met ED$_{50}$ > 400 (po)	Bell et al. (1968b)
Cl	H	NH$_2$	C$_6$H$_5$	Met ED$_{50}$ 7.8 (po); MES ED$_{50}$ 13 (po)	Bell et al. (1968b)
Cl	H	NH$_2$	2-ClC$_6$H$_5$	Met ED$_{50}$ 3.0 (po); MES ED$_{50}$ 3.5 (po)	Bell et al. (1968b)

(continued)

511

TABLE XLIII—Continued

X	R	R_1	Ar	Activity	Reference
Cl	H	NHMe	C_6H_5	Met ED_{50} > 40 (po); MES ED_{50} > 40 (po)	Bell *et al.* (1968b)
Cl	H	NC_4H_8O	C_6H_5	Met ED_{50} 17 (po); MES ED_{50} > 400 (po)	Bell *et al.* (1968b)
Cl	H	$NHCH_2CH_2NMe_2$	C_6H_5	Met ED_{50} 54 (po); MES ED_{50} > 400 (po)	Bell *et al.* (1968b)
Cl	H	NEt_2, Me	C_6H_5	Met ED_{50} > 127 (po); MES ED_{50} > 127 (po)	Bell *et al.* (1968b)
Cl	H	NC_5H_5Cl	C_6H_5	Met ED_{50} > 127 (po)	Bell *et al.* (1968b)
Cl	H	NHCHO	C_6H_5	Met ED_{50} 38 (po)	Bell *et al.* (1968b)
Cl	H	NHCOMe	C_6H_5	Met ED_{50} 500 (po)	Bell *et al.* (1968b)
Cl	H	NHCOMe	$2\text{-}ClC_6H_5$	Met ED_{50} > 400 (po)	Bell *et al.* (1968b)
Cl	H	NMeCOMe	C_6H_5	Met ED_{50} > 400 (po)	Bell *et al.* (1968b)
Cl	H	$NHCOCH_2CH_2C_6H_5$	C_6H_5	Met ED_{50} > 127 (po)	Bell *et al.* (1968b)
Cl	H	$NHCOC_6H_5$	C_6H_5	Met ED_{50} > 40 (po)	Bell *et al.* (1968b)
Cl	H	NHCOMe	CH_3	Met ED_{50} > 127 (po)	Bell *et al.* (1968b)
Cl	H	$NHCO_2Et$	C_6H_5	Met ED_{50} > 400 (po)	Bell *et al.* (1968b)
Cl	CO_2Et	$NHCO_2Et$	C_6H_5	Met ED_{50} > 400 (po)	Bell *et al.* (1968b)
Cl	H	CO_2Et	C_6H_5	Met ED_{50} 2.4 (po); MES ED_{50} 13 (po)	Bell *et al.* (1968b)
Cl	H	CO_2Et, OH	C_6H_5	Met ED_{50} 6.2 (po); MES ED_{50} 86 (po)	Bell *et al.* (1968b)
Cl	H	CO_2Et, OMe	C_6H_5	Met ED_{50} 40 (po); MES ED_{50} > 127 (po)	Bell *et al.* (1968b)
Cl	H	CO_2Et, OEt	C_6H_5	Met ED_{50} 40 (po); MES ED_{50} > 40 (po)	Bell *et al.* (1968b)

With n = 1

X	R	R_1	Ar	Activity	Reference
Cl	R	R_1	Ar	Active	Reeder and Sternbach (1964a)

	R₁				
H	H	C_6H_5	Active		Ning and Sternbach (1972a)
Cl	Me	H	C_6H_5	Met ED$_{50}$ 3.1 (po)	Childress and Gluckman (1964)

E. 1,3-Dihydro-2H-1,4-benzodiazepin-2-ones

Compound	Activity	Reference
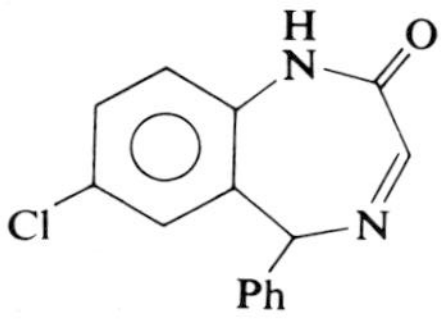 (structure)	Met ED$_{50}$ 21	Bell et al. (1968a)

F. Benzodiazepine-2,5-diones

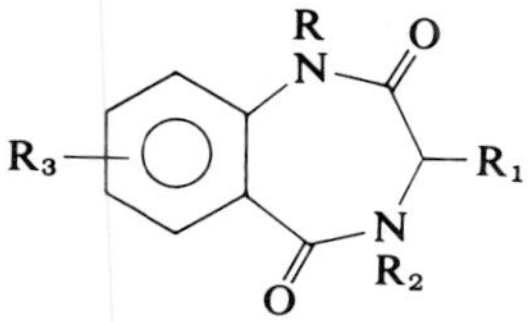

R	R₁	R₂	R₃	Activity	Reference
$(CH_2)_n NMe_2$	H	Ar	H	Active	Sumitomo Chemical Co., Ltd. (1969)
Ar	R₁	R₂	R₃	Active	Weber et al. (1969)
R	H	H	R₃	Active	Bauer et al. (1973b)
Ar	H	COR₄	R₃	Active	Bauer et al. (1974b)

(continued)

513

TABLE XLIII—*Continued*

G. 2,3-Dihydro-1H-1,4-benzodiazepines

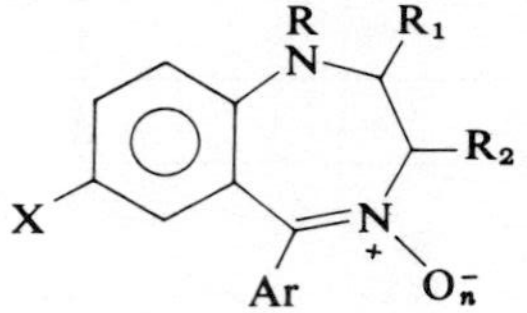

With n = 0; $R_1 = R_2 = H$

X	R	Ar	Activity	Reference
Cl	Me	C_6H_5	Active	Oklobdziji et al. (1973)
Cl	C(=X)NHR$_3$	C_6H_5	Active	Metlesics and Sternbach (1974)
CF$_3$O	H	C_6H_5	MES ED > 50	McEvoy (1968)
C(OH)R$_3$R$_4$	Me	Ar	Active	Ning and Sternbach (1972c)
Cl	R	Ar	Active	Okamoto et al. (1972)
Cl	Me	Ar	Active	Earley et al. (1974)
Cl	R	C_6H_5	Active	Hellerbach and Zanetti (1974)
X	R	Ar	Active	Shimizu and Yamanaka (1975)
RCO	R	Ar	Active	Wehrli et al. (1971)
MeCO	Me	C_6H_5	Active	Wehrli et al. (1974)
Cl	Me	C_6H_5	Active	Krva (1975)
Cl	CH$_2$CF$_3$	Ar	Active	Steinman (1971)
H	Me	C_6H_5	Met, 100% protn. at 25	Marmo et al. (1971)
	(medazepam)		Met ED$_{50}$ 5 (po); MES ED$_{50}$ 46 (po)	Ferrini et al. (1974)
			Met ED$_{50}$ 9.2 (ip)	Nakanishi et al. (1973e)
Cl	Me	C_6H_5	Met ED$_{50}$ 2.7; MES ED$_{50}$ 215	Kido et al. (1970)
			Met ED$_{50}$ 1.6 (po); MES ED$_{50}$ 37 (po)	Randall et al (1969)
			Met ED$_{50}$ 6.7 (po); MES ED$_{50}$ 37.6 (po)	Sternbach and Randall (1966)
Cl	H	C_6H_5	Met ED$_{50}$ 4 (po); MES ED$_{50}$ 19 (po)	Sternbach and Randall (1966)
			Met ED$_{50}$ 0.9 (po); MES ED$_{50}$ 9.8 (po)	Childress and Gluckman (1964)

X	R	R_1	Ar	Activity	Reference
NO_2	H		C_6H_5	Met ED_{50} 1.4 (po)	Childress and Gluckman (1964)
MeCO	Me		C_6H_5	Met ED_{50} 25	Wehrli et al. (1971)
CF_3	H		C_6H_5	Met ED_{50} 3.7 (po); MES ED_{50} 30 (po)	Sternbach and Randall (1966)
NO_2	Me		C_6H_5	Met ED_{50} 4.9 (po); MES ED_{50} 400 (po)	Sternbach and Randall (1966)
Cl	$CH_2CH_2NEt_2$		C_6H_5	Met ED_{50} 17 (po); MES ED_{50} 150	Sternbach and Randall (1966)
Cl	CH_2CF_3		C_6H_5	Met ED_{50} 5-10 (po)	Steinman et al. (1973)
Cl	CH_2CF_3		2-ClC_6H_4	Met ED_{50} 0.5 (po)	Steinman et al. (1973)
Cl	CH_2CF_3		2-FC_6H_4	Met ED_{50} 1 (po)	Steinman et al. (1973)
H	CH_2CF_3		2-FC_6H_4	Met ED_{50} > 100 (po)	Steinman et al. (1973)
NO_2	CH_2CF_3		2-FC_6H_4	Met ED_{50} 2.5 (po)	Steinman et al. (1973)
NO_2 (9-NO_2)	CH_2CF_3		2-FC_6H_4	Met ED_{50} > 100 (po)	Steinman et al. (1973)
Cl (9-NO_2)	CH_2CF_3		2-FC_6H_4	Met ED_{50} > 100 (po)	Steinman et al. (1973)
Br	CH_2CF_3		2-FC_6H_4	Met ED_{50} 0.15 (po)	Steinman et al. (1973)
N_3	Me		C_6H_5	Met ED_{50} 6.5 (po); MES ED_{50} 45 (po)	Ning et al. (1973)
With n = 1; $R_1 = R_2 = H$					
Cl	H		C_6H_5	Met ED_{50} 4 (po); MES ED_{50} 12.7 (po)	Childress and Gluckman (1964)
Cl	H		2-ClC_6H_4	Met ED_{50} 4 (po); MES ED_{50} 9 (po)	Childress and Gluckman (1964)
Cl	MeCO		C_6H_5	Met ED_{50} 78 (po); MES ED_{50} 150 (po)	Childress and Gluckman (1964)
Cl	CH_2CF_3		2-ClC_6H_4	Met ED_{50} > 30 (po)	Steinman et al. (1973)
Cl	CH_2CF_3		2-FC_6H_4	Met ED_{50} 36 (po)	Steinman et al. (1973)

X	R	R_1	Ar	Activity	Reference
With n = 0; $R_2 = H$					
X	R	CH_2R_3	Ar	Active	Milkowski et al. (1973)
Cl	Me	CH_2OR_3	Thio, Fur	Active	Milkowski et al. (1974)
Cl	Me	R_1	Ar	Active	Ning and Schwartz (1975)
Cl	CH_2CF_3	SEt	C_6H_5	Active	Steinman (1974)
X	R	CH_2R_3	Thio, Fur	Active	Kali-chemie Pharma (1974)
Cl	H	SCH_2CH_2OH	C_6H_5	Met ED_{50} 3.2	Coffen and Fryer (1974b)
Cl	H	$CONH_2$	C_6H_5	Met ED_{50} 4.6	Coffen and Fryer (1974a)

(continued)

TABLE XLIII—*Continued*

With n = 0; R₁ = H

X	R	R_2	Ar	Activity	Reference
X	R	R_2	Ar	Active	Archer (1964); Broger et al. (1972); Ishizumi et al. (1973); Reeder and Sternbach (1963), (1964b,c)
X	H	R_2	Ar	Active	Reeder and Sternbach (1965)
X	R	R_2	2-Pyr	Active	Fryer et al. (1968)
NO_2	H	$CONHR_3$	C_6H_5	Active	Fryer and Sternbach (1974)
Cl	CH_2CF_3	OCOMe	$2\text{-}ClC_6H_4$	Met ED_{50} > 30 (po)	Steinman et al. (1973)

H. 1,3,4,5-Tetrahydro-2H-1,4-benzodiazepin-2-ones

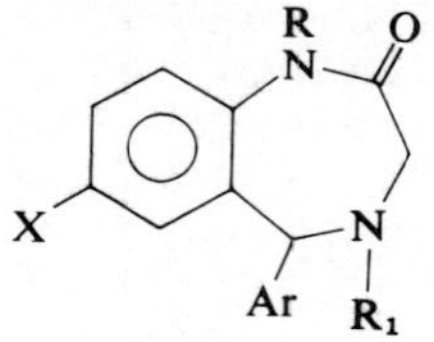

X	R	R_1	Ar	Activity	Reference
MeO	H	Me	C_6H_5	Active	Fryer and Sternbach (1970)
Cl	R	H	Ar	Active	Hoffman-La Roche & Co. (1964b)
CN	Me	H	C_6H_5	Active	Hoffman-La Roche & Co. (1965b)
X	R	R_1	Ar	Active	Ishizumi et al. (1974)
MeCO	H	R_1	C_6H_5, R_3	Active	Ning and Sternbach (1972a)
X	R	OH (3-R_3)	Ar	Active	Reeder and Sternbach (1964a)
X	R	R_2 (3-R_3)	Ar	Active	Reeder and Sternbach (1964a)
Cl	H	H	C_6H_5	Met ED_{50} 6.8 (po); MES ED_{50} 40 (po)	Sternbach and Randall (1966)
				Met ED_{50} 12.9; MES ED_{50} 173	Swinyard and Castellion (1966)
				Met ED_{50} 5.2 (po); MES ED_{50} 13 (po)	Childress and Gluckman (1964)

X	R	R₁	R₂	Ar		Reference
Cl	Me	H		C$_6$H$_5$	Met ED$_{50}$ 15 (po); MES ED$_{50}$ 12.5 (po)	Sternbach and Randall (1966)
Cl	Me	H (± form)		C$_6$H$_5$	Met ED$_{50}$ 2.4 (ip); MES ED$_{50}$ 24.2 (ip)	Palosi et al. (1973)
Cl	Me	H (+ form)		C$_6$H$_5$	Met ED$_{50}$ 3.5 (ip); MES ED$_{50}$ 20.3 (ip)	Palosi et al. (1973)
Cl	Me	H (− form)		C$_6$H$_5$	Met ED$_{50}$ 1.75 (ip) MES ED$_{50}$ 16.2 (ip)	Palosi et al. (1973)
CF$_3$	H	H		C$_6$H$_5$	Met ED$_{50}$ 18 (po); MES ED$_{50}$ 43 (po)	Sternbach and Randall (1966)
H	H	H		C$_6$H$_5$	Met ED$_{50}$ 29 (po)	Childress and Gluckman (1964)
Cl	Me	Me		C$_6$H$_5$	Met ED$_{50}$ 8 (po)	Childress and Gluckman (1964)
Cl	(CH$_2$)$_2$NEt$_2$			2-FC$_6$H$_4$	Met ED$_{50}$ 100 (po); MES ED$_{50}$ 200 (po)	Sternbach et al. (1965)
Cl	H		(CH$_2$)$_2$NEt$_2$	2-FC$_6$H$_4$	Met ED$_{50}$ 14 (po); MES ED$_{50}$ 133 (po)	Sternbach et al. (1965)
Cl	Me		Me	2-FC$_6$H$_4$	Met ED$_{50}$ 800 (po); MES ED$_{50}$ 353 (po)	Sternbach et al. (1965)
Cl	H		(CH$_2$)$_3$NHMe	2-FC$_6$H$_4$	Met ED$_{50}$ 400 (po); MES ED$_{50}$ 533 (po)	Sternbach et al. (1965)
Cl	H		(CH$_2$)$_3$NMe$_2$	2-FC$_6$H$_4$	Met ED$_{50}$ > 400 (po); MES ED$_{50}$ 300 (po)	Sternbach et al. (1965)
Cl	H		(CH$_2$)$_3$NEt$_2$	2-FC$_6$H$_4$	Met ED$_{50}$ > 400 (po); MES ED$_{50}$ 300 (po)	Sternbach et al. (1965)

I. 1,2,3,4-Tetrahydro-5H-1,4-benzodiazepines

(Structure: 1,2,3,4-tetrahydro-5H-1,4-benzodiazepine nucleus bearing R on N, R$_1$ at the 2-position, R$_2$ on N, Ar at the 5-position, and X on the fused benzene ring.)

X	R	R$_1$	R$_2$	Ar	Activity	Reference
X	R	R$_1$	R$_2$	Ar	Active	Archer et al. (1963, 1964); Reeder and Sternbach (1963, 1964b,c, 1965)
X	(CH$_2$)$_n$NR$_3$CONH$_2$	R$_1$	R$_2$	R$_4$, R$_5$	Active	Earley et al. (1968)
NO$_2$	ME	H	H	(2-thiazolyl ring, S and N)	Active	Broger et al. (1972)

(continued)

TABLE XLIII—*Continued*

Compound	Activity	Reference
	Met ED$_{50}$ 6	Coffen and Fryer (1974b)

J. 1,4-Benzodiazepines with additional rings

Compound	Activity	Reference
	Active	Hester (1972c)
	Active	Hester (1972a)
	Active	Hester (1972a)
	Active	Hester (1972a)
	Active	Hester (1971)

	Active	Hester (1973b)
	Active	Hester (1972b)
	Active	Hester (1973a, 1974)
	$n = 1, 2$: active	Derieg et al. (1968)
	$n = 1, 2$: active	Derieg et al. (1973)
	Active	Upjohn Co. (1975)
	Active	Gagneux et al. (1974a)

(continued)

TABLE XLIII—*Continued*

R	R_1	R_2	n	Activity	Reference
R	R_1	H	1	Active	Tawada et al. (1974)
Cl	R_1	H	0	Met, active	Gagneux et al. (1972, 1973a)
R	$CONR_3R_4$	H	0	Active	Gagneux et al. (1973b)
Cl	CH_2NH_2	H	0	Active	Gagneux et al. (1974b)
R	$CONR_3R_4$	R_2	0	Active	Kuwada et al. (1974b)

R	R_1	R_2	n	Ar	Activity	Reference
R	Me	R_2	0	Ar	Active	Ning and Sternbach (1974b)
R	Me	R_2	1	Ar	Active	Ning and Sternbach (1974b)
Cl	R_1	H	1	C_6H_5	Active	Meguro and Kuwata (1974a)
R	R_1	H	0	Ar	Active	Meguro and Kuwata (1971)

Cl	H	H	0	C_6H_5	MES ED_{50} 4.6 (po); Met ED_{50} 2.2 (po)	Nakajima et al. (1971)
Cl	Me	H	0	C_6H_5	MES ED_{50} 1.6; Met ED_{50} 0.25	Nakajima et al. (1971)
R	$(CH_2)_nR_3$	H	0	Ar	Active	Allgeier and Gagneux (1972a, 1973a)
R	$(CH_2)_nR_3$	H	1	Ar	Active	Allgeier and Gagneux (1972a, 1973a)
R	R_1	R_2	0	Ar	Met, active	Allgeier and Gagneux (1972b)
Cl	R_1	H	0	Ar	Active	Allgeier and Gagneux (1974a)
Cl	$CH_2NR_3R_4$	H	0	Ar	Active	Allgeier and Gagneux (1974b, 1975a)
R	R_1	H	0	Ar	Active	Kuwada et al. (1974a)
R	R_1	OR_3	0	Ar	Active	Meguro and Kuwada (1974c,d,e)
R	R_1	R_2	0	Ar	Active	Kuwada et al. (1975)
Cl	CH_2R_3	H	0	C_6H_5	Active	Allgeier and Gagneux (1975b)
Cl	R_1	H	0	Ar	Active	Ciba-Geigy (1974)
R	Me	R_2	0	Ar	Active	Walser and Sternbach (1974)
R	Me	R_2	1	Ar	Active	Walser and Sternbach (1974)
Cl	$CH(OEt)_2$	Me	0	C_6H_5	Active	Allgeier and Gagneux (1975c)
Cl	Me	H	0	C_6H_5	MES ED_{50} 25 (ip); Met ED_{50} 0.2 (ip)	Hester et al. (1971)
Cl	Et	H	0	C_6H_5	MES ED_{50} > 6 (ip); Met ED_{50} 1.0 (ip)	Hester et al. (1971)
Cl	n-Pr	H	0	C_6H_5	MES ED_{50} > 25 (ip); Met ED_{50} 3.1 (ip)	Hester et al. (1971)
Cl	C_6H_5	H	0	C_6H_5	MES ED_{50} > 100 (ip); Met ED_{50} 63 (ip)	Hester et al. (1971)
Cl	$C_6H_5CH_2$	H	0	C_6H_5	MES ED_{50} 200 (ip); Met ED_{50} > 50 (ip)	Hester et al. (1971)
Cl	CO_2Et	H	0	C_6H_5	MES ED_{50} > 200 (ip); Met ED_{50} 8.0 (ip)	Hester et al. (1971)
Cl	H	H	0	C_6H_5	MES ED_{50} > 25 (ip); Met ED_{50} 0.6 (ip)	Hester et al. (1971)
H	Me	H	0	C_6H_5	MES ED_{50} > 25 (ip); Met ED_{50} 1.1 (ip)	Hester et al. (1971)
CF_3	Me	H	0	C_6H_5	MES ED_{50} > 0.8 (ip); Met ED_{50} 0.2 (ip)	Hester et al. (1971)
NO_2	Me	H	0	C_6H_5	MES ED_{50} 3.6 (ip); Met ED_{50} 0.25 (ip)	Hester et al. (1971)
SMe	Me	H	0	C_6H_5	MES ED_{50} 7.9 (ip); Met ED_{50} 1.6 (ip)	Hester et al. (1971)
Cl	Me	H	0	$2\text{-}FC_6H_4$	MES ED_{50} 20 (ip); Met ED_{50} 0.03 (ip)	Hester et al. (1971)
Cl	Me	H	0	$2\text{-}ClC_6H_4$	MES ED_{50} 50 (ip); Met ED_{50} 0.03 (ip)	Hester et al. (1971)
NO_2	Me	H	0	$2\text{-}ClC_6H_4$	MES ED_{50} 28 (ip); Met ED_{50} 0.023 (ip)	Hester et al. (1971)
Cl	Me	H	0	$2,6\text{-}F_2C_6H_3$	MES ED_{50} 16 (ip); Met ED_{50} 0.022 (ip)	Hester et al. (1971)
H	Me	H	0	$2\text{-}ClC_6H_4$	MES ED_{50} > 100 (ip); Met ED_{50} 0.55 (ip)	Hester et al. (1971)

TABLE XLIII—*Continued*

Compound	Activity	Reference
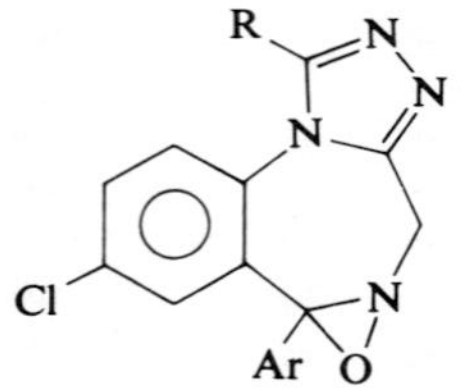	Active	Allgeier and Gagneux (1973a)
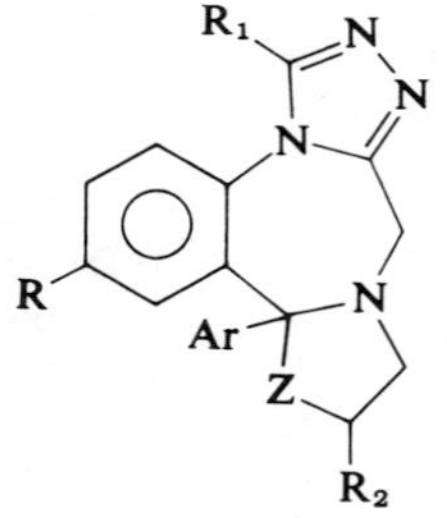	Z = O, NH, CH$_2$O: active	Meguro et al. (1972)
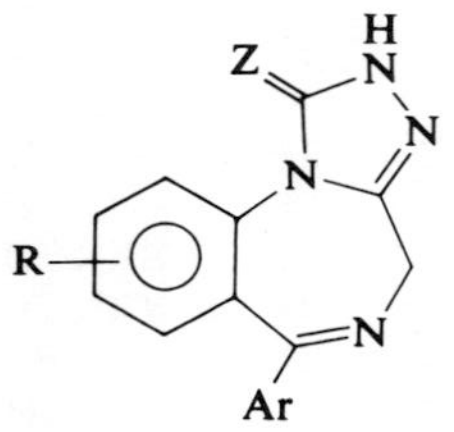	Active	Meguro and Kuwada (1974b)

522

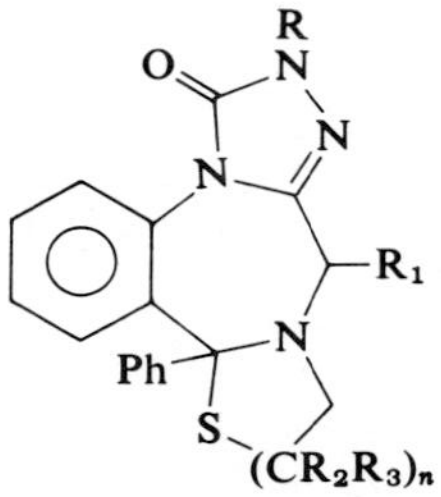

Kuwada *et al.* (1974d)

Kuwada *et al.* (1974e)

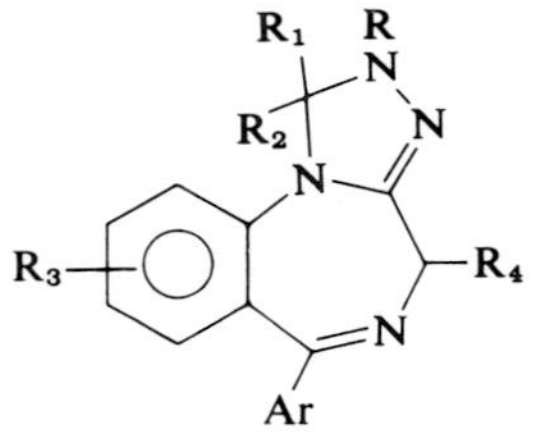

Coffen and Fryer (1974a)

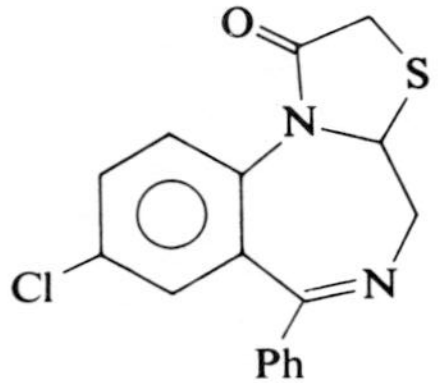

Fryer and Walser (1973)

(continued)

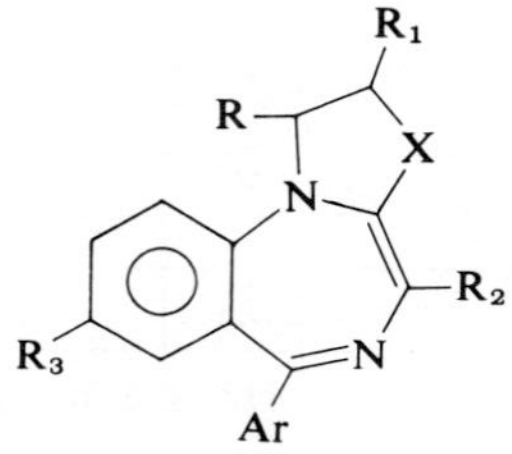

Active

Active

Met ED_{50} 137

Active

TABLE XLIII—Continued

Compound	Activity	Reference
	MES ED_{50} > 200 (ip); Met ED_{50} > 50 (ip)	Hester and Rudzik (1974)
	MES ED_{50} 4.6 (po); Met ED_{50} 2.2 (po)	Saji et al. (1973)
	MES ED_{50} > 50 (ip); Met ED_{50} 23 (ip)	Moffett and Rudzik (1973)

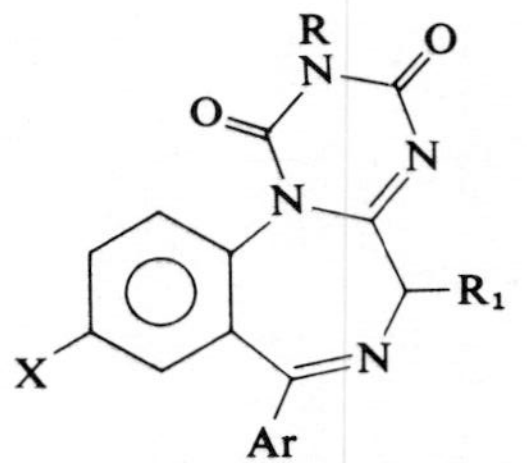

R	R_1	Ar	X	Activity	Reference
H	H	C_6H_5	Cl	MES ED_{50} > 100 (ip); Met ED_{50} 14 (ip)	Moffett and Rudzik (1973)
Me	H	C_6H_5	Cl	MES ED_{50} 40 (ip); Met ED_{50} 2.8 (ip)	Moffett and Rudzik (1973)
H	H	$2\text{-}ClC_6H_4$	Cl	MES ED_{50} > 50 (ip); Met ED_{50} 3.1 (ip)	Moffett and Rudzik (1973)
Me	Me	$2\text{-}ClC_6H_4$	Cl	MES ED_{50} > 100 (ip); Met ED_{50} 11 (ip)	Moffett and Rudzik (1973)
H	H	$2\text{-}ClC_6H_4$	H	MES ED_{50} > 100 (ip); Met ED_{50} > 100 (ip)	Moffett and Rudzik (1973)

Compound	Activity	Reference
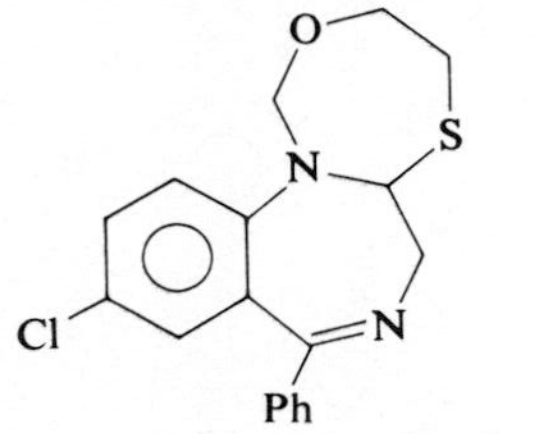	Met ED_{50} 5.4	Coffen and Fryer (1974a)
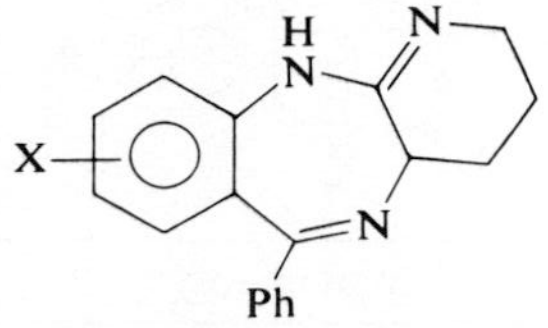	Active	Murakami et al. (1973)

(continued)

525

TABLE XLIII—*Continued*

Compound	Activity	Reference
	Active	Field *et al.* (1970)
	Active	Takahashi (1974)
	Active	Takahashi (1974)
	Active	Duncan and Helsley (1971)

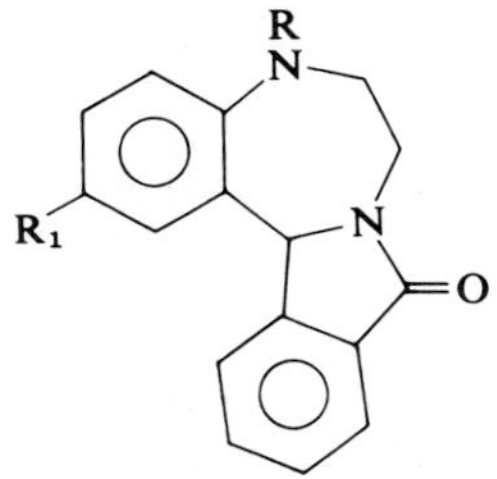	Active	Hardtmann and Ott (1970)
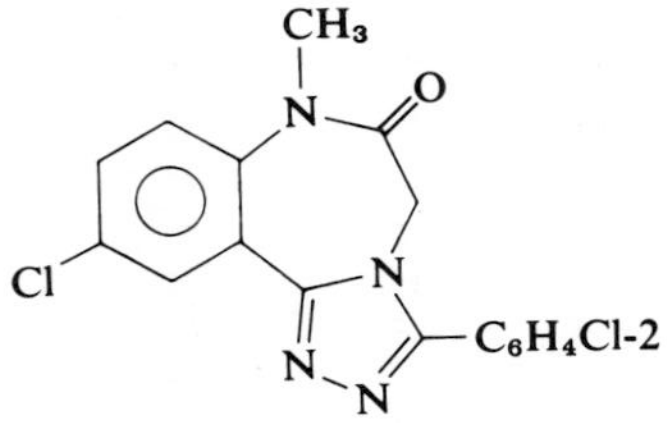	Active	Kathawala (1975b)
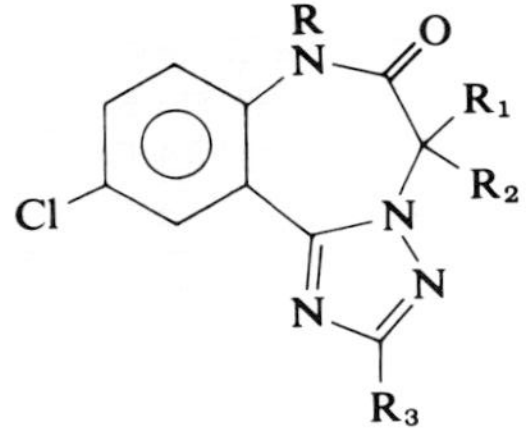	Active	Kathawala (1975a)
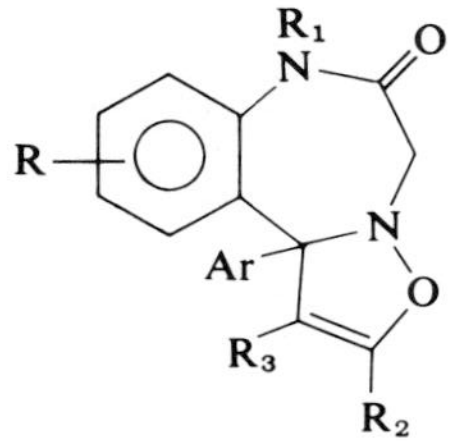	Active	Takashima et al. (1974b)

(continued)

527

TABLE XLIII—*Continued*

X	R	Ar	R_1	R_2	Activity	Reference
X	H	Ar	H	H	Active	Tachikawa et al. (1972)
Cl	$CH_2CH_2NEt_2$	$2\text{-}FC_6H_4$	H	H	Active	Derieg et al. (1972)
HONH	CH_2OCH_3	$2\text{-}ClC_6H_4$	H	H	Met ED_{50} 3.1 (sc)	Fryer and Walser (1975b)
Cl	H	$2\text{-}ClC_6H_4$	Me	H	Met ED_{50} 0.75 (po); MES ED_{50} 25 (po)	Kamioka et al. (1972)
Cl	H	C_6H_5 (oxazolazepam)	H	H	Met ED_{50} 5.3 (po); MES ED_{50} 38 (po)	Takagi et al. (1971); Takagi et al. (1971)
Cl	H	C_6H_5	H	H	Met ED_{50} 4.9 (po); MES ED_{50} 26 (po)	Takagi et al. (1971)
Cl	H	C_6H_5	H	Me	Met ED_{50} 1.9 (po); MES ED_{50} 17 (po)	Takagi et al. (1971)
Cl	H	C_6H_5	H	Et	Met ED_{50} 2.0 (po); MES ED_{50} 22 (po)	Takagi et al. (1971)
Br	H	C_6H_5	H	H	Met ED_{50} 3.1 (po); MES ED_{50} 18 (po)	Takagi et al. (1971)
Br	H	C_6H_5	H	H	Met ED_{50} 1.7 (po); MES ED_{50} 17 (po)	Takagi et al. (1971)
Br	H	C_6H_5	Me	Me	Met ED_{50} 5.2 (po); MES ED_{50} 27 (po)	Takagi et al. (1971)
NO_2	H	C_6H_5	H	H	Met ED_{50} 1.4 (po); MES ED_{50} 32 (po)	Takagi et al. (1971)
NO_2	H	C_6H_5	H	Me	Met ED_{50} 0.47 (po); MES ED_{50} 18 (po)	Takagi et al. (1971)
NO_2	H	C_6H_5	Me	H	Met ED_{50} 2.6 (po); MES ED_{50} 30 (po)	Takagi et al. (1971)
Cl	Me	C_6H_5	H	H	Met ED_{50} 6.2 (po)	Takagi et al. (1971)
Br	Me	C_6H_5	H	H	Met ED_{50} 5.6 (po); MES ED_{50} 50 (po)	Takagi et al. (1971)
NO_2	Me	C_6H_5	H	H	Met ED_{50} 1.6 (po); MES ED_{50} 28 (po)	Takagi et al. (1971)
Cl	Me	C_6H_5	Me	H	Met ED_{50} 7.5 (po); MES ED_{50} 170 (po)	Takagi et al. (1971)
Br	Me	C_6H_5	Me	H	Met ED_{50} 10 (po); MES ED_{50} 114 (po)	Takagi et al. (1971)
NO_2	Me	C_6H_5	Me	H	Met ED_{50} 6.3 (po); MES ED_{50} 55 (po)	Takagi et al. (1971)
Cl	H	$2\text{-}ClC_6H_4$	H	H	Met ED_{50} 0.75 (po); MES ED_{50} 26 (po)	Takagi et al. (1971)

				Activity	Reference
Br	2-ClC$_6$H$_4$	H	H	Met ED$_{50}$ 0.47 (po); MES ED$_{50}$ 7.0 (po)	Takagi et al. (1971)
Cl	2-FC$_6$H$_4$	H	H	Met ED$_{50}$ 0.42 (po); MES ED$_{50}$ 16 (po)	Takagi et al. (1971)
Cl	2-ClC$_6$H$_4$	Me	H	Met ED$_{50}$ 1.4 (po); MES ED$_{50}$ 63 (po)	Takagi et al. (1971)
Br	2-ClC$_6$H$_4$	Me	H	Met ED$_{50}$ 1.0 (po); MES ED$_{50}$ 25 (po)	Takagi et al. (1971)
Cl	2-ClC$_6$H$_4$	H	Me	Met ED$_{50}$ 0.83 (po); MES ED$_{50}$ 33 (po)	Takagi et al. (1971)
Cl	2-FC$_6$H$_4$	H	Me	Met ED$_{50}$ 0.71 (po); MES ED$_{50}$ 19 (po)	Takagi et al. (1971)
Br	2-ClC$_6$H$_4$	H	Me	Met ED$_{50}$ 0.70 (po); MES ED$_{50}$ 10 (po)	Takagi et al. (1971)
Cl	2-ClC$_6$H$_4$	Me	Me	Met ED$_{50}$ 5.0 (po); MES ED$_{50}$ 158 (po)	Takagi et al. (1971)
Br	2-ClC$_6$H$_4$	Me	Me	Met ED$_{50}$ 3.9 (po); MES ED$_{50}$ 107 (po)	Takagi et al. (1971)
Cl	2-ClC$_6$H$_4$	H	Me	Met ED$_{50}$ 0.38 (po); MES ED$_{50}$ 9.1 (po)	Takagi et al. (1971)
Cl	2-FC$_6$H$_4$	H	Me	Met ED$_{50}$ 0.27 (po); MES ED$_{50}$ 16 (po)	Takagi et al. (1971)
Br	2-ClC$_6$H$_4$	H	Me	Met ED$_{50}$ 0.4 (po); MES ED$_{50}$ 9.4 (po)	Takagi et al. (1971)
Cl	2-ClC$_6$H$_4$	H (5-Me)	H	Met ED$_{50}$ 1.7 (po); MES ED$_{50}$ 28 (po)	Takagi et al. (1971)
Br	2-ClC$_6$H$_4$	H (5-Me)	H	Met ED$_{50}$ 1.0 (po); MES ED$_{50}$ 40 (po)	Takagi et al. (1971)

Compound	Activity	Reference
(structure: MeCO-substituted benzo-fused diazepine with N, O ring and F-phenyl; labeled R, N, O, F)	Active	Earley et al. (1972)
(structure: R$_1$, R$_2$, R$_3$, R$_4$, X, N, S, Ar, R, O substituted fused ring system)	Active	Kuwada et al. (1975)

(continued)

529

TABLE XLIII—*Continued*

Compound	Activity	Reference
	Met ED_{50} 8.5 (po); MES ED_{50} 58 (po)	Takagi *et al.* (1971)
	Active	Gschwend (1974)
	Active	Coyne and Cusic (1968, 1970)
	Active	Niigata *et al.* (1974b); Wander (1964)

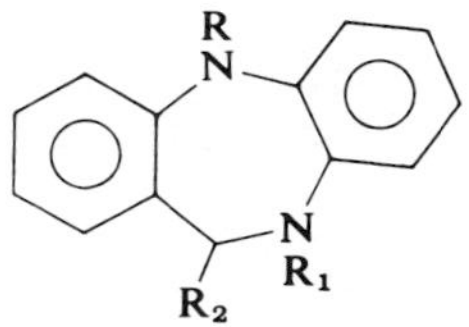

Wander (1964)

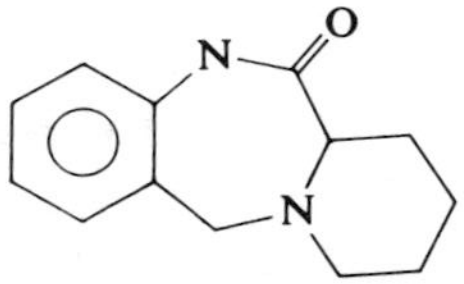

Active

Doebel and Pfenninger (1965)

Active

K. 1,4- (Fused heteroring) diazepines

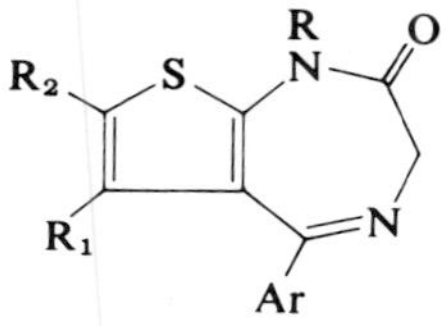

R_1	R_2	R	Ar	Activity	Reference
R_1	R_2	H	Ar	Active	Madronero-Pelaez et al. (1974)
R_1	R_2	R	Ar	Active	Nakanishi et al. (1971 b,c,d, 1972c,)
R_1	R_2	R	Pyr	Active	Nakanishi et al. (1972b)
H	Cl	Me	$2\text{-}FC_6H_4$	Active	Hirohashi et al. (1972, 1973a,b, 1974a–d)

(continued)

531

TABLE XLIII—*Continued*

R$_1$	R$_2$	R	Ar	Active	Activity	Reference
H	Cl	H	2-ClC$_6$H$_4$	Met	ED$_{50}$ 1.5	Hirohashi *et al.* (1972)
H	Me	H	C$_6$H$_5$	Met	ED$_{50}$ 17 (ip)	Nakanishi *et al.* (1973d)
			2-ClC$_6$H$_4$	Met,	100% protn. at 4 (po)	Tinney *et al.* (1974)
H	Me	H	2-ClC$_6$H$_4$	Met	ED$_{50}$ 0.9 (ip)	Nakanishi *et al.* (1973d)
H	Et	H	C$_6$H$_5$	Met	ED$_{50}$ 3.1 (ip); MES ED$_{50}$ 12 (ip)	Nakanishi *et al.* (1973d)
H	Et	H	2-FC$_6$H$_4$	Met	ED$_{50}$ 0.3 (ip); MES ED$_{50}$ 3.9 (ip)	Nakanishi *et al.* (1973d)
H	Et	H	2-ClC$_6$H$_4$	Met	ED$_{50}$ 3.3 (ip); MES ED$_{50}$ 7.0 (ip)	Nakanishi *et al.* (1973d)
H	Et	H	2-BrC$_6$H$_4$	Met	ED$_{50}$ 3.6 (ip)	Nakanishi *et al.* (1973d)
H	Et	H	2-MeC$_6$H$_4$	Met	ED$_{50}$ 8 (ip)	Nakanishi *et al.* (1973d)
H	Et	H	2-MeOC$_6$H$_4$	Met	ED$_{50}$ 17 (ip)	Nakanishi *et al.* (1973d)
H	*i*-Pr	H	2-ClC$_6$H$_4$	Met	ED$_{50}$ 10 (ip)	Nakanishi *et al.* (1973d)
H	*n*-Bu	H	C$_6$H$_5$	Met	ED$_{50}$ > 160 (ip)	Nakanishi *et al.* (1973d)
Me	Me	H	C$_6$H$_5$	Met	ED$_{50}$ 15 (ip)	Nakanishi *et al.* (1973d)
			2-ClC$_6$H$_4$	Met,	100% protn. at 32 (po)	Tinney *et al.* (1974)
Me	Me	H	2-ClC$_6$H$_4$	Met	ED$_{50}$ 47 (ip)	Nakanishi *et al.* (1973d)
Me	Me	H	3-CF$_3$C$_6$H$_4$	Met	ED$_{50}$ > 169 (ip)	Nakanishi *et al.* (1973d)
Me	*n*-Pr	H	C$_6$H$_5$	Met	ED$_{50}$ > 160 (ip)	Nakanishi *et al.* (1973d)
i-Pr	H	H	C$_6$H$_5$	Met	ED$_{50}$ 130 (ip)	Nakanishi *et al.* (1973d)
H	Me	Me	C$_6$H$_5$	Met	ED$_{50}$ > 160 (ip)	Nakanishi *et al.* (1973d)
H	Me	Me	2-ClC$_6$H$_4$	Met	ED$_{50}$ 2.1 (ip)	Nakanishi *et al.* (1973d)
H	Et	Me	C$_6$H$_5$	Met	ED$_{50}$ 10 (ip)	Nakanishi *et al.* (1973d)
H	Et	Me	2-FC$_6$H$_4$	Met	ED$_{50}$ 0.4 (ip); MES ED$_{50}$ 4.6 (ip)	Nakanishi *et al.* (1973d)
H	Et	Me	2-ClC$_6$H$_4$	Met	ED$_{50}$ 0.5 (ip); MES ED$_{50}$ 8.0 (ip)	Nakanishi *et al.* (1973d)
H	Et	Me	2-ClC$_6$H$_4$	Met	ED$_{50}$ 0.5 (po); MES ED$_{50}$ 7.4 (po)	Nakanishi *et al.* (1972a)
H	Et	Me	2-ClC$_6$H$_4$	Met	ED$_{50}$ 0.5 (ip)	Nakanishi *et al.* (1973e)
H	Et	Me	2-BrC$_6$H$_4$	Met	ED$_{50}$ 0.3 (ip)	Nakanishi *et al.* (1973d)
Me	Me	Me	C$_6$H$_5$	Met	ED$_{50}$ 15 (ip)	Nakanishi *et al.* (1973d)

		Ar	Activity	Reference
Me	Me	$2\text{-}ClC_6H_4$	Met ED_{50} 12.5 (ip)	Nakanaishi et al. (1973d)
Me	Me	$4\text{-}ClC_6H_4$	Met ED_{50} > 160 (ip)	Nakanishi et al. (1973d)
Me	H	C_6H_5	Met, 100% protn. at 32 (po)	Tinney et al. (1974)
Me	H	2-Thiop	Met, 100% protn. at 16 (po)	Tinney et al. (1974)
H	H	C_6H_5	Met, 100% protn. at 250 (po)	Tinney et al. (1974)
Et	Me	C_6H_5	Met, 100% protn. at 250 (po)	Tinney et al. (1974)
Me	H	C_6H_5	Met, 100% protn. at 125 (po)	Tinney et al. (1974)
Me	H	C_6H_5	Met, 100% protn. at 63 (po)	Tinney (1970)
$(CH_2)_4$	R	Ar	Active	
$(CH_2)_3$	H	C_6H_5	Met ED_{50} 30 (ip)	Nakanishi et al. (1973d)
			Met, 100% protn. at 16 (po)	Tinney et al. (1974)
$(CH_2)_4$	H	C_6H_5	Met ED_{50} 35 (ip)	Nakanishi et al. (1973d)
			Met, 100% protn. at 63	Tinney (1971)
			Met, 100% protn. at 8 (po)	Tinney et al. (1974)
$(CH_2)_4$	H	$2\text{-}ClC_6H_4$	Met ED_{50} 20 (ip)	Nakanishi et al. (1973d)
			Met, 100% protn. at 250 (po)	Tinney et al. (1974)
$(CH_2)_4$	H	$4\text{-}ClC_6H_4$	Met ED_{50} 160 (ip)	Nakanishi et al. (1973d)
$(CH_2)_4$	H	$2\text{-}MeOC_6H_4$	Met ED_{50} 80 (ip)	Nakanishi et al. (1973d)
			Met, 100% protn. at 125 (po)	Tinney et al. (1974)
$(CH_2)_4$	H	$3\text{-}CF_3C_6H_4$	Met ED_{50} > 160 (ip)	Nakanishi et al. (1973d)
$CH_2CH_2CH\text{-}MeCH_2$	H	C_6H_5	Met ED_{50} 80 (ip)	Nakanishi et al. (1973d)
$(CH_2)_5$	H	C_6H_5	Met ED_{50} > 160 (ip)	Nakanishi et al. (1973d)
$(CH_2)_4$	Me	C_6H_5	Met ED_{50} 15 (ip)	Nakanishi et al. (1973d)
			Met, 100% protn. at 8 (po)	Tinney et al. (1974)
$(CH_2)_4$	Me	$2\text{-}ClC_6H_4$	Met ED_{50} 3.7 (ip)	Nakanishi et al. (1973d)
$(CH_2)_4$	Me	$2\text{-}MeOC_6H_4$	Met ED_{50} 16 (ip)	Nakanishi et al. (1973d)
$(CH_2)_4$	Me	$3\text{-}CF_3C_6H_4$	Met ED_{50} > 160 (ip)	Nakanishi et al. (1973d)
$(CH_2)_5$	Me	C_6H_5	Met ED_{50} > 160 (ip)	Nakanishi et al. (1973d)
$(CH_2)_4$	$CH_2CH=CH_2$	C_6H_5	Met ED_{50} > 160 (ip)	Nakanishi et al. (1973d)
$(CH_2)_4$	$CH_2C\equiv CH$	C_6H_5	Met ED_{50} > 160 (ip)	Nakanishi et al. (1973d)

(continued)

TABLE XLIII—*Continued*

R₁	R₂	R	Ar	Activity	Reference
$(CH_2)_4$		n-Bu	C_6H_5	Met $ED_{50} > 160$ (ip)	Nakanishi *et al.* (1973d)
$(CH_2)_4$		$C_6H_5CH_2$	C_6H_5	Met $ED_{50} > 160$ (ip)	Nakanishi *et al.* (1973d)
$(CH_2)_4$		H	2-FC_6H_4	Met, 100% protn. at 16 (po)	Tinney *et al.* (1974)
$(CH_2)_4$		H	2-MeC_6H_4	Met, 100% protn. at 250 (po)	Tinney *et al.* (1974)
$(CH_2)_4$		H	3-MeOC_6H_4	Met, 100% protn. at 63 (po)	Tinney *et al.* (1974)
$(CH_2)_4$		H	2-Thiop	Met, 100% protn. at 125	Tinney (1971)
$(CH_2)_4$		H	2-Fur	Met, 100% protn. at 63 (po)	Tinney *et al.* (1974)
$(CH_2)_4$ (3-Me)		H	C_6H_5	Met, 100% protn. at 250 (po)	Tinney *et al.* (1974)
$(CH_2)_4$ (N₄-O)		Me	C_6H_5	Met, 100% protn. at 63 (po)	Tinney *et al.* (1974)
$(CH_2)_4$ (3-OH)		Me	C_6H_5	Met, 100% protn. at 63 (po)	Tinney *et al.* (1974)

Compound	Activity	Reference
(thienotriazolodiazepine structure with X)	X = CH=CH, N=N, C(=O)O: active	Nakanishi *et al.* (1974a)
(thienotriazolodiazepinone structure)	Active	Nakanishi *et al.* (1974b)

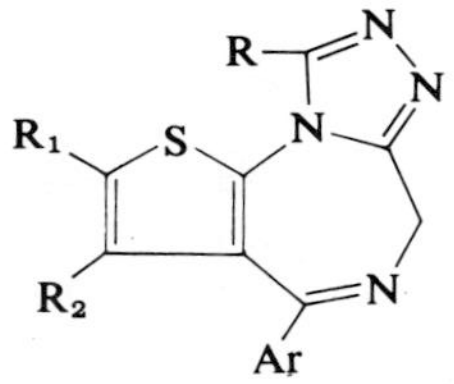

Nakanishi *et al.* (1972e)

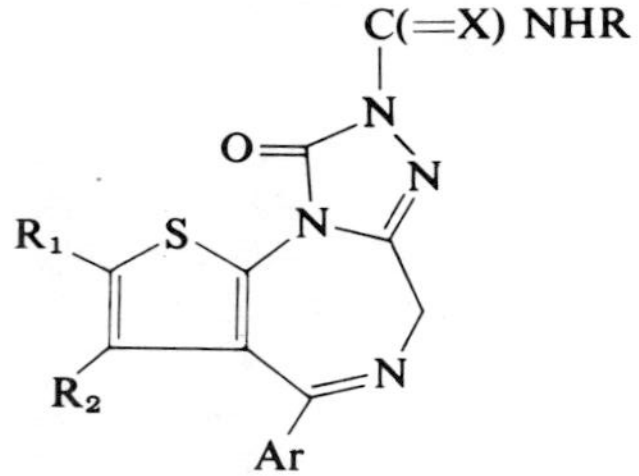

Active

Nakanishi *et al.* (1974g)

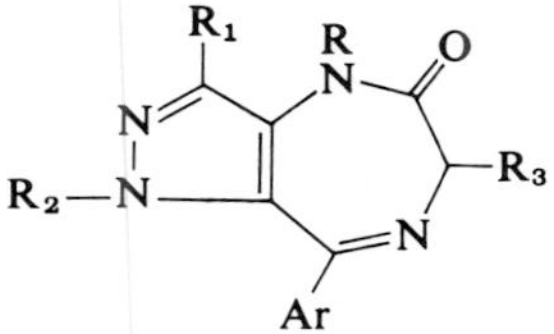

Active

C(=X) NHR

R	R₁	R₂	R₃	Ar	Activity	Reference
R	R₁	R₂	H	Ar	Active	DeWald and Nordin (1969, 1971)
R	Me	R₂	H	2-Thio-p	Active	L'Italien and Nordin (1971)
H	Me	Me	H	C_6H_5	Met, 100% protn. at 8	DeWald and Butler (1971); DeWald *et al.* (1973)
Me	Me	Me	H	C_6H_5	Met, 100% protn. at 32	DeWald and Butler (1971); DeWald *et al.* (1973)

(*continued*)

TABLE XLIII—*Continued*

R	R₁	R₂	R₃	Ar	Activity	Reference
CH₂CF₃	Me	Me	H	C₆H₅	Met, 100% protn. at 250	DeWald *et al.* (1973)
H	Me	Me	H	4-FC₆H₄	Met, 100% protn. at > 500	DeWald *et al.* (1973)
H	Me	Me	H	2-Thiop	Met, 100% protn. at 64	DeWald *et al.* (1973)
H (pyrazapon)	Me	Et	H	C₆H₅	Met, 100% protn. at 4	DeWald and Butler (1971); DeWald *et al.* (1973)
ME	Me	Et	H	C₆H₅	Met, 100% protn. at 16	DeWald *et al.* (1973)
Et	Me	Et	H	C₆H₅	Met, 100% protn. at > 500	DeWald *et al.* (1973)
(CH₂)₃NMe₂	Me	Et	H	C₆H₅	Met, 100% protn. at > 500	DeWald *et al.* (1973)
(CH₂)₂NEt₂	Me	Et	H	C₆H₅	Met, 100% protn. at > 500	DeWald *et al.* (1973)
H	Me	Et	Me	C₆H₅	Met, 100% protn. at 64	DeWald *et al.* (1973)
H	Me	Et	H	4-MeC₆H₄	Met, 100% protn. at > 500	DeWald *et al.* (1973)
H	Me	Et	H	4-MeOC₆H₄	Met, 100% protn. at > 500	DeWald *et al.* (1973)
H	Me	Et	H	4-ClC₆H₄	Met, 100% protn. at > 500	DeWald *et al.* (1973)
H	Me	Et	H	3-NO₂C₆H₄	Met, 100% protn. at 500	DeWald *et al.* (1973)
H	Me	Et	H	2-CF₃C₆H₄	Met, 100% protn. at 16	DeWald *et al.* (1973)
H	Me	Et	H	2-Thiop	Met, 100% protn. at 16	DeWald *et al.* (1973)
H	Me	n-Pr	H	C₆H₅	Met, 100% protn. at 8	DeWald *et al.* (1973)
Me	Me	n-Pr	H	C₆H₅	Met, 100% protn. at 16–32	DeWald *et al.* (1973)
H	Me	i-Pr	H	C₆H₅	Met, 100% protn. at 32	DeWald *et al.* (1971)
Me	Me	i-Pr	H	C₆H₅	Met, 100% protn. at 63	DeWald *et al.* (1973)
H	Et	Me	H	C₆H₅	Met, 100% protn. at > 250	DeWald *et al.* (1973)
Me	Et	Me	H	C₆H₅	Met, 100% protn. at 16	DeWald *et al.* (1973)
H	Et	Et	H	C₆H₅	Met, 100% protn. at 16	DeWald *et al.* (1973)
Me	Et	Et	H	C₆H₅	Met, 100% protn. at 32	DeWald *et al.* (1973)
H	Me	Et	OCOMe	C₆H₅	Met, 100% protn. at 32	Nordin (1971a)
Me	Me	Et	OCOMe	C₆H₅	Met, 100% protn. at 32	Nordin (1971a)
H	Me	Me	OCOMe	C₆H₅	Met, 100% protn. at 32	Nordin (1971a)

				Activity	Reference
H	Me	Et	C$_6$H$_5$	Met, 100% protn. at 16	Nordin (1971a)
Me	Me	Et	C$_6$H$_5$	Met, 100% protn. at 32	Nordin (1971a)
H	Me	Me	C$_6$H$_5$	Met, 100% protn. at 16	Nordin (1971a)
H (N—O)	Me	Et	C$_6$H$_5$	Met, 100% protn. at 32	Nordin (1971b)
Me (N—O)	Me	Et	C$_6$H$_5$	Met, 100% protn. at 63	Nordin (1971b)
H (N—O)	Me	Me	C$_6$H$_5$	Met, 100% protn. at 63	Nordin (1971b)
Me (N—O)	Me	Me	C$_6$H$_5$	Met, 100% protn. at 63	Nordin (1971b)

Compound	Activity	Reference
	Active	Nordin (1975)

R	R$_1$	R$_2$	Activity	Reference
Et	H	H	Met, 100% protn. at 16	Nordin (1972)
Me	H	H	Met, 100% protn. at 63	Nordin (1972)
Pr	H	H	Met, 100% protn. at 32	Nordin (1972)
Pr	Me	H	Met, 100% protn. at 32	Nordin (1972)
Pr	H	Me	Met, 100% protn. at 32	Nordin (1972)

(continued)

TABLE XLIII—*Continued*

R	R_1	Ar	Activity	Reference
H	Me	C_6H_5	Met, 100% protn. at 125	DeWald et al. (1973)
Me	Me	C_6H_5	Met, 100% protn. at 32	DeWald et al. (1973)
Et	Me	C_6H_5	Met, 100% protn. at 250	DeWald et al. (1973)
H	Et	C_6H_5	Met, 100% protn. at 32	DeWald et al. (1973)
Me	Et	C_6H_5	Met, 100% protn. at 32	DeWald et al. (1973)
H	i-Pr	C_6H_5	Met, 100% protn. at > 500	DeWald et al. (1973)
H	Me		Met, 100% protn. at 500	DeWald et al. (1973)

R	R_1	R_2	Ar	Activity	Reference
Me	Me	Me	C_6H_5	Met, 100% protn. at 8 (po)	DeWald and Butler (1971)
Me	Me	Me	$2\text{-}FC_6H_4$	Met, 100% protn. at 2	DeWald and Butler (1971)
Et	Me	Me	C_6H_5	Met, 100% protn. at 4	DeWald and Butler (1971)
Me	Me	Me	$2\text{-}ClC_6H_4$	Met, 100% protn. at 4	DeWald and Butler (1971)
Et	Me	H	C_6H_5	Met, 100% protn. at 8	DeWald and Butler (1971)

TABLE XLIII—*Continued*

Compound	Activity	Reference
	Active	Butler (1973)
	Active	Nordin (1975)
	Active	von Bebenburg and Offermanns (1974b)
	Active	von Bebenburg and Offermanns (1974a)
	Active	Field *et al.* (1975)

(continued)

TABLE XLIII—*Continued*

L. 1,5-Benzodiazepines

Ar	R	R$_1$	R$_2$	Activity	Reference
C$_6$H$_5$	H	H	Cl	MES ED$_{50}$ 32	Bauer *et al.* (1973a)
C$_6$H$_5$	H	H	CF$_3$	MES ED$_{50}$ 27; Met ED$_{50}$ 7	Bauer *et al.* (1973a)
C$_6$H$_5$	H	H	NO$_2$	MES ED$_{50}$ 29; Met ED$_{50}$ 8	Bauer *et al.* (1973a)
C$_6$H$_5$	H	H	Br	MES ED$_{50}$ 37	Bauer *et al.* (1973a)
C$_6$H$_5$	H	H	F	MES ED$_{50}$ 160	Bauer *et al.* (1973a)
2-FC$_6$H$_4$	H	H	Cl	MES ED$_{50}$ 165	Bauer *et al.* (1973a)
2-ClC$_6$H$_4$	H	H	Cl	MES ED$_{50}$ 100	Bauer *et al.* (1973a)
C$_6$H$_5$	H	i-C$_3$H$_7$	CF$_3$	MES ED$_{50}$ 88	Bauer *et al.* (1973a)
C$_6$H$_5$	H	t-C$_4$H$_9$	Cl	MES ED$_{50}$ > 342	Bauer *et al.* (1973a)
C$_6$H$_5$	H	Me	NO$_2$	MES ED$_{50}$ 270; Met ED$_{50}$ > 90	Bauer *et al.* (1973a)
C$_6$H$_5$	H	Me	CF$_3$	MES ED$_{50}$ 47	Bauer *et al.* (1973a)
C$_6$H$_5$	H	CH$_2$CH=CH$_2$	Cl	MES ED$_{50}$ 185	Bauer *et al.* (1973a)
C$_6$H$_5$	Me	Me	CF$_3$	MES ED$_{50}$ 41	Bauer *et al.* (1973a)
C$_6$H$_5$	Me	Me	NO$_2$	MES ED$_{50}$ 219; Met ED$_{50}$ 6	Bauer *et al.* (1973a)
C$_6$H$_5$	H	Me	Cl	MES ED$_{50}$ 41	Bauer *et al.* (1973a)
C$_6$H$_5$	H	Et	CF$_3$	MES ED$_{50}$ 44	Bauer *et al.* (1973a)
C$_6$H$_5$	H	(CH$_2$)$_2$OH	NO$_2$	MES ED$_{50}$ > 340	Bauer *et al.* (1973a)
C$_6$H$_5$	H	(CH$_2$)$_3$OEt	Cl	MES ED$_{50}$ > 360	Bauer *et al.* (1973a)
C$_6$H$_5$	H	COMe	Cl	MES ED$_{50}$ 36	Bauer *et al.* (1973a)
C$_6$H$_5$	H	COMe	CF$_3$	MES ED$_{50}$ 58; Met ED$_{50}$ 24	Bauer *et al.* (1973a)
C$_6$H$_5$	H	CO$_2$Et	Cl	MES ED$_{50}$ 68; Met ED$_{50}$ 30	Bauer *et al.* (1973a)

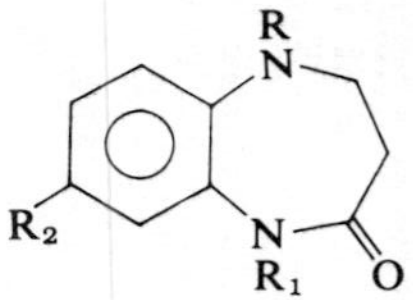

R	R_1	R_2	Activity	Reference
$CH_2CH=CH_2$	C_6H_5	NO_2	MES ED_{50} > 320	Bauer et al. (1974d)
H	$2\text{-}NO_2C_6H_4$	CF_3	MES ED_{50} 40	Bauer et al. (1974d)
H	$2\text{-}ClC_6H_4$	NO_2	MES ED_{50} > 280	Bauer et al. (1974d)
n-Bu	C_6H_5	Br	MES ED_{50} 100	Bauer et al. (1974d)
CHO	C_6H_5	CF_3	MES ED_{50} 66	Bauer et al. (1974d)
CHO	C_6H_5	NO_2	MES ED_{50} 311	Bauer et al. (1974d)
$CH_2CH=CHCH_3$	C_6H_5	NO_2	MES ED_{50} > 310	Bauer et al. (1974d)
H	Et	CN	MES ED_{50} 110	Bauer et al. (1974d)
n-Pr	C_6H_5	CF_3	MES ED_{50} 342	Bauer et al. (1974d)
Me	C_6H_5	NO_2	MES ED_{50} 200	Bauer et al. (1974d)
Miscellaneous	Miscellaneous	Miscellaneous	Active	Bauer et al. (1972b)
Miscellaneous	Aromatic	Cl	Active	Bub et al. (1972a,b)

Compound	Activity	Reference
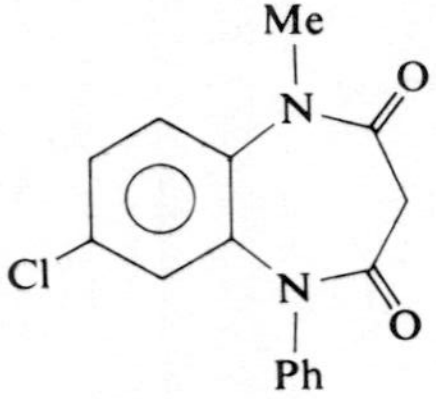	Met ED_{50} 1.6 (po); MES ED_{50} 23 (po)	Barzaghi et al. (1973)
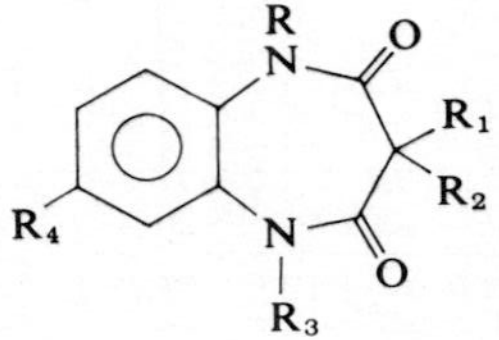 Active		Bauer et al. (1972a); Weber et al. (1972)

(continued)

541

TABLE XLIII—*Continued*

Compound	Activity	Reference
	Active	Hauptmann *et al.* (1968)
	Active	Hester (1971)
	Active	Hester (1971)
	Active	Hester (1972b)
	Active	Hester (1972c)

Structure	Activity	Reference
(structure)	Active	Hester (1973b)
(structure)	Active	Eiden and Heja (1975)
(structure)	Active	Bauer et al. (1974a)
(structure)	Active	Bauer et al. (1974c)

[a] This compound is used as a standard in many papers, and the listing here is not complete.

TABLE XLIV   TRIAZEPINE DERIVATIVES

X	R	Activity	Reference
H	H	Active	Sulkowski and Childress (1965)
Cl	H	Met $ED_{50} > 400$ (ip)	Kohl *et al.* (1974)
Cl	Me	Met ED_{50} 280	Kohl *et al.* (1974)
Cl	C_6H_5	Met $ED_{50} > 400$	Kohl *et al.* (1974)

Compound	Activity	Reference
	Active	Hester (1975)

TABLE XLV   THIADIAZEPINE DERIVATIVES[a]

R	R_1	MES ED_{50} (ip)	Met ED_{50} (ip)
Me	Me	> 150	> 150
Me	Et	> 150	> 250
Me	*n*-Pr	> 150	> 150
Me	*i*-pr	> 150	> 150
Me	*n*-Bu	> 150	> 150
Me	C_6H_4	> 150	> 150
Me	$4\text{-}NO_2C_6H_4$	> 150	> 150
n-C_6H_{13}	Me	> 100	> 100
n-C_6H_{13}	Et	> 300	> 300
n-C_6H_{13}	*n*-Pr	287	405
n-C_6H_{13}	*i*-Pr	375	> 500
n-C_6H_{13}	*n*-Bu	183	294
n-C_6H_{13}	*n*-C_5H_{11}	378	386
n-C_6H_{13}	EtS	> 500	> 500

[a] Data from Fernandez-Tome *et al.* (1972).

(XIV)   (XV)   (XVI)

variety of alternative methods. Medazepam (**XVI**) has also been oxidized to
XV. Nitrazepam (**XVII**) has been prepared by nitration and from 2-amino-5-
nitrobenzophenone by ring closure methods. Oxazepam (**XVIII**) has been
prepared by a variety of reactions involving ring closure, ring contraction,

(XVII)   (XVIII)

and rearrangement of demoxepam. By far the largest variety of 1,4-benzo-
diazepines have been prepared by routes involving ring closure of substituted
2-aminobenzophenones.

The first of the benzodiazepines to see clinical use as an anticonvulsant
agent was chlordiazepoxide (**XIV**), but this drug has now been largely
replaced by other benzodiazepines. Table XLIII can be referred to for the
structure–activity relationships of the wide variety of 1,4-benzodiazepines and
related compounds which have been reported.

In addition to the data in the table, chlordiazepoxide prevented clinical and
electroencephalogram (EEG) convulsant effects of metrazole in epileptic and
normal monkeys (Chusid and Kopeloff, 1962). Metabolism studies of chlordiazepoxide show that the concentration of the *N*-demethyl metabolite most
closely parallels the pattern of anticonvulsant activity (Coutinho *et(al.*, 1969).
Some evidence exists that chronic administration of chlordiazepoxide leads
to tolerance, possibly caused by an increase in the rate of metabolism (Goldberg *et al.*, 1967). In a comparative study of metrazole-induced seizures in the
cat nitrazepam was found to be more potent that diazepam, which in turn
was more potent than chlordiazepoxide, and this appears to also be true
clinically (Straw, 1968).

Mechanism of action studies have been carried out on diazepam (**XV**) and
clonazepam (**XIX**) in the cat and monkey (Guerrero-Figueroa *et al.*, 1969a,b;
Guerrero-Figueroa and Gallant, 1971). The metabolism of diazepam in

rabbits is reported to give a variety of benzophenones (Jommi *et al.*, 1964), while in rats and mice it is metabolized to *N*-demethyldiazepam, *N*-methyloxazepam, and oxazepam (**XVIII**) (Marcucci *et al.*, 1968). The metabolism and anticonvulsant activity of diazepam differ in newborn versus adult animals (Marcucci *et al.*, 1973b). The anticonvulsant activity of deuterated *N*-demethyldiazepam is of much shorter duration than that of the undeuterated compound and appears to result in a lesser accumulation of oxazepam in the brain (Marcucci *et al.*, 1973a).

(**XIX**)

In addition to the data in Table XLIII, diazepam prevented clinical and EEG convulsant effects of metrazole in epileptic and normal monkeys and was more effective in this regard than was chlordiazepoxide (Kopeloff and Chusid, 1967). A comparative study of diazepam and chlordiazepoxide on electrical activity of the rabbit brain also indicates a greater effectivity for diazepam, although the two drugs had a marked analogy in the mode and level of action (Arrigo *et al.*, 1965). Diazepam in the mouse significantly reduced the frequency and severity of seizures by metrazole and electric shock, although the anticonvulsant doses were also observed to decrease locomotor activity, depress the righting reflex, and produce sedation (Hudson, and Wolpert, 1970). Based on studies in the cat, diazepam has a generalized depressant action on the epileptogenic structures throughout the brain and also depresses rather selectively the reticular facilitatory neurons involved in the regulation of postural tone throughout the gamma efferent loop (Hernandez-Peon *et al.*, 1964).

Clinically, diazepam appears to be an excellent short-term anticonvulsant drug (Sawyer *et al.*, 1968), and it has been suggested that the pragmatic use of diazepam in whatever clinical circumstances status epilepticus occurs or is suspected appears to be justified (Wilson, 1968).

Clonazepam (**XIX**), which has recently been approved by the Federal Drug Administration, has a broad spectrum of anticonvulsant activity in animals with excellent chronic tolerance and no fetotoxic effects. It probably acts by potentiating inhibitory mechanisms in those subcortical brain structures that are responsible for the propagation of seizure activity (Blum *et al.*, 1973). Clonazepam reduced the frequency and amplitude of rhinencephalic electrical discharges in normal rabbits and also inhibited the epileptic manifestations of brain waves following electrical stimulation of the amygdala (DiRocco *et al.*, 1974a, b). Clonazepam consistently blocks the evoked paroxysms and the associated clinical discharges at a dose ten times less than that of diazepam with an equally low toxicity. The immediate action of clonazepam on spontaneous epileptic paroxysms is particularly striking in relation to generalized attacks and in status epilepticus (Poire and Royer, 1969).

Nitrazepam (**XVII**) has been the subject of a favorable clinical study as an anticonvulsant drug on 50 patients (Liske and Forster, 1963). Oxazepam (**XVIII**) has shown favorable anticonvulsant action in the cat (Bertolini *et al.*, 1969). In a comparative study lorazepam (**XX**) exhibits an antimetrazole activity three to twelve times higher than that of oxazepam, while the brain concentration necessary to obtain a comparable degree of activity is three to four times lower for lorazepam than for oxazepam (Marcucci *et al.*, 1972). Temazepam (**XXI**) has marked antiepileptic properties as determined by an

(**XX**)   (**XXI**)

electroencephalographic method in rabbits, and its activity is reported as being more marked and more pronounced than that of other 1,4-benzodiazepines (Mille *et al.*, 1969).

The disposition and anticonvulsant activity of bromozepam in mice has been reported (Schwarz *et al.*, 1975).

Oxazolazepam (**XXII**), a benzodiazepinooxazole in clinical practice for a variety of psychoneurotic, mental, and neurological disorders, has been the subject of a review and compares favorably as an anticonvulsant with some of the clinically used benzodiazepines (Takagi *et al.*, 1971). Another heterobenzodiazepine (**XXIII**) exhibits greater antimaximal electroshock action than nitrazepam and diazepam (Saji *et al.*, 1973). A number of triazolobenzodiazepines have also been reported to have useful anticonvulsant properties (Hester *et al.*, 1971). Prazapon (**XXIV**), a pyrazolodiazepinone, is effective

(XXII)   (XXIII)   (XXIV)

against metrazole-induced convulsions, but much tolerance develops to it in the course of daily treatments (Poschel *et al.*, 1974).

Some of the 1,5-benzodiazepines studied have an anticonvulsant action in the same order of magnitude as that of the 1,4-benzodiazepine, chlordiazepoxide (Bauer *et al.*, 1973a; Barzaghi *et al.*, 1973).

REFERENCES

Aeberli, P., Gogerty, J., and Houlihan, W. J. (1967). *J. Med. Chem.* **10**, 636.

Agarwal, V. K., Gupta, T. K., and Parmar, S. S. (1972). *J. Med. Chem.* **15**, 1000.

Agarwal, V. K., Chaturvedi, A. K., Gupt, T. K., Parmar, S. S., and DeBoer, B. (1974). *J. Med. Chem.* **17**, 378.

Ahmad, A. (1967). *Indian J. Med. Res.* **55**, 994.

Ahmad, A., Patnaik. G. K., and Vohra, M. M. (1966). *Indian J. Exp. Biol.* **4**, 154.

Ainsworth, C., Easton, N. R., Livezey, M., Morrison, D. E., and Gibson, W. R. (1962). *J. Med. & Pharm. Chem.* **5**, 383.

Akkerman, A. M., Kofman, H., and deVries, G. (1965). Netherlands Patent 105,432; *Chem. Abstr.* **62**, 6495 (1965).

Albertson, N. F. (1968). U.S. Patent 3,382,249.

Allen, G. R., Jr., DeVries, V. G., Greenblatt, E. N., Littell, R., McEvoy, F. J., and Moran, D. B. (1973). *J. Med. Chem.* **16**, 949.

Allgeier, H., and Gagneux, A. (1972a). German Patent 2,156,472; *Chem. Abstr.* **77**, 88554g (1972).

Allgeier, H., and Gagneux, A. (1972b). German Patent 2,201,210; *Chem. Abstr.* **77**, 126711r (1972).

Allgeier, H., and Gagneux, A. (1973a). German Patent 2,308,280; *Chem. Abstr.* **79**, 137206x (1973).

Allgeier, H., and Gagneux, A. (1973b). German Patent 2,323,371; *Chem. Abstr.* **80**, 83084f (1974).

Allgeier, H., and Gagneux, A. (1974a). German Patent 2,357,795; *Chem. Abstr.* **81**, 91593g (1974).

Allgeier, H., and Gagneux, A. (1974b). Swiss Patent 544,764; *Chem. Abstr.* **80**, 96032n (1974).

Allgeier, H., and Gagneux, A. (1975a). Swiss Patent 558,803; *Chem. Abstr.* **82**, 156399r (1975).

Allgeier, H., and Gagneux, A. (1975b). Swiss Patent 561,723; *Chem. Abstr.* **83**, 97411j (1975).

Allgeier, H., and Gagneux, A. (1975c). Swiss Patent 562,822; *Chem. Abstr.* **83**, 193411e (1975).

Almirante, L., and Murmann, W. (1967). British Patent 1,076,089; *Chem. Abstr.* **68**, 87295a (1968).

Almirante, L., Polo, L., Mugnaini, A., Provinciali, E., Rugarli, P., Biancotti, A., Gamba A., and Murmann, W. (1965). *J. Med. Chem.* **8**, 305.

Almirante, L., Polo, L., Mugnaini, A., Provinciali, E., Rugarli, P., Gamba, A., Olivi, A., and Murmann, W. (1966). *J. Med. Chem.* **9**, 29.

Almirante, L., Mugnaini, A., Rugarli, P., Gamba, A., Zefelippo, E., DeToma, N., and Murmann, W. (1969). *J. Med. Chem.* **12**, 122.

Amann, A., Koenig, H., Giertz, H., Kretzschmar, R., and Chieme, P. (1974). German Patent 2,306,543; *Chem. Abstr.* **81**, 136150d (1974).

Amann, A., Koenig, H., Thieme, P. C., and Giertz, H. (1975). German Patent 2,408,288; *Chem. Abstr.* **83**, 193341g (1975).

American Home Products. (1968). British Patent 1,126,245; *Chem. Abstr.* **70**, 115007v (1969).

Andronati, S. A., Vikhyaev, Y. I., Klygul, T. A., and Bogatskii, A. V. (1970). *Fiziol. Akt. Veshchestva* **5**, 117; *Chem. Abstr.* **81**, 3901c (1974).

Anton-Jay, F. (1971). German Patent 2,125,427; *Chem. Abstr.* **76**, 108285e (1972).

Applegath, F., and France, R. A. (1958). U.S. Patent 2,857,392.

Archer, S., and Schulenberg, J. W. (1972a). U.S. Patent 3,676,444.

Archer, S., and Schulenberg, J. W. (1972b). U.S. Patent 3,682,926.

Archer, S., and Schulenberg, J. W. (1972c). U.S. Patent 3,684,813.

Archer, G. A., and Sternbach, L. H. (1964). U.S. Patent 3,131,178.

Archer, G. A., and Sternbach, L. H. (1966). U.S. Patent 3,236,838.

Archer, G. A., Metlesics, W., Reeder, E., and Sternbach, L. H. (1963). Belgian Patent 620,773; *Chem. Abstr.* **59**, 10094 (1963).

Archer, G. A., Sternbach, L. H., and Mueller, M. (1964). Belgian Patent 634,438; *Chem. Abstr.* **61**, 4382 (1964).

Archer, G. A., Stempel, A., Sternbach, L. H., Felix, A. M., and Fryer, I. R. (1970). German Patent 1,929,910; *Chem. Abstr.* **72**, 100769n (1970).

Archibald, J. L., and Freed, M. E. (1969). U.S. Patent 3,471,499.

Archibald, J. L., and Freed, M. E. (1971). U.S. Patent 3,577,423.

Arena, F., Manna, F., Stein, M. L., and Parente, L. (1975). *Farmaeo, Ed. Sci.* **30**, 380.

Aries, R. (1975). French Patent 2,240,224; *Chem. Abstr.* **83**, 131650y (1975).

Aron-Samuel, J. M. D., and Sterne, J. J. (1969). South African Patent 69/00,641; *Chem. Abstr.* **72**, 100767k (1970).

Arora, R. B., Gupta, L., Bagchi, N., and Singh, M. (1972). *Indian J. Exp. Biol.* **10**, 315; *Chem. Abstr.* **78**, 52726w (1973).

Arrigo, A., Jann, G., and Tonali, P. (1965). *Arch. Int. Pharmacodyn. Ther.* **154**, 364.

Asami, Y., Otsuka, M., Hirohashi, T., Inabu, S., and Yamamoto, H. (1974). *Arzneim.-Forsch.* **24**, 1563 (1974).

Asami, Y., Otsuka, M., Akatsu, M., Kitagawa, S., Inaba, S., and Yamamoto, H. (1975). *Arzneim.-Forsch.* **25**, 534.

Ashford, A., Brown, G. R., Palmer, P. J., Ross, J. W., Trigg, R. B., and Ward, R. J. (1971). *Arzneim.-Forsch.* **21**, 937.

Azimov, M. M., Kamilov, I. K., and Polievstsev, N. P. (1966). *Farmakol. Farmakoter. Alkaloidov Glikozidov*, p. 5; *Chem. Abstr.* **67**, 42381p (1967).

Babbini, M., DeMarchi, F., Montanaro, N., Strocchi, P., and Torrielli, M. V. (1969). *Arzneim.-Forsch.* **19**, 1931.

Babington, R. G., and Horovitz, Z. P. (1973). *Arch. Int. Pharmacodyn. Ther.* **202**, 106.

Baker, K. M., Csetenyi, J., Frigerio, A., Morselli, P. L., Parravicini, F., and Pifferi, G. (1973). *J. Med. Chem.* **16**, 703.

Barron, D. I., Hall, G. H., Natoff, I. L., Ridley, H. F., Spickett, R. G. W., and Vallance, D. K. (1965). *J. Med. Chem.* **8**, 836.

Barthwal, J. P., Tandon, S. K., Agarwal, V. K., Dixit, K. S., and Parmar, S. S. (1973). *J. Pharm. Sci.* **62**, 613.

Barzaghi, F., Fournex, R., and Mantegazza, P. (1973). *Arzneim.-Forsch.* **23**, 683.

Bass, W. B., Gray, J. E., and Larson, E. J. (1959). *Toxicol. Appl. Pharmacol.* **1**, 426.

Batulin, Y. M. (1968). *Farmakol. Toksikol.* (*Moscow*) **31**, 533; *Chem. Abstr.* **70**, 2236a (1969).

Batulin, Y. M., Klimko, V. T., Klygul, T. A., Chupriyanova, N. E., Vikhlyaev, Y. I., and Skoldinov, A. P. (1968). *Khim.-Farm. Zh.* **2**, 3; *Chem. Abstr.* **70**, 11628g (1969).

Bauer, A., Weber, K. H., Minck, K., and Dannenberg, P. (1972a). German Patent 2,103,744; *Chem. Abstr.* **77**, 140179e (1972).

Bauer, A., Weber, K. H., and Unruh, M. (1972b). *Arch. Pharm.* (*Weinheim, Ger.*) **305**, 557.

Bauer, A., Dannenberg, P., Weber, K. H., and Minck, K. (1973a). *J. Med. Chem.* **16**, 1011.

Bauer, A., Weber, K. H., Dannenberg, P., and Kuhn, F. J. (1973b). German Patent 2,165,311; *Chem. Abstr.* **79**, 92301f (1973).

Bauer, A., Weber, K. H., Dannenberg, P., and Kuhn, F. J. (1974a). German Patent 2,231,560; *Chem. Abstr.* **80**, 96043s (1974).

Bauer, A., Weber, K. H., Dannenberg, P., and Kuhn, F. J. (1974b). German Patent 2,257,171; *Chem. Abstr.* **81**, 91591e (1974).

Bauer, A., Weber, K. H., Dannenberg, P., and Kuhn, F. J. (1974c). German Patent 2,318,673; *Chem. Abstr.* **82**, 57747w (1975).

Bauer, A., Weber, K. H., Merz, H., Zeile, K., Giesemann, R., and Dannenberg, P. (1974a). U.S. Patent 3,816,409.

Beiersdorf, A. G. (1974). Belgian Patent 814,400.

Bell, S. C. (1965a). U.S. Patent 3,176,009.

Bell, S. C. (1965b). French Patent M 3314; *Chem. Abstr.* **63**, 13299 (1965).

Bell, S. C. (1968). U.S. Patent 3,418,315.

Bell, S. C., and Gochman, C. (1971). U.S. Patent 3,631,061.

Bell, S. C., Childress, S. J., and Sulkowski, T. S. (1964a). French Patent 1,378,343; *Chem. Abstr.* **62**, 10454 (1965).

Bell, S. C., Wei, P. H. L., and Gochman, C. (1964b). Belgian Patent 643,913; *Chem. Abstr.* **63**, 9971 (1965).

Bell, S. C., McCaully, R. J., and Childress, S. J. (1968a). *J. Med. Chem.* **11**, 172.

Bell, S. C., McCaully, R. J., Gochman, C., Childress, S. J., and Gluckman, M. I. (1968b). *J. Med. Chem.* **11**, 457.

Bellus, D. (1973). German Patent 2,259,222; *Chem. Abstr.* **79**, 78787n (1973).

Berger, L., Stempel, A., Sternbach, L. H., Wenis, E., Fryer, R. I., and Schmidt, R. A. (1962). Belgian Patent 619,101; *Chem. Abstr.* **59**, 10092 (1963).

Bergstrom, W. K., Carzoli, R. F., Lombroso, C., Davidson, D. T., and Wallace, N. M. (1952). *Am. J. Dis. Child.* **84**, 771.

Berlin, A., Belfrage, P., and Magno, R. (1974). *Acta Pharm. Suec.* **11**, 645.

Bernardi, L., Coda, S., Pegrassi, L., and Suchowsky, G. K. (1969). French Patent CAM 279; *Chem. Abstr.* **75**, 154980e (1971).

Bernardi, L., Bonsignori, A., Coda, S., and Suchowsky, G. K. (1970). German Patent 1,958,515; *Chem. Abstr.* **73**, 77279n (1970).

Bernstein, J., and Losee, K. A. (1966). U.S. Patent 3,238,200.

Bertolini, M., Canger, R., and Pietropolli-Charmet, G. (1969). *Arzneim.-Forsch.* **19**, 742.

Beton, J. L. (1974). British Patent 1,346,176; *Chem. Abstr.* **80**, 146211t (1974).

Bhargava, P. N., and Shyam, R. (1974). *Curr. Sci.* **43**, 33.

Bhargava, P. N., and Singh, S. N. (1971). *Indian J. Pharm.* **33**, 36; *Chem. Abstr.* **75**, 63678w (1971).

Bianchi, C., and David, A. (1960). *J. Pharm. Pharmacol.* **12**, 501.

Bicking, J. B. (1959). U.S. Patent 2,917,511.

Blom, S. (1962). *Lancet* **1**, 839.

Blum, J. E., Haefely, W., Jalfre, M., Polc, P., and Scharer, K. (1973). *Arzneim.-Forsch.* **23**, 377.

Boch, J., and Molle, J. (1974). French Patent 2,181,559; *Chem. Abstr.* **80**, 108368s (1974).

Boemches, H. (1973). German Patent 2,252,378; *Chem. Abstr.* **79**, 42575c (1973).

Boemches, H. (1974). German Patent 2,334,273; *Chem. Abstr.* **80**, 108590h (1974).

Bogatskii, A. V., Vikhlyaev, Y. I., Andronati, S. A., Klygul, T. A., Chumachenko, T. K., and Zhilina, Z. I. (1970). *Khim.-Farm. Zh.* **4**, 5.

Bogatskii, A. V., Vikhlyaev, Y. I., Andronati, S. A., Klygul, T. A., and Zhilina, Z. I. (1973). *Khim. Geterotsikl. Soedin.* p. 1558.

Boido, V., and Boidocanu, C. (1973). *Ann. Chim. (Rome)* **63**, 593.

Boido, V., and Sparatore, F. (1974). *Farmaco, Ed. Sci.* **29**, 526.

Boissier, J. R., Dumont, C., and Ratouis, R. (1967). *Therapie* **22**, 129.

Boissier, J. R., Simon, P., Zaczinska, M., and Fichelle, J. (1972a). *Therapie* **27**, 325.

Boissier, J. R., Zebrowska-Lupina, I., and Simon, P. (1972b). *Arch. Int. Pharmacodyn. Ther.* **196**, 330.

Boltze, K. H., Dell, H. D., Lehwald, H., Lorenz, D., and Ruberg-Schweer, M. (1963). *Arzneim.-Forsch.* **13**, 688.

Boltze, K. H., Lorenz, D., Hurden, K., and Ruberg-Schweer, M. (1965). U.S. Patent 3,194,806.

Bonati, F., and Rosati, G. (1965). *Arch. Ital. Sci. Farmacol.* **15**, 45.

Bondavalli, F., Longobardi, M., and Schenone, P. (1975). *Farmaco, Ed. Sci.* **30**, 391.

Bonola, G., DaRe, P., Magistretti, M. J., Massarani, E., and Setnikar, I. (1968). *J. Med. Chem.* **11**, 1136.

Boswell, R. F., Jr., Helsley, G. C., Duncan, R. L., Jr., Funderburk, W. H., and Johnson, D. N. (1974). *J. Med. Chem.* **17**, 1000.

Breen, M. P., Bojanowski, E. M., Cipolle, R. J., Dunn, W. J., III, Frank, E., and Gearien, J. E. (1973). *J. Pharm. Sci.* **62**, 847.

Breuer, H., and Roesch, A. (1971). *Arzneim.-Forsch.* **21**, 238.

Breuer, H., Hoehn, H., and Roesch, E. (1967). German Patent 1,232,152; *Chem. Abstr.* **67**, 3098g (1967).

Broger, E., Field, G. F., and Sternbach, L. H. (1972). German Patent 2,223,648; *Chem. Abstr.* **78**, 43533d (1973).

Brown, S. S., and Goenechea, S. (1973). *Clin. Pharmacol. Ther.* **14**, 314.

Brunaud, M., Navarro, J., Salle, J., and Siou, G. (1970). *Arzneim.-Forsch.* **20**, 123.

Brust, B., Fryer, R. I., and Sternbach, L. H. (1966). Belgian Patent 668,701; *Chem. Abstr.* **65**, 5446 (1966).

Brust, B., Fryer, R. I., and Sternbach, L. H. (1970). U.S. Patent 3,536,649.

Bub, O., Friedrich, L., Hofmann, H. P., Kreiskolt, H., and Zimmermann, F. (1972). German Patent 2,052,840; *Chem. Abstr.* **77**, 34599g (1972).

Bub, O., Friedrich, L., Hofmann, H. P., Kreiskott, H., and Zimmermann, F. (1972b). German Patent 2,052,841; *Chem. Abstr.* **77**, 48528v (1972).

Buguet, G., Fauran, C., Douzon, C., and Raynaud, G. (1974). French Patent 2,215,949; *Chem. Abstr.* **82**, 156324n (1975).

Burroughs Wellcome & Co. (1965). British Patent 981,458; *Chem. Abstr.* **63**, 4308 (1965).

Butler, D. E. (1973). U.S. Patent 3,770,762.

Buzas, A., Dehnel, A., Egnell, C., Bourillert, F., Linee, P., and Simon, J. C. (1972). *Chim. Ther.* **7**, 135.

Calanda-Stiftung. (1963). British Patent 924,589; *Chem. Abstr.* **59**, 11424 (1963).

Cameron, M. D. (1958). U.S. Patent 2,844,590.

Carboni, S., Dasettimo, A., Bertini, D., Ferrarini, P. L., Livi, O., and Tonetti, I. (1975). *Farmico, Ed. Sci.* **30**, 185.

Challier, J. L., Jeanmart, C., Messer, M. N., and Simon, P. (1972). German Patent 2,162,011; *Chem. Abstr.* **77**, 114432n (1972).

Challier, J. L., Jeanmart, C., and Messer, M. N. (1973). German Patent 2,251,559; *Chem. Abstr.* **79**, 32100e (1973).

Charonnat, R., Lechat, P., and Chareton, J. (1956). *Therapie* **11**, 261.

Charonnat, R., Lechat, P., and Chareton, J. (1957). *Therapie* **12**, 68.

Charonnat, R., Lechat, P., Chareton, J., and Boime, A. (1958). British Patent 792,158; *Chem. Abstr.* **52**, 20199 (1958).

Chase, G. O. (1975). U.S. Patent 3,886,141.

Chaturvedi, A. K., and Parmar, S. S. (1972a). *Curr. Sci.* **41**, 253.

Chaturvedi, A. K., and Parmar, S. S. (1972b). *Indian J. Pharm.* **34**, 72.

Chaturvedi, A. K., Parmar, S. S., Bhatnagar, S. C., Mistra, G., and Nigam, S. K. (1974). *Res. Commun. Chem. Pathol. Pharmacol.* **9**, 11.

Chaturvedi, A. K., Barthwal, J. P., Parmar, S. S., and Stenberg, V. I. (1975). *J. Pharm. Sci.* **64**, 454.

Chaudhari, S. K., Verma, M., Chaturvedi, A. K., and Parmar, S. S. (1975). *J. Pharm. Sci.* **64**, 614.

Chemische Werke Albert. (1965). Belgian Patent 643,289; *Chem. Abstr.* **63**, 1790 (1965).

Chen, G., and Bohner, B. (1961). *Proc. Soc. Exp. Biol. Med.* **106**, 632.

Chesnokov, V. P., Konshin, M. E., Zalesov, V. S., and Kudryashova, V. K. (1973). *Khim.-Farm. Zh.* **7**, 20; *Chem. Abstr.* **80**, 47803f (1974).

Childress, S. C., and Gluckman, M. I. (1964). *J. Pharm. Sci.* **53** 577.

Chladt, J., and Braunlich, H. (1965). *Acta Biol. Med. Ger.* **15**, 79.

Chodnekar, M. S., and Blum, J. E. (1968). *J. Med. Chem.* **11**, 1023.

Chou, C., Chou, K., and Chi, J. Y. (1966). *Yao Hsueh Hsueh Pao* **13**, 438; *Chem. Abstr.* **67**, 1850x (1967).

Chou, K., and Tu, T. H. (1965). *Yao Hsueh Hseuh Pao* **12**, 362; *Chem. Abstr.* **64**, 11739 (1966).

Christmas, A. J., and Maxwell, D. R. (1970). *Neuropharmacology* **9**, 17.

Chusid, J. G., and Kopeloff, L. M. (1962). *Proc. Soc. Exp. Biol. Med.* **109**, 546.

Ciba-Geigy A.G. (1974). Netherlands Patent 73/10,900; *Chem. Abstr.* **83**, 79295v (1975).

Clark, R. L., and Pessolano, A. A. (1957). U.S. Patent 2,806,853.

Clark, R. L., and Pessolano, A. A. (1960). U.S. Patent 2,933,503.

Clarkson, R. (1964). British Patent 950,529; *Chem. Abstr.* **60**, 15884 (1964).

Classe, V., and Mos, G. H. M. (1967). U.S. Patent 3,304,304.

Close, W. J., and Spielman, M. A. (1961). *Med. Chem.* (*N. Y.*) **5**, 1.

Coffen, D. L., and Fryer, R. I. (1974a). U.S. Patent 3,849,399.

Coffen, D. L., and Fryer, R. I. (1974b). U.S. Patent 3,850,948.

Coffen, D. L., and Fryer, R. I. (1975). U.S. Patent 2,436,146.

Cohnen, E. (1974). German Patent 2,321,786; *Chem. Abstr.* **82**, 73035t (1975).

Cohnen, E. (1975). German Patent 2,335,147; *Chem. Abstr.* **82**, 156393j (1975).

Coscia, L., DeNatale, G., and Causa, P. (1968). *Boll. Chim. Farm.* **107**, 261.

Cotrel, C., Jeanmart, C., and Messer, M. N. (1972). German Patent 2,141,634; *Chem. Abstr.* **77**, 5526a (1972).

Cotrel, C., Jeanmart, C., and Messer, M. N. (1973a). German Patent 2,300,491; *Chem. Abstr.* **79**, 92284c (1973).

Cotrel, C., Jeanmart, C., and Messer, M. N. (1973b). German Patent 2,301,069; *Chem. Abstr.* **79**, 92024t (1973).

Cotrel, C., Crisan, C., Jeanmart, C., and Messer, M. N. (1974). German Patent 2,423,650 *Chem. Abstr.* **82**, 112103k (1975).

Coutinho, C. B., Cheripko, J. A., and Carbone, J. J. (1969). *Biochem. Pharmacol.* **18**, 303.

Coyne, W. E., and Cusic, J. W. (1968). *J. Med. Chem.* **11**, 1158.

Coyne, W. E., and Cusic, J. W. (1970). U.S. Patent 3,534,019.

Craig, C. R. (1967). *Arch. Int. Pharmacodyn. Ther.* **165**, 328.

Crowther, A. F., and Smith, L. H. (1966). British Patent 1,028,812; *Chem. Abstr.* **65**, 7145 (1966).

Cusic, J. W., and Levon, E. F. (1964). U.S. Patent 3,159,635.

Cusic, J. W., and Levon, E. F. (1965). U.S. Patent 3,178,422.

Cusic, J. W., and Yonan, P. S. (1968). French Patent CAM 235; *Chem. Abstr.* **74**, 76449b (1071).

Cusic, J. W., Ellefson, C. R., and Levon, E. F. (1973). U.S. Patent 3,773,759.

Cusic, J. W., Ellefson, C. R., and Levon, E. F. (1974). German Patent 2,342,007; *Chem. Abstr.* **80**, 133475g (1974).

Danielsson, B., Kronberg, L., and Ljungner, F. (1968). *Acta Pharm. Suec.* **5**, 77.

Daruwala, A. B., Gearien, J. E., Dunn, W. J., III, Benoit, P. S., and Bauer, L. (1974). *J. Med. Chem.* **17**, 819.

Davis, M. A., and Dobson, T. A. (1969). U.S. Patent 3,487,075.

Davis, M. A., and Dobson, T. A. (1972). U.S. Patent 3,641,038.

Davis, M. A., Winthrop, S. O., Thomas, R. A., Herr, F., Charest, M. P., and Gaudry, R. (1964). *J. Med. Chem.* **7**, 88.

Deak, G., Doda, M., Gall, K., Gyorgy, L., and Pfeiffer, K. (1972). German Patent 2,225,669; *Chem. Abstr.* **78**, 84277s (1973).

DeAngelis, L., Traversa, U., and Vertua, R. (1974a). *Curr. Ther. Res., Clin. Exp.* **16**, 324.

DeAngelis, L., Traversa, U., and Vertua, R. (1974b). *Pharmacol. Res. Commun.* **6**, 61.

Delschlager, H., Behrendt, W. A., and Hoffmann, H. (1973). *Arzneim.-Forsch.* **23**, 802.

DeMarchi, F., and Tamagnone, G. (1971). U.S. Patent 3,625,962.

DeMarchi, F., and Torrielli, M. V. (1968). *Chim. Ther.* **3**, 430.

DeMarchi, F., Tamagnone, G. F., and Torrielli, M. V. (1971). *J. Pharm. Sci.* **60**, 1757.

Demerson, C. A., Philipp, A. H., Humbler, L. G., Kraml, M. J., Charest, M. P., Tom, H., and Vavra, I. (1974). *J. Med. Chem.* **17**, 1140.

DeRidder, R. (1970). U.S. Patent 3,538,111.

Derieg, M. E., Fryer, R. I., and Sternbach, L. H. (1968). South African Patent 67/06,526; *Chem. Abstr.* **70**, 87862z (1969).

Derieg, M. E., Earley, J. V., Fryer, R. I., and Sternbach, L. H. (1972). South African Patent 71/05,419; *Chem. Abstr.* **77**, 152244k (1972).

Derieg, M. E., Fryer, R. I., and Sternbach, L. H. (1973). German Patent 2,260,448; *Chem. Abstr.* **79**, 92298k (1973).

DeWald, H. A. (1969). German Patent 1,927,429; *Chem. Abstr.* **72**, 55526t (1970).

DeWald, H. A. (1971). U.S. Patent 3,557,095.

DeWald, H. A., and Butler, D. E. (1971). U.S. Patent 3,558,605.

DeWald, H. A., Nordin, I. C., L'Italien, Y. J., and Parcell, R. F. (1973). *J. Med. Chem.* **16**, 1346.

Dickinson, W. B. (1972). U.S. Patent 3,682,962.

DiRocco, C., Maira, G., Meglio, M., and Rossi, G. (1974a). *Riv. Neurol.* **44**, 146.

DiRocco, C., Maira, G., Meglio, M., and Rossi, G. F. (1974b). *Riv. Neurol.* **44**, 155.

Dobrescu, D., and Coeugniet, E. (1971). *Ann. Pharm. Fr.* **29**, 501.

Dobrescu, D., Cicotti, A., and Salceanu, M. (1974). *Farmacia (Bucharest)* **22**, 65; *Chem. Abstr.* **82**, 11300s.

Dobson, T. A., and Davis, M. A. (1970a). U.S. Patent 3,491,088.

Dobson, T. A., and Davis, M. A. (1970b). U.S. Patent 3,493,560.

Dobson, T. A., and Davis, M. A. (1971). U.S. Patent 3,597,433.

Doebel, K. J., and Pfenninger, H. (1965). French Patent 1,389,526; *Chem. Abstr.* **63**, 620 (1965).

Dojtschinov, D. I. (1970). German Patent 2,144,060; *Chem. Abstr.* **77**, 52361c (1972).

Druey, J., and Eichenberger, K. (1957). U.S. Patent 2,782,195.

Dua, P. R., Kohli, R. P., and Bharagava, K. P. (1967). *Indian J. Med. Sci.* **21**, 318.

Duchene-Marullaz, P., Lakatos, C., DeMarchi, F., and Torrielli, M. V. (1967). *Farmaco, Ed. Prat.* **22**, 506.

Dufour, C. (1973). German Patent 2,263,026; *Chem. Abstr.* **79**, 78623f (1973).

Duncan, R. L., Jr., and Helsley, G. C. (1971). German Patent 2,051,230; *Chem. Abstr.* **75**, 36163t (1971).

Dwivedi, C., and Parmar, S. S. (1972). *Curr. Sci.* **41**, 487.

Dwivedi, C., Gupta, T. K., and Parmar, S. S. (1972). *J. Med. Chem.* **15**, 553.

Earley, J. V., and Fryer, R. I. (1975). U.S. Patent 3,868,363.

Earley, J. V., Fryer, R. I., and Sternbach, L. H. (1968). South African Patent 68/02,239; *Chem. Abstr.* **72**, 21722p (1970).

Earley, J. V., Fryer, R. I., and Sternbach, L. H. (1971). German Patent 2,030,669; *Chem. Abstr.* **74**, 88077s (1971).

Earley, J. V., Fryer, R. I., and Sternbach, L. H. (1972). German Patent 2,163,641; *Chem. Abstr.* **77**, 126703q (1972).

Earley, J. V., Fryer, R. I., and Walser, A. (1973). German Patent 2,249,447; *Chem. Abstr.* **79**, 5372p (1973).

Earley, J. V., Fryer, R. I., and Walser, A. (1974). U.S. Patent 3,838,116.

Easton, N. (1961). U.S. Patent 2,973,367.

Eberle, M. K. (1975). U.S. Patent 3,859,285.

Edmonds, H. L., Stark, L. G., and Hollinger, M. A. (1974a). *Exp. Neurol.* **45**, 377.

Edmonds, H. L., Stark, L. G., and Rinne, S. (1974b). *Proc. West. Pharmacol. Soc.* **17**, 77.

Edmonds, H. L., and Stark, L. G. (1974). *Neuropharmacology* **13**, 269.

Eiden, F., and Heja, G. (1975). German Patent 2,343,528; *Chem. Abstr.* **83**, 43395p (1975).

Elpern, B., and Bandurco, V. T. (1972). U.S. Patent 3,651,067.

Engelbrecht, H. J., and Lenke, D. (1960). German (East) Patent 19,629; *Chem. Abstr.* **55**, 22346 (1961).

Engelmeier, M. P. (1960). *Dtsch. Med. Wochenschr.* **85**, 2207.

English, A., Koch, K., and Zimmermann, R. (1971). German Patent 1,302,662; *Chem. Abstr.* **74**, 141745m.

Ermili, A., Roma, G., Mazzei, M., Balbi, A., Cuttica, A., and Passerini, N. (1974a). *Farmaco, Ed. Sci.* **29**, 225.

Ermili, A., Roma, G., Mazzei, M., Ambrosini, A., and Passerini, N. (1974b). *Farmaco, Ed. Sci.* **29**, 237.

Fanshawe, W. J., and Safir, S. R. (1974). U.S. Patent 3,857,843.

Farbenfabriken Bayer A. G. (1969). French Patent M6753; *Chem. Abstr.* **74**, 76347s (1971).

Farbwerke Hoechst A. G. (1969). French Patent M7358; *Chem. Abstr.* **75**, 151811q (1971).

Fauran, C., Douzon, C., Huguet, G., Raynaud, G., and Gouret, C. (1971a). German Patent 2,111,775; *Chem. Abstr.* **76**, 34235q (1972).

Fauran, C., Eberle, J., Raynaud, G., Gouret, C., Thomas, J., and Huguet, G. (1971b). South African Patent 71/02,214; *Chem. Abstr.* **77**, 88472d (1972).

Fauran, C., Turin, M., Raynaud, G., and Thomas, J. (1972). German Patent 2,202,046; *Chem. Abstr.* **77**, 140139s (1972).

Fauran, C., Eberle, J., Raynaud, G., Gouret, C., Thomas, J., and Huguet, G. (1973a). U.S. Patent 3,726,900.

Fauran, C., Turin, M., Huguet, G., Raynaud, G., and Pourrias, B. (1973b). German Patent 2,328,384; *Chem. Abstr.* **80**, 83007h (1974).

Fauran, C., Eberle, J., LeCloarec, A. Y., Raynaud, G., and Sargent, M. (1974a). French Patent 2,186,251; *Chem. Abstr.* **81**, 3938v (1974).

Fauran, C., Turin, M., Gouret, C., and Raynaud, G. (1974b). French Patent 2,190,429; *Chem. Abstr.* **81**, 13384a (1974).

Fauran, C., Douzon, C., Raynaud, G., and Pourrias, B. (1974c). French Patent 2,215,223; *Chem. Abstr.* **82**, 73003f (1975).

Fauran, C., Douzon, C., Hugnet, G., Raynaud, G., and Gouret, C. (1974d). French Patent 2,226,165; *Chem. Abstr.* **82**, 156266v (1975).

Fauran, C., Eberle, J., Raynaud, G., and Bailly, Y. J. (1974e). German Patent 2,350,207; *Chem. Abstr.* **81**, 13528a (1974).

Fauran, C., Raynaud, G., and Thomas, J. M. (1974f). U.S. Patent 3,796,703.

Fauran, C., Eberle, J., Raynaud, G., and Bailly, Y. J. (1975). U.S. Patent 3,878,207.

Fernandez-Tome, M. P., Madronero, R., del Rio, J., and Vega, S. (1972). *J. Med. Chem.* **15**, 887.

Ferrari, W., and Sandrini, M. (1973). *Riv. Farmacol. Ter.* **4**, 97a.

Ferrini, R., Miragoli, G., and Taccardi. B. (1974). *Arzneim.-Forsch.* **24**, 2029.

Ferrosan, A. K. (1965). Netherlands Patent 6,408,661; *Chem. Abstr.* **63**, 4263 (1965).

Field, G. F., and Sternbach, L. H. (1971a). U.S. Patent 3,555,022.

Field, G. F., and Sternbach, L. H. (1971b). German Patent 2,062,927; *Chem. Abstr.* **76**, 59670r (1972).

Field, G. F., and Sternbach, L. H. (1972). South African Patent 70/08,348; *Chem. Abstr.* **78**, 72231j (1973).

Field, G. F., and Sternbach, L. H. (1973). British Patent 1,332,697; *Chem. Abstr.* **80**, 37186t (1974).

Field, G. F., and Sternbach, L. H. (1975a). Swiss Patent 561,189; *Chem. Abstr.* **83**, 114502j (1975).

Field, G. F., and Sternbach, L. H. (1975b). Swiss Patent 561,190; *Chem. Abstr.* **83**, 114501h (1975).

Field, G. F., and Sternbach, L. H. (1975c). Swiss Patent 561,191; *Chem. Abstr.* **83**, 114503k (1975).

Field, G. F., and Sternbach, L. H. (1975d). Swiss Patent 561,703; *Chem. Abstr.* **83**, 97409q (1975).

Field. G. F., and Sternbach, L. H. (1975e). Swiss Patent 561,704; *Chem. Abstr.* **83**, 97408p (1975).

Field, G. F., and Sternbach, L. H. (1975f). Swiss Patent 561,705; *Chem. Abstr.* **83**, 97407n (1975).

Field, G. F., and Sternbach, L. H. (1975g). Swiss Patent 561,706; *Chem. Abstr.* **83**, 97406m (1975).

Field, G. F., Ning, R. Y. F., and Sternbach, L. H. (1970). German Patent 1,950,595; *Chem. Abstr.* **72**, 132806p (1970).

Field, G. F., Sternbach, L. H., and Walser, A. (1975). U.S. Patent 3,880,840.

Fiordalisi, F. M. (1963). U.S. Patent 3,079,397.

Fiordalisi, F. M. (1965). U.S. Patent 3,166,475.

Flugel, F., Bente, D., and Itil, T. (1960). *Dtsch. Med. Wochenschr.* **85**, 2199.

Fontanella, L., Occelli, E., Testa, F., and Cignarella, G. (1972). *Farmaco, Ed. Sci.* **27**, 755.

Fouche, J., and Leger, A. (1971). French Patent 2,069,831; *Chem. Abstr.* **77**, 34370a (1972).

Fouche, J., and Leger, A. (1972). French Patent 2,092,877; *Chem. Abstr.* **77**, 101405f (1972).

Frank, E., Gearien, J., Megahy, M., and Pokorny, C. (1971). *J. Med. Chem.* **14**, 551.

Freed, M. E., and Archibald, J. L. (1969). U.S. Patent 3,462,441.

Freedman, J., and Judd, C. I. (1972). U.S. Patent 3,637,747.

Friebel, H., and Sommer, S. (1960). *Dtsch. Med. Wochenschr.* **85**, 2192.

Fryer, R. I., and Sternbach, L. H. (1970). U.S. Patent 3,501,474.

Fryer, R. I., and Sternbach, L. H. (1974). U.S. Patent 3,795,702.

Fryer, R. I., and Walser, A. (1973). German Patent 2,250,425; *Chem. Abstr.* **79**, 18774w (1973).

Fryer, R. I., and Walser, A. (1975a). U.S. Patent 3,865,815.

Fryer, R. I., and Walser, A. (1975b). U.S. Patent 3,868,362.

Fryer, R. I., Schmidt, R. A., and Sternbach, L. H. (1963). U.S. Patent 3,100,770.

Fryer, R. I., Schmidt, R. A., and Sternbach, L. H. (1968). U.S. Patent 3,403,161.

Fujimoto, M. (1975). Japanese Patent 75/41,872; *Chem. Abstr.* **83**, 193089f (1975).

Gagneux, A., Heckendorn, R., and Meier, R. (1972). German Patent 2,159,527; *Chem. Abstr.* **77**, 101690v (1972).

Gagneux, A., Heckendorn, R., and Meier, R. (1973a). German Patent 2,234,620; *Chem. Abstr.* **78**, 124624r (1973).

Gagneux, A., Heckendorn, R., and Meier, R. (1973b). German Patent 2,304,307; *Chem. Abstr.* **79**, 126535c (1973).

Gagneux, A., Heckendorn, R., and Meier, R. (1974a). Germant Patent 2,363,515; *Chem. Abstr.* **82**, 4322x (1975).

Gagneux, A., Hechendorn, R., and Meier, R. (1974b). Swiss Patent 551,993; *Chem. Abstr.* **82**, 43479y (1975).

Ganellin, C. R., Loynes, J. M., Ridley, H. F., and Spickett, R. G. W. (1967). *J. Med. Chem.* **10**, 826.

Garattini, S., Mussini, E., and Randall, L. O. (1973). "The Benzodiazepines." Raven, New York.

Gardner, D. V., and Tickle, R. W. (1972). German Patent 2,222,926; *Chem. Abstr.* **78**, 43273u (1973).

Gardner, J. N., and Willey, G. L. (1964). U.S. Patent 3,149,129.

J. R. Geigy, A.-G. (1962). British Patent 908,788; *Chem. Abstr.* **59**, 10011 (1963).

J. R. Geigy, A.-G. (1966). Netherlands Patent 6,605,741; *Chem. Abstr.* **66**, 65507c (1967).

Georges, G., Herold, M., and Cahn, J. (1958). *Therapie* **13**, 689.

Germane, S., Voitenko, A. D., and Kastrons, J. (1975). *Khim.-Farm. Zh.* **9**, 28; *Chem. Abstr.* **83**, 498g (1975).

Gesler, R. M., and Surrey, A. R. (1958). *J. Pharmacol. Exp. Ther.* **122**, 517 (1958).

Ghosal, S., Dutta, S. K., and Bhattacharya, S. K. (1972). *J. Pharm. Sci.* **61**, 1274.

Gilbert, E. E., and Rumanowski, E. J. (1971). U.S. Patent 3,592,822.

Gilbert, J. C., Gray, P., and Heaton, G. M. (1971). *Biochem. Pharmacol.* **20**, 240.

Gittos, M. W., James, J. W., and Wiggins, L. F. (1967). British Patent 1,088,846; *Chem. Abstr.* **68**, 105193x (1968).

Giurgea, C. E. (1972). German Patent 2,152,233; *Chem. Abstr.* **77**, 52322r (1972).

Gladenko, I. N., and Fortushnyi, V. A. (1964). *Farmakol. Toksikol. (Moscow)* **27**, 555; *Chem. Abstr.* **62**, 4490 (1965).

Glasser, A. C., Diamond, L., and Combs, G. (1971). *J. Pharm. Sci.* **60**, 127.

Gluckman, M. I. (1971). *Arzneim.-Forsch.* **21**, 1049.

Godefroi, E. F. (1962). U.S. Patent 3,040,048.

Godefroi, E. F., and Platje, J. T. J. (1972). *J. Med. Chem.* **15**, 336.

Goldberg, M. E., Manian, A. A., and Efron, D. H. (1967). *Life Sci.* **6**, 481.

Goldman, L., and Williams, R. P. (1956). U.S. Patent 2,756,232.

Golik, U. (1975). *Tetrahedron Lett.* p. 1327.

Goodman, L. S. (1956). U.S. Patent 2,744,852.

Gootjes, J., Funcke, A. B. H., and Timmerman, H. (1972). *Arzneim.-Forsch.* **22**, 632.

Gordon, M., Pachter, I. J., and Wilson, J. W. (1963). *Arzneim.-Forsch.* **13**, 802.

Greenblatt, D. J., and Shader, R. I. (1974). "Benzodiazepines in Clinical Practice." Raven, New York.

Greenwood, D. T., Mallion, K. B., Todd, A. H., and Turner, R. W. (1975). *J. Med. Chem.* **18**, 573.

Griot, R. G. (1966). U.S. Patent 3,271,404.

Gschwend, H. W. (1974). U.S. Patent 3,853,851.

Guczoghy, L., Puklics, M., Kelemen, G., and Leszkovsky, G. (1972). U.S. Patent 3,639,415.

Guerrero-Figueroa, R., and Gallant, D. M. (1971). *Curr. Ther. Res.* **13**, 747.

Guerrero-Figueroa, R., Rye, M. M., and Heath, R. G. (1969a). *Curr. Ther. Res.* **11**, 27.

Guerrero-Figueroa, R., Rye, M. M., and Heath, R. G. (1969b). *Curr. Ther. Res.* **11**, 40.

Gujral, M. L., Sareen, K. N., and Kohli, R. P. (1957). *Indian J. Med. Res.* **45**, 207.

Gupta, A. K., Dwivedi, C., Gupta, T. K., Parmar, S. S., and Cornatzer, W. E. (1974). *J. Pharm. Sci.* **63**, 1227.

Gupta, A. K., Dwivedi, C., Gupta, T. K., Parmar, S. S., and Harbison, R. D. (1975). *J. Pharm. Sci.* **64**, 1001.

Gupta, L., Arora, R. B., and Singh, M. (1972). *Indian J. Exp. Biol.* **10**, 456.

Gupta, L., Arora, R. B., and Singh, M. (1973). *Indian J. Exp. Biol.* **11**, 243.

Gupta, T. K., Kumar, R., Ali, B., and Parmar, S. S. (1973). *Jpn. J. Pharmacol.* **23**, 5.

Gy, E., and Gyar, T. G. (1974a). British Patent 1,354,246; *Chem. Abstr.* **81**, 105320e (1974).

Gy, E., and Gyar, T. G. (1974b). German Patent 2,406,490; *Chem. Abstr.* **81**, 135992t (1974).

Hadley, M. S. (1973). German Patent 2,253,900; *Chem. Abstr.* **79**, 31873x (1973).

Hallmann, G., Schoetensach, W., and Blechschmidt, W. (1962). German Patent 1,122,073; *Chem. Abstr.* **56**, 15516 (1962).

Hammann, W. C. (1960). U.S. Patent 2,945,857.

Hardie, W. R., Hidalgo, J., Halverstadt, I. F., and Allen, R. E. (1966). *J. Med. Chem.* **9**, 127.

Hardtmann, G. E., and Ott, H. (1970). U.S. Patent 3,506,647.

Hardtmann, G. E., and Ott, H. (1972). U.S. Patent 3,663,698.
Hardtmann, G. E., and Ott, H. (1974). U.S. Patent 3,829,422.
Harper, N. J., Hussey, C. W. T., Peel, M. E., Ritchie, A. C., and Waring, J. M. (1967). *J. Med. Chem.* **10**, 819.
Hasegawa, G., and Kotani, A. (1974). Japanese Patent 74/49,959; *Chem. Abstr.* **81**, 77923h.
Hashimoto, Y. (1967). Japanese Patent 10,922; *Chem. Abstr.* **68**, 24550f (1968).
Hauptmann, K., Weber, K. H., Zeile, K., Danneberg, P., and Giesemann, R. (1968). South African Patent 68/00,803; *Chem. Abstr.* **70**, 106579f (1969).
Hayashi, S. (1973). Japanese Patent 73/48,464; *Chem. Abstr.* **79**, 92198c (1973).
Helferich, B. (1959). U.S. Patent 2,917,512.
Hellerbach, J., and Walser, A. (1970). German Patent 2,005,508; *Chem. Abstr.* **73**, 131050w (1970).
Hellerbach, J., and Walser, A. (1970). German Patent 2,137,994; *Chem. Abstr.* **76**, 113260x (1972).
Hellerbach, J., and Walser, A. (1973). German Patent 2,238,579; *Chem. Abstr.* **78**, 136349p (1973).
Hellerbach, J., and Zanetti, G. (1974). Swiss. Patent 551,986; *Chem. Abstr.* **81**, 105589z (1974).
Hellerbach, J., Szente, A., and Walser, A. (1972). U.S. Patent 3,657,223.
Hellerbach, J., Hoffmann, H., and Zanetti, G. (1974). German Patent 2,347,455; *Chem. Abstr.* **81**, 13568p (1974).
Helsley, G. C. (1970). German Patent 2,017,255; *Chem. Abstr.* **74**, 99863w (1971).
Helsley, G. C. (1971). German Patent 2,048,589; *Chem. Abstr.* **75**, 35777j (1971).
Helsley, G. C., Duncan, R. L., Jr., Funderburk, W. H., and Johnson, D. N. (1969). *J. Med. Chem.* **12**, 1098.
Herbertz, G. (1974). German Patent 2,236,796; *Chem. Abstr.* **80**, 120915a (1974).
Hernandez-Peon, R., Rojas-Ramirez, J. A., O'Flaherty, J. J., and Mazzuchelli-O'Flaherty, A. L. (1964). *Int. J. Neuropharmacol.* **3**, 405.
Hernestam, S. E. H., Sterner, N. O., and Lassen, J. B. (1971). Swedish Patent 332,984; *Chem. Abstr.* **77**, 151964h (1972).
Hernestam, S. E. H., Sterner, N. O., and Lassen, J. B. (1974). U.S. Patent 3,816,433.
Hester, J. B., Jr. (1971). U.S. Patent 3,579,503.
Hester, J. B., Jr. (1972a). U.S. Patent 3,642,820.
Hester, J. B., Jr. (1972b). U.S. Patent 3,642,821.
Hester, J. B., Jr. (1972c). U.S. Patent 3,651,083.
Hester, J. B., Jr. (1973a). U.S. Patent 3,714,149.
Hester, J. B., Jr. (1973b). U.S. Patent 3,734,919.
Hester, J. B., Jr. (1974). U.S. Patent 3,793,328.
Hester, J. B., Jr. (1975). U.S. Patent 3,880,878.
Hester, J. B., Jr., and Rudzik, A. D. (1974). *J. Med. Chem.* **17**, 293.
Hester, J. B., Jr., Rudzik, A. D., and Kamdar, B. V. (1971). *J. Med. Chem.* **14**, 1078.
Heusner, A., Zeile, K., and Danneberger, P. (1969). U.S. Patent 3,462,434.
Hindley, N. C., and McClymont, T. M. (1975). British Patent 1,390,277; *Chem. Abstr.* **83**, 79300t (1975).
Hindley, N. C., McClymont, T. M., and Chase, G. O. (1973). South African Patent 72/04,577; *Chem. Abstr.* **79**, 126536d (1973).
Hirai, S., and Kawata, K. (1974). German Patent 2,341,537; *Chem. Abstr.* **80**, 133414m (1974).
Hirata, Y., Murakami, M., Takahashi, K., and Takeda, M. (1974). Japanese Patent 74/95,964; *Chem. Abstr.* **82**, 97877p (1975).

Hirohashi, T., Sato, H., Inaba, S., and Yamamoto, H. (1972). German Patent 2,155,403; *Chem. Abstr.* **77**, 101688a (1972).

Hirohashi, T., Sato, H., Inaba, S., and Yamamoto, H. (1973a). Japanese Patent 73/49,786; *Chem. Abstr.* **79**, 105304m (1973).

Hirohashi, T., Sato, H., Inaba, S., and Yamamoto, H. (1973b). Japanese Patent 73/75,591; *Chem. Abstr.* **80**, 121014t (1974).

Hirohashi, T., Sato, H., Inaba, S., and Yamamoto, H. (1974a). Japanese Patent 74/81,378; *Chem. Abstr.* **82**, 57749y (1975).

Hirohashi, T., Sato, H., Inaba, S., and Yamamoto, H. (1974b). Japanese Patent 74/81,385; *Chem. Abstr.* **82**, 57750s (1975).

Hirohashi, T., Sato, H., Inaba, S., and Yamamoto, H. (1974c). Japanese Patent 74/81,386; *Chem. Abstr.* **82**, 57748x (1975).

Hirohashi, T., Sato, H., Inaba, S., and Yamamoto, H. (1974d). Japanese Patent 74/81,387; *Chem. Abstr.* **82**, 140206q (1975).

Hisano, T., Ichikawa, M., Kito, G., and Nishi, T. (1972). *Chem. Pharm. Bull.* **20**, 2575.

Hitchings, G. H., Ledig, K. W., and West, R. A. (1962). U.S. Patent 3,037,980.

Hoffmann-LaRoche & Co. (1964a). Netherlands Patent 6,401,335; *Chem. Abstr.* **62**, 5288 (1965).

Hoffmann-LaRoche & Co. (1964b). Netherlands Patent 6,406,381; *Chem. Abstr.* **63**, 13298 (1965).

Hoffmann-LaRoche & Co. (1965a). Netherlands Patent 6,413,180; *Chem. Abstr.* **63**, 14890 (1965).

Hoffmann-LaRoche & Co. (1965b). Netherlands Patent 6,414,904; *Chem. Abstr.* **64**, 2114 (1966).

Hoffmann-LaRoche & Co. (1965c). Netherlands Patent 6,500,817; *Chem. Abstr.* **64**, 5122 (1966).

Hoffmann-LaRoche & Co. (1966a). Netherlands Patent 6,510,538; *Chem. Abstr.* **65**, 733 (1966).

Hoffmann-LaRoche & Co. (1966b). Netherlands Patent 6,510,539; *Chem. Abstr.* **65**, 732 (1966).

Hoffmann-LaRoche & Co. (1974). Austrian Patent 315,861; *Chem. Abstr.* **83**, 28295n (1975).

Hoffmann, K., Sury, E., and Tagmann, E. (1956). U.S. Patent 2,742,475.

Hofmann, C. M. (1956). U.S. Patent 2,748,125.

Holland, G. F., Funderburk, W. H., and Finger, K. F. (1963). *J. Med. Chem.* **6**, 307.

Hollister, R. P., and Julien, R. M. (1974). *Proc. West. Pharmacol. Soc.* **17**, 103.

Houlihan, W. J., and Nadelson, J. (1972). German Patent 2,148,513; *Chem. Abstr.* **77**, 19452k (1972).

Hudson, R. D., and Wolpert, M. K. (1970). *Arch. Int. Pharmacodyn. Ther.* **186**, 388.

Huguet, G., Fauran, C., Douzon, C., Raynaud, G., and Gouret, C. (1972). French Patent 2,121,442; *Chem. Abstr.* **78**, 136262e (1973).

Hurmer, R., and Vernin, J. (1967). *Therapie* **22**, 1325.

Hurmer, R., and Vernin, J. (1969). French Patent CAM 0254; *Chem. Abstr.* **77**, 19673h (1972).

Imperical Chemical Industries Ltd. (1964). Belgian Patent 637,802; *Chem. Abstr.* **62**, 10422 (1965).

Inaba, S., Izumi, T., Hirohashi, T. Akatsu, M., Sakai, S., and Yamamoto, H. (1971). German Patent 2,016,385; *Chem. Abstr.* **74**, 100117g (1971).

Inaba, S., Akatsu, M., Sakai, S., Yamamoto, H., Hirohashi, T., and Izumi, T. (1974). Japanese Patent 74/03,995; *Chem. Abstr.* **81**, 152290e (1974).

Irwin, W. J., Wheeler, D. L., and Harper, N. J. (1972). *J. Med. Chem.* **15**, 445.

Ishizumi, K., Mori, K., Okamoto, T., Akase, T., Izumi, T., Akatsu, M., Kume, Y., Inaba, S., and Yamamoto, H. (1973). German Patent 2,204,484; *Chem. Abstr.* **79**, 137208z (1973).

Ishizumi, K., Mori, K., Inaba, S., and Yamamoto, H. (1974). Japanese Patent 74/41,392; *Chem. Abstr.* **81**, 91596k (1974).

Jacob, R. M., and Joseph, N. M. (1959). British Patent 874,096; *Chem. Abstr.* **56**, 10165 (1962).

Jacobson, C. R., D'Adamo, A., and Cosgrove, C. E. (1972). U.S. Patent 3,663,564.

Jain, P. C., Kapoor, V., Anand, N., Ahmad, A., and Patnaik, G. K. (1967). *J. Med. Chem.* **10**, 812.

Jain, P. C., Kapoor, V., Anand, N., Patnaik, G. K., Ahmad, A., and Vohra, M. M. (1968). *J. Med. Chem.* **11**, 87.

Jansen, A. B. A., Hollywood, J., and Wilson, A. B. (1974). U.S. Patent 3,823,148.

Janssen, P. A. J. (1961). U.S. Patent 2,973,365.

Jaunin, R., and Hellerbach, J. (1972). German Patent 2,150,075; *Chem. Abstr.* **77**, 48523q (1972).

Jaunin, R., and Hellerbach, J. (1975a). Swiss Patent 599,190; *Chem. Abstr.* **82**, 171113m (1975).

Jaunin, R., and Hellerbach, J. (1975b). Swiss Patent 559,191; *Chem. Abstr.* **82**, 171112k (1975).

Jaunin, R., and Hellerbach, J. (1975c). Swiss Patent 559,192; *Chem. Abstr.* **83**, 28294m (1975).

Jaunin, R., and Hellerbach, J. (1975d). Swiss Patent 559,193; *Chem. Abstr.* **83**, 10184r (1975).

Jeanmart, C., Leger, A., and Messer, M. N. (1974). German Patent 2,360,362; *Chem. Abstr.* **81**, 105528d (1974).

Jommi, G., Manitto, P., and Silanos, M. A. (1964). *Arch. Biochem. Biophys.* **108**, 334.

Joshi, K. C., Singh, V. K., Mehta, D. S., Sharma, R. C., and Gupta, L. (1975). *J. Pharm. Sci.* **64**, 1428.

Judd, C. I., and Biel, H. (1963). French Patent 1,315,372; *Chem. Abstr.* **58**, 12575 (1963).

Julien, R. M. (1973). *Proc. West. Pharmacol. Soc.* **16**, 126.

Julou, L., Courvoisier, S., Bardone, M. C., Ducrot, R., Fournel, J., and Leau, O. (1957). *C. R. Seances Soc. Biol. Ses. Fil.* **151**, 864.

Kajfez, F., Kovac, T., and Sunjic, V. (1975). German Patent 2,264,794; *Chem. Abstr.* **83**, 10181n (1975).

Kaku, T., Kuboto, K., Murakami, H., and Asada, I. (1964). *Yakugaku Zasshi* **84**, 983; *Chem. Abstr.* **62**, 6467 (1965).

Kali-Chemie Pharma GMBH. (1974). German Patent 2,314,488.

Kalish, R., Steppe, T. V., and Walser, A. (1975). *J. Med. Chem.* **18**, 222.

Kamioka, T., Takagi, H., Kobayashi, S., and Suzuki, Y. (1972). *Arzneim.-Forsch.* **22**, 884.

Kano, H., and Takahashi, S. (1974). Japanese Patent 74/41,272; *Chem. Abstr.* **81**, 152209k (1974).

Karamchand Premchand Private Ltd. (1972). French Patent 2,131,843; *Chem. Abstr.* **78**, 147986v (1973).

Karamchand Premchand Private Ltd. (1973). British Patent 1,298,603; *Chem. Abstr.* **80**, 27277j (1974).

Kariss, J., and Newmark, H. L. (1963). U.S. Patent 3,116,203.

Kariss, J., and Newmark, H. L. (1964). U.S. Patent 3,123,529.

Karmas, G. (1960a). U.S. Patent 2,928,842.

Karmas, G. (1960b). U.S. Patent 2,931,814.

Karmas, G., and Mallory, R. A. (1959). U.S. Patent 2,883,392.

Karmas, G., and Oroshnik, W. (1960). U.S. Patent 2,926,170.

Kathawala, F. G. (1974). U.S. Patent 3,856,808.

Kathawala, F. G. (1975a). U.S. Patent 3,862,137.

Kathawala, F. G. (1975b). U.S. Patent 3,869,450.

Kato, H., and Koshinaka, E. (1974a). German Patent 2,356,999; *Chem. Abstr.* **81**, 37573n (1974).

Kato, H., and Koshinaka, E. (1974b). Japanese Patent 74/72,284; *Chem. Abstr.* **83**, 114507g (1975).

Kato, H., Nishikawa, T., and Mori, T. (1974). German Patent 2,355,420; *Chem. Abstr.* **81**, 120694y (1974).

Kato, H., Nishikawa, T., and Mori, T. (1975a). Japanese Patent 75/62,984; *Chem. Abstr.* **83**, 179152q (1975).

Kato, H., Nishikawa, T., and Mori, T. (1975b). Japanese Patent 75/62,985; *Chem. Abstr.* **83**, 164230q (1975).

Kato, H., Nishikawa, T., and Mori, T. (1975c). Japanese Patent 75/62,989; *Chem. Abstr.* **83**, 179142m (1975).

Keasling, H. H., and Moffett, R. B. (1971). *J. Med. Chem.* **14**, 1106.

Keasling, H. H., Willette, R. E., and Szmuszkovicz, J. (1964). *J. Med. Chem.* **7**, 94.

Keller, O., Steiger, N., and Sternbach, L. H. (1962). Belgian Patent 616,024; *Chem. Abstr.* **58**, 10222 (1963).

Keller, O., Steiger, N., and Sternbach, L. H. (1963). Belgian Patent 632,685; *Chem. Abstr.* **62**, 577 (1965).

Keller, O., Steiger, N., and Sternbach, L. H. (1964a). U.S. Patent 3,121,074.

Keller, O., Steiger, N., and Sternbach, L. H. (1964b). U.S. Patent 3,121,045.

Keller, O., Steiger, N., and Sternbach, L. H. (1964c). U.S. Patent 3,121,103.

Keller, O., Steiger, N., and Sternbach, L. H. (1964d). U.S. Patent 3,121,114.

Khaldarov, K. K., and Lebedeva, L. D. (1973). *Dokl. Akad. Nauk Tadzh. SSR* **16**, 64; *Chem. Abstr.* **79**, 364c (1973).

Kido, R., Hirose, K., Sato, H., and Fujito, A. (1970). *Oyo Yakuri* **4**, 185; *Chem. Abstr.* **76**, 81137u (1972).

Kim, D. H., and Santilli, A. A. (1970). U.S. Patent 3,517,007.

Kishimoto, T., Kaneda, Y., and Umio, S. (1974a). Japanese Patent 74/56,987; *Chem. Abstr.* **81**, 120500g (1974).

Kishimoto, T., Kouchi, H., and Umio, S. (1974b). Japanese Patent 74/56,988; *Chem. Abstr.* **81**, 120497m (1974).

Kitano, S., Sugiyama, M., and Yagi, S. (1973). Japanese Patent 73/37,034; *Chem. Abstr.* **80**, 120974u (1974).

Klupp, H., and Kahling, J. (1965). *Arzneim.-Forsch.* **15**, 359.

Kohl, H., Desai, P. D., Dohadwalla, A. N., and deSouza, N. J. (1974). *J. Pharm. Sci.* **63**, 838.

Koo, C. M. C., Pattison, T. W., and Herbst, D. R. (1970). U.S. Patent 3,516,987.

Kopeloff, L. M., and Chusid, J. G. (1967). *Int. J. Neuropsychiatry* **3**, 469.

Kopicova, Z., Sedivy, Z., Hradil, F., and Protiva, M. (1972). *Collect. Czech. Chem. Commun.* **37**, 1371.

Kornet, M. J., Thorstenson, J. H., and Lubawy, W. C. (1974). *J. Pharm. Sci.* **63**, 1090.

Kovac, T., Kajfez, F., Sunjic, V., and Oklobdzja, M. (1974). *J. Med. Chem.* **17**, 766.

Kovaleva, A. E., and Lazebnik, L. B. (1966). *Farmakol. Toksikol. (Moscow)* **29**, 518; *Chem. Abstr.* **66**, 9763x (1967).

Kozhevnikov, Y. V., Petyunin, P. A., Kharchenko, N. E., and Grishina, V. M. (1970). *Khim.-Farm. Zh.* **4**, 25.

Kozhevnikov, Y. V., Pilat, N. V., Kharchenko, N. E., and Zalesov, V. S. (1975). *Khim.-Farm. Zh.* **9**, 20.
Kreighbaum, W. E., and Scarborough, H. C. (1964). *J. Med. Chem.* **7**, 310.
Kreighbaum, W. E., and Scarborough, H. C. (1965). U.S. Patent 3,177,202.
Kretzschmar, R., and Meyer, H. J. (1969). *Arch. Int. Pharmocodyn. Ther.* **177**, 261.
Krva, Z. T. (1975). British Patent 1,385,612; *Chem. Abstr.* **83**, 43398s (1975).
Kuch, H., Schmitt, K., Seidl, G., and Hoffman, I. (1973). U.S. Patent 3,725,404.
Kumar, R., Gupta, T. K., and Parmar, S. S. (1970). *J. Prakt. Chem.* **312**, 201.
Kunstmann, R., and Kaiser, J. (1975). German Patent 2,352,702; *Chem. Abstr.* **83**, 164005v (1975).
Kutter, E., Austel, V., Kaehling, J., and Ziegler, H. (1974). German Patent 2,237,770; *Chem. Abstr.* **80**, 120794k (1974).
Kuwada, Y., Natsugari, H., and Meguro, K. (1973a). German Patent 2,261,777; *Chem. Abstr.* **79**, 78860f (1973).
Kuwada, Y., Natsugari, H., and Meguro, K. (1973b). Japanese Patent 73/99,191; *Chem. Abstr.* **80**, 96049y (1974).
Kuwada, Y., Meguro, K., and Tawada, H. (1974a). Japanese Patent 74/85,095.
Kuwada, Y., Tawada, H., and Meguro, K. (1974b). Japanese Patent 74/108,096; *Chem. Abstr.* **82**, 140204n (1975).
Kuwada, Y., Souda, T., and Meguro, K. (1974c). Japanese Patent 74/109,396; *Chem. Abstr.* **83**, 10173m (1975).
Kuwada, Y., Souda, T., and Meguro, K. (1974d). Japanese Patent 74/126,699; *Chem. Abstr.* **83**, 28293k (1975).
Kuwada, Y., Souda, T., and Meguro, K. (1974e). Japanese Patent 74/134,698; *Chem. Abstr.* **83**, 28291h (1975).
Kuwada, Y., Meguro, K., and Maguoka, Y. (1975). Japanese Patent 75/18,498; *Chem. Abstr.* **83**, 97403b (1975).
Laboratoire Millot. (1964), French Patent M 2649; *Chem. Abstr.* **61**, 16073 (1964).
Laboratoires Dausse S. A., and Société B.M.C. (1969). French Patent 1,559,568; *Chem. Abstr.* **72**, 43431u (1970).
Laborit, H., Wermuth, C. G., Weber, B. P., Delbarre, B., Chekler, C., Baron, C., and Rosengarten, H. (1965). *Agressologie* **6**, 415.
Lamdan, S., Gaozza, C. H., Sicardi, S., and Izquierdo, J. A. (1970). *J. Med. Chem.* **13**, 742.
Lechat, P. (1966). *Acta Psychiatr. Scand., Suppl.* **42**, 15.
Lechat, P., Streichenberger, G., Boime, A., and Lemeignan, M. (1965). *Ann. Pharm. Fr.* **23**, 369.
Lemke, T. L., Hester, J. B., and Rudzik, A. D. (1972). *J. Pharm. Sci.* **61**, 275.
Lepetit S. p. A. (1959). British Patent 815,188; *Chem. Abstr.* **54**, 1553 (1960).
Leszkovszky, G., Erdely, I., and Tardos, L. (1965). *Acta Physiol. Acad. Sci. Hung.* **27**, 81.
Leszkovszky, G. P., and Tardos, L. (1970). *Acta Physiol. Acad. Sci. Hung.* **37**, 319.
LeVon, E. F., and Cusic, J. W. (1963). Belgian Patent 623,058; *Chem. Abstr.* **60**, 9291 (1964).
Lietz, W., and Matthies, H. (1964). *Acta Biol. Med. Ger.* **13**, 591.
Linares, H. (1972). German Patent 2,159,678; *Chem. Abstr.* **77**, 88351p (1972).
Lindberg, V. H. (1966). *Acta Pharm. Suec.* **3**, 161.
Lindberg, V. H. (1971a). *Acta Pharm. Suec.* **8**, 39.
Lindberg, V. H. (1971b). *Acta Pharm. Suec.* **8**, 647.
Lindberg, V. H., Pedersen, J., and Ulff, B. (1967). *Acta Pharm. Suec.* **4**, 269.
Lindberg, V. H., Bexell, G., Pedersen, J., and Ross, S. (1970). *Acta Pharm. Suec.* **7**, 423.

Lindberg, V. H., Bexell, G., and Ulff, B. (1971). *Acta Pharm. Suec.* **8**, 49.

Linder, J. (1973). German Patent 2,254,564; *Chem. Abstr.* **79**, 42533n (1973).

Linder, J. (1974). French Patent 2,222,089; *Chem. Abstr.* **82**, 156352v (1975).

Liske, E., and Forster, F. M. (1963). *J. New Drugs* **3**, 241.

L'Italien, Y. J., and Nordin, I. C. (1971). U.S. Patent 3,553,209.

Livingston, S., Villamater, C., Sakata, Y., and Pauli, L. L. (1967a). *J. Am. Med. Assoc.* **200**, 204.

Livingston, S., Villamater, C., and Sakata, Y. (1967b). *Dis. Nerv. Syst.* **28**, 259.

Lopresti, R. J., and Safir, S. R. (1958). U.S. Patent 2,852,523.

Lukes, J. J., and Nieforth, K. A. (1975). *J. Med. Chem.* **18**, 351.

Lunsford, C. D. (1965). German Patent 1,198,368; *Chem. Abstr.* **63**, 14867 (1965).

Lutz, A. H., and Schnider, O. (1959). U.S. Patent 2,916,498.

Lutz, A. H., and Schnider, O. (1961). Swiss Patent 356,771; *Chem. Abstr.* **56**, 14242 (1962).

Madronero-Palaez, R., Del Rio-Zambrana, J., Garcia-Topia, A., Martinez-Roldan, C., Fernandez, M. B., and Vila-CoroBarrachina, A. (1974). German Patent 2,319,174; *Chem. Abstr.* **82**, 4321w (1975).

Maffii, G. (1959). *Farmaco, Ed. Sci.* **14**, 176.

Maffii, G., Testa, E., and Ettorre, R. (1958). *Farmaco, Ed. Sci.* **13**, 187.

Marcucci, F., Guaitani, A., Kvetina, J., Mussini, E., and Garattini, S. (1968). *Eur. J. Pharmacol.* **4**, 467.

Marcucci, F., Mussini, E., Airoldi, L., Guaitani, A., and Garattini, S. (1972). *J. Pharm. Pharmacol.* **24**, 63.

Marcucci, F., Mussini, E., Martelli, P., Guaitani, A., and Garattini, S. (1973a). *J. Pharm. Sci.* **62**, 1900.

Marcucci, F., Mussini, E., Airoldi, L., Guaitani, A., and Garattini, S. (1973b). *Biochem. Pharmacol.* **22**, 3051.

Marmo, E., Imperatore, A., Amelio, A., and Caputi, A. P. (1971). *Gazz. Int. Med. Chir.* **76**, 1149.

Marshall, F. J. (1958). *J. Org. Chem.* **23**, 503.

Martinez-Roldan, C., and Fernandez, M. (1973). South African Patent 72/07,621; *Chem. Abstr.* **80**, 47850u (1974).

Martinez-Roldan, C., and Fernandez, M. (1974a). British Patent 1,346,014; *Chem. Abstr.* **80**, 133260h (1974).

Martinez-Roldan, C., and Fernandez, M. (1974b). U.S. Patent 3,830,821.

Martinez-Roldan, C., Fernandez, M., Castellano, B., and Jose, M. (1974). German Patent 2,329,895; *Chem. Abstr.* **80**, 95743h (1974).

Maruyama, I., Nakao, M., Sasajima, K., and Yanagihara, I. (1975). German Patent 2,264,668; *Chem. Abstr.* **82**, 170956b (1975).

Maruyama, S., Otorii, T., Kojima, T., Ishida, T., and Matsuda, K. (1965). *Niigata Igakkai Zasshi* **79**, 598; *Chem. Abstr.* **64**, 11732 (1966).

Maruyama, S., Kusumi, K., Katano, Y., Kawai, Y., and Matsuda, K. (1967a). *Niigata Igakkai Zasshi* **81**, 479.

Maruyama, S., Kusumi, K., Katano, Y., Kawai, Y., and Matsuda, K. (1967b). *Niigata Igakkai Zasshi* **81**, 600.

Maruyama, S., Kusumi, K., Katano, Y., Kawai, Y., and Matsuda, K. (1968). *Niigata Igakkai Zasshi* **82**, 547.

Mashimo, K., Miyazaki, M., and Tanaka, T. (1974a). Japanese Patent 74/81,374; *Chem. Abstr.* **82**, 16707q (1975).

Mashimo, K., Miyazaki, M., and Tanaka, T. (1974b). Japanese Patent 74/81,399; *Chem. Abstr.* **82**, 16807 (1975).

Mathes, W., and DaVanzo, J. P. (1963). French Patent M 2092; *Chem. Abstr.* **60**, 9252 (1964).

Mazzanti, L. (1960). *Riv. Neurobiol.* **6**, 69.

McEvoy, F. J., and Allen, G. R., Jr. (1970). French Patent M 7666; *Chem. Abstr.* **76**, 127028q (1972).

McEvoy, F. J., Greenblatt, E. N., Osterberg, A. C., and Allen, G. R., Jr. (1968). *J. Med. Chem.* **11**, 1248.

Meguro, K., and Kuwata, Y. (1971). German Patent 1,955,349; *Chem. Abstr.* **74**, 88078t (1971).

Meguro, K., and Kuwata, Y. (1974a). Japanese Patent 73/43,754; *Chem. Abstr.* **81**, 49709z (1974).

Meguro, K., and Kuwada, Y. (1974b). Japanese Patent 74/21,156; *Chem. Abstr.* **82**, 140195k (1975).

Meguro, K., and Kuwada, Y. (1974c). Japanese Patent 74/35,636; *Chem. Abstr.* **83**, 10177r (1975).

Meguro, K., and Kuwada, Y. (1974d). Japanese Patent 74/35,637; *Chem. Abstr.* **83**, 10176q (1975).

Meguro, K., and Kuwada, Y. (1974e). Japanese Patent 74/35,638; *Chem. Abstr.* **83**, 10178s (1975).

Meguro, K., Kuwada, Y., and Tawada, H. (1972). German Patent 2,153,519; *Chem. Abstr.* **77**, 88557k (1972).

Meguro, K., Tawada, H., and Kuwada, Y. (1974). Japanese Patent 74/24,074; *Chem. Abstr.* **83**, 164188g (1975).

Mehta, V. L., and Malhotra, C. L. (1966). *J. Pharm. Pharmacol.* **18**, 536.

Melone, G., Vecchi, A., and Maffii, G. (1961). British Patent 870,888; *Chem. Abstr.* **56**, 482 (1962).

Melson, F. (1962). *Acta Biol. Med. Ger.* **8**, 381.

Mennear, J. H., and Rudzik, A. D. (1966). *J. Pharm. Pharmacol.* **18**, 833.

Mennear, J. H., and Rudzik, A. D. (1968). *Life Sci.* **7**, 1265.

Mercier, J., Schmitt, J., Aurousseau, M., Etzensperger, P., and Bonifay, D. (1957). *Arch. Int. Pharmacodyn. Ther.* **113**, 53.

E. Merck, A.-G. (1965). French Patent M 3091; *Chem. Abstr.* **62**, 16209 (1965).

Metlesics, W., and Sternbach, L. H. (1974). U.S. Patent 3,812,103.

Meyer, H. J., and Kretzschmar, R. (1969). *Arzneim.-Forsch.* **19**, 617.

Mikhalev, A. I., Kudryashova, V. K., Konshin, M. E., and Zalesov, V. S. (1975). *Khim.-Farm. Zh.* **9**, 15.

Milkowski, W., Budden, R., Funke, S., Hueschens, R., Liepmann, H. G., Stuehmer, W., and Zengner, H. (1973). German Patent 2,221,558; *Chem. Abstr.* **80**, 27306t (1974).

Milkowski, W., Funke, S., Stuehmer, W., Hueschens, R., Liepmann, H. G., Zeugner, H., and Budden, R. (1974). German Patent 2,314,993; *Chem. Abstr.* **82**, 4325a (1975).

Mille, T., Pastorino, G., and Arrigo, A. (1969). *Arzneim.-Forsch.* **19**, 730.

Miller, C. A. (1958). U.S. Patent 3,004,037.

Millichap, J. G., Pitchford, G. L., and Millichap, M. G. (1968). *Proc. Soc. Exp. Biol. Med.* **127**, 1187.

Misra, R. S., Barthwal, J. P., Parmar, S. S., and Brumleve, S. J. (1974). *J. Pharm. Sci.* **63**, 401.

Misra, V. S., and Prakash, S. (1974). *Indian J. Pharm.* **36**, 142.

Mitchell, C. L. (1964). *Toxicol. Appl. Pharmacol.* **6**, 23.

Mochizuki, K., Ishibashi, K., and Miyaji, Y. (1974). Japanese Patent 74/31,672; *Chem. Abstr.* **81**, 49577e (1974).

Moffett, R. B. (1968a). U.S. Patent 3,412,091.
Moffett, R. B. (1968b). *J. Med. Chem.* 11, 1251.
Moffett, R. B. (1974). U.S. Patent 3,847,935.
Moffett, R. B., and Hester, J. B. (1972). *J. Med. Chem.* 15, 1243.
Moffett, R. B., and Rudzik, A. D. (1971). *J. Med. Chem.* 14, 588.
Moffett, R. B., and Rudzik, A. D. (1972). *J. Med. Chem.* 15, 1079.
Moffett, R. B., and Rudzik, A. D. (1973). *J. Med. Chem.* 16, 1256.
Morita, K., and Kawashima, T. (1973). Japanese Patent 73/08,631; *Chem. Abstr.* 79, 31953y (1973).
Morselli, P. L., Green, M., and Garattini, S. (1971). *Biochem. Pharmacol.* 20, 2043.
Motovilov, P. E., and Kozhevnikov, S. P. (1968). *Farmakol. Toksikol. (Moscow)* 31, 205.
Mucci, P., Bertolini, A., and Sternieri, E. (1965). *Boll. Soc. Ital. Biol. Sper.* 41, 1391.
Mueller, M., and Schmiedel, R. (1964). *Med. Exp.* 11, 149.
Murakami, M., Inukui, N., and Nakano, K. (1973). Japanese Patent 73/43,520; *Chem. Abstr.* 80, 133501n (1974).
Mussini, E., Marcucci, F., Fanelli, R., Guaitani, A., and Garattini, S. (1972). *Biochem. Pharmacol.* 21, 127.
Nacci, V., Filacchioni, G., Porretta, G. C., Stefancich, G., and Guaitani, A. (1973). *Farmaco, Ed. Sci.* 28, 494.
Nagar, S., and Parmar, S. S. (1971). *Indian J. Pharm.* 33, 61.
Nagar, S., Agarwal, V. K., and Parmar, S. S. (1972). *Curr. Sci.* 41, 215.
Nagar, S., Singh, H. H., Sinha, J. N., and Parmar, S. S. (1973). *J. Med. Chem.* 16, 178.
Naka, K., Sugiyama, M., and Wishibori, S. (1972). German Patent 2,164,104; *Chem. Abstr.* 77, 126666e (1972).
Naka, K., Sugiyama, M., and Wishibori, S. (1974). U.S. Patent 3,787,413.
Nakajima, R., Saji, Y., Chiba, S., and Nagawa, Y. (1970). *Takeda Kenkyusho Ho* 29, 153.
Nakajima, R., Take, Y., Moriya, R., Saji, Y., Yui, T., and Nagawa, Y. (1971). *Jpn. J. Pharmacol.* 21, 497.
Nakanishi, M., and Kobayashi, R. (1974). Japanese Patent 74/31,986; *Chem. Abstr.* 82, 139962b (1975).
Nakanishi, M., and Taira, T. (1973). Japanese Patent 73/43,743; *Chem. Abstr.* 81, 13404g (1974).
Nakanishi, M., Araki, K., Tahara, T., and Shiroki, M. (1971). German Patent 2,107,356; *Chem. Abstr.* 75, 129847j (1971).
Nakanishi, M., Tsumagari, T., Takigawa, Y., Shuto, S., Kenjo, T., and Fukuda, T. (1972a). *Arzneim.-Forsch.* 22, 1905.
Nakanishi, M., Shiroki, M., Tahara, T., and Araki, K. (1972b). German Patent 2,144,105; *Chem. Abstr.* 76, 140907v (1972).
Nakanishi, M., Tahara, T., and Araki, K. (1972c). German Patent 2,160,671; *Chem Abstr.* 77, 88555h (1972).
Nakanishi, M., Oe, T., and Tashiro, C. (1972d). German Patent 2,217,154; *Chem. Abstr.* 78, 29814q (1973).
Nakanishi, M., Tahara, T., Araki, K., and Shiroki, M. (1972e). German Patent 2,229,845; *Chem. Abstr.* 78, 84416m (1973).
Nakanishi, M., Arimura, K., and Tsumagari, T. (1973a). German Patent 2,302,383; *Chem. Abstr.* 79, 105270x (1973).
Nakanishi, M., Araki, K., Tahara, T., and Shiroki, M. (1973b). Japanese Patent 73/39,491; *Chem. Abstr.* 79, 53385s (1973).
Nakanishi, M., Shiroki, M., Tahara, T., and Araki, K. (1973c). Japanese Patent 73/39,496; *Chem. Abstr.* 79, 53387u (1973).

Nakanishi, M., Tahara, T., Araki, K., Shiroki, M., Tsumagari, T., and Takigawa, Y. (1973d). *J. Med. Chem.* **16**, 214.

Nakanishi, M., Yasuda, H., and Tsumagari, T. (1973e). *Life Sci.* **13**, 467.

Nakanishi, M., Araki, K., Tahara, T., and Shiroki, M. (1974a). German Patent 2,331,540; *Chem. Abstr.* **80**, 96036s (1974).

Nakanishi, M., Araki, K., Tahara, T., and Shiroki, M. (1974b). Japanese Patent 74/56,997; *Chem. Abstr.* **81**, 120715f (1974).

Nakanishi, M., Arimura, K., and Tsumagari, T. (1974c). Japanese Patent 74/87,697; **82**, 156350t (1975).

Nakanishi, M., Arimura, K., and Tsumagari, T. (1974d). Japanese Patent 74/87,698; *Chem. Abstr.* **82**. 156351u (1975).

Nakanishi M., Arimura, K., and Tsumagari, T. (1974e). Japanese Patent 74/88,896; *Chem. Abstr.* **82**, 125415p (1975).

Nakanishi, M., Arimura, K., and Tsumagari, T. (1974f). Japanese Patent 74/88,897; *Chem. Abstr.* **82**, 125414n (1975).

Nakanishi, M., Araki, K., Tahara, T., and Shiroki, M. (1974g). Japanese Patent 74/117,495; *Chem. Abstr.* **83**, 164250w (1975).

Nakanishi, M., Yokobe, T., Arai, T., and Abe, M. (1974h). Japanese Patent 74/134,677; *Chem. Abstr.* **83**, 10180m (1975).

Nakanishi, M., Yokobe, T., Arai, T., and Abe, M. (1975). Japanese Patent 75/41,860; *Chem. Abstr.* **83**, 193312y (1975).

Nedelec, L., and Frechet, D. (1973). German Patent 2,305,496; *Chem. Abstr.* **79**, 115455a (1973).

Nedelec, L., Frechet, F., and Cariou, M. (1973a). French Patent 2,174,771; *Chem. Abstr.* **80**, 82718d (1974).

Nedelec, L., Guillaume, J., and Allais, A. (1973b). German Patent 2,310,012; *Chem. Abstr.* **79**, 137115s (1973).

Neumeyer, J. L., Weinhardt, K. K., Carrano, R. A., and McCurdy, D. H. (1973). *J. Med. Chem.* **16**, 808.

Niigata, K., Murakami, M., and Tametani, H. (1974a). Japanese Patent 74/13,192; *Chem. Abstr.* **80**, 108588p (1974).

Niigata, K., Murakami, M., and Nozaki, Y. (1974b). Japanese Patent 74/51,289; *Chem. Abstr.* **81**, 120510k (1974).

Ning, R. Y. F., and Schwartz, M. A. (1975). German Patent 2,436,147; *Chem. Abstr.* **83**, 43393m (1975).

Ning, R. Y. F., and Sternbach, L. H. German Patent 2,163,522; *Chem. Abstr.* **77**, 126705s (1972).

Ning, R. Y. F., and Sternbach, L. H. (1972b). German Patent 2,163,642; *Chem. Abstr.* **77**, 140181z (1972).

Ning, R. Y. F., and Sternbach, L. H. (1972c). U.S. Patent 3,682,892.

Ning, R. Y. F., and Sternbach, L. H. (1973a). German Patent 2,260,446; *Chem. Abstr.* **79**, 78858m (1973).

Ning, R. Y. F., and Sternbach, L. H. (1973b). U.S. Patent 3,781,353.

Ning, R. Y. F., and Sternbach, L. H. (1974a). U.S. Patent 3,823,166.

Ning, R. Y. F., and Sternbach, L. H. (1974b). German Patent 2,335,282; *Chem. Abstr.* **80**, 121020s (1974).

Ning, R. Y. F., Sternbach, L. H., Pool, W., and Randall, L. O. (1973). *J. Med. Chem.* **16**, 879.

Noda, K., Nakagawa, A., Yamazaki, S., and Ide, H. (1974). Japanese Patent 74/21,681; *Chem. Abstr.* **81**, 77955v (1974).

Nordin, I. C. (1971a). U.S. Patent 3,553,207.

Nordin, I. C. (1971b). U.S. Patent 3,553,210.

Nordin, I. C. (1972). U.S. Patent 3,700,657.

Nordin, I. C. (1975). U.S. Patent 3,886,143.

Nordin, I. C., and Dewald, H. A. (1975). U.S. Patent 3,886,144.

Ochiai, T., Ishida, R., Ryuichi, N., Seiichi, I., and Ichizo, K. Y. (1972). *Jpn. J. Pharmacol.* **22**, 431; *Chem. Abstr.* **78**, 11554v (1973).

O'Dell, T. B., Napoli, M. D., and Mirsky, J. H. (1963). *Arch. Int. Pharmacodyn. Ther.* **58**, 83.

Okamoto, T., Akase, T., Izumi, T., Akatsu, M., Kume, Y., Inaba, S., and Yamamoto, H. (1972). German Patent 2,151,540; *Chem. Abstr.* **77**, 126709w (1972).

Okamoto, T., Kobayashi, T., and Yamamoto, H. (1974). Japanese Patent 74/45,874; *Chem. Abstr.* **83**, 9836y (1975).

Oklobdziji, M., Japell, M., Ostroversnik, S., and Jerman, P. (1973). German Patent 2,316,121; *Chem. Abstr.* **80**, 14966h (1974).

Olin Mathieson Chemical Corp. (1964). French Patent 1,367,738; *Chem. Abstr.* **62**, 1672 (1965).

Orcutt, J. A., Prytherch, J. P., Konicov, M., and Michaelson, S. M. (1964). *Arch. Int. Pharmacodyn. Ther.* **152**, 121.

Oroshnik, W. (1959). U.S. Patent 2,878,263.

Osumi, Y., Ban, T., Kamiya, S., and Shimamoto, K. (1967). *Acta Sch. Med. Univ. Kioto* **40**, 76; *Chem. Abstr.* **73**, 2307m (1970).

Ottaviano, G., and Pasqua, L. (1959). *Atti Accad. Gioenia Sci. Nat. Catania* **12**, 29.

Otto, N. (1970). *Arzneim.-Forsch.* **20**, 1497.

Owen, J. E., Jr., Swanson, E. E., and Meyers, D. B. (1958). *J. Am. Pharm. Assoc.* **47**, 70

Pala, G., and Sguanci, A. (1960). *Arch. Ital. Sci. Farmacol.* **10**, 70.

Pala, G., Donetti, A., Mantegani, A., and Sale, A. O. (1971). *J. Med. Chem.* **14**, 174.

Palosi, E., Trodgi, L., Rohricht, J., Szporny, L., and Kisfauldy, L. (1973). *Acta Pharm. Hung.* **43**, 218; *Chem. Abstr.* **80**, 128165b (1974).

Paragamian, V. (1970). U.S. Patent 3,502,647.

Parke Davis & Co. (1959). British Patent 823,265; *Chem. Abstr.* **54**, 5697 (1960).

Parke Davis & Co. (1961). British Patent 871,327; *Chem. Abstr.* **56**, 462 (1962).

Parmar, S. S., Rastogi, V. K., Gupta, T. K., and Arora, R. C. (1970). *Jpn. J. Pharmacol.* **20**, 325.

Parmar, S. S., Dwivedi, C., Chaudhari, A., and Gupta, T. K. (1972a). *J. Med. Chem.* **15**, 99.

Parmar, S. S., Gupta, A. K., Singh, H. H., and Gupta, T. K. (1972b). *J. Med. Chem.* **15**, 999.

Parmar, S. S., Misra, R. S., Chaudhari, A., and Gupta, T. K. (1972c). *J. Pharm. Sci.* **61**, 1322.

Parmar, S. S., Chaturvedi, A. K., Chaudhary, A., and Brumleve, S. J. (1974a). *J. Pharm. Sci.* **63**, 356.

Parmar, S. S., Joshi, P. C., Ali, B., and Cornatzer, W. E. (1974b). *J. Pharm. Sci.* **63**, 872.

Parmar, S. S., Pandey, B. R., Dwivedi, C., and Harbison, R. D. (1974c). *J. Pharm. Sci.* **63**, 1152 (1974)

Parravicini, F., Monguzzi, R., Banfi, S., and Pifferi, G. (1975). *Eur. J. Med. Chem.— Chim. Ther.* **10**, 252.

Pelczarska, A. (1969). *Arch. Immunol. Ther. Exp.* **17**, 118.

Pelz, K., and Protiva, M. (1967). *Collect. Czech. Chem. Commun.* **32**, 2840.

Perez de la Mora, M., and Tapia, R. (1973). *Biochem. Pharmacol.* **22**, 2635.

Pesson, M. (1969). British Patent 1,173,942; *Chem. Abstr.* **72**, 55474z (1970).

Pesson, M. (1972). U.S. Patent 3,681,330.

Pfeifer, S., and Pohlmann, H. (1974). *Acta Pharm. Suec.* **11**, 645.

Pfirrmann, R. W., and Hofstetter, E. (1972). German Patent 2,139,072; *Chem. Abstr.* **76**, 140503k (1972).

Phillippe, J. (1973). German Patent 2,239,311; *Chem. Abstr.* **78**, 124572t (1973).

Philips' Gloeilampenfabrieken. (1965). Netherlands Patent 64/03,115; *Chem. Abstr.* **64**, 5114 (1966).

Philips' Gloeilampenfabrieken. (1970). Netherlands Patent 68/10,133; *Chem. Abstr.* **72**, 121354p (1970).

Pieper, H., Krueger, G., Keck, J., Noll, K. R., and Kaehling, J. (1974a). German Patent 2,234,150; *Chem. Abstr.* **80**, 108589q (1974).

Pieper, H., Krueger, G., Keck, J., and Noll, K. (1974b). German Patent 2,304,095; *Chem. Abstr.* **81**, 136197z (1974).

Pieper, H., Krueger, G., Keck, J., and Noll, K. R. (1974c). German Patent 2,311,714; *Chem. Abstr.* **82**, 4323y (1975).

Pieper, H., Krueger, G., Keck J., Noll, K., and Kaehling, J. (1974d). German Patent 2,324,962; *Chem. Abstr.* **83**, 10175p (1975).

Pieper, H., Kruegger, G., Keck, J., and Noll, K. R. (1974e). German Patent 2,326,657; *Chem. Abstr.* **83**, 10174n (1975).

Pifferi, G., Consonni, P., Banfi, S., and Diena, A. (1969). *J. Med. Chem.* **12**, 261.

Podesva, C., and Vagi, K. (1975). U.S. Patent 3,842,094.

Poire, R., and Royer, J. (1969). *Electroencephalogr. Clin. Neurophysiol.* **27**, 106.

Polevoi, L. G., Kudrin, A. N., Grandberg, I. I., and Kost, A. N. (1968). *Izv. Timiryazevsk. Skh. Akad.* p. 192.

Portoghese, P. S., Pazdernik, T. L., Kuhn, W. L., Hite, G., and Shafiee, A. (1968). *J. Med. Chem.* **11**, 12.

Poschel, B. P. H., McCarthy, D. A., Chen, G., and Ensor, C. R. (1974). *Psychopharmacologia* **35**, 257.

Prince, A. K. (1965). *Biochem. Pharmacol.* **15**, 411.

Protiva, M., Seidlova, V., Svatek, E., Kakac, B., and Holubek, J. (1972). *Collect. Czech. Chem. Commun.* **37**, 2081.

Protiva, M., Kopicova, Z., Sedivy, Z., and Hradil, F. (1974a). Czech Patent 151,751; *Chem. Abstr.* **82**, 140186h (1975).

Protiva, M., Kopicova, Z., Sedivy, Z., and Hradil, F. (1974b). Czech Patent 151,759; *Chem. Abstr.* **82**, 140183e (1975).

Quick, C. M. (1973). U.S. Patent 3,726,981.

Raffauf, H. J. (1960). *Dtsch. Med. Wochenschr.* **85**, 2203.

Rajsner, M., Metysova, J., Nemec, J., and Protiva, M. (1975). *Collect. Czech. Chem. Commun.* **40**, 1218.

Ram, V. J., and Pandey, H. N. (1974). *J. Indian Chem. Soc.* **51**, 634.

Ramsby, S. I., Ogren, S. O., Ross, S. B., and Stjernstrom, N. E. (1973). *Acta Pharm. Suec.* **10**, 285.

Randall, L. O., Schallek, W., Scheckel, C., Banziger, R., and Moe, R. A. (1968). *Arzneim.-Forsch.* **18**, 1542.

Randall, L. O., Scheliek, W., Sternbach, L. H., and Ning, R. Y. (1976). "Psychopharmacological Agents" (M. Gordon, ed.), Vol. 3. Academic Press, New York.

Rastogi, V. K., Agarwal, V. K., Sinha, J. N., Chaudhari, A., and Parmar, S. S. (1974). *Can. J. Pharm. Sci.* **9**, 108.

Ratouis, R. (1972). U.S. Patent 3,679,802.

Ratouis, R., and Boissier, J. R. (1971). German Patent 2,048,547; *Chem. Abstr.* 75, 40404q (1971).

Rauh, C. E., and Gray, W. D. (1968). *J. Pharmacol. Exp. Ther.* 161, 329.

Raynaud, G., and Gouret, C. (1972). *Ann. Pharm. Fr.* 30, 735.

Razdan, R. K., and Mehta, A. C. (1973). South African Patent 72/05,019; *Chem. Abstr.* 79, 126312c (1973).

Reeder, E., and Sternbach, L. H. (1962). U.S. Patent 3,051,701.

Reeder, E., and Sternbach, L. H. (1963). U.S. Patent 3,109,843.

Reeder, E., and Sternbach, L. H. (1964a). U.S. Patent 3,136,815.

Reeder, E., and Sternbach, L. H. (1964b). U.S. Patent 3,141,890.

Reeder, E., and Sternbach, L. H. (1964c). U.S. Patent 3,144,439.

Reeder, E., and Sternbach, L. H. (1965). U.S. Patent 3,222,359.

Reeder, E., Sternbach, L. H., Steiger, N., Keller, O., and Stempel, A. (1962). German Patent 1,136,709; *Chem. Abstr.* 59, 12827 (1963).

Regnier, G., Canevari, R., LeDouarec, J. C., and Laubie, M. (1972). *Bull. Chim. Ther.* 7, 192.

Rice, L. N., Freed, M. E., and Hertz, E. (1965). U.S. Patent 3,218,326.

Robichaud, R. C., Gylys, J. A., Sledge, K. L., and Hillyard, I. W. (1970). *Arch. Int, Pharmacodyn. Ther.* 185, 213.

Roderick, W. R., Platte, H. J., and Pollard, C. B. (1966). *J. Med. Chem.* 9, 181.

Roehnert, H., and Carstens, E. (1973). German Patent 2,307,174; *Chem. Abstr.* 79, 136999w (1973).

Roussel-UCLAF. (1974). French Patent 2,224,146; *Chem. Abstr.* 83, 79097g (1975).

Roussinov, K. S. (1966). *C. R. Acad. Bulg. Sci.* 19, 985.

Rudzik, A. D., and Mennear, J. H. (1966). *Life Sci.* 5, 747.

Rusinov, K. (1966). *C. R. Acad. Bulg. Sci.* 19, 985.

Rusinov, K. S. (1968). *Izv. Inst. Fiziol., Bulg. Akad. Nauk.* 11, 141.

Russel, J. H. (1971). Swiss Patent 510,684; *Chem. Abstr.* 76, 14375q (1972).

Saeter, P. E., and Lindberg, U. H. A. (1968). U.S. Patent 3,401,172.

Safir, S. R., and Hlavka, J. J. (1956a). U.S. Patent 2,750,383.

Safir, S. R., and Hlavka, J. J. (1956b). U.S. Patent 2,762,804.

Safir, S. R., and Hlavka, J. J. (1956c). U.S. Patent 2,762,805.

Saji, Y., Mizuno, K., and Nagawa, Y. (1973). *Takeda Kenkyusho Ho* 32, 172.

Sakai, S., Inukai, T., Hara, Y., and Kitagawa, S. (1971). *Oyo Yakuri* 5, 581.

Sakai, S., Kitagawa, S., and Yamamoto, H. (1972). *Arzneim.-Forsch.* 22, 534.

Sakamoto, T. (1968). *Yonaga Igaku Zasshi* 19, 325; *Chem. Abstr.* 70, 76389z (1969).

Sallay, S. I. (1966). U.S. Patent 3,274,188.

Sallay, S. I. (1970). U.S. Patent 3,498,989.

Sam, J. (1961). U.S. Patent 2,978,458.

Sandoz, Ltd. (1965). Netherlands Patent 64/08,293; *Chem. Abstr.* 64, 2089 (1966).

Sandrini, M. (1965). *Farmacol. Riv. Ter.* 6, 327.

Sandrini, M., and Ferrari, W. (1973). *Riv. Farmacol. Ter.* 4, 319.

Santilli, A. A., and Osdene, T. S. (1970). U.S. Patent 3,534,058.

Sareen, K. N., Kohli, R. P., Amma, M. K. P., and Gujral, M. L. (1962). *Indian J. Physiol. Pharmacol.* 6, 87.

Sasajima, K., Ono, K., Nakao, M., Maruyama, I., Takayama, M., Katayama, S., Katsabe, J., Inaba, S., and Yamamoto, H. (1974). Japanese Patent 74/102,680; *Chem. Abstr.* 82, 155796f (1975).

Sasajima, K., Ono, K., Nakao, M., Maruyama, I., Takayama, M., Katayama, S., Katsabe, J., Inaba, S., and Yamamoto, H. (1975). Japanese Patent 75/05,385; *Chem. Abstr.* **83**, 28114c (1975).

Satzinger, G. (1967). German Patent 1,249,876; *Chem. Abstr.* **68**, 21966p (1968).

Satzinger, G. (1968). German Patent 1,271,118; *Chem. Abstr.* **69**, 77283b (1968).

Sawyer, G. T., Webster, D. D., and Schut, L. J. (1968). *J. Am. Med. Assoc.* **203**, 913.

Saxena, V. C., Bapat, S. K., and Dhawan, B. N. (1969). *Jpn. J. Pharmacol.* **19**, 477.

Schenone, P., Longobardi, M., and Bondavalli, F. (1975). *Farmaco, Ed. Sci.* **30**, 456.

Schindler, O. (1968). South African Patent 67/06,763; *Chem. Abstr.* **70**, 47297n (1969).

Schindler, O. (1970). U.S. Patent 3,541,088.

Schindler, W. (1960). U.S. Patent 2,948,718.

Schindler, W., and Blattner, H. (1966). Swiss Patent 408,021; *Chem. Abstr.* **66**, 28688s (1967).

Schindler, W., and Prins, D. (1964). Swiss Patent 375,722; *Chem. Abstr.* **61**, 6998 (1964).

Schmitt, J. (1966). French Patent 1,455,048; *Chem. Abstr.* **66**, 95096k (1967).

Schmitt, J., Comoy, P., Suquet, M., Callet, G., LeMeur, J., Clim, T., Brunaud, M., Mercier, J., Salle, J., and Siou, G. (1969). *Chim. Ther.* **4**, 239.

Scholler, W. A. (1958). German Patent 1,035,144; *Chem. Abstr.* **55**, 3625 (1961).

Schumann, E. L. (1965). U.S. Patent 3,167,563.

Schumann, E. L., Roberts, E. M., and Claxton, G. P. (1964). U.S. Patent 3,123,618.

Schwan, T. J., Honkomp, L. J., Castellion, A. W., and Burns, R. H. (1972). German Patent 2,214,474; *Chem. Abstr.* **78**, 4279f (1973).

Schwartz, M. A., Pool, W. R., Hane, D. L., and Postma, E. (1974). *Drug Metab. Dispos.* **2**, 31.

Scrollini, F., Caliari, S., Romano, A., and Torchio, P. (1975). *Arzneim.-Forsch.* **25**, 934.

Scudi, J. V., Reisner, D. B., and Childress, S. J. (1960a). U.S. Patent 2,947,754.

Scudi, J. V., Reisner, D. B., and Childress, S. J. (1960b). U.S. Patent 2,947,755.

Shapiro, S. L., Parrino, V. A., and Freedman, L. (1959). *J. Am. Chem. Soc.* **81**, 3996.

Shapiro, S. L., Freedman, L., and Parrino, V. A. (1960a). U.S. Patent 2,937,172.

Shapiro, S. L., Parrino, V. A., and Freedman, L. (1960b). *J. Org. Chem.* **25**, 384.

Shapiro, S. L., Parrino, V. A., and Freedman, L. (1960c). *J. Am. Pharm. Assoc., Sci. Ed.* **49**, 737.

Sharma, V. N., Singh, K. P., and Rathore, D. S. (1967). *Indian J. Med. Res.* **55**, 897.

Sharma, V. N., Vyas, D. S., and Madan, B. R. (1968). *Indian J. Med. Res.* **56**, 887.

Shenoy, V. D. (1974a). British Patent 1,359,287; *Chem. Abstr.* **81**, 120712c (1974).

Shenoy, V. D. (1974). British Patent 1,359,289; *Chem. Abstr.* **81**, 120711b (1974).

Shimizu, S., and Yamanaka, T. (1975). Japanese Patent 75/18,492; *Chem. Abstr.* **83**, 97402g (1975).

Shiroki, M., Tahara, T., and Araki, K. (1974). Japanese Patent 74/69,667; *Chem. Abstr.* **81**, 152238u (1974).

Shoeb, A., Anwer, F., Kapil, R. S., Popli, S. P., Dua, P. R., and Dhawan, B. N. (1973). *J. Med. Chem.* **16**, 425.

Sianesi, E., DaRe, P., Setnikar, I., and Massarani, E. (1973a). U.S. Patent 3,770,733.

Sianesi, E., Redaelli, R., Magistretti, M. J., and Massarani, E. (1973b). *J. Med. Chem.* **16**, 1133.

Sindelar, K., Svatek, E., Kakac, B., Hradil, F., and Protiva, M. (1972). *Collect. Czech. Chem. Commun.* **37**, 1195.

Singh, H. H., Nagar, S., and Parmar, S. S. (1972). *Curr. Sci.* **41**, 527.

Singh, J. M. (1969). *J. Med. Chem.* **12**, 962.

Singh, J. M. (1970). *J. Med. Chem.* **13**, 1018.

Singh, K. P., and Bhandari, D. S. (1973). *Arzneim.-Forsch.* **23**, 973.

Singh, K. P., Mahawar, M. M., Rathore, D. S., and Bhandari, D. S. (1969). *Indian J. Med. Res.* **57**, 1729.

Singh, S. P., Auyong, T. K., and Parmar, S. S. (1974a). *J. Pharm. Sci.* **63**, 960.

Singh, S. P., Chaudhari, A., Barthwal, J. P., and Parmar, S. S. (1974b). *J. Pharm. Sci.* **63**, 1948.

Singh, S. P., Chaudhari, A., Parmar, S. S., and Cornatzer, W. E. (1974c). *Can. J. Pharm. Sci.* **9**, 110.

Singh, S. P., Misra, R. S., Parmar, S. S., and Brumleve, S. J. (1975). *J. Pharm. Sci.* **64**, 1245.

Skinner, G. S., and Bicking, J. B. (1957). U.S. Patent 2,786,838.

Skinner, G. S., and Elmslie, J. S. (1959). *J. Org. Chem.* **24**, 1702.

Société des Usines Chimiques Rhone-Poulenc. (1958). British Patent 804,193; *Chem. Abstr.* **53**, 15111 (1959).

Société des Usines Chimiques Rhone-Poulenc. (1959a). French Patent 1,172,514; *Chem. Abstr.* **56**, 463 (1962).

Société des Usines Chimiques Rhone-Poulenc. (1959b). French Patent Addn. 71,322; *Chem. Abstr.* **56**, 4735 (1962).

Société d'Etudes Scientifiques et Industrielles de l'Ille-de-France. (1966). French Patent M 4500; *Chem. Abstr.* **68**, 95871a (1968).

Société d'Exploitation des Laboratoires Bottu. (1961). French Patent M 18; *Chem. Abstr.* **57**, 15251 (1962).

Somasekhara, S., Dighe, V. S., and Gokhale, S. V. (1972). *Indian J. Pharm.* **34**, 121.

Soncin, E. (1961). *Rass. Clin. Ter. Sci. Affini* **60**, 83; *Chem. Abstr.* **56**, 1970 (1962).

Song, J., Horton, R. L., MacGregor, P. T., and Markley, F. X. (1962). U.S. Patent 3,024,243.

Squires, R. F., and Lassen, J. B. (1968). *Biochem. Pharmacol.* **17**, 369.

Stefanova, D., Daleva, L., Kolchagova, R., and Zhelyazkor, L. (1972). *Tr. Nauchnoizsled. Khim.-Farm. Inst.* **8**, 129; *Chem. Abstr.* **79**, 38438t (1973).

Steiner, W. G., and Himwich, H. E. (1963). *Arch. Int. Pharmacodyn Ther.* **142**, 1.

Steinman, M. (1971). German Patent 2,115,906; *Chem. Abstr.* **76**, 34318u (1972).

Steinman, M. (1972). German Patent 2,138,773; *Chem. Abstr.* **77**, 5545f (1972).

Steinman, M. (1974). U.S. Patent 3,856,787.

Steinman, M., Topliss, J. G., Alekel, R., Wong, Y. S., and York, E. E. (1973). *J. Med. Chem.* **16**, 1354.

Sterling Drug Inc. (1959). British Patent 815,203; *Chem. Abstr.* **53**, 20099 (1959).

Sternbach, L. H., and Ning, R. Y. (1975). U.S. Patent 3,873,525.

Sternbach, L. H., and Randall, L. O. (1966). *Symp. CNS Drugs, Hyderabad, India*, p. 53.

Sternbach, L. H., and Saucy, G. (1964). U.S. Patent 3,120,521.

Sternbach, L. H., and Stempel, A. (1969). U.S. Patent 3,450,695.

Sternbach, L. H., Reeder, E., Keller, O., and Metlesics, W. (1961). *J. Org. Chem.* **26**, 4488.

Sternbach, L. H., Stempel, A., Sach, G. S., Saucy, G., and Smith, F. A. (1962a). Belgian Patent 615,194; *Chem. Abstr.* **59**, 12827 (1963).

Sternbach, L. H., Saucy, G., Keller, O., and Steiger, N. (1962b). Belgian Patent 616,023; *Chem. Abstr.* **58**, 10222 (1963).

Sternbach, L. H., Fryer, R. I., Feller, O., Metlesics, W., Sach, G., and Steiger, N. (1963). *J. Med. Chem.* **6**, 261.

Sternbach, L. H., Archer, G. A., Earley, J. V., Fryer, R. I., Reeder, E., Wasylew, N., Randall, L. O., and Banziger, R. (1965). *J. Med. Chem.* **8**, 815.

Sternbach, L. H., Sancilio, F. D., and Blount, J. F. (1974). *J. Med. Chem.* **17**, 374.
Stille, G., Braun, W., and Walter, M. (1957). *Arzneim.-Forsch.* **7**, 225.
Straw, R. N. (1968). *Arch. Int. Pharmacodyn. Ther.* **175**, 464.
Sulkowski, T. S. (1962). U.S. Patent 3,066,145.
Sulkowski, T. S. (1967). Belgian Patent 646,221; *Chem. Abstr.* **63**, 9972 (1965).
Sulkowski, T. S. (1967). U.S. Patent 3,336,306.
Sulkowski, T. S. (1969). U.S. Patent 3,423,421.
Sulkowski, T. S., and Childress, S. J. (1965). U.S. Patent 3,176,008.
Sulkowski, T. S., and Mascitti, A. A. (1969). U.S. Patent 3,466,297.
Sullivan, H. R., Jr. (1965). U.S. Patent 3,222,365.
Sumitomo Chemical Co., Ltd. (1963a). French Patent M 2087; *Chem. Abstr.* **61**, 1719 (1964).
Sumitomo Chemical Co., Ltd. (1963b). French Patent M 2088; *Chem. Abstr.* **61**, 1718 (1964).
Sumitomo Chemical Co., Ltd. (1969). French Patent M 6621; *Chem. Abstr.* **74**, 76458d (1971).
Sumitomo Chemical Co., Ltd. (1974a). Japanese Patent 74/35,280.
Sumitomo Chemical Co., Ltd. (1974b). Japanese Patent 74/45,876.
Sumitomo Chemical Co., Ltd. (1974c). Austrian Patent 314,544; *Chem. Abstr.* **83**, 28298r (1975).
Sumitomo Chemical Co., Ltd. (1975). Japanese Patent 75/2,517.
Sunjic, V., Kuftinec, J., and Kajfez, F. (1975). *Arzneim.-Forsch.* **25**, 340.
Surrey, A. R. (1964). U.S. Patent 3,155,655.
Surrey, A. R., and Webb, W. G. (1967). U.S. Patent 3,328,415.
Swift, J. G., Dickens, E. A., and Becker, B. A. (1960). *Arch. Int. Pharmacodyn. Ther.* **128**, 112.
Swinyard, E. A., and Castellion, A. W. (1966). *J. Pharmacol. Exp. Ther.* **151**, 369.
Szmuszkovicz, J., and Anthony, W. C. (1961a). U.S. Patent 2,978,459.
Szmuszkovicz, J., and Anthony, W. C. (1961b). U.S. Patent 2,984,670.
Tachikawa, R., Miyadera, T., Terada, A., Kawano, Y., Takagi, H., and Kamioka, T. (1972). German Patent 2,156,518; *Chem. Abstr.* **77**, 62034n (1972).
Tajana, A., and Pozzi, R. (1971). *J. Med. Chem.* **14**, 1017.
Takagi, H., Ban, T., Takashima, H., and Takashima, T. (1960). *Nippon Yakurigaku Zasshi* **56**, 1421; *Chem. Abstr.* **56**, 899 (1962).
Takagi, H., Kamioka, T., Kobayashi, S., Suzuki, Y., and Tachikawa, R. (1970). *Nippon Yakurigaku Zasshi* **66**, 107; *Chem. Abstr.* **75**, 18261u (1971).
Takagi, H., Kobayashi, S., and Kamioka, T. (1971). *Annu. Rep. Sankyo Res. Lab.* **23**, 1.
Takahashi, S. (1974). Japanese Patent 74/124,061; *Chem. Abstr.* **83**, 10044v (1975).
Takahashi, S. (1975a). Japanese Patent 75/46,662; *Chem. Abstr.* **83**, 193281n (1975).
Takahashi, S. (1975b). Japanese Patent 75/46,664; *Chem. Abstr.* **83**, 19328q (1975).
Takashima, Y., Hirohashi, T., Ishizumi, K., Akatsu, M., Inaba, S., and Yamamoto, H. (1974a). Japanese Patent 74/93,395; *Chem. Abstr.* **82**, 140214r (1975).
Takashima, Y., Hirohashi, T., Ishizumi, K., and Akatsu, M. (1974b). Japanese Patent 74/116,097; *Chem. Abstr.* **83**, 28292j (1975).
Takayama, M., Nakao, M., Katayama, S., Tanaka, Y., Inaba, S., and Yamamoto, H. (1973a). Japanese Patent 73/34,180; *Chem. Abstr.* **79**, 31925r (1973).
Takayama, M., Nakao, M., Katayama, S., Tanaka, Y., Inaba, S., and Yamamoto, H. (1973b). Japanese Patent 73/48,479; *Chem. Abstr.* **79**, 105092r (1973).
Takeda Chemical Industries, Ltd. (1973). German Patent 1,966,616; *Chem. Abstr.* **79**, 32119t (1973).

Takeda Chemical Industries, Ltd. (1974). Austrian Patent 315,169; *Chem. Abstr.* **82,** 31330e (1975).

Takiura, K., Yuki, H., and Yoshida, S. (1973). Japanese Patent 73/34,741; *Chem. Abstr.* **80,** 120757a (1974).

Tamagnone, G. F., Torrielli, M. V., and DeMarchi, F. (1974). *J. Pharm. Pharmacol.* **26,** 566.

Tashbaev, K. I., and Sultanov, M. B. (1965). *Farmakol. Alkaloidov* No. 2, 197.

Tawada, H., Meguro, K., and Kuwata, Y. (1974). Japanese Patent 74/21,157; *Chem. Abstr.* **82,** 140196m (1975).

Tenconi, F., Tagliabue, R., and Molteni, L. (1974). German Patent 2,339,790; *Chem. Abstr.* **80,** 133492k (1974).

Testa, E. (1960). British Patent 853,954; *Chem. Abstr.* **55,** 12432 (1961).

Testa, E., and Fontanella, L. (1957). British Patent 829,663; *Chem. Abstr.* **56,** 1429 (1962).

Testa, E., Fontanella, L., and Maffii, G. (1961). British Patents 872,447 and 872,449; *Chem. Abstr.* **56,** 453–4 (1962).

Testa, E., Fontanella, L., and Maffii, G. (1962). U.S. Patent 3,037,019.

Testa, E., Fontanella, L., and Maffii, G. (1963). U.S. Patent 3,094,518.

Testa, E., Fontanella, L., and Maffii, G. (1968). South African Patent 67/07,088; *Chem. Abstr.* **70,** 57602x (1969).

Theobald, W., Wilhelmi, G., and Krupp, P. (1967). *Pain, Proc. Int. Sym.,* p. 239.

Thomas, J. (1974). German Patent 2,403,357; *Chem. Abstr.* **81,** 136153g (1974).

Thyagarajan, G., Sidhu, G. S., and Zaheer, S. H. (1963). *Indian J. Chem.* **1,** 252 (1963).

Tinney, F. J. (1970). German Patent 2,005,276; *Chem. Abstr.* **73,** 131051x (1970).

Tinney, F. J. (1971). U.S. Patent 3,558,606.

Tinney, F. J., Sanchez, J. P., and Nogas, J. A. (1974). *J. Med. Chem.* **17,** 624. (1974)

Topliss, J. G. (1972). U.S. Patent 3,641,147.

Torchiana, M. L., Lotti, V. J., and Stone, C. A. (1973). *Eur. J. Pharmacol.* **21,** 343.

Trepanier, D. L. (1969). U.S. Patent 3,420,826.

Trepanier, D. L., Krieger, P. E., and Eble, J. N. (1965). *J. Med. Chem.* **8,** 802.

Trepanier, D. L., Sprancmanis, V., and Eble, J. N. (1966a). *J. Med. Chem.* **9,** 753.

Trepanier, D. L., Wagner, E. R., Harris, G., and Rudzik, A. D. (1966b). *J. Med. Chem.* **9,** 881.

Troponwerke Dinklage & Co. (1964). French Patent M 2581; *Chem. Abstr.* **61,** 14691 (1964).

Tsujikawa, T., Takei, S., Tsushima, S., Tsuda, T., Tsukamura, K., Sirakawa, K., Chiba, S., Nagawa, Y., and Yui, T. (1975a). *J. Pharm. Soc. Jpn.* **95,** 499.

Tsujikawa, T., Tsukamura, K., Takei, S., Sirakawa, K., Chiba, S., Nagawa, Y., and Yui, T. (1975b). *J. Pharm. Soc. Jpn.* **95,** 512.

Tursunova, S. A., Tushbaev, K. I., and Sutanov, M. B. (1968). *Dokl. Akad. Nauk Uzb. SSR* **25,** 34; *Chem. Abstr.* **72,** 41440y (1970).

Umio, S., and Ueda, I. (1972a). Japanese Patent 72/33,357; *Chem. Abstr.* **77,** 164541t (1972).

Umio, S., and Ueda, I. (1972b). Japanese Patent 72/33,358; *Chem. Abstr.* **77,** 164540s (1972).

Union Chimique-Chemische Bedryven Société Anon. (1966). Netherlands Patent 6,509,994; *Chem. Abstr.* **65,** 13671 (1966).

Upjohn Co. (1975). British Patent 1,402,810; *Chem. Abstr.* **83,** 179150m (1975).

Vander Burg, W. J. (1975). German Patent 2,443,057; *Chem. Abstr.* **83,** 58823a (1975).

vanderStelt, C., Hofman, P. S., and Funcke, A. B. H. (1971). *Arzneim.-Forsch.* **21,** 1415.

vanderStelt, C., Hofman, P. S., Funcke, A. B. H., and Timmerman, H. (1972). *Arzneim.-Forsch.* **22**, 133.

vanProosdij-Hartzema, E. G., Kok, K., and deJongh, D. K. (1958). *Arch. Int. Pharmacodyn. Ther.* **115**, 332.

Vejdelek, Z. J., Nemec, J., and Protiva, M. (1973a). *Collect. Czech. Chem. Commun.* **38**, 2768.

Vejdelek, Z. J., Kakac, B., Nemec, J., and Protiva, M. (1973b). *Collect. Czech. Chem. Commun.* **38**, 2989 (1973).

Vejdelek, Z. J., Newec, J., Sedivy, Z., Tuma, L., and Protiva, M. (1974). *Collect. Czech. Chem. Commun.* **39**, 2276.

Verma, M., Chaturvedi, A. K., Chaudhari, A., and Parmar, S. S. (1974). *J. Pharm. Sci.* **63**, 1740.

Vikhlyaev, Y. I., Ilinskii, B. I., Raevskii, K. S., Batulia, Y. M., Grandberg, I. I., and Kost, A. N. (1962). *Farmakol. Toksikol.* (*Moscow*) **25**, 27.

Viscontini, M., and Adank, K. (1962). German Patent 1,141,285; *Chem. Abstr.* **59**, 1593 (1963).

Viterbo, R., Brancaccio, G., and Perri, G. C. (1972). German Patent 2,202,788; *Chem. Abstr.* **77**, 140021x (1972).

Vohra, M. M., Pradhan, S. N., Jain, P. C., Chatterjee, S. K., and Anand, N. (1965). *J. Med. Chem.* **8**, 296.

von Bebenburg, W., and Offermanns, H. (1974a). German Patent 2,416,608; *Chem. Abstr.* **82**, 43481t (1975).

von Bebenburg, W., and Offermanns, H. (1974b). German Patent 2,419,386; *Chem. Abstr.* **82**, 73038w (1975).

Walser, A., and Fryer, R. I. (1974). *J. Med. Chem.* **17**, 1228.

Walser, A., and Sternbach, L. H. (1974). German Patent 2,335,281; *Chem. Abstr.* **80**, 96042r (1974).

Dr. A. Wander, A.-G. (1964). British Patent 961,106; *Chem. Abstr.* **61**, 13332 (1964).

Waring, W. S., and Whittle, B. A. (1969). *J. Pharm. Pharmacol.* **21**, 520.

Wasson, B. K., and Parker, J. M. (1963). U.S. Patent 3,099,662.

Watanabe, K., Goto, Y., and Yoshitomi, K. (1973). *Chem. Pharm. Bull.* **21**, 1700.

Watanabe, T., Sugiyama, M., and Yagi, T. (1973a). Japanese Patent 73/33,753; *Chem. Abstr.* **80**, 120972s (1974).

Watanabe, T., Sugiyama, M., and Yagi, T. (1973b). Japanese Patent 73/33,754; *Chem. Abstr.* **80**, 120968v (1974).

Weaver, L. C., Jones, W. R., and Kerley, T. L. (1963). *Arch. Int. Pharmacodyn. Ther.* **143**, 119.

Weber, K. H., Zeile, K., Danneberg, P., and Giesmann, R. (1969). German Patent 1,810,423; *Chem. Abstr.* **72**, 43753b (1970).

Weber, K. H., Minck, K., Bauer, A., and Danneberg, P. (1972). German Patent 2,103,745; *Chem. Abstr.* **77**, 140177c (1972).

Weber, R. O., Soeder, A., and Boksay, I. (1974). German Patent 2,240,665; *Chem. Abstr.* **82**, 171046s (1975).

Wehrli, P. A., Fryer, R. I., and Sternbach, L. H. (1971). U.S. Patent 3,553,206.

Wehrli, P. A., Fryer, R. I., and Sternbach, L. H. (1974). Swiss Patent 549,036; *Chem. Abstr.* **81**, 25702r (1974).

Wei, P. H. L., and Bell, S. C. (1970). U.S. Patent 3,509,156.

Wei, P. H. L., and Bell, S. C. (1972). U.S. Patent 3,644,401.

Wei, P. H. L., and Bell, S. C. (1973). U.S. Patent 3,714,147.

Weiss, B., and Ewing, C. G. T. (1959). *Am. J. Pharm.* **131**, 307.

Wellcome Foundation Ltd. (1964). British Patent 960,613; *Chem. Abstr.* **61**, 5664 (1964).

Welstead, J. W., Jr. (1972a). South African Patent 71/07,494; *Chem. Abstr.* **78**, 97732m (1973).

Welstead, J. W., Jr. (1972b). German Patent 2,157,309; *Chem. Abstr.* **77**, 101687z (1972).

Whittle, B. A., and Young, E. H. P. (1963). *J. Med. Chem.* **6**, 378.

Wilson, P. J. E. (1968). *Br. J. Clin. Pract.* **22**, 21.

Winn, M., Razdan, R. K., Dalzell, H. C., and Krei, J. R. (1975). German Patent 2,441,205; *Chem. Abstr.* **83**, 28106b (1975).

Winter, D., and Sanvard, S. (1965). *Stud. Cercet. Fiziol.* **10**, 425; *Chem. Abstr.* **64**, 13267 (1966).

Wirth, W., Hoffmeister, F., Friebel, H., and Sommer, S. (1960). *Dtsch. Med. Wochenschr.* **85**, 2195.

Witkowska, M. (1972). *Arch. Immunol. Ther. Exp.* **20**, 787.

Wohlfarth-Ribbentrop, A., and Schaumann, W. (1969). *Arzneim.-Forsch.* **19**, 2012.

Wolf, M. (1968a). U.S. Patent 3,394,143.

Wolf, M. (1968b). U.S. Patent 3,415,840.

Woodbury, D. M., and Kemp, J. W. (1970). *Pharm. Neuropsychophiatr.* **3**, 201.

Wright, W. B., Jr. (1956). U.S. Patent 2,767,191.

Wright, W. B., Jr., and Brabander, H. J. (1970). German Patent 1,936,721; *Chem. Abstr.* **73**, 120496 (1970).

Wunderlich, H., Femmer, K., Lugenhein, W., Carstens, E., and Fuerst, H. (1964). German (East) Patent 31,787; *Chem. Abstr.* **63**, 11581 (1965).

Yale, H. L. (1968). *J. Med. Chem.* **11**, 396.

Yamamoto, H., Inaba, S., Hirohashi, T., Yamamoto, M., Ishizumi, K., Akatsu, M., Maryama, I., Kume, R., Mori, K., and Izumi, T. (1972). German Patent 2,141,443; *Chem. Abstr.* **76**, 140916x (1972).

Yamamoto, H., Inaba, S., Hirohashi, T., Yamamoto, M., Ishizumi, K., Akatsu, M., Maryama, I., Kume, R., Mori, K., and Izumi, T. (1973a). Japanese Patent 73/43,513; *Chem. Abstr.* **80**, 133493m (1974).

Yamamoto, H., Inaba, S., Hirohashi, T., Yamamoto, M., Ishizumi, K., Akatsu, M., Maryama, I., Kume, R., Mori, K., and Izumi, T. (1973b). Japanese Patent 73/43,514; *Chem. Abstr.* **80**, 133500m (1974).

Yamamoto, H., Inaba, S., Okamoto, T., Hirohashi, T., Ishizumi, K., Yamamoto, M., Maruyama, I., Mori, K., and Kobayashi, T. (1974a). Japanese Patent 74/04,225; *Chem. Abstr.* **81**, 63692v (1974).

Yamamoto, H., Inaba, S., Okamoto, T., Hirohashi, T., Ishizumi, K., Yamamoto, M., Maruyama, I., Mori, K., and Kobayashi, T. (1974b). Japanese Patent 74/45,876; *Chem. Abstr.* **83**, 10185s (1975).

Yamamoto, H., Saito, O., Inaba, S., Inukai, T., Kobayashi, K., Faukumaru, T., Koga, Y., Honma, T., and Asami, Y. (1975). *Arzneim.-Forsch.* **25**, 795.

Yissum Research Development Co. (1968). French Patent M 5678; *Chem. Abstr.* **71**, 102006q (1969).

Young, E. H. P. (1966). British Patent 1,031,082.

Zakirov, V. B., and Kamilov, I. K. (1967). *Farmakol Alkaloidov Glikozidov*, p. 107; *Chem. Abstr.* **69**, 94881n (1968).

Zenitz, B. L. (1964). U.S. Patent 3,124,586.

Zilbermints, L. G. (1964). *Izv. Estestvennonauchn. Inst. Permsk. Gos. Univ.* **14**, 141; *Chem. Abstr.* **64**, 1220 (1966).

8

NONCYCLIC ANTICONVULSANTS

Wallace J. Murray and Lemont B. Kier

ABBREVIATIONS USED IN THE TABLES

Unless otherwise noted, the activities are expressed in milligrams per kilogram.

ES-A   The threshold procedure described by Putnam and Merritt (1937). Interrupted direct current or 60-cycle alternating current (half-wave or full wave). Occipital-mouth electrodes. Stimulus applied for 10 seconds to cats. Results expressed as follows: 0, no protection; +, elevation of threshold by 5–15 mA; 2+, elevation of threshold by 20–30 mA; 3+, elevation of threshold by 30–50 mA; 4+, elevation of threshold above 50 mA.

ES-Ba   The supramaximal shock procedure of Toman, Swinyard, and Goodman (1946). Sixty-cycle alternating current or rectangular current of 100 pulses/second. Corneal electrodes. Stimulus of three to five times threshold value applied for 0.2–0.3 second to mice. Results are expressed as follows: 0, no protection; +, incomplete protection with side effects; 2+, complete protection with side effects; 3+, complete protection without side effects.

MES   Drug administered orally to mice. Method essentially according to Swinyard *et al.* (1952) with ED_{50} (when given) determined graphically.

LD_{50} Lethal dose computed graphically; acute toxicity in 50% of experimental animals.

ED_{50} Results determined graphically as by method of Litchfield and Wilcoxon (1949). Effective dose in 50% of experimental animals.

Met-A   The method of Chen and Ensor (1950). Metrazole given in dose of 93 mg/kg subcutaneously to rats. Results expressed as follows: 0, no protection; +, 2/5 animals protected; 2+, 3/5 animals protected; 3+, 4/5 animals protected; 4+, 5/5 animals protected.

Met-B   The method of Toman *et al.* (1952). Metrazole administered in dose of 100 mg/kg subcutaneously to mice. Results expressed as follows: 0, no protection; +, incomplete protection with side effects; 2+, complete protection with side effects; 3+, complete protection without side effects.

Met   No seizure after subcutaneous pentylenetetrazole in mice or rats according to Swinyard *et al.* (1952). Drug administered po. ED_{50} determined graphically.

act.   No other data given. Most often a patent or an abstract.

inact. Inactive

sl. act. Slightly active

I. GENERAL

In their comprehensive review of anticonvulsant drugs studied prior to 1959 Close and Spielman include a variety of chemical classes. Among the compounds of the noncyclic chemical classes only a small number of compounds possessed significant anticonvulsant activity. Many of these compounds could be characterized as generalized central nervous system (CNS) depressants and thus seemingly lacked specificity in their action. Some, however, were highly active and led to further studies during the subsequent one and a half decades. Tables I–VI summarize the structures and activities of the most active of the noncyclic anticonvulsants listed by Close and Spielman.

There does not appear to be a common denominator among these agents in terms of structure and, with few exceptions, none were clinically valuable anticonvulsant agents. Except for the alcohols, all contain carbonyls and, except for the ketones, all might be considered amide- or imidelike compounds.

Among the alcohols, the tertiary and polyfunctional alcohols are the most active against seizures. Compounds such as 2-(*p*-chlorophenyl)-3-methyl-2,3-butanediol (phenaglycodol, **1**), marketed as a sedative, or 2,2-diethyl-propane-1,3-diol (diethylpropanediol, **2**), marketed as a spasmolytic, are among the most active at high doses. These compounds are more effective as antispasmodic agents or skeletal muscle relaxants than as anticonvulsants.

(1)   (2)

TABLE I   ACYLUREAS[a]

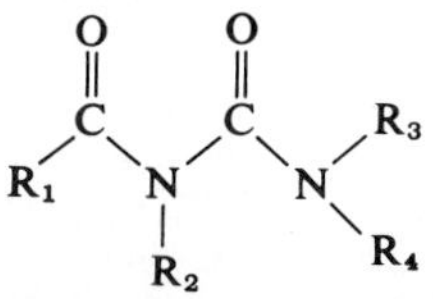

R_1	R_2	R_3	R_4	Activity
$C_6H_5CH_2$—	H—	H—	H—	ES-A, 4+/200; ES-Ba, 3+; Met-A, 4+/400
$C_6H_5CH(CH_3)$—	H—	H—	H—	ES-Ba, 3+
$C_6H_5CH(C_2H_5)$—	H—	H—	H—	ES-Ba, 3+
$C_6H_5CH_2$—	CH_3—	H—	H—	ES-Ba, 3+; Met-B, 3+
$C_6H_5CH_2$—	CH_3—	CH_3—	H—	ES-Ba, 3+
$(C_2H_5)_2CBr$—	H—	H—	H—	Met-A, 4+
$(i\text{-}C_3H_7)_2C(C_2H_5)$—	H—	H—	H—	Met-B, 3+

[a] Data from Close and Spielman (1961).

TABLE II   UREAS[a]

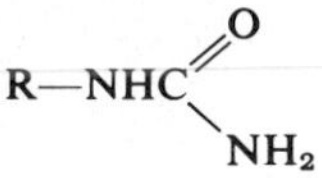

R	Activity
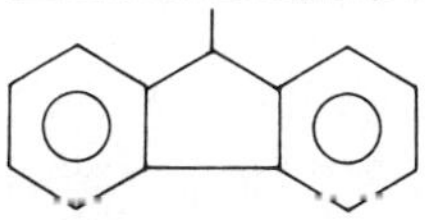	ES-Ba, 3+
$(C_6H_5)_2CH$—	ES-Ba, 3+

[a] Data from Close and Spielman (1961).

TABLE III   CARBAMATES[a]

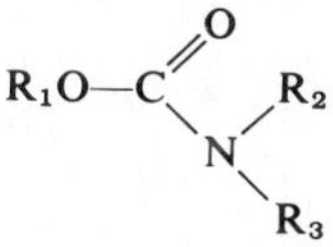

R_1	R_2	R_3	Activity
C_2H_5—	CH_3—	H—	Met-A, 4+
$C_6H_5CH_2$—	H—	H—	ES-A, 4+

[a] Data from Close and Spielman (1961).

TABLE IV   BIURETS[a]

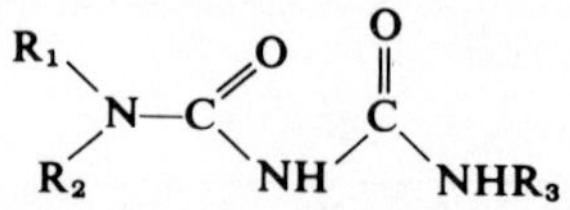

R_1	R_2	R_3	Activity
$C_6H_5CH_2-$	H—	H—	ES-Ba, 3+
$C_6H_5CHCH_3-$	H—	H—	ES-Ba, 3+

[a] Data from Close and Spielman (1961).

TABLE V   AMIDES[a]

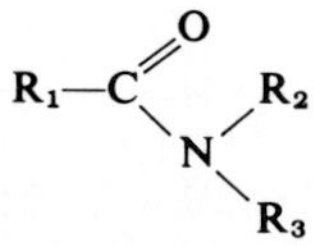

R_1	R_2	R_3	Activity
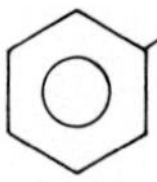 CH=CH—	H—	H—	ES-A, 3+ ; Met-A, 3+
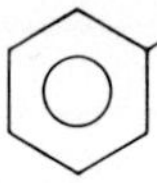 CH=CH—	CH_3-	CH_3-	Met-A, 4+
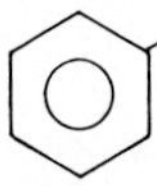 CH_2CH_2-	CH_3-	CH_3-	Met-A, 3+
CH_3-	$(C_6H_5)_2CH-$	H—	ES-Ba, 3+
CH_3CH- | OH	CH_3-	H—	Met-A, 4+
$(CH_3)_2C-$ | OH	CH_3-	H—	Met-A, 4+
$(C_6H_5)_2C-$ | OH	CH_3-	H—	ES-A, 3+
OH | $C_6H_5C-CH_2-$ | CH_3	CH_3-	H—	Met-A, 4+

[a] Data from Close and Spielman (1961).

TABLE VI   KETONES[a]

Compound	Activity
$C_6H_5CH{=}CHC{\overset{O}{\underset{CH_3}{\diagup\diagdown}}}$	ES-A, 3+
$C_6H_5C{\overset{O}{\underset{n\text{-}C_3H_7}{\diagup\diagdown}}}$	ES-A, 4+
$C_6H_5C{\overset{O}{\underset{i\text{-}C_3H_7}{\diagup\diagdown}}}$	ES-A, 4+
$C_6H_5C{\overset{O}{\underset{n\text{-}C_5H_{11}}{\diagup\diagdown}}}$	ES-A, 4+
$C_6H_5{-}C{\overset{O}{\underset{C_6H_5}{\diagup\diagdown}}}$	ES-A, 4+(3+)
$p\text{-}(i\text{-}C_5H_{11})C_6H_5C{\overset{O}{\underset{CH_3}{\diagup\diagdown}}}$	ES-A, 3+
$C_6H_5CH_2{-}C{\overset{O}{\underset{CH_2C_6H_5}{\diagup\diagdown}}}$	ES-A, 4+
$C_6H_5\overset{O}{\overset{\|}{C}}{-}\overset{O}{\overset{\|}{C}}{-}\overset{O}{\overset{\|}{C}}{-}CH_3$	ES-A, 4+
$C_6H_5\overset{O}{\overset{\|}{C}}CH_2\overset{O}{\overset{\|}{C}}CH_3$	ES-A, 4+
$p\text{-}HO{-}C_6H_5\overset{O}{\overset{\|}{C}}CH_3$	ES-A, 4+
(3-methoxy-4-hydroxyphenyl) $CH{=}CH\overset{O}{\overset{\|}{C}}{-}CH_3$	ES-A, 3+

[a] Data from Close and Spielman (1961).

Experimentally, ketones appear to be potent anticonvulsants. One plausible explanation for the activity of these agents may lie in their mode of metabolism. It is generally assumed that one of the physiological conditions that prevents the onset of seizures is systemic acidosis. The alcohols and ketones are principally metabolized to acid metabolites and if present in large enough amounts may lead to an acidotic state. It seems plausible that this may be the mode of action of these agents.

Beginning in 1948 many noncyclic variants of active cyclic anticonvulsant compounds were synthesized and tested. Many of these studies led to highly active compounds, but by and large most compounds synthesized were inactive or not as active as their barbiturate, hydantoin, or succinimide analogues. Furthermore, many of the compounds that showed activity in clinical trials and were subsequently approved for therapeutic use turned out to have undesirable side effects ranging from the innocuous, such as sedation, to the more serious, such as development of blood dyscrasias, personality changes, and drug-induced hepatic disorders.

The rationale behind the development of these compounds lay in the search for some common pharmacophoric pattern of anticonvulsant compounds. Using the fact that all of the active cyclic anticonvulsants of that time possessed an amide, imide, or urea subunit as part of their structure, noncyclic compounds possessing some variant of this fragment (3) were investigated. Probably the most familiar compounds examined in this regard were the phenylacylureas.

(3)

II. UREA DERIVATIVES

By considering 2-phenylbutyrylurea (4) as an open-chain model of phenobarbital (5) less a carbonyl carbon connection, Spielman *et al.* (1948) looked at a number of noncyclic compounds bearing structural resemblance to the anticonvulsant barbiturates. Subsequent testing of the anticonvulsant properties of these compounds revealed that phenylacetylurea (phenacemide, 6) was a potent anticonvulsant against seizures induced by maximal electroshock (MES) and metrazole (Met).

Phenylacetylurea was introduced as a therapeutic agent in 1951. However, dangerous side effects including personality changes (suicidal tendencies,

(4)   (5)   (6)

depression, aggressiveness), hepatic damage, and blood dyscrasias have led to its limited use. It is still used when patients have become refractory to other agents and is useful particularly in psychomotor epilepsy.

Ethylphenacemide (2-phenylbutyrylurea, pheneturide, 4) was shown to be active against electroshock but not metrazole seizures (Spielman, 1948; Orloff *et al.*, 1951; Sorel, 1957). Clinically, it has been effective in grand mal and petit mal, and reportedly good results have been obtained in psychomotor epilepsy.

A variety of disubstituted phenylbutyrylureas were synthesized and tested for anticonvulsant activities (Table VII). Their anticonvulsant activity in guinea pigs was less than that of pheneturide itself (Gold-Curbert and Toribia, 1963).

TABLE VII   DISUBSTITUTED
UREIDES[a]

R	Activity
H—	MES, act.
CH_3—	MES, act.
C_2H_5—	MES, act.
C_6H_5—	MES, inact.
p-C_2H_5—O—C_6H_4—	MES, inact.
o-CH_3—C_6H_4—	MES, act.
m-CH_3—C_6H_4—	MES, inact.
p-$CH_3C_6H_4$—	MES, inact.
p-CH_3O—C_6H_4—	MES, inact.
p-Cl—C_6H_4—	MES, inact.
o-Cl—C_6H_4—	MES, inact.
m-Cl—C_6H_4—	MES, inact.
p-Br—C_6H_4—	MES, inact.
p-$(CH_3)_2N$—C_6H_4—	MES, act.

[a] Data from Gold-Curbert and Toribia, (1963).

TABLE VIII STRUCTURE–ACTIVITY RELATIONSHIP OF THE PHENYL-
ACYLUREAS[a]

R_1	R_2	R_3	R_4	Results
Phenyl-	H—	H—	H—	Maximum activity for all types of experimental epileptic seizures, MES or Met
Phenyl-	H—	CH_3—	H—	Met protection increased
Phenyl-	CH_3—	H—	H—	Increased sedation; no change in anticonvulsant activity over phenacemide
Phenyl-	H—	H—	CH_3—	Reduced anticonvulsant activity
Phenyl-	H—	CH_3—	CH_3—	Elimination of Met protection
Phenyl-	C_2H_5—	H—	H—	Increased MES protection, decreased Met protection, and increased sedation
Phenyl-	Phenyl-	H—	H—	No activity

[a] From Mercier (1973).

Mercier (1973) has summarized the structure–activity relationship of the phenylacylureas, as shown in Table VIII.

The diphenyl analogue reported as having no anticonvulsant activity is the acylurea counterpart of diphenylhydantoin (DPH). The inactivity of this compound has been used as evidence that DPH is not transformed metabolically to diphenylacetylurea (Swinyard and Toman, 1950; Hazard *et al.*, 1951).

The 2-chloro and 2-bromo derivatives of phenacemide have also been synthesized. These compounds reportedly possess more activity than phenacemide in suppressing MES and Met seizures while having decreased toxicity (Job *et al.*, 1954). The 2-chloro derivative chlorphenacemide (phenyl-α-chloroacetylurea, **7**) was selected for clinical trials. Although the compound was shown to be superior to phenacemide in both its lack of toxicity and its

(7)

TABLE IX PHENYLUREAS

R	Activity	Reference
H—	MES, act.; Met-B, act.	Georgiev, 1965, 1967
	ES-Ba, 2+ ; Met-B, 0	Close and Spielman, 1961
2-CH$_3$—	MES, act.	Georgiev et al., 1964
3-CH$_3$—	MES, act.	Georgiev et al. (1964)
4-CH$_3$—	MES, act.	Georgiev et al. (1964)
2-C$_2$H$_5$—	Met-B, 1+	Georgiev and Vasileva, 1965
2-CH$_3$O—	Met-B, act.	Georgiev, 1967
3-CH$_3$O—	MES, act.	Georgiev, 1965a
4-CH$_3$O—	Met-B, act.	Georgiev (1965a)
2-C$_2$H$_5$O—	ES-Ba, 1+	Georgiev (1965a)
4-C$_2$H$_5$O—	Met-B, 1+	Georgiev (1965a)
3,4-(CH$_3$)$_2$—	Met-B, 1+	Georgiev (1965a)
2-Cl—	Met-B, 1+	Georgiev (1965a)
4-Cl—	Met-B, 1+	Georgiev (1965a)
2-OH—	ES-Ba, 2+ ; Met-B, 1+	Georgiev et al. (1964)
3-OH—	ES-Ba, 2+ ; Met-B, 1+	Georgiev et al. (1964)
2-H$_2$NCONH—	ES-Ba, 1+	Georgiev et al. (1964)
3-H$_2$NCONH—	ES-Ba, 1+	Georgiev et al. (1964)
4-H$_2$NCONH—	ES-Ba, 1+	Georgiev et al. (1964)

usefulness in the three major types of epilepsy, nothing further has been reported for chlorphenacemide. The drug has been marketed in Austria.

A number of other urea derivatives have also been tested and found to have anticonvulsant activity. Close and Spielman reported that aliphatic-substituted ureas gave maximal activity with branched six-carbon side chains. If both nitrogens of the urea were substituted, inactive compounds resulted. When aromatic substituents were used, the compounds having the greatest activity appeared to be those having a diphenylbenzyl (**8**) or a carbazole (**9**) nucleus. These compounds reportedly gave high activity against electroshock convulsions in mice and had no side effects. They were ineffective in guarding against Met-induced seizures.

(8)   (9)

A number of substituted phenylureas (10) were studied by Georgiev (1965a, b, 1967; Georgiev *et al.*, 1964; Georgiev and Vasileva, 1965). These compounds are compiled in Table IX. He found that these compounds offered no advantage over phenacemide or phenylurea. Substitution on the ring with electron-donating groups (*o*-methoxy, *m*-methoxy, *o*-ethoxy, *o*-amino, and 3,4-dimethyl) produced compounds with higher acute toxicity, manifested by markedly suppressed CNS activity. These compounds possessed anticonvulsant action equal to phenacemide but were less active than sodium barbital

(10)

and diphenylhydantoin (Georgiev, 1965a). The compounds exerted their strongest effect in suppressing Met seizures and were much less active in suppressing MES seizures. The substituted urea showing the strongest anticonvulsant effect was *m*-tolylurea.

Rousinov (1967) studied the anticonvulsive activity of phenylurea, *m*-tolylurea, and phenacemide on thiosemicarbazide convulsions. He found that the ED_{50} of *m*-tolylurea (75 mg/kg) was best, followed by that of phenacemide (90 mg/kg) and phenylurea (145 mg/kg).

Lazarova (1970) tested the anticonvulsant activity of 14 aryl-substituted ureas (Table X). When tested for acute toxicity in mice and rats, 2,3-dimethyl- and 2,5-dimethylphenylurea were determined to be least toxic, and *o*-phenylenediurea was the most toxic. *m*-Tolylurea, 2,4-dimethylurea, and *p*-tolylurea were the most active compounds in preventing Met convulsions in rats, equaling ethosuximide in potency. *o*-Phenylenediurea showed the greatest inhibiting effect against MES in rats and mice.

When urea is substituted with aliphatic cyclic groups, the resulting compounds are reportedly comparable in potency to trimethadione and diphenylhydantoin in preventing seizures in rats and dogs (Echague and Lim, 1962). Thus, 1-methylcyclohexylurea is active against Met seizures while 1-methylcyclopentylurea and 1-ethylcyclohexylurea are effective against both Met and MES convulsions (Table XI). All three possess sedative–hypnotic properties.

If the second nitrogen in phenylurea is substituted with alkyl groups of a propyl or larger size, inactive compounds result (Dobychina and Pechenkin, 1966) (Table XII).

Carbamazepine (11) may also be considered as a urea derivative. It has been found to be useful in controlling psychomotor seizures (Livingston *et al.*,

TABLE X   PHENYLUREAS

$$R-NHC\underset{NH_2}{\overset{O}{\diagup}}$$

R	Activity
	MES, act.
	Met, act.
	Met, act.
	Met, act.
	Met, act.
	Met, act.
	MES, act.

[a] Data from Lazarova (1970).

TABLE XI ALIPHATIC CYCLIC UREAS

$$R-NHC\overset{O}{\underset{NH_2}{<}}$$

R	Activity
1-Methylcyclohexyl-	Met, act.
1-Methylcyclopentyl-	Met, act; MES, act.
1-Ethylcyclopentyl-	Met, act.; MES, act.

[a] Data from Echague and Lim (1962).

TABLE XII N^2-SUBSTITUTED PHENYLUREAS[a]

$$\text{(phenyl)}-NHC\overset{O}{\underset{NHR}{<}}$$

R	Activity
$i\text{-}C_3H_7-$	inact.
$i\text{-}C_4H_9-$	inact.
$n\text{-}C_4H_9-$	inact.
4-Piperidyl-	inact.
3-Piperidyl-	inact.

[a] Data from Dobychina and Pechenkin (1966).

1967) and in other epileptic patients (Cereghino *et al.*, 1974). The dibenzoxazepine amide (12), being similar in structure to carbamazepine, provided electroshock protection equivalent to carbamazepine and one-half that of diphenylhydantoin but was ineffective against metrazole convulsions (Babington and Horovitz, 1973).

(11)   (12)

III. CARBAMATES

Carbamates such as meprobamate (13) and the acetylenic compounds methylpentynol carbamate (14) and carbimate (1-phenylpropyn-2-ol carbamate) (15) have been used as anticonvulsants. However, the duration of

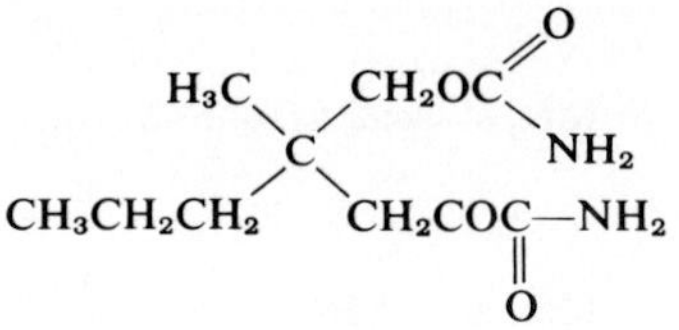

(13)

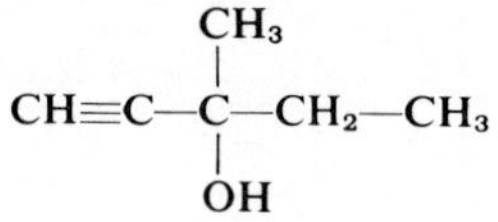

(14)

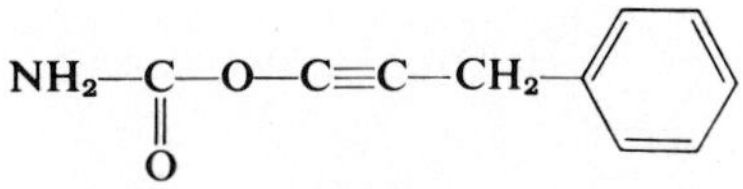

(15)

action of these compounds is very short, and this has led to their discontinuance as therapeutic agents. The search for additional anticonvulsant carbamates continued through the 1960's. Daleva and Nikolova (1964) and Nikolova (1965) reported that several esters of carbamic acid were effective against all experimentally induced convulsions but were most effective in

TABLE XIII   CARBAMATES

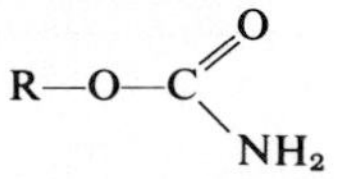

R	Activity	Reference
CH_3—	Met, inact.	Daleva and Nikolova (1964)
	MES, inact.	Nikolova (1965)
C_3H_7—	MES, act.	Nikolova (1965)
C_4H_9—	MES, act.	Nikolova (1965)
i-C_4H_9—	MES, act.	Nikolova (1965)
n-C_5H_{11}—	Met, act.	Daleva and Nikolova (1964)
i-C_5H_{11}—	Met, act.	Daleva and Nikolova (1964)
Cyclopentyl-	MES, act.	Nikolova (1965)
Cyclohexyl-	Met, act.	Daleva and Nikolova (1964)
Benzyl-	Met, act.	Daleva and Nikolova (1964)
n-C_7H_{15}—	MES, act.	Nikolova (1965)
n-C_8H_{17}—	MES, inact.	Nikolova (1965)
	Met, inact.	Daleva and Nikolova (1964)
i-C_8H_{17}—	MES, inact.	Nikolova (1965)

TABLE XIV   CARBAMATES

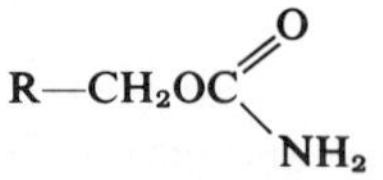

$$R-CH_2OC\underset{NH_2}{\overset{O}{\diagup}}$$

R	Activity
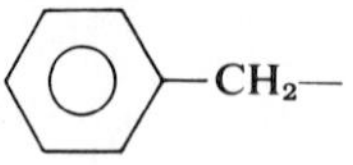 ⬡—CH_2—	Met, sl. act.; $LD_{50} > 2$
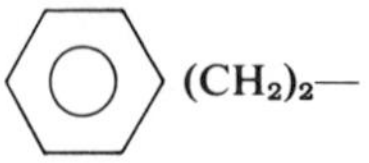 ⬡ $(CH_2)_2$—	Met, act.; LD_{50} 1.2
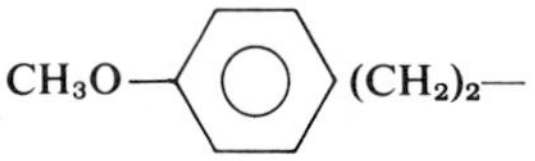 CH_3O—⬡ $(CH_2)_2$—	Met, sl. act.; $LD_{50} > 2$
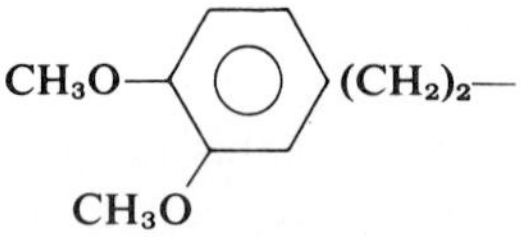 CH_3O—⬡ $(CH_2)_2$— CH_3O	Met, sl. act.; LD_{50} 1.3
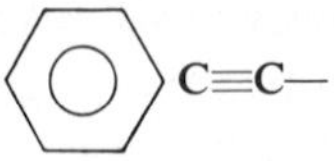 ⬡ $C\equiv C$—	Met, inact.; LD_{50} 0.8
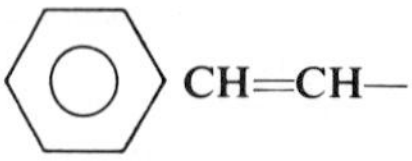 ⬡ $CH=CH$—	LD_{50} 1.0

a Data from Boissier *et al.* (1962).

preventing electroshock convulsions (Table XIII). The activity increased as substitution went from the methyl to amyl esters and decreased with the higher analogues. The anticonvulsant action of some phenylpropanol and phenylpropenol carbamates has also been reported (Bossier *et al.*, 1962, Table XIV). Methyl α-phenylethylcarbamate (**16**) possesses anticonvulsive properties against electroshock and has no sedative–hypnotic effects. It does, however, potentiate the action of narcotics (Joultry, 1963). Cyclohexane and cyclohexane dicarbamates (Table XV) possess anticonvulsant and sedative action.

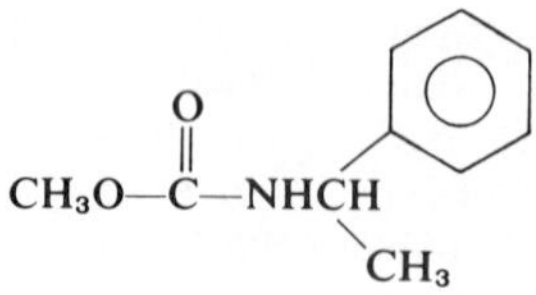

$$CH_3O-\overset{O}{\overset{\|}{C}}-NHCH\underset{CH_3}{}$$

(**16**)

$$ROC\overset{O}{\diagup}NHCH_2CH_2CH_2OC\underset{NHR^1}{\overset{O}{\diagup}}$$

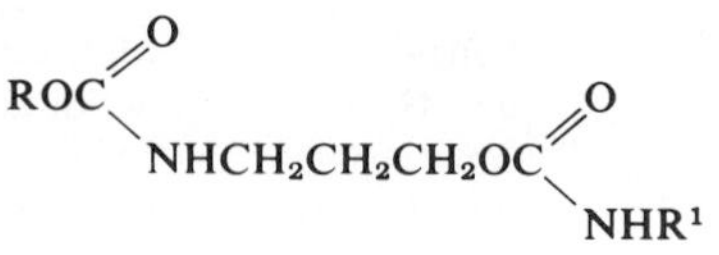

(**17**)

TABLE XV   CYCLOALKYL DICARBAMATES[a]

R	R_1	R_2	Activity
H—	H—	*i*-Pr—	No data
H—	Me—	Me—	No data
Me—	H—	*i*-Pr—	No data

[a] Lincoln (1963), British Patent 932,965 (1963).

TABLE XVI   CARBAMOYLALKYL CARBAMATES[a]

R	R_1	Activity
C_2H_5—	C_4H_9—	MES, act.
C_2H_5—	C_5H_{11}—	MES, act.

[a] Data from Yamamoto *et al.* (1963).

In addition to these single carbamate compounds, carbamoylalkyl carbamates (**17**) were found to possess muscle relaxant and anticonvulsant properties (Table XVI). They are said to be superior to mephenesin and meprobamate in preventing paralytic electroshock in mice but lack antichemoshock activity.

IV. CARBOXYLIC ACIDS AND AMIDES

Structurally, the simplest compounds possessing anticonvulsant properties are carboxylic acids and their amides. Merritt and Putnam (1945) showed that diphenylacetic acid (**18**) was very effective in preventing electroshock seizures in cats. Sterically hindered amides, especially α-hydroxyamides, were found to be efficacious in both Met and MES seizure prevention (Table XVII).

TABLE XVII   AMIDES

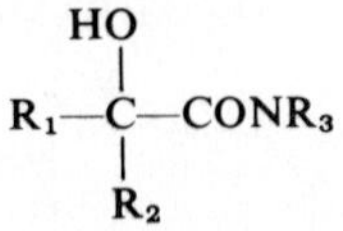

$$HO$$
$$R_1-\overset{\displaystyle |}{\underset{\displaystyle |}{C}}-CONR_3$$
$$R_2$$

R_1	R_2	R_3	Activity	Reference
CH_3-	$H-$	CH_3-	Met, 4+	Long (1952)
CH_3-	CH_3-	CH_3-	Met, 4+	Long (1952)
C_6H_5-	$H-$	C_6H_5-	ES-Ba, 3+	Merritt and Putnam (1945)

Meunier *et al.* (1963) and Lebreton *et al.* (1964) studied the experimental antiepileptic properties of *n*-dipropylacetic acid (Depakine, Valproate sodium, DPA, **19**). This open-chain acid has been marketed as an anticonvulsant in Europe since the mid-1960's and is currently undergoing clinical trials in the United States. The sodium salt at a dose of 200 mg/kg in rats, mice, and

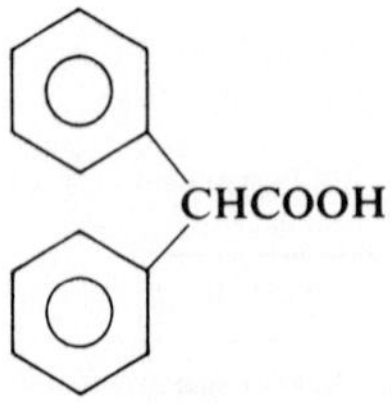

(18) 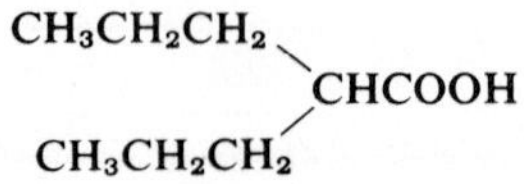   **(19)**

rabbits protects against Met (Meunier *et al.*, 1963) and MES convulsions (Godin *et al.*, 1969). The LD_{50} was found to be 800 mg/kg. Among other straight-chain acids studied by Carraz (1967) (Table XVIII) unsaturated straight-chain acids and α-keto acids appear to have no effect on metrazole seizures. Compounds having substitution at the α-carbon are the most active. There seems to be a dramatic dropoff in activity when one goes from di-*n*-propyl acetate (100%) to di-*n*-butyl acetate (0%). If the efficacy of DPA were dependent solely on its lipophilic properties or partitioning ability, one would not expect such a dramatic change in activity with only a two-carbon change. The aryl-substituted acetic acid **20** was also found to have electroshock protective action (Rozkowski *et al.*, 1972).

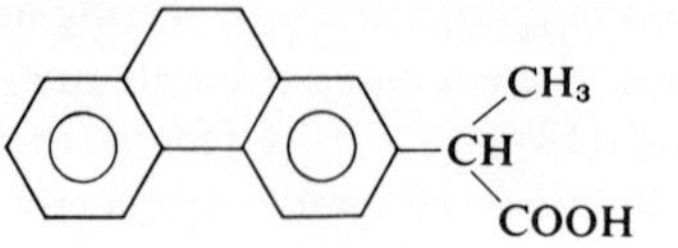

(20)

TABLE XVIII   CARBOXYLIC ACIDS[a]

$$R_2-\underset{\underset{R_3}{\overset{|}{\,}}}{\overset{\overset{R_1}{|}}{C}}-COOH$$

R_1	R_2	R_3	Activity[b]
$n\text{-}C_3H_7-$	$n\text{-}C_3H_7-$	$H-$	100
$i\text{-}C_6H_{13}-$	$H-$	$H-$	100
C_2H_5-	C_2H_5-	$H-$	80
CH_3-	CH_3-	C_2H_5-	80
CH_3-	CH_3-	CH_3-	80
CH_3-	CH_3-	$H-$	20
$n\text{-}C_4H_9-$	$n\text{-}C_4H_9-$	$H-$	0
$i\text{-}C_3H_7-$	$H-$	$H-$	0
$CH_2{=}CH-$	$H-$	$H-$	0

Compound	Activity[b]
$CH_3CH{=}CHCOOH$	0
$CH_3CH{=}\underset{\underset{CH_3}{\overset{|}{\,}}}{C}COOH$	0
$CH_3CH_2\overset{\overset{O}{\overset{\|}{\,}}}{C}\diagdown_{COOH}$	0
$CH_3(CH_2)_2\overset{\overset{O}{\overset{\|}{\,}}}{C}\diagdown_{COOH}$	0
$CH_3(CH_2)_3\overset{\overset{O}{\overset{\|}{\,}}}{C}\diagdown_{COOH}$	0

[a] Data from Carraz (1967).
[b] Percent mice surviving an ip injection of 80 mg/kg pentylenetetrazole compared to 200 mg/kg of di-*n*-propylacetic acid.

The amide of dipropylacetic acid (Depamide) was found by Carraz *et al.* (1964) to be as effective as the acid at one-half the dose. Interestingly, the incorporation of an amine onto the dipropylamide structure gives compounds with strong convulsive effects (Table XIX). If the amide nitrogen is disubstituted with an isopropyl group a narcotic effect at 100 mg/kg in mice is noted. It was not determined if the convulsant effect of the amine-substituted amides could be reversed by treatment with Depamide or Depakine.

TABLE XIX   DIPROPYLAMIDE
AMINES[a]

$$(C_3H_7)_2CHC\overset{\displaystyle O}{\underset{\displaystyle NHR}{}}$$

R	Activity
—$(CH_2)_3N(C_2H_5)_2$	Convulsant
—$(CH_2)_2N(i\text{-}C_3H_7)_2$	Convulsant
—$CH_2N(CH_3)_2$	Convulsant
—$(i\text{-}C_3H_7)_2$	Narcotic

[a] Data from Carraz *et al.* (1964).

Earlier studies with amides have shown them to have anticonvulsant properties (Close and Spielman, 1961), but generally their strong sedative properties have prevented their coming to clinical trial. N-Benzyl-3-chloro-propionamide (beclamide, **21**) was found to have high anticonvulsant action and low toxicity in experimental animals, but its use clinically resulted in very variable results. The drug was later withdrawn from usage. Fenaclone (N-phenylethyl-β-chloropropionamide, **22**), which might be considered a homologue of beclamide, was found to prevent audiogenic, MES, and Met

(21)   (22)

convulsions (Toreva, 1967). It is currently being used in the Soviet Union to treat grand mal epilepsy (Maskovskij, 1972). Atrolactamide (2-phenyl-2-hydroxypropionamide, Themisone, **23**) was evaluated clinically and found to be effective in grand mal, but development of several nervous, cutaneous, and blood complications forced it to be withdrawn (Mercier, 1973).

Benzilamide (**24**) α-methoxydiphenylacetamide (**25**), and N-ethyldiphenyl-acetamide (**26**) were found to prevent MES convulsions with minimal side effects. This formed the basis for their clinical testing as anticonvulsant agents (Zalesov, 1964).

(23)

(24)   **(25)**   **(26)**

Amides of aryl-substituted benzoic acid also possess anticonvulsant activity. Decimemide (3,5-dimethoxy-4-*n*-deciloxybenzamide, **27**) is reported to be more than twice as effective as phenacemide in preventing both electroshock and Met seizures in mice and rats (J. Borsey, S. Elek, S. Polgári, and I. Schäfer, private communication, 1968). The LD_{50} was 3 gm/kg in mice and 1.7 gm/kg in rats. When decimemide was administered orally an ED_{50} of 4.2 mg/kg was obtained for inhibition of electroshock convulsions, while for

(27)

Met inhibition the ED_{50} was 24 mg/kg. The values for phenacemide to inhibit these convulsions was 19 and 48 mg/kg, respectively. Clinical trials have shown decimemide to have a marked antiepileptic effect in the treatment of temporal (psychomotor) epilepsy and to be beneficial in grand mal seizures.

Horrom (1963) studied the tranquilizing and anticonvulsant activities of a number of amides of 3,4,5,-trisubstituted benzoic acid and found them to be useful agents (Table XX).

Diphenylacetic acid amides were studied by Johnsen *et al.* (1962) (Table XXI). They found that *N*-benzyl-2-hydroxy- and *N*-benzyl-2-acetoxydiphenyl-acetamides (**28, 29**) showed anti-Met activity, and **28** abolished the convulsive actions of electroshock.

Davis *et al.* (1964) and Funcke and Zandberg (1970) found that cyheptamide (**30**) has anticonvulsant properties, although it is not as potent as sodium phenobarbital or carbamazepine (**11**) (Table XXII). Cyheptamide, however, exhibited considerably less neurotoxicity than the other two agents and because of this Funcke and Zandberg claim cyheptamide to be superior. They studied other tricyclic amides (Table XXII) and found the amide **31** to be a good anticonvulsant as well.

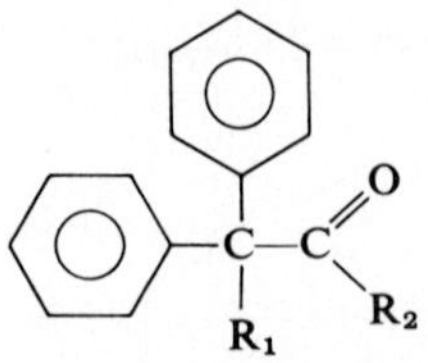

(28) $R_1 = $ —OH, $R_2 = $ —NHCH$_2$

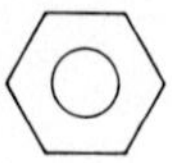

(29) $R_2 = $ —OCOCH$_3$, $R_2 = $ —NHCH$_2$

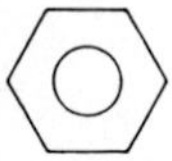

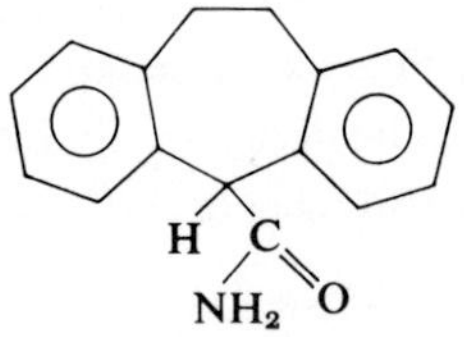

(30)

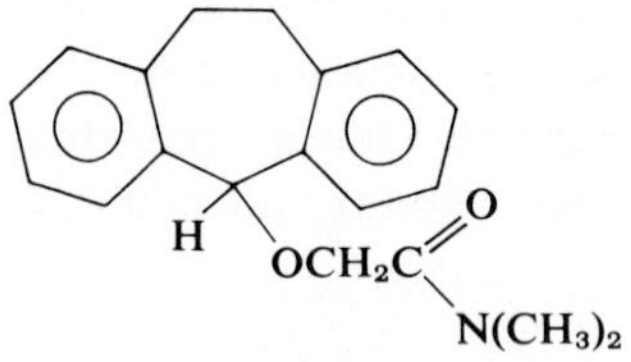

(31)

TABLE XX   TRISUBSTITUTED BENZOIC ACID AMIDES[a]

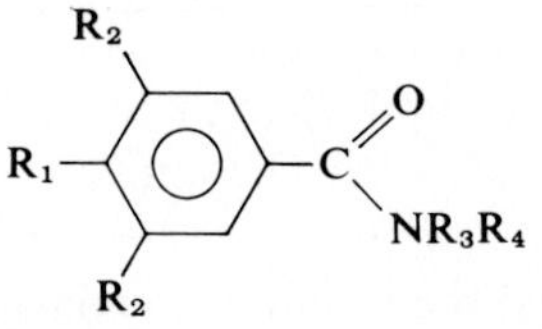

R_1	R_2	R_3	R_4	Activity
NH$_2$—	Cl—	H—	Cyclopropyl-	No data
NH$_2$—	Br—	H—	Cyclopropyl-	No data
N(CH$_3$)$_2$—	Cl—	H—	C$_3$H$_7$	No data
NH$_2$—	Cl—	H—	t-C$_4$H$_9$—	No data
NH$_2$—	Cl—	H—	CH$_2$CH=CH$_2$—	No data
NH$_2$—	Cl—	H—	CH$_2$C≡CH—	No data
NH$_2$—	Cl—	C$_3$H$_7$—	C$_3$H$_7$—	No data
NH$_2$—	Cl—	i-C$_3$H$_7$—	i-C$_3$H$_7$—	No data
NH$_2$—	Cl—	H—	—CH$_2$—(cyclopropyl)	No data
NH$_2$—	Cl—	H—	Cyclobutyl-	No data
NH$_2$—	Cl—	Cyclopropyl—	(CH$_2$)$_2$OH	No data

[a] Data from Horrom (1963).

TABLE XXI DIPHENYLACETIC ACID AMIDES[a]

$$(C_6H_5)_2-\overset{\displaystyle |}{\underset{\displaystyle R_1}{C}}-C\overset{\displaystyle O}{\underset{\displaystyle R_2}{\diagup}}$$

R_1	R_2	Activity
Cl—	—NHCH$_2$C$_6$H$_5$	Met, inact.; MES, inact.
Cl—	—N(CH$_3$)CH$_2$C$_6$H$_5$	Met, inact.; MES, inact.
—OH	—NHCH$_2$C$_6$H$_5$	Met, act.; MES, inact.
—OH	—N(CH$_3$)CH$_2$C$_6$H$_5$	Met, inact.; MES, inact.
—OCOCH$_3$	—NHCH$_2$C$_6$H$_5$	Met, sl. act.; MES, act.
—OC$_2$H$_5$N(CH$_3$)$_2$	—NHCH$_2$C$_6$H$_5$	Met, inact.; MES, inact.
—NHCH$_2$C$_6$H$_5$	—NH$_2$	Met, inact; MES, inact.
—NHCH$_2$C$_6$H$_5$	—NHCH$_2$C$_6$H$_5$	Met, inact.; MES, inact.

[a] Data from Johnsen *et al.* (1962).

TABLE XXII AMIDES[a]

Compound	Activity (ED$_{50}$)
Sodium phenobarbital	MES, 17.8; Met, 3.6
Carbamazepine	MES, 18.8; Met, 11.5
	MES, 33; Met, 14.5
	MES, 125; Met, 620

[a] Data from Funcke and Zandberg (1970).

The amide lidocaine (**32**) when given intravenously in doses of 1–2 mg/kg in cats suppressed electroencephalogenic manifestations of epileptic seizures (Bernhard and Bohm, 1954). In man intravenous lidocaine temporarily halts grand mal and status epilepticus. In doses higher than 2 mg/kg convulsions ensue. Since convulsions are known to result when amines are incorporated into the dipropylacetamide structure, it would be interesting to determine the result if the amine nitrogen were replaced with a methylene group.

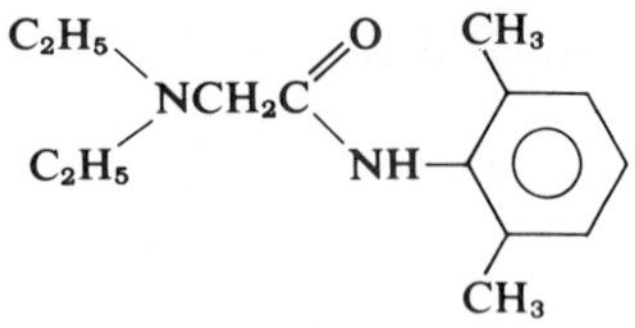

$$C_2H_5\diagdown\!\!\!$$

(structure, compound 32)

(32)

V. SULFONAMIDES

Sulfonamides are also known to have anticonvulsant activity (Close and Spielman, 1961; Mercier, 1973). Acetazolamide **(33)** received the attention of earlier studies. The mode of action of acetazolamide and other sulfonamides is believed to reside in their ability to inhibit carbonic anhydrase activity (Millichap *et al.*, 1955; Nishimura, 1963; Tanimukai *et al.*, 1965) with a passive mechanism involving a buildup of excess carbon dioxide, which inhibits nerve transmission (Nishimura *et al.*, 1963). The metabolic acidosis

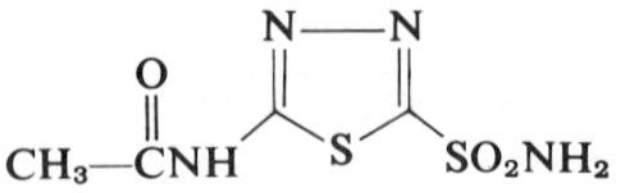

(structure, compound 33)

(33)

produced by inhibition of renal carbonic anhydrase may play a secondary role. Acetazolamide has been successfully used in the treatment of moderately severe grand mal; however, there are reports of it being ineffective in adult epileptics and children with petit mal (Spinks and Waring, 1961). In Europe it is used principally for psychomotor therapy and usually as an adjunct medication or with other antiepileptic drugs. Tolerance to the pharmacological action of the drug develops quickly, which also limits its effectiveness.

N^5-Alkyl- and N^5-acylsulfonamide derivatives of acetazolamide have been prepared (Table XXIII). The isopropyl and butyryl derivatives are active, whereas the methyl, *tert*-butyl, and acetyl derivatives are not. Activity of these compounds is thought to be dependent on the ease with which the N^5 substituent is removed from the acetazolamide nucleus.

6-Ethoxybenzthiazole-2-sulfonamide (ethoxzolamide, **34**), another carbamic anhydrase inhibitor, controls both grand mal and petit mal seizures.

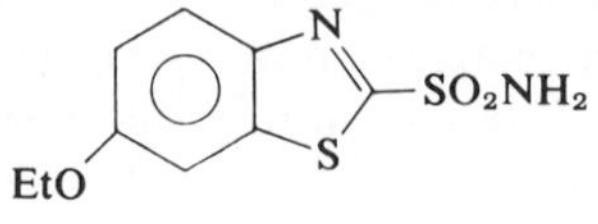

(structure, compound 34)

(34)

TABLE XXIII   ACETAZOLAMIDE
DERIVATIVES[a]

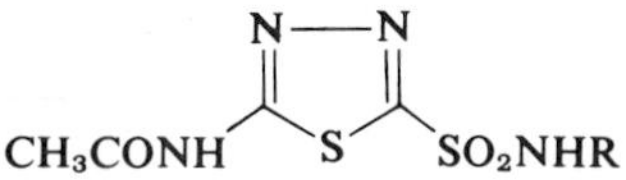

$$CH_3CONH \overset{N-N}{\underset{S}{\diagup \diagdown}} SO_2NHR$$

R	Activity
—CH(CH$_3$)$_2$	act.
—COC$_3$H$_7$	act.
—CH$_3$	inact.
t-C$_4$H$_9$—	inact.
—COCH$_3$	inact.

[a] Data from Spinks and Waring
(1961).

Control of psychomotor epilepsy was less significant (Solomon and Hirans,
1959; Merlis, 1960).

The structure–activity relationship of 4-substituted benzenesulfonamides
has been described (Keasling *et al.*, 1965) (Table XXIV). The anticonvulsant
effect as measured by protection against MES seizures, thiosemicarbazide
lethality, or strychnine lethality revealed that the 4-CF$_3$ analogue (**35**) was the

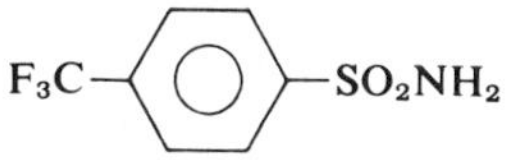

$$F_3C - \langle \bigcirc \rangle - SO_2NH_2$$

(**35**)

most potent anticonvulsant (MES, ED$_{50}$ = 23 mg/kg; thiosemicarbazide
lethality, ED$_{50}$ = 79 mg/kg). However, the authors concluded that, in terms
of the ratio of activity to lethality, the 4-Br compound was most effective.
Simple *N*-alkyl substitution did not seem to abolish activity but did increase
toxicity. If the substituent were *n*-butyl or larger, activity was lost. With the
exception of the *N,N*-dimethyl derivative, disubstituted compounds are
inactive. Just as with N^5 substitution on acetazolamide (Spinks and Waring,
1961), the activity of *N*-substituted compounds is believed to be dependent on
biotransformation to the nonsubstituted —SO$_2$NH$_2$ compound.

Holland *et al.* (1963) studied the anticonvulsant activity of a series of
N-substituted-3- and -4-benzenedisulfonamides (**36**) (Table XXV and XXVI).

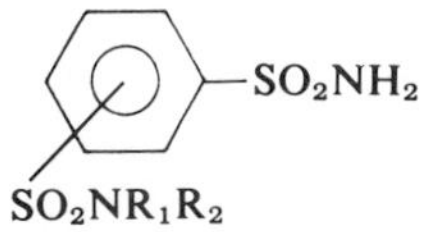

$$\langle \bigcirc \rangle - SO_2NH_2$$
$$SO_2NR_1R_2$$

(**36**)

TABLE XXIV   4-SUBSTITUTED BENZENESULFONAMIDES[a]

R_1	R_2	R_3	Activity
H—	H—	H—	LD_{50} 1000; MES, 89
4-F—	H—	H—	LD_{50} 562; MES, 113
4-Cl—	H—	H—	LD_{50} 233; MES, 45
4-Br—	H—	H—	LD_{50} 1000; MES, 36
4-I—	H—	H—	LD_{50} 933; MES, 62
4-CF$_3$—	H—	H—	LD_{50} 533; MES, 23
4-COOH—	H—	H—	LD_{50} > 1000
4-NH$_2$—	H—	H—	LD_{50} > 1000
4-OCH$_3$—	H—	H—	LD_{50} > 1000; MES, 142
4-CN—	H—	H—	LD_{50} 650; MES, 28
4-CH$_3$—	H—	H—	LD_{50} > 1000; MES 142
4-COCH$_3$—	H—	H—	LD_{50} > 1000
4-CH$_2$CN—	H—	H—	LD_{50} 100
4-SO$_2$CH$_3$—	H—	H—	LD_{50} 767
4-SOCH$_3$—	H—	H—	LD_{50} > 1000; MES, 146
4-SCH$_3$—	H—	H—	LD_{50} > 1000
4-Br—	H—	—OH	LD_{50} 1000; MES, 45
4-Br—	H—	—OCH$_3$	LD_{50} > 1000; MES, 126
4-Br—	CH$_3$—	—OH	LD_{50} 562
4-Br—	H—	CH$_3$—	LD_{50} 562; MES, 56
4-Br—	H—	—CH$_2$CH$_3$	LD_{50} 562; MES, 45
4-Br—	H—	—(CH$_2$)$_2$CH$_3$	LD_{50} 562; MES, 77
4-Br—	H—	—CH$_2$CH=CH$_2$	LD_{50} 178; MES, 56
4-Br—	H—	i-C$_3$H$_7$—	LD_{50} 562; MES, 50
4-Br—	H—	—(CH$_2$)$_3$CH$_3$	LD_{50} 562
4-Br—	H—	—CH$_2$C$_6$H$_5$	LD_{50} > 1000
4-Br—	H—	—CH$_2$CH$_2$C$_6$H$_5$	LD_{50} > 1000
4-Br—	H—		LD_{50} > 1000
4-Br—	H—		LD_{50} 237
4-Br—	H—		LD_{50} > 1000
4-Br—	CH$_3$—	CH$_3$—	LD_{50} 1000; MES, 89
4-Br—			LD_{50} > 1000

TABLE XXIV—*Continued*

R$_1$	R$_2$	R$_3$	Activity
4-Br—	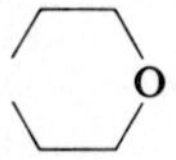 (ring) O		LD$_{50}$ > 1000
4-Br—	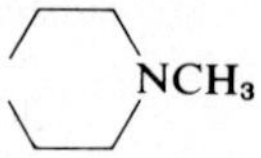 (ring) NCH$_3$		LD$_{50}$ 562

[a] Data from Keasling *et al.* (1965).

TABLE XXV *N*-SUBSTITUTED -4-BENZENEDISULFONAMIDES[a]

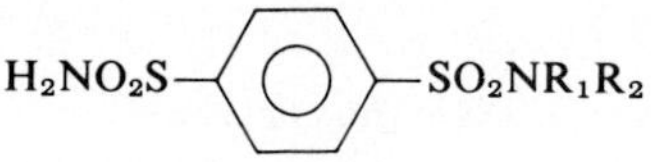

$$H_2NO_2S-\langle\bigcirc\rangle-SO_2NR_1R_2$$

R$_1$	R$_2$	Activity
H—	C$_2$H$_5$—	MES, < 30
H—	i-C$_3$H$_7$—	MES, < 30
H—	—(CH$_2$)$_3$OCH$_3$	MES, < 30
H—	—CH$_2$C$_6$H$_5$	MES, < 30
C$_2$H$_5$—	C$_2$H$_5$—	MES, < 30
—(CH$_2$)$_6$—	—(CH$_2$)$_6$—	MES, < 30
—(CH$_2$)$_2$O(CH$_2$)$_2$—	—(CH$_2$)$_2$O(CH$_2$)$_2$—	MES, < 30
H—	—CH$_3$	MES, 30–135
H—	—(CH$_2$)$_2$Br	MES, 30–135
H—	—(CH$_2$)$_3$Br	MES, 30–135
H—	n-C$_3$H$_7$—	MES, 30–135
H—	n-C$_4$H$_9$—	MES, 30–135
H—	n-C$_5$H$_{11}$—	MES, 30–135
H—	—CH$_2$CH=CH$_2$	MES, 30–135
H—	—CH$_2$C(CH$_3$)=CH$_2$	MES, 30–135
H—	C$_6$H$_5$—	MES, 30–135
H—	p-ClC$_6$H$_4$—	MES, 30–135
H—	o-ClC$_6$H$_4$—	MES, 30–135
CH$_3$—	—CH$_2$-o-ClC$_6$H$_4$	MES, 30–135
CH$_3$—	—CH$_2$-p-ClC$_6$H$_4$	MES, 30–135
H—	—H	MES, 135–250
H—	—(CH$_2$)$_2$COOH	MES, 135–250
H—	—(CH$_2$)$_3$COOH	MES, 135–250
H—	—CH$_2$CONH$_2$	MES, 135–250
H—	—CH$_2$CONHNH$_2$	MES, 135–250
H—	—CH$_2$-p-ClC$_6$H$_4$	MES, 135–250

(continued)

TABLE XXV—*Continued*

R_1	R_2	Activity
H—	—CH(CH$_3$)CH$_2$C$_6$H$_5$	MES, 135–250
H—	—CH$_2$COOH	MES, 250–500
H—	—CH$_2$CONHC$_3$H$_7$	MES, 250–500
H—	—CH$_2$COOC$_2$H$_5$	MES, 250–500
H—	m-CF$_3$C$_6$H$_4$—	MES, 250–500
—CH$_2$C$_6$H$_5$	—CH$_2$C$_6$H$_5$	MES, 250–500
H—	—(CH$_2$)$_2$C$_6$H$_5$	MES, 250–500
H—	C$_7$H$_{15}$—	MES, > 500
H—	p-(CH$_3$)$_2$NC$_6$H$_4$—	MES, > 500
H—	1-C$_{10}$H$_7$—	MES, > 500

[a] Data from Holland *et al.* (1963).

TABLE XXVI *N*-SUBSTITUTED
-3-BENZENEDISULFONAMIDES[a]

H_2NO_2S ... $-SO_2NR_1R_2$

R_1	R_2	Activity
H—	i-C$_3$H$_7$	MES, 30–135
H—	—CH$_2$C$_6$H$_5$	MES, 135–250
H—	H—	MES, 250–500
H—	—(CH$_2$)$_2$Br	MES, > 500
H—	m-CF$_3$—C$_6$H$_4$	MES, > 500
H—	—CH(CH$_3$)CH$_2$C$_6$H$_5$	MES, > 500

[a] Data from Holland *et al.* (1963).

Many of these compounds have an ED$_{50}$ of less than 30 mg/kg, and therefore, are more active than acetozolamide or ethoxzolamide. *N*-Alkylated substituents (ethyl, cycloalkyl, arylalkyl) appear to have a favorable effect on anticonvulsant action as measured by MES. Increasing the size of lipophilic groups above a seven-carbon substituent decreases activity. Replacing R_1 and R_2 with polar substituents such as acids, amides, or esters also decreases activity. In all cases, the 1,4-disulfonamide pattern is more active than the 1,3 pattern. The authors studied the *in vitro* activity of the *N*-substituted benzenedisulfonamides on carbonic anhydrase activity but could draw no correlation between enzyme inhibition and anticonvulsant activity. They point out that *in vivo* carbonic anhydrase inhibition would be a better measure since *in vitro* activity does not ensure adequate concentration of drug to accumulate in the brain. When they measured the carbonic anhydrase inhibition in rat brains after administration of acetazolamide, benzthiazide (37), and the most active of their compounds (*N*-isopropyl-4-benzenedisulfonamide, 38), the results suggested that there was a correlation between *in vivo* carbonic anhydrase activity and the anticonvulsant activity of the compounds.

(37)   (38)

The *N*-isopropyl analogue was tested further and found to protect mice not only from electroshock convulsions but also from Met seizures. It had no effect against strychnine. Table XXVII summarizes the comparative data of *N*-isopropyl-4-benzenedisulfonamide and other anticonvulsant agents. Against electroshock the *N*-isopropylbenzenedisulfonamide is less potent than diphenylhydantoin and equipotent to phenobarbital. It appears to be slightly more effective than trimethadione in suppressing Met seizures.

2-Substituted sulfonamides were examined for CNS and anticonvulsant activity by Raffa *et al.* (1963, 1964, 1965) (Table XXVIII). They found that all the compounds showed marked inhibitory action against Met or MES seizures.

Sulthiame [*N*-(4′-sulfamylphenyl)-1,4-butansultam, 39] is a sulfonamide carbonic anhydrase inhibitor whose action is not totally abolished if the

(39)

sulfonamide group is removed (Tanimukai *et al.*, 1965). It is said to be particularly effective in psychomotor epilepsy but to have little or no effect in petit mal. In other forms of epilepsy it has been used in combination with reduced doses of other anticonvulsants.

The activity of sulthiame and its analogues has been examined (Table XXIX) (Friebel and Sommer, 1960; Wirth *et al.*, 1960). The tonic phase of MES seizures in rats is abolished and pentylenetetrazole convulsions are inhibited. It is nonsedative and weakly diuretic.

N-Alkyl cyclic sulfonamides (sultams) do not apparently have any useful pharmacological property. Although the aryl-substituted sultams show anticonvulsant activity, they are sedating and lower the body temperature. The unsaturated ring increases the anticonvulsant properties but also increases toxicity. Other *N*- substituents, or substitution at other positions in the sultam ring, led to less active compounds or raised the toxicity. Additional variations on the sultam structure produced no compound possessing greater activity than sulthiame (Table XXX) (Behnisch *et al.*, 1963).

TABLE XXVII COMPARISON OF *N*-ISOPROPYL-4-
BENZENEDISULFONAMIDE WITH
OTHER ANTICONVULSANTS

Compound	Activity
N-Isopropyl-4-benzenedisulfonamide	MES, 21; Met, 171
Acetazolamide	MES, 134; Met, weak
Ethoxzolamide	MES, 65; Met, 354
Diphenylhydantoin	MES, 6.6
Trimethadione	Met, 218
Phenobarbital	MES, 24

[a] Data from Holland *et al.* (1963).

TABLE XXVIII 2-SUBSTITUTED SÚLFONAMIDES[a]

R_1	R_2	Activity
$-NO_2$	$-CO$-p-ClC_6H_5	Met, act.; MES, act.
$-NO_2$	$-CO$-m,p-$Cl_2C_6H_4$	Met, act.; MES, act.
$-NO_2$	$-CO$-m-Br—C_6H_5	Met, act.; MES, act.
$-NO_2$	$-CO$-p-Br—C_6H_5	Met, act.; MES, act.
$-NO_2$	$-CO$-p-CH_3O—C_6H_5	Met, act.; MES, act.
$-NO_2$	$-CO$-o,m,p-$(CH_3O)_3C_6H_3$	Met, act.; MES, act.
$-NO_2$	$-CO$— (thiophene)	Met, act.; MES, act.
$-NH_2$	$-CO$-p-ClC_6H_5	Met, act.; MES, act.
$-NH_2$	$-CO$-m,p-$Cl_2C_6H_4$	Met, act.; MES, act.
$-NH_2$	$-CO$-m-Br—C_6H_5	Met, act.; MES, act.
$-NH_2$	$-CO$-p-Br—C_6H_5	Met, act.; MES, act.
$-NH_2$	$-CO$-p-CH_3O—C_6H_5	Met, act.; MES, act.
$-NH_2$	$-CO$-o,m,p-$(CH_3O)_3C_6H_3$	Met, act.; MES, act.
$-NH_2$	$-CO$— (thiophene)	Met, act.; MES, act.

[a] Data from Raffa *et al.* (1965).

TABLE XXIX SULTHIAME ANALOGUES

Compound	Activity
H_2N—⬡—N(SO$_2$) ring	LD_{50} 720; MES, 105; Met, 0
⬡ with H_2N meta, —N(SO$_2$) ring	LD_{50} > 5000; MES, 155; Met, 0
CH_3O—⬡(H_2N)—N(SO$_2$) ring	LD_{50} 4560; MES, ~500; Met, 0
C_2H_5O—⬡(H_2N)—N(SO$_2$) ring	LD_{50} ~ 2000; MES, 248; Met, ~300
C_4H_9O—⬡(H_2N)—N(SO$_2$) ring	LD_{50} > 2000; MES, 500; Met, 306
pyridine—N(SO$_2$) ring	LD_{50} ~ 1000; MES, 470; Met, 340
⬡—CH_2—N(SO$_2$) ring	LD_{50} > 2200; MES, 220; Met, ~400
H_2N—⬡—N(SO$_2$) ring with H_3C and —CH_3	LD_{50} 550; MES, 66; Met, ~150
H_2N—⬡—N(SO$_2$) five-membered ring	LD_{50} 1200; MES, 260; Met, 0

[a] Data from Friebel and Sommer (1960).

TABLE XXX   SULFONAMIDES[a]

R_1	R_2	R_3	R_4	Activity
H—	H—	—SO_2NH_2	H—	No data
H—	H—	—SO_2NHCH_3	H—	No data
H—	H—	—$SO_2NHC_4H_9$	H—	No data
H—	H—	—$SO_2NH(CH_3)$	H—	No data
H—	H—	—SO_2N⟨⟩	H—	No data
H—	H—	—$SO_2NHC_6H_4$-p-SO_2NHCH_3	H—	No data
H—	H—	—SO_2NHCH-p-$SO_2NH(CH_3)$	H—	No data
H—	H—	—$SO_2NHCOCH_3$	H—	No data
H—	Cl—	—SO_2NH_2	H—	No data
CH_3O—	H—	—SO_2NH_2	CH_3—	No data
H—	SO_2NH_2—	H—	H—	No data
H—	SO_2NH_2—	Cl—	H—	No data
Cl—	H—	H—	—SO_2NH_2	No data
H—	H—	—$CH_2SO_2NH_2$	H—	No data
H—	H—	—SO_2CH_3	H—	No data
H—	H—	—$SO_2C_2H_5$	H—	No data
H—	H—	—SO_2-i-C_3H_7	H—	No data
H—	H—	—$SO_2CH_2C_6H_5$	H—	No data
H—	H—	—SO_2CH_2Cl	H—	No data

[a] Data from Behnisch *et al.* (1963).

VI. HYDRAZONES

Generally, anticonvulsants have been categorized on the basis of their similarity in structure to ureides. However, two types of compounds studied recently do not fit this pattern. Craig (1967) studied derivatives of the hydrazones of benzhydrylpiperazines (**40**) (Table XXXI) and benzhydrylpiperidines (**41**) (Table XXXII) and found them to be highly active compounds. In doses of ca. 1 mg/kg orally they abolish the tonic phase of MES convulsions. They have no effect in preventing Met seizures.

The piperazine derivatives cinnarizine (**42**) and flunarizine (**43**) possess a multitude of pharmacological and clinical activities (Desmedt *et al.*, 1975).

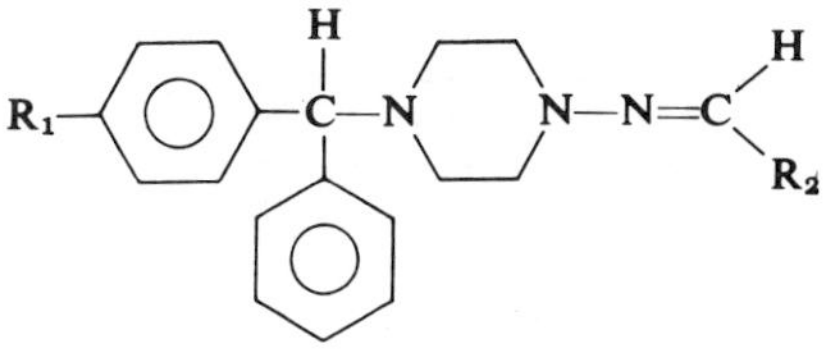

(40)

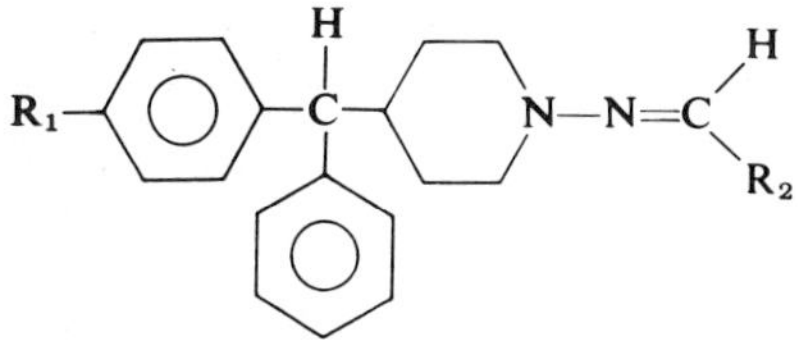

(41)

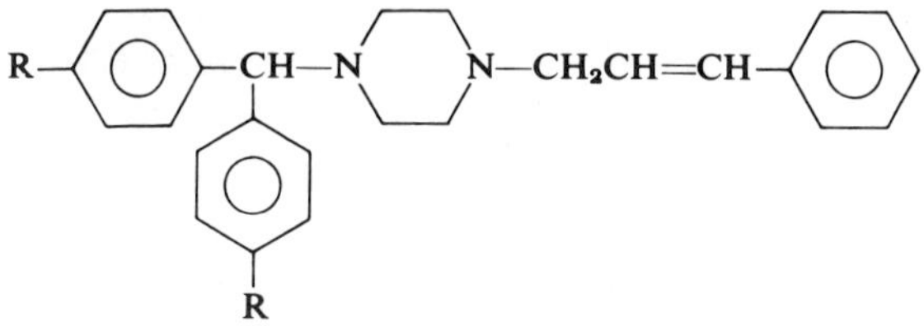

(42) R = —H
(43) R = —F

In addition to their effectiveness in allergic disorders, labyrinthic disorders, and cerebrovascular disturbances, they are found to possess anticonvulsant properties as well (Table XXXIII). They are not as potent as phenobarbital or diphenylhydantoin in suppressing MES seizures but are more effective than diphenylhydantoin and equipotent to phenobarbital in preventing Met convulsions. The compounds have a delayed onset of action, perhaps indicating the conversion to a metabolite which is the active compound. Flunarazine had the longest duration of action and slowest onset of the compounds studied.

TABLE XXXI   BENZHYDRYLPIPERAZINE HYDRAZONES[a]

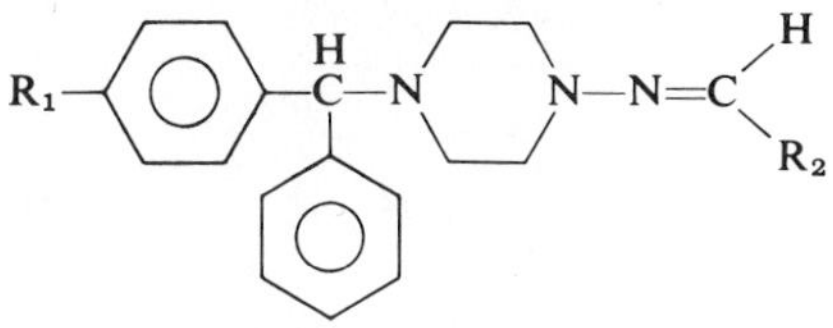

R_1	R_2	Activity
H—	—C_6H_5	MES, > 50
Cl—	—C_6H_5	MES, 44
H—	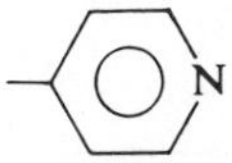	MES, 4.9

(continued)

TABLE XXXI—*Continued*

R₁	R₂	Activity
Cl—		MES, 16
H—		MES, 6.2
Cl—		MES, 3.7
H—		MES, 10
Cl—		MES, 3.7
Cl—		MES, 8.2
Cl—		MES, 6.2
H—		MES, 2.9
CH₃—		MES, 5.5
Br—		MES, 39
Br—		MES, 4.2

ᵃ Data from Craig (1967).

TABLE XXXII   BENZHYDRYLPIPERADINE HYDRAZONES[a]

R_1⟨○⟩—CH—⟨ ⟩N—N=CHR$_2$

R_1	R_2	Activity
H—		MES, 8.4
H—		MES, 27
Cl—		MES, 10.8
Cl—		MES, 28

[a] Data from Craig (1967).

TABLE XXXIII   CINNARIZINE AND FLUNARIZINE[a]

Compound	Activity
Sodium phenobarbital	MES, 13.2; Met, 4.10
Diphenylhydantoin	MES, 7.0; Met, 19.30
Cinnarizine	MES, 49.0; Met, 9.84
Flunarizine	MES, 20.9; Met, 6.04

[a] Data from Desmedt *et al.* (1975).

VII. STRUCTURE–ACTIVITY RELATIONSHIPS

Until recently any discussions of structure–activity relationships in anti-convulsants were summarized by emphasizing the common structural features of nearly all active antiepileptic agents. These discussions centered on the dicarboximide function (44) and/or the disubstituted quaternary carbon groups, which are features common to most of the anticonvulsant agents. No

(44)

attempt was made to relate the common structural characteristics of these anticonvulsive agents to some biological substance, biological pathway, or biological receptor implicated in the etiology of convulsions or epilepsy (Kier, 1971; Halpern and Julien, 1972; Julien and Halpern, 1972).

γ-Aminobutyric acid (GABA, **45**) was first identified in brain tissues in 1950 (Awapara *et al.*, 1950; Roberts and Frankel, 1950; Udenfriend, 1950). In the late 1950's Hayashi (Hayashi and Hagai, 1956; Hayashi, 1959) demonstrated that GABA applied directly to the canine motor cortex could inhibit localized epileptic discharges. However, only recently has sufficient evidence

(45)

become available which strongly supports a biochemical and physiological role of GABA in neurotransmission and especially its possible relationship to epilepsy.

Recent evidence suggests that GABA is an inhibitory neurotransmitter in cerebral tissues (DeFeudis, 1975; Meldrum, 1975; Roberts, 1974). The site of the inhibitory function of GABA is considered to be the cerebral cortex or cerebellum (Roberts and Hammerschlag, 1972). In particular the inhibitory cells of the cerebellum (Purkinje, Basket, Stellate and Golgi) use GABA as transmitter (Kuriyama *et al.*, 1966; McLaughlin *et al.*, 1974). The biochemical sequence of glutamate $\rightarrow$ GABA acting as a neurotransmitting mechanism roughly parallels the biogenic amine neurotransmitting mechanisms. These mechanisms all involve a precursor amino acid (tyrosine, tryptophan, or glutamate) whose first transformation step is a decarboxylation reaction (DOPA, serotonin, or GABA). The product thus formed may be the neurotransmitter, e.g., serotonin or GABA, or another series of reactions may be required to obtain the neurotransmitter, e.g., DOPA $\rightarrow$ norepinephrine. Figure 1 summarizes the hypothesized neurotransmitting scheme for GABA.

γ-Aminobutyric acid is produced at the end of the presynaptic fiber by decarboxylation of glutamic acid. Glutamic acid decarboxylase (GAD) is the enzyme responsible for this conversion (Weinstein *et al.*, 1963; Salganicoff and DeRobertis, 1965; Kuriyama *et al.*, 1968; Perez de la Mora *et al.*, 1973).

The site of GABA uptake is not known but it is known to be a high-affinity

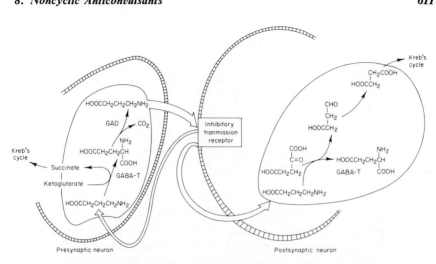

Fig. 1. The hypothesized neurotransmitting scheme for GABA.

uptake system (Logan and Snyder, 1971; Bennett *et al.*, 1973). It is tempting to speculate that uptake may occur in the presynaptic fiber, thus recycling the GABA precursor, glutamate (Kravitz, 1967).

Early studies showed that GABA applied directly to the motor cortex had a localized antiepileptic effect (Hayashi and Nagai, 1956; Hayashi, 1959). If one assumes the biochemical sequence pictured above to be correct, then there are a number of ways to alter GABA levels. To decrease levels of GABA or cause an apparent decrease in GABA levels one might inhibit the GABA synthesizing enzyme, GAD, or block the access of GABA to the inhibitory transmission receptor. To increase GABA levels one might block the uptake of GABA into neurons or inhibit the inactivating enzyme, GABA-T.

Since GAD is a pyridoxal phosphate-dependent enzyme it can be inhibited by a variety of agents that interfere with pyridoxal (Meldrum, 1975). However, it is difficult to draw any conclusions from some of these studies because some of the agents that inhibit GAD also have inhibitory effects on GABA-T. However, in those systems where decreased GABA levels can be attributed to GAD inhibition, convulsant effects are produced. The seizures induced by GAD inhibition appear to be principally sensory-induced epilepsy, e.g., audiogenic seizures (Lehmann, 1964) or photosensitive epilepsy (Meldrum and Balzamo, 1972).

Bicuculline (**46**) competes with GABA for specific inhibitory transmission receptor sites (Curtis *et al.*, 1971a, b; Stranghan *et al.*, 1971; Hill and Simmonds, 1973; Hill *et al.*, 1973). Kier and George (1973) found structural similarities between the onium group and carboxylate oxygen of bicuculline

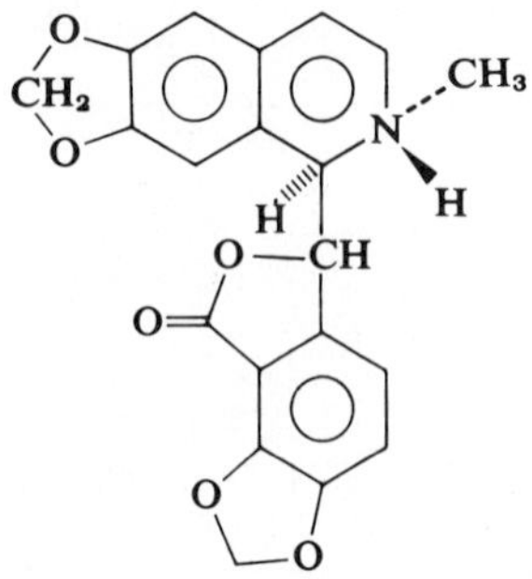

Wallace J. Murray and Lemont B. Kier

(46)

and the amino and carboxylate groups of GABA. They surmise that these similarities lead to bicuculline's role as a competitive antagonist. The receptor-blocking actions of bicuculline lead to its convulsant properties. Picrotoxin seems to have the same action (Hill *et al.*, 1973). Benzylpenicillin (**47**) is another antagonist of GABA having potent local convulsant action (Curtis *et al.*, 1972; Hill *et al.*, 1973).

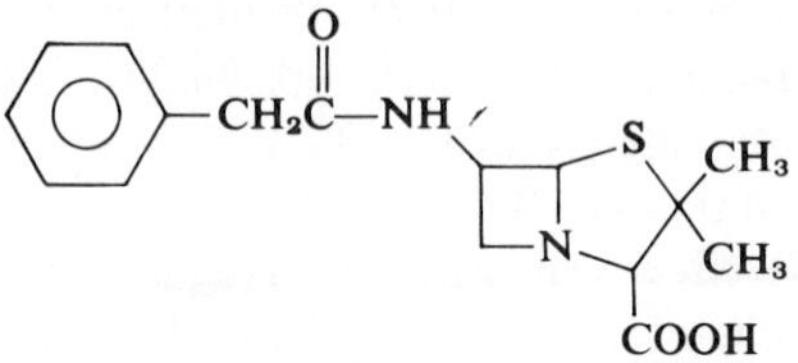

(47)

Curtis and Watkins (1965) have reviewed the pharmacology of amino acids related to GABA. They report that many amino acids structurally similar to GABA depress cortical activity of cats and mice and raise the threshold of chemical- and electroshock-induced seizures in dogs. Among the amino acids that in addition to GABA have this action are taurine (**48**), 3-amino-1-propanesulfonic acid (homotaurine, **49**) and γ-amino-β-hydroxybutyric acid (β-hydroxy-GABA, **50**). They report the order of activity as homotaurine > β-hydroxy-GABA > GABA > taurine.

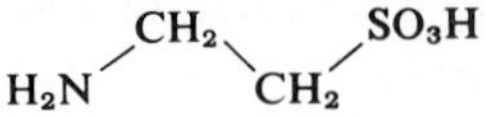

(48) 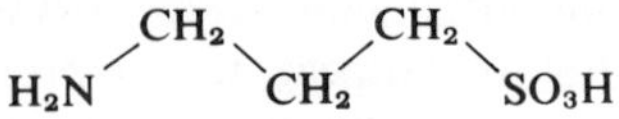   **(49)**

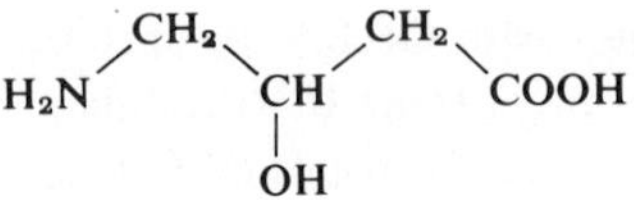

(50)

TABLE XXXIV COMPOUNDS FOUND TO HAVE GABA-LIKE BIOLOGICAL EFFECTS

Compound	Activity	Reference
$^-OOCC{\equiv}CCH_2NH_3^+$ (4-Aminotetrolic acid)	Competitive inhibition of GABA-T and GABA uptake in cerebral cells	Beart *et al.* (1972a,b, 1973)
(*trans*-4-Aminocrotonic acid)	Competitive inhibition of GABA-T	Beart and Johnston (1973a)
(*cis*-3-Aminocyclohexane-carboxylic acid)	Competitive inhibition of uptake in cerebral cells	Beart *et al.* (1972b)
$^-OOCCH_2CH_2NHNH_3^+$ (Hydrazinopropionic acid)	Competitive inhibitor of GABA-T	Van Gelder (1968)
$^-O_3SCH_2CH_2CH_2NH_3^+$ (Homotaurine)	GABA-like CNS effects	Curtis *et al.* (1967)
(Imidazoleacetic acid)	GABA-like CNS effects	Anderson *et al.* (1972)

Straight-chain analogues of GABA exhibit depressant or anticonvulsant effects in a variety of test systems. Table XXXIV summarizes the anticonvulsant effect of these straight-chain analogues.

X-ray studies and theoretical calculations have been performed on GABA, GABA-mimetic agents, and competitive antagonists of GABA (Curtis *et al.*, 1970; Kier and Truitt, 1970; Tonita, 1966; Brehm *et al.*, 1972; Kier and George, 1973). These studies have led to the proposal that the pharmacophoric pattern necessary for GABA-like action requires a fully extended zwitterionic molecule in which the distance between the onium group and the oxygen atoms of the carboxylate is ideally 5–6 Å (**51**) (Kier *et al.*, 1970).

Structure–activity studies on GABA analogues support this hypothesized pharmacophore (Beart *et al.*, 1971, 1972a,b; Beart and Johnson, 1973a,b; Van Gelder, 1968; Curtis *et al.*, 1967; Anderson *et al.*, 1972). Table XXXIV gives the name, structure, and nature of GABA activity of these compounds. When these were subjected to molecular orbital calculations, all had a

5.8 Å

(51)

predicted conformation comparable to that of the fully extended GABA (Kier *et al.*, 1974).

In partial support of the hypothesis that increased levels of GABA in the brain lead to decreased epileptiform activity is the finding that the open-chain anticonvulsant acid, di-*n*-propylacetic acid, increases GABA levels. Godin *et al.* (1969) and Simler *et al.* (1973) report that di-*n*-propylacetic acid inhibits the enzyme GABA-T, blocking the transformation of GABA to glutamate, which leads to GABA buildup. Other than dipropyl acetate no work has been performed with other acids or sterically hindered amides having anticonvulsant activity correlating GABA levels or the effect on GABA-T activity.

Other GABA analogues have also been synthesized and tested. Khaunina (1964, 1968) showed that GABA substituted at the β position gave compounds more centrally active than α-substituted analogues. β-Phenyl-γ-aminobutyric acid (52) reduced motor activity, potentiated narcosis, and antagonized

(52) R = H
(53) R = Cl

H_2N—CH_2—CH—CH_2—$COOH$

thiosemicarbazide convulsions. Metrazole convulsions were not antagonized.

Substitution of a *p*-chloro group on **52** gives baclofen (Liorsal, **53**). This compound has been found to be clinically effective against spasticity (Birkmayer *et al.*, 1967; Burke *et al.*, 1971; Knutsson *et al.*, 1973; McLellan, 1973). Bein (1972) found that baclofen antagonizes metrazole or thiosemicarbazide convulsions in mice but is not effective in counteracting electroshock convulsions.

In addition to its antispasmodic action baclofen has been found in a number of instances to provoke seizures in epileptic patients (Pinto *et al.*, 1972; Bein, 1972) and to cause sustained epileptiform activity in baboons with photosensitive epilepsy (Meldrum, 1975). On the basis of the GABA-mediator model this dual action might be explained on the one hand by GAD inhibition giving GABA insufficiency and epileptiform activity and on the other hand by GABA-T inhibition giving increased GABA levels and an antispasticity response. No study has been done showing the effects of baclofen on these two enzymatic systems.

Interestingly, the four prominent structural classes of antiepileptics, the hydantoins (54), the oxazolidinediones (55), the succinimides (56), and the barbiturates (57), are known to be metabolized to compounds resembling GABA. The rupturing of five-membered rings at the 1–5 bond results in the closely related carboximide acids 58, 59, and 60. Ring opening at the barbiturate 1–6 bond leads to formation of a carboxide acid (61) (see reactions 1 and 2). Metabolic ring opening is known to be a minor metabolic pathway for barbiturates (Mark, 1963; Tsukamota *et al.*, 1956). Studies *in vitro* show that at neutral pH barbiturates open exclusively at the 1–6 bond to give malonuric acids (61) (Maulding *et al.*, 1972). The hydantoic acid 58 has been reported to be formed during metabolism of diphenylhydantoin (Nakamura *et al.*, 1966). The oxazolidinedione ring (55) is known to be cleaved to the acid (59) in the liver (Butler, 1953). The succinimides (56) such as the 5-phenyl, 5-ethyl derivative are known to be metabolized to the amide acids (60) (Glazko *et al.*, 1954).

When these open-chain acids are submitted to molecular orbital calculation (Aldrich and Kier, 1973), it is found that the extended conformation is

$$\text{(1)}$$

54:X = NH, hydantoins   58:X = NH
55:X = O, oxazolidinediones   59:X = O
56:X = CH$_2$, Succinimides   60:X = CH$_2$

$$\text{(2)}$$

(57)   (61)

preferred. These conformations fit the GABA pharmacophore predicted by Kier and Truitt (1970). The metabolite acids also bear close resemblance to the anticonvulsant α-disubstituted acids such as dipropylacetic acid. For these reasons the possibility that these metabolites may have anticonvulsant activity via GABA-like effects merits attention.

REFERENCES

Aldrich, H. S., and Kier, L. B. (1975). In "Molecular and Quantum Pharmacology, Proceedings of the 7th Jerusalem Symposium" (E. D. Bergman and P. Pullman, eds.), p. 229. Reidel, Publ., Dordrecht, Netherlands.

Anderson, E. G., Haas, H. L., and Hosli, L. (1972). *Experientia* **28**, 741.

Awapara, J., Landua, A. J., Fuerst, R., and Seale, B. (1950). *J. Biol. Chem.* **187**, 35.

Babington, R. G., and Horovitz, Z. P. (1973). *Arch. Int. Pharmacodyn. Ther.* **202**, 100.

Beart, P. M., and Johnston, G. A. R. (1973a). *Brain Res.* **49**, 459.

Beart, P. M., and Johnston, G. A. R. (1973b). *J. Neurochem.* **20**, 319.

Beart, P. M., Curtis, D. R., and Johnston, G. A. R. (1971). *Nature (London), New Biol.* **234**, 78.

Beart, P. M., Uhr, M. L., and Johnston, G. A. R. (1972a). *J. Neurochem.* **19**, 1849.

Beart, P. M., Johnston, G. A. R., and Uhr, M. L. (1972b). *J. Neurochem.* **19**, 1855.

Behnisch, R., Hoffmeister, F., Horstmann, H., Schranfstatter, F., and Wirth, W. (1963). *Med. Chem. (Lererkusen, Ger.)* **7**, 296.

Bein, H. J. (1972). In "Spasticity—A Topical Survey" (W. Birkmayer, ed.), p. 76. Huber, Bern.

Bennett, J. P., Logan, W. J., and Snyder, S. H. (1973). *J. Neurochem.* **21**, 1533.

Bernard, C. G., and Bohm, E. (1954). *Experientia* **10**, 474.

Birkmayer, W., Danielcyzk, W., and Weiler, G. (1967). *Wien. Med. Wochenschr.* **117**, 7.

Bossier, J. P., Datonis, D., Dumont, C., and Pagny, J. (1962). *Therapie* **17**, 713.

Brehm, L., Hjeds, H., and Krogsgaard-Larsen, P. (1972). *Acta Chem. Scand.* **26**, 1298.

Burke, D., Andrews, C., and Knowles, L. (1971). *J. Neurol. Sci.* **14**, 199.

Butler, T. C. (1953). *J. Pharmacol. Exp. Ther.* **108**, 11.

Carraz, C. L. (1967). *Aggressologie* **8**, 13.

Carraz, G., Boucherle, A., Lebreton, S., Benoit-Guyod, J. L., and Boitard, M. (1964). *Therapie* **19**, 917.

Cereghino, J. J., Brock, J. T., Van Meter, J. C., Penry, J. K., Smith, L. D., and White, B. G. (1974). *Neurology* **24**, 401.

Chen, G., and Ensor, C. R. (1950). *Arch. Neurol. Psychiatry* **63**, 56.

Close, W. J., and Spielman, M. A. (1961). *Med. Chem. (N.Y.)* **5**, 1.

Craig, C. R. (1967). *Arch. Int. Pharmacodyn. Ther.* **165**, 328.

Curtis, D. R., and Watkins, J. C. (1965). *Pharmacol. Rev.* **17**, 347.

Curtis, D. R., Hosli, L., and Johnston, G. A. R. (1967). *Nature (London)* **215**, 1502.

Curtis, D. R., Duggan, A. W., Felix, D., and Johnston, G. A. R. (1970). *Nature (London)* **226**, 1222.

Curtis, D. R., Duggan, A. W., Felix, D., and Johnston, G. A. R. (1971a). *Brain Res.* **32**, 69.

Curtis, D. R., Duggan, A. W., Felix, D., Johnston, G. A. R., and McLennan, H. (1971b). *Brain Res.* **33**, 57.

Curtis, D. R., Game, C. J. A., Johnston, G. A. R., McCulloch, R. M., and MacLachlin, R. M. (1972). *Brain Res.* **43**, 242.

Daleva, L., and Nikolova, M. (1964). *Farmatsiya (Moscow)* **14**, 13.

Davis, M. A., Winthrop, S. O. Thomas, R. A., Herr, F., Charest, M. P., and Gaudry, R. (1964). *J. Med. Chem.* **7**, 88.

DeFeudis, F. V. (1975). *Annu. Rev. Pharmacol.* **15**, 105.

Desmedt, L. K. C., Niemegeers, C. J. E., and Janssen, P. A. J. (1975). *Arzneim.-Forsch.* **25**, 1408.

Dobychina, N. S., and Pechenkin, A. G. (1966). *Izv. Tomsk. Politekh. Inst.* **5**, 85.

Echague, E. S., and Lim, R. K. S., (1962). *J. Pharmacol. Exp. Ther.* **138**, 224.

Friebel, H., and Sommer, S. (1960). *Dtsch. Med. Wochenschr.* **85**, 2192.

Funcke, A. B. H., and Zandberg, P. (1970). *Arzneim.-Forsch.* **20**, 1896.

Georgiev, V. (1965a). *Izv. Inst. Fiziol. Bulg. Akad. Nauk.* **9**, 115.

Georgiev, V. (1965b). *Compt. Rend. Acad. Bulgare Sci.* **18**, 883.

Georgiev, V. (1967). *Eksp. Med. Morfol.* **6**, 205.

Georgiev, V., and Vasileva, O. (1965). *Izv. Inst. Fiziol. Bulg. Akad. Nauk.* **9**, 105.

Georgiev, V., Rousinov, K., and Vasileva, O. (1964). *Izv. Inst. Fiziol. Bulgar. Akad. Nauk.* **7**, 233.

Glazko, A. J., Dill, W. A., Wolf, L. M., and Miller, C. A. (1954). *J. Pharmacol. Exp. Ther.* **111**, 413.

Godin, Y., Heiner, L., Mark, J., and Mandel, P. (1969). *J. Neurochem.* **16**, 869.

Gold-Curbert, P., and Toribia, H. (1963). *Arch. Sci.* **16**, 405.

Halpern, L. M., and Julien, R. M. (1972). *Epilepsia* **13**, 377.

Hayashi, T. (1959). *J. Physiol. (London)* **145**, 570.

Hayashi, T., and Nagai, K. (1956). *Abstr. Commun., Int. Physiol. Congr., 20th*, p. 410.

Hazard, R., Cheymol, J., Chabrier, P., and Smarzewska, K. (1951). *Therapie* **6**, 129.

Hill, R. G., and Simmonds, M. A. (1973). *Br. J. Pharmacol.* **48**, 1.

Hill, R. G., Simmonds, M. A., and Straughan, D. W. (1973). *Br. J. Pharmacol.* **49**, 37.

Holland, G. F., Funderburk, W. H., and Finger, K. F. (1963). *J. Med. Chem.* **6**, 307.

Horrom, B. W. (1963). U.S. Patent 3,066,167; *Chem. Abstr.* **58**, 11284 (1963).

Job, C., Lindinger, H., and Zellner, H. (1954). *Wien. Med. Wochenschr.* **104**,911.

Johnsen, U. F., Jacobsen, C. R., LaForge, R. A., and Hanna, C. (1962). *J. Pharm. Sci.* **51**, 799.

Joultry, A. (1963). French Patent M12; *Chem. Abstr.* **58**, P1400c (1963).

Julien, R. M., and Halpern, L. M. (1972). *Epilepsia* **13**, 387.

Keasling, H. H., Schumann, E. L., and Veldkamp, W. (1965). *J. Med. Chem.* **8**, 548.

Khaunina, R. A. (1964). *Farmakol. Toksikol. (Moscow)* **27**, 399.

Khaunina, R. A. (1968). *Farmakol. Toksikol. (Moscow)* **31**, 302.

Kier, L. B. (1971). "Molecular Orbital Theory in Drug Research," p. 246. Academic Press, New York.

Kier, L. B., and George, J. M. (1973). *Experientia* **29**, 501.

Kier, L. B., and Truitt, E. B. (1970). *Experientia* **26**, 988.

Kier, L. B., George, J. M., and Holtje, H.-D. (1974). *J. Pharm. Sci.* **63**, 1435.

Knutsson, E., Lindblom, U., and Martensson, A. (1973). *Brain* **96**, 29.

Kravitz, E. A. (1967). "The Neurosciences" (G. C. Quarton, T. Malnechuk, and F. O. Schmitt, ed.), p. 433. The Rockefeller University Press, New York.

Kuriyama, K., Haber, B., Sisken, B., and Roberts, E. (1966). *Proc. Natl. Acad. Sci. U.S.A.* **55**, 846.

Lazarova, M. (1970). *Dokl. Bolg. Akad. Nauk.* **23**, 599.

Lebreton, S., Carraz, G., Beriel, H., and Mennier, H. (1964). *Therapie* **19**, 457.

Lehmann, A. (1964). *Agressologie* **5**, 311.

Lincoln, J. (1963). British Patent 932,965; *Chem. Abstr.* **60**, 427f (1964).

Litchfield, J. T., Jr., and Wilcoxon, F. (1949). *J. Pharmacol. Exp. Ther.* **96**, 99.

Livingston, S., Villamater, C., Sakata, Y., and Pauli, L. L. (1967). *J. Am. Med. Assoc.* **200**, 204.

Logan, W. J., and Snyder, S. H. (1971). *Nature (London)* **234**, 297.

Long, L. M. (1952). *Abstr. 121st Meeting Am. Chem. Soc., 1952*, p. 8J.

McLaughlin, B. J., Wood, J. G., Saito, K., Barber, R., Vaughn, J. E., Roberts, E., and Wu, J.-Y. (1974). *Brain Res.* **76**, 377.

McLellan, D. L. (1973). *J. Neurol., Neurosurg. Psychiatry* **36**, 555.

Mark, L. C. (1963). *Clin. Pharmacol. Ther.* **4**, 504.

Maskovskij, M. D. (1972). *Lek. Stredstva Past. Part I*, p. 117.

Maulding, H. V., Nazareno, J., Polesuk, J., and Michaelis, A. (1972). *J. Pharm. Sci.* **61**, 1389.

Meldrum, B. S. (1975). *Int. Rev. Neurobiol.* **17**, p. 1.

Meldrum, B. S., and Balzamo, E. (1972). *Proc. Conf. Exp. Med. Surg. Primates, 3rd, 1970*, Part II, p. 282.

Mercier, J. (1973). *Int. Encycl. Pharmacol. Ther.* Vol. 1, p. 203.

Merlis, S. (1960). *Neurology* **10**, 210.

Merritt, H. H., and Putnam, T. R. J. (1945). *Epilepsia* **3**, 51.

Meunier, G., Carraz, G., Mennier, Y., Eymard, P., and Aimard, M. (1963). *Therapie* **18**, 435.

Millichap, J. G., Woodbury, D. M., and Goodman, L. S. (1955). *J. Pharmacol. Exp. Ther.* **115**, 251.

Nakamura, K., Masuda, Y., Nakatsuji, K., and Hiroka, T. (1966). *Naunyn-Schmiedebergs Arch. Pharmakol. Exp. Pathol.* **254**, 406.

Nikolova, M. (1965). *Farmatsiya (Moscow)* **15**, 32.

Nishimura, T. (1963). *Psychiatr. Neurol. Jpn.* **65**, 523.

Nishimura, T., Tanimukai, H., and Nichinuma K. (1963). *J. Neurochem.* **10**, 257.

Orloff, M. J., Feldman, P. E., Shaiova, C. H., and Pfeiffer, C. C. (1951). *Neurology* **1**, 377.

Perez de la Mora, M., Feria-Velasco, A., and Tapia, R. (1973). *J. Neurochem.* **20**, 1575.

Pinto, O. de S., Polikar, M., and Loustalof, P. (1972). "Spasticity—A Topical Survey" (W. Birkmayer, ed.), p. 192. Huber, Bern.

Putnam, T. J., and Merritt, H. H. (1937). *Science* **85**, 525.

Raffa, L., DiBella, M., and DiBella, L. (1963). *Farmaco, Ed. Sci.* **18**, 530.

Raffa, L., DiBella, M., DiBella, L., and Conti, G. (1964). *Farmaco. Ed. Sci.* **19**, 425.

Raffa, L., DiBella, M., DiBella, L., and Lolli, M. G. (1965). *Farmaco, Ed. Sci.* **20**, 786.

Roberts, E. (1974). *Biochem. Pharmacol.* **23**, 2637.

Roberts, E., and Frankel, S. (1950). *J. Biol. Chem.* **187**, 55.

Roberts, E., and Hammerschlag, R. (1972). *In* "Basic Neurochemistry" (R. W. Albers *et al.*, eds.), p. 131. Little, Brown, Boston, Massachusetts.

Rousinov, K. S. (1967). *C. R. Acad. Bulg. Sci.* **20**, 1233.

Rozkowski, A. P., Schuler, M. E., and Nelson, P. H. (1972). *J. Med. Chem.* **15**, 1336.

Salganicoff, L., and De Robertis, E. (1965). *J. Neurochem.* **12**, 187.

Simler, S., Ciesielski, L., Maitre, M., Randrianarisou, H., and Mandel, P. (1973). *Biochem. Pharmacol.* **22**, 1701.

Solomon, S., and Hirano, A. (1959). *Neurology* **9**, 167.

Sorel, L. (1957). *Confin. Neurol. (Basel)*, **17**, 16.

Spielman, M. A., Geiszler, A. O., and Close, W. J. (1948). *J. Am. Chem. Soc.* **70**, 4189.

Spinks, A., and Waring, W.S. (1961). *In* "Progress in Medicinal Chemistry" (G. P. Ellis and G. B. West, eds.), p. 261. Butterworth, London.

Stranghan, D. W., Neal, M. J., Simmonds, M. A., Collins, G. G. S., and Hill, R. G. (1971). *Nature (London)* **233**, 352.

Swinyard, E. A., and Toman, J. E. P. (1950). *J. Pharmacol. Exp. Ther.* **100**, 151.

Swinyard, E. A., Brown, W. C., and Goodman, L. S. (1952). *J. Pharmacol. Exp. Ther.* **106**, 319.

Tanimukai, H., Inui, M., Harigucki, S., and Kaneko, Z. (1965). *Biochem. Pharmacol.* **14**, 961.

Toman, J. E. P., Swinyard, E. A., and Goodman, L. S. (1976). *J. Neurophysiol.* **9**, 231.

Toman, J. E. P., Everett, G. M., and Richards, R. K. (1952). *Tex. Rep. Biol. Med.* **10**, 96.

Tonita, K. (1966). *Jpn. J. Brain Physiol.* **61**, 1.

Toreva, D. (1967). *Farmakol. Toksikol. (Moscow)* **30**, 301.

Tsukamoto, H. (1956). *Pharm. Bull.* **4**, 371.

Udenfriend, S. (1950). *J. Biol. Chem.* **187**, 65.

Van Gelder, N. M. (1968). *J. Neurochem.* **15**, 747.

Weinstein, H., Roberts, E., and Kakefuda, T. (1963). *Biochem. Pharmacol.* **12**, 503.

Wirth, W., Hoffmeister, F., Friebel, H., and Sommer, S. (1960). *Dtsch. Med. Wochenschr.* **85**, 2195.

Yamamoto, I., Inoki, R., and Otori, K. (1963). *Nippon Yakurigaku Zasshi* **59**, 242.

Zalesov, V. S. (1964). *Farm. Zh. (Kiev)* **19**, 19.

SUBJECT INDEX

A

A 7
B 8
C 9
D 0
E 1
F 2
G 3
H 4
I 5
J 6